DIAGNOSTIC ELECTROCARDIOGRAPHY AND VECTORCARDIOGRAPHY

DIAGNOSTIC ELECTROCARDIOGRAPHY AND VECTORCARDIOGRAPHY

Third Edition

H. HAROLD FRIEDMAN, M.D.
F.A.C.P., F.A.C.C., F.C.C.P.

Clinical Professor of Medicine,
University of Colorado School of Medicine;
Attending Physician and Director of the Electrocardiographic Laboratory,
Rose Medical Center, Denver;
Attending Physician and Electrocardiographer,
St. Joseph Hospital, Denver;
Electrocardiographer,
St. Luke's Hospital, Denver;
Consulting Cardiologist, Denver General Hospital

McGRAW-HILL BOOK COMPANY
New York   St. Louis   San Francisco   Auckland   Bogotá
Guatemala   Hamburg   Johannesburg   Lisbon   London
Madrid   Mexico   Montreal   New Delhi   Panama   Paris   San Juan
São Paulo   Singapore   Sydney   Tokyo   Toronto

DIAGNOSTIC ELECTROCARDIOGRAPHY AND VECTORCARDIOGRAPHY

Copyright © 1985, 1977, 1971 by McGraw-Hill, Inc. All rights reserved. Printed in the United States of America. Except as permitted under the United States Copyright Act of 1976, no part of this publication may be reproduced or distributed in any form or by any means, or stored in a data base or retrieval system, without the prior written permission of the publisher.

1 2 3 4 5 6 7 8 9 0   DOCDOC   8 9 8 7 6 5 4

ISBN 0-07-022427-7

This book was set in Optima by Monotype Composition Company, Inc; the editors were Beth Ann Kaufman and Steven Tenney; the production supervisor was Avé McCracken; R. R. Donnelley & Sons was printer and binder.

Library of Congress Cataloging in Publication Data

Friedman, H. Harold (Henry Harold), date
Diagnostic electrocardiography and vectorcardiography.

Includes bibliographies and index.
1. Electrocardiography.   2. Vectorcardiography.
I. Title.   [DNLM: 1. Electrocardiography.   2. Vector-
cardiography.   WG 140 F911o]
RC683.5.E5F68   1985   616.1'207547   84-9739
ISBN 0-07-022427-7

To
My Wife Charlotte, and to Our Children,
Alan, Marsha, and Betsy

CONTENTS

Preface   ix

1   Electrophysiology   1
2   Anatomy and Physiology of the Conduction System of the Heart   21
3   Basic Considerations in Electrocardiography   35
4   The Derivation of the Electrocardiogram and Vectorcardiogram   50
5   The Normal Electrocardiogram   57
6   The Normal Vectorcardiogram   111
7   Abnormalities of the T Wave or Vector   119
8   Abnormalities of the S-T Segment or Vector   122
9   Atrial Abnormalities   128
10   Ventricular Hypertrophy, or Enlargement   140
11   Ventricular Conduction Defects   177
12   The Preexcitation, or Wolff-Parkinson-White (W-P-W) Syndrome   226
13   Myocardial Infarction   241
14   Transient Myocardial Ischemia and Injury; Exercise
Electrocardiography   307
15   Pericarditis   320
16   Effect of Certain Drugs on the Electrocardiogram   328
17   Effect of Electrolyte Abnormalities on the Electrocardiogram   338
18   Pulmonary Disease   351
19   Right Axis Deviation   359
20   Left Axis Deviation   364
21   Miscellaneous Disorders   369

22 The Normal Electrocardiogram in Infants and Children   383
23 The Electrocardiogram in Congenital Heart Disease   388
24 The Arrhythmias   403
25 Tabular Outline of the Differential Diagnosis of Various
        Electrocardiographic Abnormalities   619

Appendix   627

Index   647

PREFACE

The scope and aims of the third edition of "Diagnostic Electrocardiography and Vectorcardiography" remain the same as those of the previous editions: to provide a practical textbook, concise enough for the beginner but comprehensive enough to furnish detailed information and serve as a ready reference for the more advanced student and the electrocardiographic interpreter. As in the previous editions, conventional electrocardiography, vectorelectrocardiography, and oscilloscopic vectorcardiography are incorporated and integrated within the text to help the reader bridge the gap between them.

The entire text is revised, updated, and expanded. Several chapters are enlarged to provide more complete coverage of the subject matter. New illustrations have been added; others, removed. Obsolete material, needless to state, has been deleted. Some of the more recent advances in electrocardiography included in the text are as follows: present-day concepts of the anatomy and physiology of the conduction system; the electrophysiology of the arrhythmias; torsades de pointes; current information about the mechanisms and diagnostic features of paroxysmal supraventricular tachycardia; sinus node dysfunction; detailed consideration of ventricular conduction defects; criteria for the diagnosis of right ventricular infarction; pseudoinfarction patterns; exercise electrocardiography; poor R wave progression; and such disorders as the mitral valve prolapse syndrome, pes excavatum, and the straight back syndrome.

Each chapter is reasonably complete, which leads to some repetition in the text but obviates to a great extent the need for cross references to other pages or chapters.   A complete bibliography is not given, but selected references are listed at the end of each chapter.   In choosing them, I give preference to the more recent literature and review articles.   Those who seek a more comprehensive bibliography will usually find it in the papers that have been cited.

The major emphasis throughout the book is on electrocardiographic and vectorcardiographic diagnosis.   The criteria listed in the text represent the consensus of competent authorities.   However, I attempt to indicate areas in which there is controversy or diversity of opinion or in which the diagnostic standards are not entirely adequate.

Several physicians have graciously provided illustrations in the original and in the current edition.   I am deeply indebted to Drs. Leonard S. Dreifus, Henry J. L. Marriott, Joseph Snyder, and especially to William P. Nelson and Ray Pryor for their courtesy in this regard.

All of the diagrams and drawings in the present and previous edition are the work of Ms. Sara Gustafson.   The photography was performed by Ms. Peggy Randall with the assistance of Mr. Larry Bartz.   I am grateful to them for their splendid spirit of cooperation and the technical excellence of their work.   Mr. Sheldon Luper, head of the Media Center at Rose Medical Center, kindly made the facilities of his department available to me.

I am very much indebted to Ms. Diane Yacovetta for providing considerable secretarial assistance and to her staff of technicians at Rose Medical Center for recording many of the tracings in the text and mounting them for photography.

In the preparation of this book, I have had the generous support of the administrative staff and board of trustees of Rose Medical Center.

My deepest gratitude and thanks go to my wife, Charlotte, whose patience and forbearance made the writing of this book an enjoyable task rather than a burdensome chore.   Without her understanding and encouragement, neither this nor any of my other books would have been written.

H. Harold Friedman

DIAGNOSTIC
ELECTROCARDIOGRAPHY
AND
VECTORCARDIOGRAPHY

CHAPTER 1

ELECTROPHYSIOLOGY

Knowledge of basic electrophysiologic principles is essential to a proper understanding of clinical electrocardiography and to the correct interpretation of the electrocardiogram.

A simple approach to the electrophysiology of the heart is through a consideration of the electrical properties of individual cardiac muscle fibers during the resting state and during the processes of depolarization and repolarization.

RESTING OR POLARIZED STATE (FIG. 1-1)

For the purposes of this discussion, a hypothetical cardiac muscle fiber or cell is immersed in a homogeneous volume conductor such as normal saline in order to simulate conditions as they exist within the body. When the muscle strip is at *rest,* or is in the *polarized state,* a series of positive charges line the outer surface of the cell membrane and a corresponding number of negative charges line its inner surface. Each pair of positive and negative charges is called a *dipole,* or *doublet.* Current flow between the two layers of charges is prevented by the high electrical resistance of the cell membrane during the resting state.

DEPOLARIZATION (FIG. 1-2)

Stimulation of the muscle cell causes the electrical resistance to be lowered at the site of stimulation, which permits an electric current to flow across

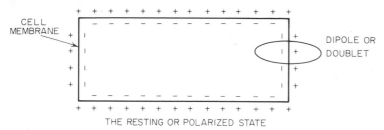

Fig. 1-1   The resting or polarized state.   Described in text.

Fig. 1-2   The process of depolarization.   Described in text.

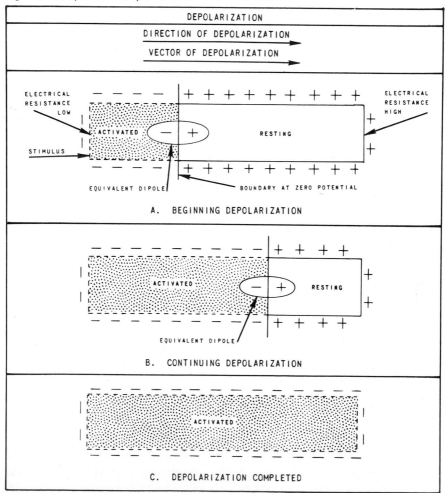

the membrane. The positive charge at this point migrates across the membrane toward the interior of the cell, and its corresponding negative charge moves to the surface of the strip. Because the muscle fiber is an excitable tissue, the stimulus is propagated through the cell without additional stimulation. Along the entire length of the muscle strip, each successive pair of positive and negative charges crosses the cell membrane until the cell is completely *activated*, or *depolarized*. At any given instant during depolarization, there is a boundary between resting and depolarized muscle. This boundary is at zero potential. The greatest positivity lies immediately in front of the zero line; the greatest negativity, immediately behind it. The depolarization process may be represented by a series of dipoles consisting of positive charges in advance of negative charges traversing the surface of the cell from the site of stimulation to the opposite end of the cell. Moreover, the whole series of dipoles may be represented by a *single equivalent dipole*. Since the cell is immersed in a homogeneous volume conductor, the flow of current creates an electric field in the conductor. Potential differences therefore exist between any points located on opposite sides of the zero line within the volume conductor.

REPOLARIZATION (FIG. 1-3)

Following depolarization, the muscle strip remains in the activated state for a brief interval and then slowly returns to the polarized state. During the time that the muscle cell remains in the activated state, no current flows, and the potential differences and the electric field disappear. Restoration of the resting state is called *repolarization*. Repolarization may take place in the same direction as depolarization (e.g., that which occurs in normal atrial muscle) or in the opposite direction from depolarization (e.g., that which occurs in normal ventricular muscle). In either case, during repolarization, the high electrical resistance of the membrane, with a layer of positive charges on the outer surface of the cell membrane and a corresponding layer of negative charges along its inner surface, is restored. The repolarization process may be represented by a series of dipoles, consisting of negative charges in advance of positive charges, traversing the surface of the cell from the site at which repolarization began to the opposite end of the cell. As in the case of depolarization, the whole series of dipoles may be represented by a single equivalent dipole. The flow of current during repolarization creates an electric field in the surrounding medium. Potential differences therefore exist between any points located on opposite sides of the zero line within the conductor.

LEADS (FIG. 1-4)

A *galvanometer* may be used to record the electrical potentials produced by a muscle strip during depolarization and repolarization. This instrument

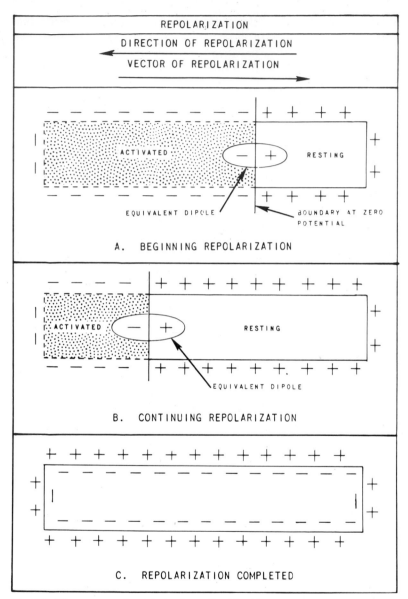

Fig. 1-3 The process of repolarization. Described in text.

has two terminals: one is connected to a positive electrode, and the other to a negative electrode. The galvanometer records the difference in potential between the two electrodes. An *electrocardiograph,* which is essentially a modified galvanometer, operates in similar fashion. When the electrodes are placed at different points in an electrical field, they form a *lead.* A hypothetical line joining the sites of the two electrodes is called the *axis of the lead*.   *Bipolar leads* are those in which both positive and negative electrodes are located in areas of electrical potential.   *Unipolar leads* are those in which the negative electrode, called the *indifferent electrode,* is at zero potential.   The positive electrode of a unipolar lead is called the *exploring electrode.*

Bipolar leads record the potential difference between the two electrode sites but give no information concerning the electric forces actually present beneath each electrode.   Unipolar leads (which, in the strict sense, are really bipolar) similarly record the potential difference between the exploring electrode and the indifferent electrode.   However, since the latter is at zero potential, a unipolar lead, in effect, records the potential variations taking place beneath the exploring electrode.

Unipolar leads may be employed to record the electrical activity of a hypothetical muscle strip.   The graphic record of the electrical forces generated by a muscle cell is called an *electrogram.*   Similarly the graphic record of the electrical potentials produced by the heart is called an *electrocardiogram.*   By convention, in both the electrogram and the electrocardiogram, positive forces cause the inscription of upward deflections; negative forces, downward deflections.

POTENTIALS RECORDED BY UNIPOLAR LEADS DURING DEPOLARIZATION AND REPOLARIZATION

The potentials recorded by a unipolar lead during depolarization and repolarization of a muscle strip are dependent on the location of the exploring electrode, the distance between the exploring electrode and the muscle strip, and the orientation of the axis of the lead with respect to the direction of depolarization and repolarization.   These factors will now be considered.

In the discussion which follows, a hypothetical muscle strip from the left ventricle, extending from endocardium to epicardium, is immersed in a large-volume conductor.   The indifferent electrode is placed in the

Fig. 1-4 Bipolar and unipolar leads.   In bipolar leads the positive and negative electrodes are located in areas of electrical potential.   In unipolar leads, the negative electrode, because it is located at a great distance from the source of electromotive forces, is at zero potential.

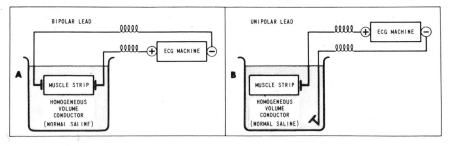

conductor at a site remote from the muscle fiber. Since in large-volume conductors electromotive force is inversely proportional to the cube of the distance between the source of the potential and the electrode, it can be assumed that the indifferent electrode is at zero potential. Exploring electrodes are placed at three points on the surface of the cell: one at each end of the cell and the third at its midportion. Each electrode is connected to a different recording channel in the galvanometer. The potential variations of the muscle cell are recorded by each lead on a moving paper or film. By standardization it is possible to determine the magnitude of the voltages from the amplitude of the deflections. Similarly, since the paper moves at a given speed, it is possible to measure the duration of the waves, complexes, and intervals. As in the case of the normal ventricular myocardium, the direction of depolarization is from endocardium to epicardium, and the direction of repolarization is from epicardium to endocardium. By convention, the deflections produced by depolarization of ventricular muscle are called *QRS complexes;* those produced by repolarization are called *T waves.*

EFFECT OF THE LOCATION OF THE EXPLORING ELECTRODE ON THE POTENTIAL VARIATIONS OF UNIPOLAR LEADS (FIG. 1-5)

Epicardial Leads

During the resting state, no current flows and the baseline remains isoelectric. When the muscle strip is stimulated, the activation process begins. An equivalent dipole with a positive charge in advance of a negative charge travels toward the electrode. The electrode, facing the positive side of the dipole, begins to record an upstroke. The positivity becomes more intense as the dipole approaches the electrode. This is represented by the gradual upward slope of the deflection. The peak of the deflection signals the arrival of the dipole at the epicardial end of the cell directly beneath the electrode. With complete activation of the muscle strip at this moment, the dipole disappears and the deflection returns precipitously to the baseline. This deflection is called an *R wave.* The muscle strip remains in the activated state for a brief period during which the entire surface of the strip has the same negative potential. During this interval, therefore, the baseline remains isoelectric. This portion of the baseline is called the *S-T segment.*

With the onset of repolarization, an equivalent dipole with a negative charge in advance of a positive charge appears at the epicardial end of the muscle strip and travels to the endocardial end in a direction away from the exploring electrode. This electrode always faces the positive side of the dipole. Since repolarization takes longer than depolarization and the magnitude of the potentials produced at any given instant is less, a small, wide, upright deflection, the T wave, is inscribed.

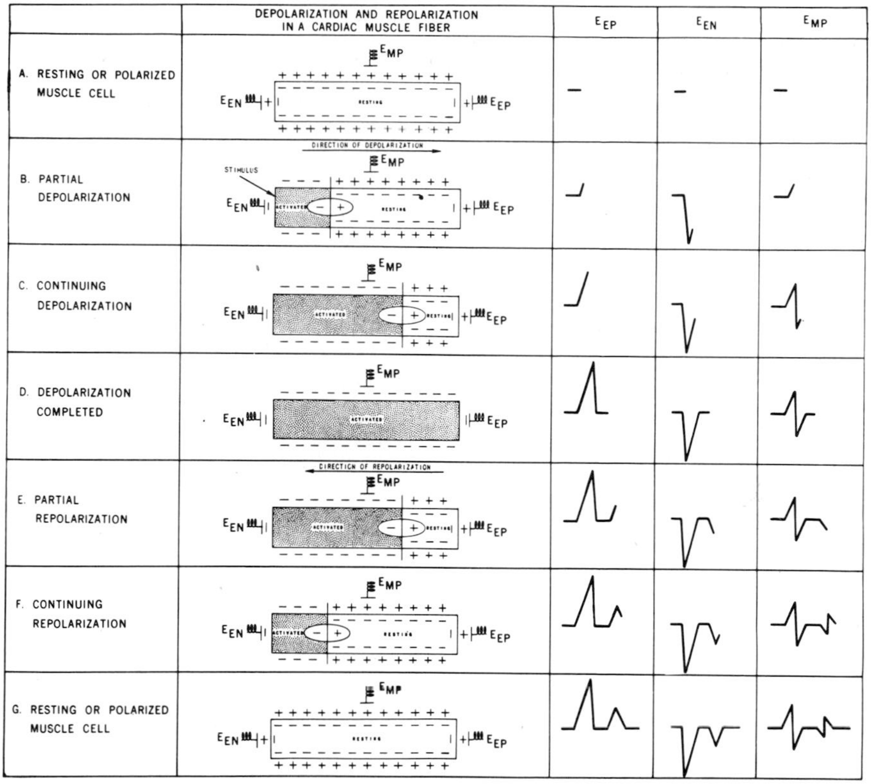

	DEPOLARIZATION AND REPOLARIZATION IN A CARDIAC MUSCLE FIBER	E_{EP}	E_{EN}	E_{MP}
A. RESTING OR POLARIZED MUSCLE CELL		—	—	—
B. PARTIAL DEPOLARIZATION				
C. CONTINUING DEPOLARIZATION				
D. DEPOLARIZATION COMPLETED				
E. PARTIAL REPOLARIZATION				
F. CONTINUING REPOLARIZATION				
G. RESTING OR POLARIZED MUSCLE CELL				

Fig. 1-5 The potentials recorded by unipolar leads during depolarization and repolarization of a cardiac muscle fiber. Described in text. E_{EP}, epicardial lead; E_{EN}, endocardial leads; E_{MP}, a lead at the midpoint of the muscle strip.

Endocardial Leads

When an exploring electrode is placed at the endocardial end of the muscle strip, the electrode faces the negative aspect of the moving dipole throughout depolarization, and a downward deflection will be recorded. The greatest negativity occurs at the onset of depolarization, since the electrode is closest to the dipole at this time. The slope of the forward limb of the deflection is, therefore, steeply downward, and its nadir is reached almost immediately. During the remainder of depolarization, the dipole moves away from the exploring electrode, so that the negativity at the electrode decreases. The hind limb of the deflection therefore shows a gradual return to the isoelectric level. This single, negative deflection is called a *QS complex*. During the time the muscle remains in the activated state, an isoelectric baseline is written. During repolarization, the electrode faces the negative aspect of the approaching dipole and a downward T wave is recorded.

Other Leads

When an exploring electrode is placed over the center of the muscle strip, the electrode faces the positive side of the approaching dipole at the onset of depolarization and an upstroke is inscribed. The upstroke continues to be written and reaches its maximum amplitude when the dipole arrives at a point directly beneath the electrode. As soon as the positive charge passes beneath the electrode, the potential becomes zero and the deflection falls abruptly from its peak to the baseline. A moment later the dipole begins to travel away from the electrode. The deflection continues sharply downward from the baseline and reaches its lowest point immediately, since the electrode now faces the negative side of the dipole. As the dipole moves away from the electrode, the negativity at the electrode decreases. The deflection thus returns gradually to the isoelectric level. This diphasic deflection is called an *RS complex*. While the muscle remains in the activated state, an isoelectric baseline is written. During repolarization, the electrode first faces the negative side of the approaching dipole and later its positive side. The T wave that is recorded is therefore diphasic.

EFFECT OF THE DISTANCE BETWEEN THE EXPLORING ELECTRODE AND THE MUSCLE STRIP ON THE POTENTIAL VARIATIONS OF UNIPOLAR LEADS (FIG. 1-6)

Since electromotive force is inversely proportional to the cube of the distance in a large-volume conductor, the potential decreases rapidly as the distance between the exploring electrode and the muscle strip increases.

Fig. 1-6 The effect of the distance between the exploring electrode and the muscle strip upon the amplitude of the deflections recorded by unipolar leads. As the exploring electrode is moved away from the muscle cell, there is a marked decrement in voltage. Compare the potentials recorded by exploring electrodes E_1 and E_2.

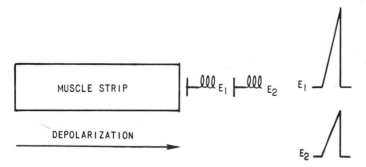

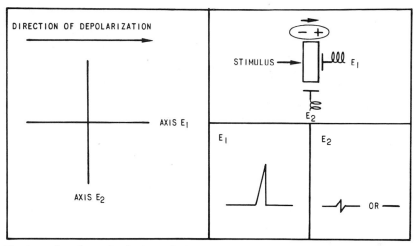

Fig. 1-7   The relationship between the lead axis and the magnitude of the deflections recorded by unipolar leads.   The axis of E_1 is parallel to the direction of deplorization, which results in a large deflection.   The E_2 axis is perpendicular to the direction of current flow.   Either no deflection or a small diphasic deflection is recorded by this lead.

RELATIONSHIP BETWEEN THE LEAD AXIS AND THE MAGNITUDE OF DEFLECTIONS RECORDED BY UNIPOLAR LEADS (FIG. 1-7)

The amplitude of a deflection is maximal when the direction of electrical forces is parallel to the axis of the lead.   As the angle between the two decreases from a straight angle to a right angle, the amplitude of the deflection becomes smaller.   When the flow of electrical forces is perpendicular to the axis of a lead, no significant deflection is recorded.

EFFECT OF SIMULTANEOUS STIMULATION OF TWO MUSCLE STRIPS ON THE POTENTIAL VARIATIONS OF UNIPOLAR LEADS (FIGS. 1-8, 1-9)

When excitation spreads simultaneously in the same direction through two identical muscle strips lying end to end, the potentials recorded by an exploring electrode placed at the outer end of the muscle fibers will be greater than that inscribed by each muscle strip alone.

When excitation spreads simultaneously in opposite directions through two identical muscle strips lying end to end, the potentials will tend to neutralize each other.   However, an exploring electrode placed at the epicardial end of the second muscle strip will record a small upright deflection because of its proximity to the positive charge of the equivalent dipole traversing the adjacent strip.   The amplitude of the deflection is lower than it would have been if the potentials in the second muscle strip had not been opposed by those produced in the first.

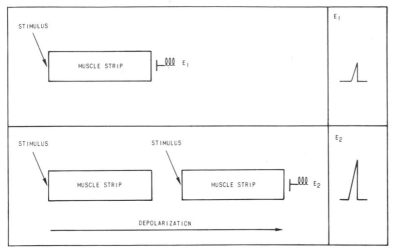

Fig. 1-8   Simultaneous stimulation of two muscle strips in the same direction results in a larger deflection than would be recorded during the deplorization of a single muscle fiber.

INTRINSIC DEFLECTION (FIG. 1-10)

The *intrinsic deflection* is the deflection that signifies activation of muscle directly beneath the exploring electrode of a unipolar lead.   All deflections preceding or following the intrinsic deflection are called *extrinsic deflections*.

FACTORS AFFECTING THE PROCESSES OF DEPOLARIZATION AND REPOLARIZATION (FIG. 1-11)

Effects of a Change in the Speed or Direction of Depolarization on the Direction of Repolarization

A change in the direction of repolarization may be secondary to a reduction in conduction velocity.   For example, if a conduction defect is present in

Fig. 1-9   Simultaneous stimulation of two muscle strips in opposite directions results in a small positive deflection recorded by exploring lead E.   Explained in text.

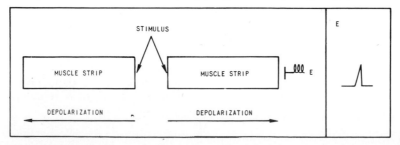

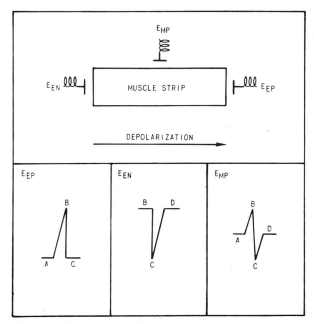

Fig. 1-10   The intrinsic deflection.   In each of the examples shown, the line *BC* is the intrinsic deflection which signifies completion of the activation process in the muscle strip directly beneath each exploring electrode.

a hypothetical muscle fiber, normal stimulation will result in the inscription of an R wave, but its duration will be increased because of the conduction delay.   Owing to the slow rate of depolarization, recovery will take place first at the endocardial end of the cell rather than at its epicardial end. The direction of repolarization will accordingly be reversed, and a negative T wave will be inscribed.

The direction of repolarization may also be altered because of a change in the direction of depolarization.   If a hypothetical muscle strip is stimulated at its epicardial end, the direction of depolarization will be reversed. Depolarization will then proceed from the epicardial to the endocardial end of the cell, which will cause a QS deflection to be written.   However, because of the altered sequence of excitation, repolarization will begin at the epicardial end of the cell and proceed toward its endocardial end.   An upright T wave will be inscribed.

A T wave change occurring because of a conduction defect or as a consequence of a change in the direction of depolarization is called a *secondary T wave change.*

Effects of a Change in the Direction of Repolarization with Depolarization Unchanged

The direction of repolarization depends not only on the direction of depolarization but significantly also on various factors which may affect

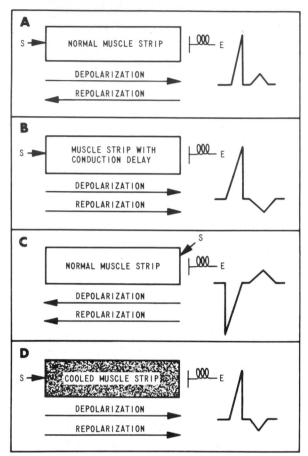

Fig. 1-11 Factors affecting the repolarization process. (A) Normal depolarization and repolarization result in upright R and T waves in an epicardial lead E. (B) Stimulation of a muscle strip with conduction delay results in an R wave of increased duration. Because of the reduced conduction velocity, repolarization begins at the endocardial end of the strip and its direction is reversed. The QRS complex is upright and the T wave is inverted. This is a secondary T wave change. (C) Stimulation of the muscle fiber in an abnormal direction causes a QS deflection of increased duration. Because of the conduction delay, recovery begins at the site of stimulation and proceeds in the same direction as depolarization. The QRS complex is inverted and the T wave is upright. This is also a secondary T wave change. (D) Cooling of the muscle strip reverses the direction of repolarization, but not of depolarization. The T wave is inverted, but the R wave remains upright. This is a primary T wave change.

the process of repolarization independently of depolarization. These include temperature changes, ischemia, drugs, and electrolytes. For example, uniform slight cooling of a hypothetical muscle strip has no effect on depolarization. The pathway of excitation is unaltered, and a normal, upright deflection is recorded by a unipolar epicardial lead. Cooling, however, causes prolongation of the period during which the muscle strip remains in the activated state, with the effect most pronounced at the epicardial end of the muscle strip where it is normally shortest and least pronounced at the endocardial end where it is normally longest.   Because of the prolonged duration of the excited state in the epicardial region, recovery occurs first in the endocardial region.   Accordingly, the direction of repolarization is reversed with concomitant reversal in the direction of the repolarization wave.   This is called a *primary T wave change,* which means that repolarization has been altered independently of depolarization.

EFFECTS OF ISCHEMIA (FIG. 1-12)

To reduce the study of the electrocardiographic changes induced by ischemia to its simplest form, reference is again made to the isolated hypothetical muscle strip extending from the endocardial surface to the epicardial surface of the left ventricle.   The muscle cell is immersed in a homogeneous volume conductor.   The exploring electrodes E_{EP} and E_{EN} are placed at the epicardial and endocardial ends of the cell, respectively. It will be recalled that normally when the muscle fiber is stimulated at its endocardial end, depolarization proceeds from this point to the epicardial

Fig. 1-12   Effects of ischemia.   Described in text.

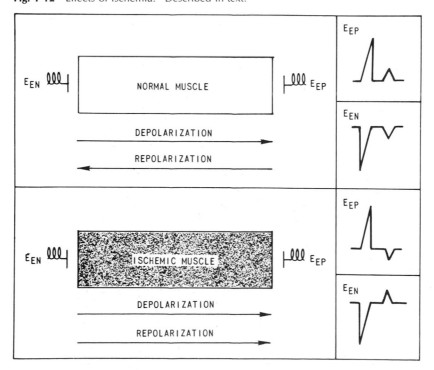

surface and repolarization proceeds in the reverse direction. This causes the electrode E_{EP} to inscribe an R wave and an upright T wave and the electrode E_{EN} to record a QS deflection and a downward T wave.

If the muscle fiber is rendered ischemic, it will be found that ischemia has no effect on the direction of depolarization, or, therefore, on the patterns inscribed by the exploring electrodes during this process. However, ischemia causes the duration of the excited state in the epicardial region, where it is normally shortest, to be prolonged. The duration of the excited state in the subendocardial region, where it is normally longest, is little affected. This results in a reversal of the order of repolarization so that its direction is now the same as that of depolarization. Thus, when the muscle cell is stimulated, the electrode E_{EP} inscribes an R wave and an inverted T wave. The electrode E_{EN} writes a QS deflection and an upright T wave. These T wave changes are primary, because the direction of repolarization is altered independently of the direction of depolarization. Ischemia is a reversible process.

EFFECTS OF SUBEPICARDIAL INJURY (FIG. 1-13)

Again, as was done in the study of myocardial ischemia, reference is made to the hypothetical muscle strip from the left ventricle suspended in a homogeneous volume conductor. Two exploring electrodes E_{EP} and E_{EN} are placed at the epicardial and endocardial ends of the cell, respectively. The epicardial one-third of the muscle strip is injured. From an electrocardiographic standpoint, this creates a situation analogous to the present in transmural myocardial injury. In other words, the patterns of transmural myocardial injury and those of subepicardial injury, for practical purposes, are identical.

When the epicardial portion of the muscle strip is injured, the resistance of the membrane in this region to the passage of electric charges is somewhat reduced. This permits some, but not all, of the positive charges on the surface of the injured segment to migrate across the membrane toward their corresponding negative charges and be neutralized. Thus, while the surface of the injured zone is still positive, its positivity is less than that of the surface of the uninjured zone. A boundary of potential difference is created at the junction between the uninjured and injured muscle. When the cell is resting, current flows from the uninjured to the injured segments across the boundary between the two. This is the current of injury. It is not possible to measure the current of injury, because it is automatically neutralized by the compensatory current of the electrocardiograph, which restores the baseline to the isoelectric level. The only electrocardiographic sign of injury is displacement of the S-T segment. How this occurs will now be elucidated.

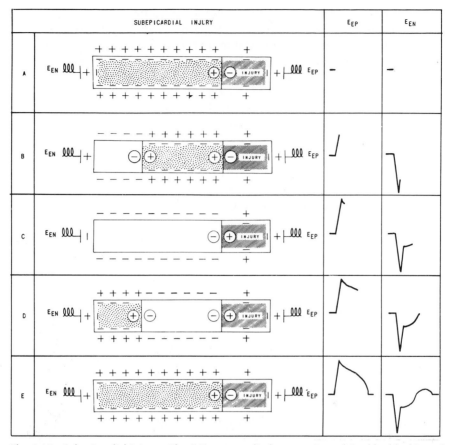

Fig. 1-13 Subepicardial injury. The S-T segment displacement is explained by blocking of the wave of excitation at the junction between uninjured and injured muscle. Described in text. E_{EP}, epicardial lead; E_{EN}, endocardial lead. *(Modified from J. M. Barker, "The Unipolar Electrocardiogram," Appleton-Century-Crofts, New York, 1952. Used by permission.)*

In the resting state, the compensatory current of the electrocardiograph neutralizes the current of injury and the baseline remains isoelectric.

When the muscle strip is stimulated at its endocardial end, an equivalent dipole begins to travel along the surface of the cell toward the electrode E_{EP} and away from the electrode E_{EN}. The former will cause the initial upstroke of an R wave; the latter, the entire downstroke of a QS deflection.

When the dipole has traversed the uninjured segment and reaches the injured segment, it is blocked at the boundary between the two. This causes the surface of the partially polarized injured zone to become relatively positive to the surface of the depolarized uninjured zone. The electrode E_{EP} inscribes the upstroke of an R wave during depolarization of the uninjured region. The peak of the R wave signals the completion of this process.   The deflection, instead of returning sharply to the baseline, remains upward because the electrode now faces the positivity of the boundary between the uninjured and injured segments.   The electrode E_{EN}, having written its maximal deflection at the onset of depolarization, continues to record the final upstroke of the QS deflection during activation of the uninjured region.   When depolarization has been completed, the deflection, which has not yet ascended to the baseline, remains beneath it because the electrode now faces the negativity of the boundary between the uninjured and injured segments.

Repolarization begins shortly thereafter, but starts at the endocardial end of the muscle strip and proceeds toward the epicardial region of the cell.   This occurs because the process causing injury has also caused ischemia of the remainder of the muscle cell.   This results in a reversal of the normal direction of repolarization   With the onset of repolarization, an equivalent dipole with a negative charge in advance of a positive charge begins to travel along the surface of the cell toward the electrode E_{EP} and away from the electrode E_{EN}.   During repolarization, the electrode E_{EP} faces the positivity of the injured zone and the increasing negativity of the repolarization wave.   This causes the deflection to return gradually to the baseline.   The electrode E_{EN} faces the negativity of the injured zone and the positivity of the repolarization wave.   The former forces are counterbalanced by the latter, so that the final component of the upstroke of the QS deflection returns gradually to the baseline.   Thus, the electrode E_{EP} inscribes a monophasic curve in which the elevated S-T segment and the T wave are merged.   The electrode E_{EN} inscribes a QS deflection and a depressed S-T segment merged with the T wave.

The degree of displacement of the S-T segment in myocardial injury is dependent upon the completeness with which the excitation wave is blocked at the junction between uninjured and injured muscle.   Complete blocking of the wave causes an epicardial lead to record the monophasic type of curve described above.   Less complete blocking results in lesser degrees of S-T segment displacement and the inscription of the intrinsic deflection (R wave) in such a lead.

It should be pointed out that there are other explanations for the displacement of the S-T segment observed in myocardial injury.   According to one hypothesis (Fig. 1-14), when a portion of a muscle strip is injured, the current of injury causes depression of the baseline in a lead overlying the injured zone.   When the current of injury is neutralized by the compensatory current from the electrocardiograph, the baseline is brought back to the isoelectric level.   However, when the muscle strip is stimulated, both the uninjured and injured zones are depolarized and the current of injury ceases to flow.   The compensatory current from the instrument is then unopposed and produces upward displacement of the S-T segment in an epicardial lead.   During repolarization, the elevated S-T segment

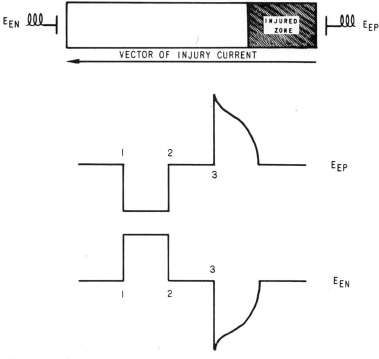

Fig. 1-14 Subepicardial injury. Alternative explanation of the mechanism of the S-T segment displacement. At 1, the muscle fiber is injured. At 2, a current from the electrocardiograph brings the baseline back to the isoelectric level. At 3, the entire muscle fiber, including uninjured and injured regions, is depolarized. The injury current ceases to flow temporarily. The S-T segment displacement is produced by the unopposed compensatory current from the electrocardiograph. E_{EP}, epicardial lead; E_{EN}, endocardial lead. The former shows an elevated S-T segment; the latter, a depressed one.

gradually returns to the baseline as the current of injury begins to flow again and neutralizes the compensatory current.

According to another hypothesis (Fig. 1-15), when the epicardial portion of a muscle strip is injured, the current of injury causes depression of the baseline in leads overlying the injured zone. This can only be observed under experimental conditions at the instant injury occurs. It is not observed in clinical practice. Were the injury current to flow constantly, downward displacement of the baseline would be continuous. This does not happen because the current of injury flows only in electrical diastole and ceases during electrical systole. Under this hypothesis, the injured as well as the uninjured zones are depolarized. There is no blocking of the excitatory wave at the boundary between the two zones as described earlier in the chapter. Following ventricular depolarization, represented by the QRS complex, the current of injury is extinguished because both the

INJURY

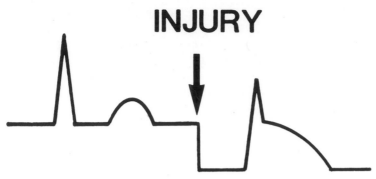

Fig. 1-15 Alternative explanation of the mechanism of S-T segment displacement in myocardial injury when both the uninjured and injured zones are depolarized. The first QRS complex is normal. The point at which injury is produced is indicated by the arrow. The baseline is depressed by the injury current. Depolarization, involving both the injured and uninjured regions, causes the inscription of the R wave of the second QRS complex. The injury current is then extinguished. As a result, the S-T segment is inscribed at the level of the original baseline. As repolarization proceeds, the current of injury is gradually reestablished and the S-T segment returns to the new baseline.

uninjured and injured areas are completely depolarized. Therefore the S-T segment is at the level of the original baseline. As repolarization proceeds there is a gradual return to the new baseline as the injury current is reestablished.

It should be noted that injury, like ischemia, is a reversible process.

EFFECTS OF SUBENDOCARDIAL INJURY (FIG. 1-16)

A hypothetical muscle strip from the left ventricle is immersed in a homogeneous volume conductor. The endocardial one-third of the strip is injured. The agent responsible for injury of the endocardial region also renders the remainder of the muscle strip ischemic. The exploring electrodes E_{EP} and E_{EN} are placed on the epicardial and endocardial ends of the cell, respectively. The patterns inscribed by each during depolarization and repolarization are recorded.

Stimulation of the muscle cell at the endocardial end has little effect on the injured segment. The stimulus, however, is conducted through to the uninjured segment. Depolarization begins at the junction between the two and proceeds in normal fashion. The electrode E_{EP} faces the positive aspect of the boundary between depolarized and resting muscle and the negative aspect of the boundary between injured and uninjured muscle. The latter forces are of lesser magnitude than the former, so that the upstroke of an R wave is inscribed. The height of the R wave is, however, less than normal, because the former forces are to some degree counterbalanced by the latter and also because the injured segment is not depolarized. The electrode E_{EN} faces the positive aspect of the boundary between injured and uninjured muscle and the negative side of the boundary between depolarized and resting muscle. At the onset of depolarization, the latter forces are maximal and counterbalance the former, so that the downstroke of a Q wave is written. During the remainder of depolarization, the negativity of the latter diminishes steadily but is always sufficient to counterbalance the positivity at the boundary between injured and uninjured muscle. Thus the upstroke of the Q wave continues to be inscribed during the remainder of depolarization.

With the completion of depolarization, the electrical forces generated by this process are extinguished. The electrode E_{EP} then faces the negative side of the boundary between the injured and uninjured muscle, and the electrode E_{EN} faces the positive side of this boundary. The electrode E_{EP} records the downstroke of the R wave, which continues beneath the

Fig. 1-16 Subendocardial injury. Described in text. E_{EP}, epicardial lead; E_{EN}, endocardial lead. *(Modified from J. M. Barker, "The Unipolar Electrocardiogram," Appleton-Century-Crofts, New York, 1952. Used by permission.)*

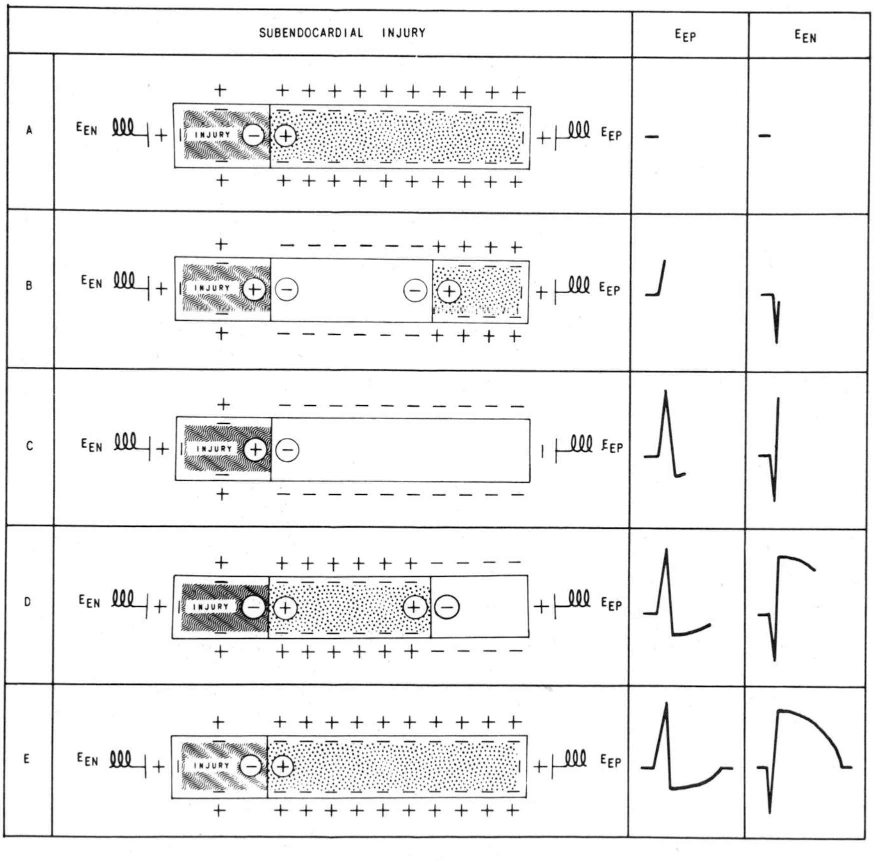

baseline; the electrode E_{EN} records the upstroke of the Q wave, which continues above the baseline.

Repolarization begins shortly thereafter and, because the uninjured muscle is ischemic, starts at the endocardial end of the muscle strip and proceeds toward its epicardial end. During repolarization, the electrode E_{EP} faces the negativity of the repolarization wave and the positive aspect of the boundary between injured and uninjured muscle. This causes the deflection to ascend gradually to the baseline. The electrode E_{EN} faces the positivity of the repolarization wave and the negative aspect of the boundary between injured and uninjured muscle. This causes the deflection to descend gradually to the baseline. In both instances the T wave is merged with the S-T segment.

SUMMARY

In anterior subepicardial ischemia, epicardial or precordial leads show T wave inversion. In anterior subendocardial ischemia, these leads show T wave elevation.

In anterior subepicardial injury, epicardial or precordial leads show S-T segment elevation, whereas when the injury is subendocardial these leads show S-T segment depression.

EFFECTS OF NECROSIS

Necrotic or dead muscle generates no electrical forces, since it is electrically inert.

COMMENT

The foregoing presentation of the cellular electrical activity of the heart is based on physical mechanisms originally proposed many years ago. The membrane theory is useful in explaining the derivation of the various components of the electrocardiogram. However, as a working concept of cellular electrophysiology it is inadequate for explaining the genesis of cardiac arrhythmias and the effect of drugs and electrolyte abnormalities on the electrocardiogram. The ionic and bioelectrical phenomena involved in the activity of cardiac muscle and the transmembrane potentials of cardiac cells are discussed in Chap. 24. The reader is referred to that section of the text for information on these subjects.

REFERENCE

Barker, J. M.: "The Unipolar Electrocardiogram," Appleton-Century-Crofts, New York, 1952.

CHAPTER 2

ANATOMY AND PHYSIOLOGY OF THE CONDUCTION SYSTEM OF THE HEART

Within the heart there exists a specialized conduction system for the initiation and propagation of the excitatory process (Figs. 2-1 to 2-4). Knowledge of this conduction system is essential to proper understanding of electrocardiography.

The excitatory process has its origin in the *sinoatrial node (SA node)*, a specialized muscular structure lying within the atrial musculature near the junction of the superior vena cava and the right atrium. Possessing the highest degree of rhythmicity of any structure within the heart, the SA node is its normal pacemaker. Because the electrical forces produced by the SA node are very small, they are not recorded in the electrocardiogram.

From the SA node the activation process spreads through both atria. Evidence suggests that atrial depolarization is not entirely radial but is asymmetric, with the internodal tracts playing a significant role in the distribution of the atrial impulse. Initially, only the right atrium is activated. Shortly thereafter, excitation spreads to the interatrial septum and to the left atrium. During the final period of atrial activation, only the left atrium is depolarized. The last region of the left atrium to be depolarized is either the tip of the left atrial appendage or its posteroinferior portion. The velocity of impulse transmission in the atria is estimated to be between 800 and 1,000 mm/s. The atrial activation time is normally 0.07 to 0.10 s.

The P wave of the electrocardiogram represents atrial depolarization. Repolarization of the atria is designated by the Tp (or Ta) wave, which is not ordinarily seen because it is usually buried in the QRS complex.

After traversing the atrial musculature, the stimulus passes into the

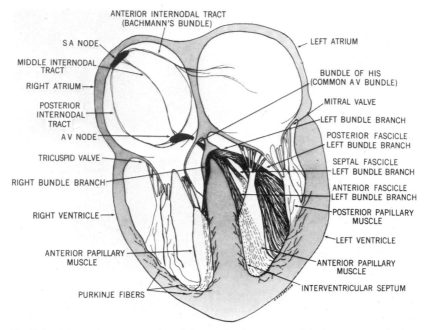

Fig. 2-1   Schematic representation of the conduction system of the heart.   Described in text.

atrioventricular node (AV node).   This structure lies within the posterobasal region of the interatrial septum between the orifice of the coronary sinus and the medial leaflet of the tricuspid valve.   The AV nodal region is divided anatomically into three areas: (1) the approaches to the AV node (superior, middle, and inferior); (2) the AV node itself; and (3) the origin of the penetrating portion of the AV bundle (His).   The approaches to the region and the node itself are subject to vagal influences, whereas the lower regions are essentially independent of these effects.   Fibers from the atria approach the AV node at all levels, including those which enter the node at its lowest portion.

Electrophysiologists have divided the AV node (Fig. 2-4) into AN (atrionodal), N (nodal), and NH (nodal-His) regions.   These may or may not coincide with the anatomic subdivisions cited above.

The bundle of His, also called the *common* or *AV bundle,* is a thin fascicle connecting the AV node with the bundle branches.   The bundle of His penetrates the central fibrous body and then courses along the lower edge of the membrane's septum toward the aortic valve, where it bifurcates into the left and right bundle branches.   The bundle of His can be considered as composed of penetrating and nonpenetrating, or branching, portions. The penetrating portion of the bundle extends from the distal end of the AV node to the point where the initial radiations of the left bundle branch are given off.   The branching portion is a continuation of the penetrating segment.   It extends from the point where the bundle begins to emit the

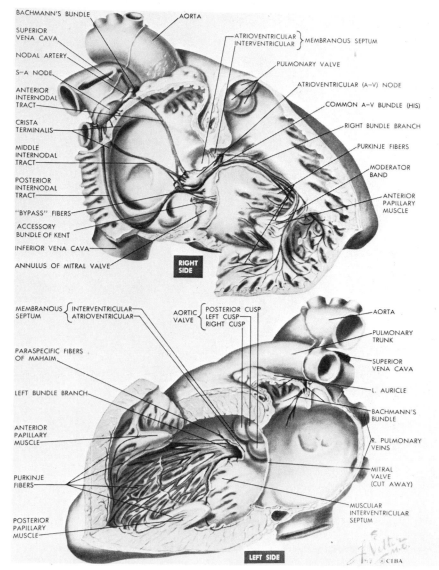

Fig. 2-2 The specialized conduction system of the heart. Subdivisions of the left bundle branch are not shown. (See also Figs. 2-1, 2-3, 11-19.) (*Copyright* 1969 *CIBA Pharmaceutical Company, Division of CIBA-GEIGY Corporation. Reproduced with permission from "The CIBA Collection of Medical Illustrations," by Frank H. Netter, M.D. All rights reserved.*)

most posterior fibers of the left bundle branch to the site which marks the origin of the right bundle branch and the most anterior fibers of the left bundle branch. Portions of the His bundle are sometimes the site of origin of the paraspecific fibers of Mahaim.

Rosenbaum et al. consider the right bundle branch to be a continuation

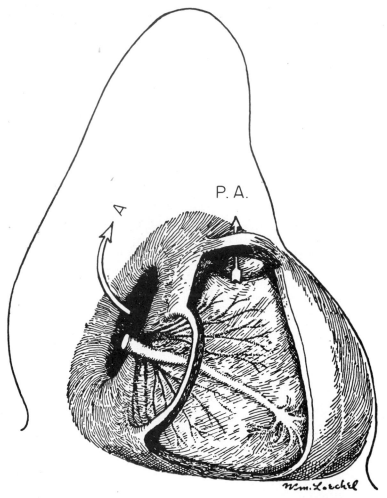

Fig. 2-3 The ventricular conduction system in humans. The free wall of the right ventricle has been partially cut away. The interventricular septum lies more or less parallel to the frontal plane of the body, with the right ventricle anterior to the left. The outflow pathways of the aorta and pulmonary artery are indicated. The common bundle branches are shown. Note the bifurcation of the left bundle branch into anterior and posterior divisions. *(From R. P. Grant, "Clinical Electrocardiography," © 1957 by McGraw-Hill, Inc., New York. Used with permission of McGraw-Hill Book Company.)*

Fig. 2-4 Schematic representation of the AN, A, and NH regions of the AV node.

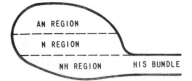

of the bundle of His after the fibers of the left bundle branch are given off. According to them the fibers of the left bundle branch arise from the main bundle in sequential fashion: first the posterior fibers and then the anterior fibers. All of them arise almost perpendicularly from the common bundle. They believe that there is no true bifurcation of the bundle of His in humans. The terminal end of the bundle, where the right bundle branch separates from the most anterior part of the left bundle branch, is called the *pseudobifurcation*. Rosenbaum and his associates have stated that within the main left bundle branch the fibers of the anterior and posterior division seem to be delineated.

The *right bundle branch* is a cordlike structure which descends subendocardially along the right side of the interventricular septum to its termination into anterior, septal, and posterior subdivisions. At present, there are no acceptable electrocardiographic criteria for recognition of lesions of these specific subdivisions of the right bundle branch in humans.

The *left bundle branch,* which runs subendocardially along the left side of the interventricular septum, is composed of multiple fascicles, and these, in turn, may be grouped into two main groups of fibers, the posterior (inferior) and anterior (superior) fascicles or divisions. The posterior group spreads inferiorly, the anterior group, superiorly. Each division consists of fine fasciculi which fan out beneath the left ventricular endocardium. More recently, it has been demonstrated that many persons also have a third division, the medial, septal, or central fascicle, which supplies the midseptal area. This fascicle arises either from the main left bundle or from the anterior or posterior radiations. All three subdivisions are widely interconnected.

Block of the anterior and posterior fascicles of the left bundle branch is recognizable electrocardiographically. However, there are no known features that would permit the electrocardiographic diagnosis of lesions of the septal fascicle.

Rosenbaum has developed the concept that the intraventricular conduction network can be regarded as a trifascicular system consisting of the right bundle branch and the two divisions of the left bundle branch.

The subdivisions of both bundle branches merge into a fascicular network (Purkinje plexus) consisting of Purkinje and transitional fibers, in the lower portions of the ventricular chambers. The Purkinje plexus is a rich network of specialized conducting fibers which penetrate the septal musculature and also cross beneath the endocardial surfaces of both ventricles to terminate in anastomoses with the ventricular muscle fibers. Except in the basal portion of the interventricular septum and in the posterobasal region of the left ventricle, where few Purkinje fibers can be found, the Purkinje fibers are widely distributed in both ventricles.

The concept that the left bundle branch divides into discrete anterior and posterior divisions and that conduction normally occurs via these fascicles has gained wide acceptance. However, it is worth emphasizing that some distinguished workers in the field accept neither the anatomic nor the electrophysiologic fascicular delineation of the left bundle branch.

The passage of the impulse through the AV node (Fig.2-4) is slow (approximately 200 mm/s). Slowing of conduction starts in the AN (atrionodal) region and reaches a maximum in the N (nodal) region. Conduction velocity increases gradually in the NH (nodal-His) region and the bundle of His and reaches a value of 1,000 to 1,500 mm/s in the latter. In the free-running Purkinje fibers, conduction velocity ranges between 3,000 and 4,000 mm/s. The nodal activation time is 0.05 to 0.13 s.

The P-R (or P-Q) interval represents the time required for an impulse to travel from the SA node to the ventricles. It is a combination of the atrial, AV nodal, and His-Purkinje conduction times (Fig. 2-5). The period between the end of the P wave and the beginning of the QRS complex, called the *P-R (or P-Q) segment,* represents conduction through part of the AV node, the bundle of His, the bundle branches, and the terminal fascicular network (Purkinje and transitional fibers).

As already indicated, the stimulus spreads rapidly from the AV node through the bundle of His, the bundle branches, and the Purkinje plexus.

The spread of the stimulus through the bundle branches initiates depolarization of the interventricular septum. According to the studies of Durrer and his coworkers on the excitation of the isolated human heart, three endocardial areas are simultaneously activated at the beginning of left ventricular excitation: (1) an area high on the anterior paraseptal wall just below the attachment of the mitral valve; (2) the central region of the left side of the interventricular septum; and (3) the posterior paraseptal area about one-third of the distance from apex to base. These investigators believe that the fibers of the anterior fascicle are responsible for activation

Fig. 2-5 Schematic representation of the relationship of activation of the specialized conducting fibers of the heart to the P wave, P-R interval, and QRST complex. The code is as follows: SN = SA node; AVN = AV node; AN = atrionodal region; N = main body of AV node; NH = nodal-His region; HIS = His bundle; BB = bundle branches; P = peripheral Purkinje fibers. *(Modified from B. F. Hoffman and D. H. Singer, Effects of Digitalis on Electrical Activity of Cardiac Fibers, Progr. Cardiovasc. Dis., 7: 226, 1964. Used by permission.)*

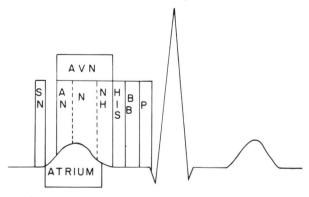

of the anterior paraseptal region and the midseptum. The activation of the posterior paraseptal region is provided by the fibers of the posterior fascicle. Uhley has suggested that the anterior branches give rise to a superiorly oriented vector, the posterior branches give rise to an inferiorly directed vector, and the septal branches give rise to a vector that is directed rightward. These findings of multiple simultaneous areas of initial septal activation represent a break with the traditional concept of a single site of early activation at the middle third of the left septal surface. Durrer and his associates in their studies found that endocardial activation of the right ventricle was found to start near the insertion of the papillary muscle 5 to 10 ms after the onset of the left ventricular cavity potential.

Figures 2-6 and 2-7 illustrate the activation of the human heart based on the work of Durrer and his associates.

Once activation has begun, depolarization waves pass from left to right from the left bundle branch and in the reverse direction from the right bundle branch. The forces tend to partially counterbalance each other, but since a much larger region of the left septum is depolarized compared with that of the right, the net direction of septal activation is from left to right. In addition to its left-to-right orientation, the overall direction of septal activation is from apex to base and from front to back.

Since conduction occurs so rapidly through the Purkinje network, and because its arborizations are profuse, both ventricular chambers are stim-

Fig. 2-6 Activation of a cross section of the human heart based on the work of Durrer. Depolarization in the walls generally proceeds from the inside outward. The earliest areas of excitation are on the left cavity anteriorly and at the septal border. The right endocardium is not excited during the first 20 ms in this section. The posterior wall is activated last. The activation times are shown in milliseconds. MV = mitral valve. *(From A. M. Scher, Excitation of the Heart: A Progress Report, in R. C. Schlant and J. W. Hurst, eds., "Advances in Electrocardiography," Grune & Stratton, New York, 1972. Used by permission.)*

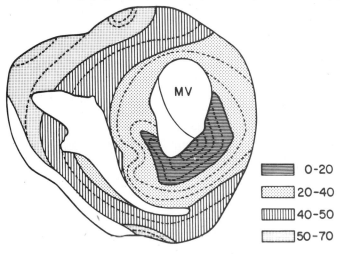

0-20
20-40
40-50
50-70

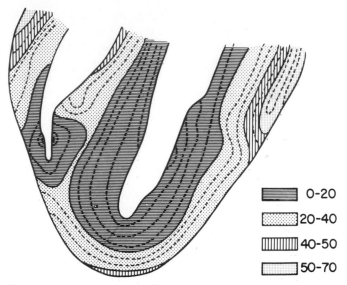

0-20
20-40
40-50
50-70

Fig. 2-7 Activation in a sagittal section of the human heart. There is extensive early activity on the left septal surface and the left mural endocardium, with much less activity on the right. The activation times are shown in milliseconds. *(From A. M. Scher, Excitation of the Heart: A Progress Report, in R. C. Schlant and J. W. Hurst, eds., "Advances in Electrocardiography," Grune & Stratton, New York, 1972. Used by permission.)*

ulated a very brief interval after depolarization of the interventricular septum has begun. This occurs first at the apex of the right ventricle, then at the apex of the left ventricle, and subsequently in the free walls of both ventricles. Within the inner layers of the myocardium there may be reversals of direction, and the excitation waves may be directed toward both the endocardium and the epicardium. In the middle and outer layers of the ventricles, depolarization proceeds centrifugally and tangentially from endocardium to epicardium. The overall direction is leftward, inferiorly, and posteriorly in the left ventricular wall. Since the free wall of the right ventricle is approximately one-third of the thickness of the free wall of the left ventricle, depolarization in the former is completed in one-third of the time required by the latter. Also, because of the larger muscle mass of the left ventricle compared with that of the right, left ventricular potentials dominate those of the right. The speed of the excitatory process in both ventricles is equal, having a rate of approxmately 300 to 400 mm/s.

The last portions of the heart to be depolarized are the posterobasal region of the left ventricle and the basal portion of the interventricular septum. The late depolarization of these regions has been attributed to the paucity of Purkinje fibers in these areas. Depolarization of the pulmonary conus in the region of the crista supraventricularis also occurs about this time, but its overall contribution to the terminal forces is probably not significant. In this final phase of ventricular activation, the forces are oriented toward the base of the heart in a posterior direction, either slightly rightward or leftward.

The QRS interval represents the intraventricular conduction time and is normally 0.06 to 0.10 s.   Ventricular repolarization is represented by the T wave.   The S-T segment represents the period of time during which the ventricles remain in the depolarized state, but repolarization begins during this interval.   The Q-T interval, representing electrical systole of the ventricles, is the time required for completion of ventricular depolarization and repolarization.   The interval from the end of the T wave to the beginning of the QRS complex represent electrical diastole of the ventricles.

NEWER CONCEPTS

The traditional concepts of supraventricular conduction, namely, that the sinus impulse spreads radially through the atria and the AV node is activated en masse by the first electrical impulse to reach it, have been challenged in the last few years.   Recent observations have suggested that the sinus impulse is not only distributed to the left atrium via special tracts but also reaches the AV node by selective pathways.   Moreover, there is evidence that there exist in the AV node dual or even multiple anatomic or physiologic pathways for the conduction of the impulse between the atria and ventricles.

James has concluded that in the human heart there are regularly three connecting pathways between the SA and AV nodes: the anterior, middle, and posterior internodal tracts (Fig. 2-8).   Fibers from these tracts also connect both atria, so that they function as interatrial as well as internodal pathways for impulse conduction.

The *anterior internodal tract* arises in the SA node and sweeps anterior to the superior vena cava into Bachmann's bundle, where it divides into two groups of fibers.   One set of fibers is connected directly with the left atrium; the other eventually makes its way via the interatrial septum to the crest of the AV node. The *middle internodal tract*, arising from the posterior margin of the SA node, courses behind the superior vena cava and reaches the crest of the AV node after traversing the interatrial septum.   Near the AV node it merges with fibers from the anterior internodal tract.   The *posterior internodal tract* follows the crista terminalis from the SA node to the Eustachian ridge and passes through the ridge to reach the posterior margin of the AV node.   Although a few fibers terminate there, the bulk of them, joined by some fibers from the anterior and middle internodal tracts, bypass the main body of the AV node.   Most of the fibers in the bypass tract reenter the lower portion of the node, some terminate at the base of the tricuspid valve, and rarely a few of them may reach the interventricular septum directly.

It has been suggested that the three internodal tracts, under both normal and abnormal conditions, separately or together, function as specific

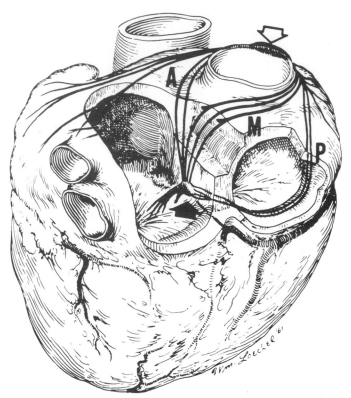

Fig. 2-8 Location and course of the three internodal tracts of the human heart. The heart is viewed from above and behind the left atrium. The open arrow indicates the SA node, while the black arrow indicates the AV node. *A*, the anterior internodal tracts and the predominant interatrial tracts, the division occurring as they course in Bachmann's bundle. These interatrial fibers were first described by Bachmann. *M*, the middle internodal tracts, first described by Wenckebach. *P*, the posterior internodal tracts, first described by Thorel. See text for further details. *(From T. N. James, Anatomy of the Conduction System of the Heart, in J. W. Hurst and R. B. Logue, eds., "The Heart," © 1966 by McGraw-Hill, Inc., New York. Used with permission of McGraw-Hill Book Company.)*

preferential pathways for impulse conduction between the SA and AV nodes. It has also been suggested that the interatrial connections of the anterior internodal tract, originally described by Bachmann, function as the preferential route for impulse conduction from the SA node to the left atrium. From the SA node to the right atrium, conduction is by radial spread of the excitation wave.

According to James, the fibers of the internodal tracts enter the AV node at two principal sites (Figs. 2-9, 2-10): (1) at its superoposterior portion (the crest), containing chiefly fibers of the anterior and middle tracts but a few of the posterior tract, and (2) along the convex surface and anteroinferior margin, composed primarily of fibers from the posterior tract which have bypassed the AV node. On entering the node, the fibers from all tracts

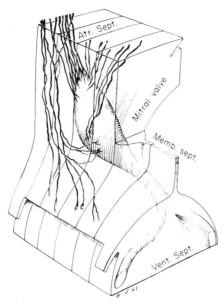

Fig. 2-9 A schematic drawing of the human AV node, illustrating its relationship to the two atrioventricular values and the interatrial and interventricular (including its membranous portion) septa. The AV bundle divides into a single right bundle branch and multiple left bundle branches, as usual. Fibers from the central interatrial septal tracts and from the Eustachian ridge enter the posterior superior margin of the node and also form bypass tracts, as described in the text. Note that some of the bypass tract fibers reenter the inferior margin of the node and some terminate at the base of the tricuspid valve; rarely, some penetrate directly into the crest of the interventricular septum. *(From T. N. James, Morphology of the Human Atrioventricular Node, with Remarks Pertinent to Its Electrophysiology, Am. Heart J., 62: 756, 1961. Used by permission.)*

divide into a network of smaller fibers. At the anteroinferior end of the node, the interlacing fibers assume a parallel course and form the bundle of His.

Some authorities, unable to demonstrate such dissectable bundles, consider still unresolved the anatomic question as to whether the discrete morphologic tracts described by James actually exist in the human heart.

Lev has reviewed the possible anatomic pathways for conduction from the atria to the ventricles in both healthy and diseased hearts. The existences of the internodal tracts of James was confirmed. The paraspecific fibers of Mahaim, consisting of short but direct connections between the AV node, the bundle of His, or the bundle branches and the interventricular septum were likewise accepted. He also verified the existence of right- and left-sided neuromuscular bridges connecting the atria and ventricles directly, called the *bundles of Kent.*

From these observations, Lev concluded that there are 11 possible pathways of conduction between the atria and ventricles. According to

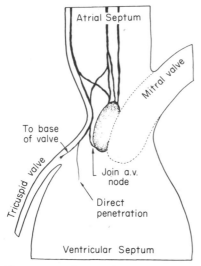

Fig. 2-10   A drawing from a representative cross section of a normal human AV node, with its relationships to the bypass tracts.   *(From T. N. James, Morphology of the Human Atrioventricular Node, with Remarks Pertinent to Its Electrophysiology, Am. Heart J., 62: 756, 1961.   Used by permission.)*

his hypothesis, subsequently elaborated by Ferrer, activation may proceed according to one of the following sequences (Fig. 2-11): (1) excitation enters the AV node at its crest and passes through the node and down the His-Purkinje system; (2) it bypasses the crest of the node, enters its lower portion, and then proceeds down the remainder of the conduction system; (3) it enters the lower AV node, bypassing the crest, and exits into the interventricular septum via Mahaim fibers; (4) it bypasses the crest, enters the lower AV node, proceeds into the bundle of His, but exits from there into the septum by way of Mahaim fibers; and (5) it bypasses the crest, enters the lower AV node, the bundle of His, and the bundle branches, but enters the left ventricle via Mahaim fibers.   Sequences 6, 7, and 8 are similar to numbers 3, 4, and 5 in that Mahaim fibers are involved, but the AV node is entered at its crest rather than at its lower portion.   Pathway 9 is identical to pathway 8 but the Mahaim tract is right-sided.   Pathways 10 and 11 represent conduction through the right- and left-sided bundles of Kent, respectively.

From these sequences, it is possible to explain the various forms of anomalous AV conduction (see Fig. 12-1).   This will be elaborated further in the section on ventricular preexcitation (the Wolff-Parkinson-White syndrome).

Sherf and James have formulated the concept of synchronized sino-ventricular conduction.   According to this hypothesis, under normal conditions an impulse leaves the SA node and descends in the internodal and interatrial tracts in a synchronized order, so that the atria and AV node

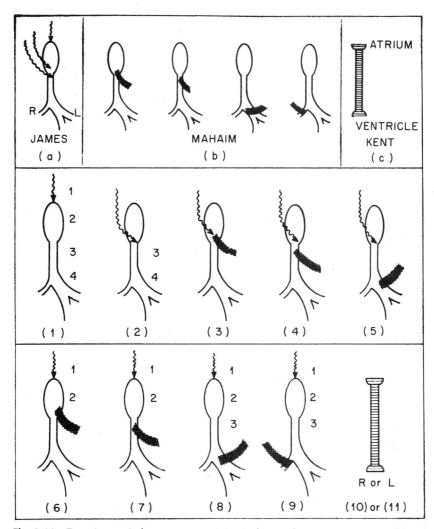

Fig. 2-11 *Top*: Anatomic bypass tracts existing in human hearts. Note (a) caudal ends of three internodal tracts, with fibers of James bypassing nodal crest; (b) four different Mahaim tracts; (c) bundle of Kent. *Bottom*: 11 possible sequences of AV conduction. *(From M. I. Ferrer, New Concepts Relating to the Preexcitation Syndrome, J.A.M.A., 201: 1038, 1967. Used by permission.)*

are depolarized in a precise fashion. The impulse is then transmitted through the His-Tawara system to the ventricles, where a similarly specific pattern of ventricular depolarization is produced. Under abnormal conditions, however, disturbances in atrial conduction or ectopic atrial rhythms may result in a different order of depolarization in the atria, the AV node, and common bundle and thus alter the sequence of ventricular activation. Asynchronous depolarization of the ventricles may also be the result of disturbances in impulse formation or conduction within the AV junction, or both. Thus the site of impulse formation and the integrity of the conduction pathways may ultimately determine the sequence of ventricular activation.

REFERENCES

Demoulin, J. C. and H. F. Kulbertus: Histopathological Examination of Concept of Hemiblock, *Brit. Heart J.*, 34: 807, 1972.

Denes, P., D. Wu, R. C. Dhingra et al.: Demonstration of Dual A-V Nodal Pathways in Patients with Paroxysmal Supraventricular Tachycardia, *Circulation*, 48: 549, 1973.

Durrer, D., R. T. van Dam, G. E. Freud et al.: Total Excitation of the Isolated Human Heart, *Circulation*, 41: 899, 1970.

Ferrer, M. I.: New Concepts Relating to the Preexcitation Syndrome, *J.A.M.A.*, 201: 1038, 1967.

Hecht, H. H. et al.: Atrioventricular and Intraventricular Conduction—Revised Nomenclature and Concepts, *Am. J. Cardiol.*, 31: 232, 1973.

James, T. N.: Anatomy of the Conduction System of the Heart, in J. W. Hurst and R. B. Logue (eds.), "The Heart," McGraw-Hill, New York, 1966.

Lev, M.: The Pre-Excitation Syndrome: Anatomic Considerations of Anomalous A-V Pathways, in L. S. Dreifus and W. Likoff (eds.), "Mechanism and Therapy of Cardiac Arrhythmias," Grune & Stratton, New York, 1966.

Rosen, K. M., A. Mehta, and R. A. Miller: Demonstration of Dual Atrio-ventricular Nodal Pathways in Man, *Am. J. Cardiol.* 33: 291, 1974.

Rosenbaum, M. B., M. V. Elizari, and J. O. Lazzari: "The Hemiblocks," Tampa Tracings, 1970.

Scher, A. M.: The Sequence of Ventricular Excitation, *Am. J. Cardiol.*, 14: 287, 1964.

―――: Excitation of the Heart: A Progress Report, in R. C. Schlant and J. W. Hurst (eds.), "Advances in Electrocardiography," Grune & Stratton, New York, 1972.

Sherf, L., and T. N. James: A New Electrocardiographic Concept: Synchronized Sinoventricular Conduction, *Dis. Chest,* 55: 127, 1969.

Truex, R. C.: Structural Basis of Atrial and Ventricular Conduction, *Cardiovasc. Clin.* 6(1): 1, 1974.

Uhley, H. N.: The Fascicular Blocks, *Cardiovasc. Clin.*, 5(3): 87, 1973.

CHAPTER 3

BASIC CONSIDERATIONS IN ELECTROCARDIOGRAPHY

THE EINTHOVEN TRIANGLE HYPOTHESIS (FIG. 3-1)

The nucleus of modern electrocardiographic theory is contained in the Einthoven triangle hypothesis.

Einthoven's triangle hypothesis includes the following assumptions: (1) the roots of the right arm, left arm, and left leg form the apices of an equilateral triangle in which the roots of the right arm, left arm, and left leg are at a relatively great distance from the heart, yet are equidistant from it and from each other; (2) the electric forces produced by the heart at any given instance can be represented by an equivalent dipole or vector at the center of the triangle; (3) the body tissues and fluids in which the triangle is located act as a homogeneous volume conductor; (4) the standard bipolar limb leads, formed by placing electrodes at each of the apices of the triangle, record the potential variations of the heart in the frontal plane of the body.

None of the foregoing assumptions is completely valid. The dipole is eccentrically placed within the torso, the heart is large in proportion to the size of the thorax, the triangle is not equilateral, the heart is not equidistant from the apices of the triangle, and the tissues of the body are not uniform in their conductivity. In spite of these deficiencies, the assumptions made by Einthoven are accurate enough to provide some insight into the genesis of the electrocardiogram.

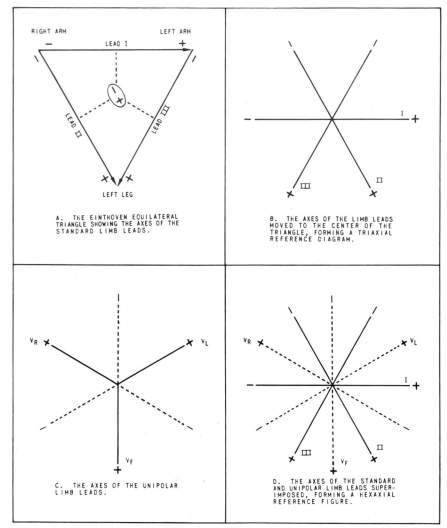

Fig. 3-1   The Einthoven equilateral triangle, the axes of the bipolar and unipolar limb leads, and the triaxial and hexaxial reference diagrams.

THE BURGER TRIANGLE (FIG. 3-2)

Burger and van Milaan showed that the Einthoven triangle is not equilateral but scalene and it does not lie entirely in the frontal plane. Moreover they demonstrated that the scalar voltage recorded by the standard leads is dependent not only on the projection of the cardiac vector on the lead axis but also on the length of the leads. Each lead is thus a vector quantity. Burger and van Milaan used the term *lead vector* to signify that a lead is a vector quantity. Basing it on the Burger triangle, Langner devised a corrected hexaxial reference diagram (Fig. 3-3) which takes into consideration the magnitude, direction, and strength of the lead vectors.   Although the improved hexaxial reference diagram is more accurate than the one based on Einthoven's triangle, it has not been adopted very widely.   It should, however, be employed whenever the scalar limb leads are to be derived from the frontal-plane vectorcardiogram.

STANDARD LIMB LEADS (FIG. 3-1)

The standard limb leads, designated leads I, II, and III, were devised by Einthoven.   By convention, lead I represents the potential of the left arm minus the potential of the right arm; lead II represents the potential of the left leg minus the potential of the right arm; and lead III represents the potential of the left leg minus the potential of the left arm.   These relationships can be expressed by the following equations:

$$Lead\ I = VL - VR$$
$$Lead\ II = VF - VR$$
$$Lead\ III = VF - VL$$

where V — potential
     R = right arm
     L = left arm
     F = left leg

Einthoven's Law

Because of the inherent relationship of the standard limb leads to each other, Einthoven stated that at any given instant during the cardiac cycle, the sum of the potentials of leads I and III equals the potential of lead II.

Fig. 3-2   The Burger triangle.   The Einthoven triangle is shown to be nonequilateral and scalene.

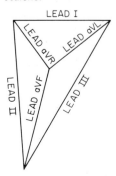

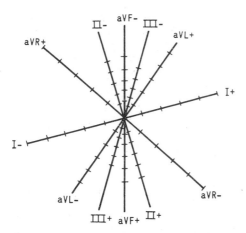

Fig. 3-3 The corrected hexaxial reference diagram of Langner. The units in each lead are different to correct for the unequal strength of the various leads.

This is Einthoven's law. It depends neither on the validity of Einthoven's hypothesis with respect to the representation of the heart as a dipole or vector nor on the validity of the Einthoven equilateral triangle hypothesis. It holds for a triangle of any shape.

The law can be stated mathematically as follows:

$$\text{Lead I} + \text{lead III} = \text{lead II}$$

Substituting, $(VL - VR) + (VF - VL) = VF - VR$

$$VF - VR = VF - VR$$

The law is useful in detecting errors in electrode placement.

The line connecting the electrode positions of each of the standard bipolar limb leads represents the axis of that lead. Each of the three lead axes constitutes one of the sides of the equilateral triangle (see Fig. 3-1). The midpoint of each lead axis divides it into positive and negative halves. Perpendiculars drawn from the midpoints of the lead axes intersect at the center of the equilateral triangle. It is at this point that the cardiac dipole is located.

The sides of the equilateral triangle (the axes of the bipolar limb leads) can be transposed to a common central point, forming the triaxial reference figure of Bayley (see Fig. 3-1), in which the axes are 60° apart. The lead I axis is 0 to ±180°, the lead II axis is +60 to −120°, and the lead III axis is +120 to −60°.

UNIPOLAR LIMB LEADS (FIGS. 3-1, 3-4)

It can be shown, if the Einthoven hypothesis is correct, that according to Kirchhoff's law, at any given instant during the cardiac cycle the sum of

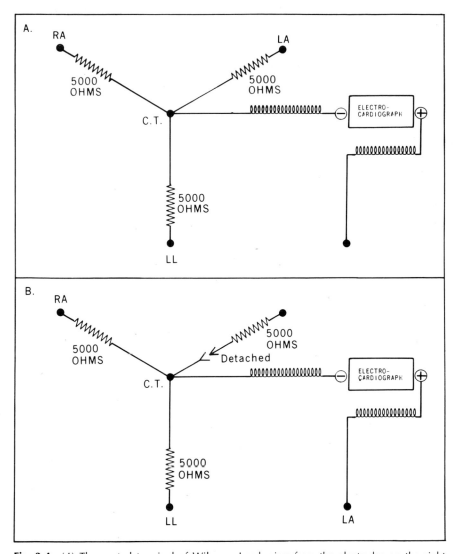

Fig. 3-4   (*A*) The central terminal of Wilson.   Lead wires from the electrodes on the right arm, left arm, and left leg are joined through equal resistances to form a central terminal which is connected to the indifferent electrodes.   (*B*) The augmented unipolar limb leads. In the example shown, unipolar lead aVL is obtained by detaching the connection between the left arm electrode and the central terminal, which remains connected to the indifferent electrode.   The exploring electrode is placed on the left arm to record this lead.

the potentials of the right arm, left arm, and left leg must be zero.   This can be represented by the equation

$$VR + VL + VF = 0$$

It then follows that if lead wires from the electrodes on each of the three extremities are connected through equal resistances to a central terminal, the potential of the central terminal must perforce be zero or nearly so throughout the cardiac cycle.   By pairing the central terminal with an exploring electrode placed upon any part of the body, a lead is obtained which records the potential variations of the exploring electrode only.   This type of lead is called a *unipolar lead* and is designated by the letter V.   It was devised by Wilson.

Unipolar leads recorded from the right arm, left arm, and left leg are called the unipolar limb leads.   They are designated by the symbols VR, VL, and VF, respectively.

It so happens, that deflections recorded by the unipolar extremity leads are inconveniently small.   To obviate this difficulty, Goldberger devised a method for increasing the amplitude of the deflections $1\frac{1}{2}$ times without affecting their form (Fig. 3-4).   This is done by breaking the connection between the central terminal and the extremity whose potential variations are being recorded.   Unipolar leads obtained by Goldberger's technique are called augmented unipolar limb leads.   They are designated by the letter a, which precedes the symbols of the unipolar extremity leads as follows: aVR, aVL, and aVF.   Goldberger also removed the resistances from the lead wires to the central terminal.   Since this procedure introduces an error, it is no longer employed, and the central terminal of Wilson is retained when augmenting the unipolar limb leads.

In the standard bipolar limb leads, the positive and negative electrodes are each attached to an extremity.   In the unipolar limb leads, the positive electrode is attached to one of the extremities, but the negative electrode is attached to the central terminal, which is at approximately zero potential. The axis for each unipolar limb lead is thus a line drawn from the extremity, where the positive electrode is placed, to the zero point of the electrical field of the heart, which is at the center of the equilateral triangle.   The axes of the three unipolar limb leads may also be drawn as a triaxial figure (see Fig. 3-1) in which the axis of lead VL or aVL is $-30°$, lead VF or aVF is $+90°$, and VR or aVR is $-150°$.   If the axes of the bipolar and unipolar limb leads are superimposed, a hexaxial reference figure is formed (Fig. 3-1).

The voltage recorded in the augmented unipolar limb leads is 87 percent of the voltage projected on the lead axis by the manifest vector, as compared to 100 percent in the bipolar extremity leads.   Therefore, the values for deflections in the augmented limb leads should be multiplied by 1.15 for greater accuracy when comparing corresponding deflections in the standard extremity leads.

RELATIONSHIP BETWEEN THE STANDARD AND THE UNIPOLAR LIMB LEADS

The mathematical relationship between the standard and unipolar extremity leads can be expressed by the following formulas:

$$I = VL - VR = \tfrac{2}{3}(aVL - aVR)$$
$$II = VF - VR = \tfrac{2}{3}(aVF - aVR)$$
$$III = VF - VL = \tfrac{2}{3}(aVF - aVL)$$
$$aVR = \tfrac{3}{2}VR = -\frac{I + II}{2}$$
$$aVL = \tfrac{3}{2}VL = \frac{I - III}{2}$$
$$aVF = \tfrac{3}{2}VF = \frac{II + III}{2}$$

PRECORDIAL LEADS (FIG. 3-5)

Before Wilson devised the central terminal, the precordial leads used were bipolar leads obtained by placing the positive electrode on the chest wall and a negative electrode on either the right arm, CR; the left arm, CL; or the left leg, CF.

These leads have been replaced by the unipolar precordial leads V, in which the negative electrode is connected to the central terminal and the

Fig. 3-5 The location of the precordial leads. Described in text.

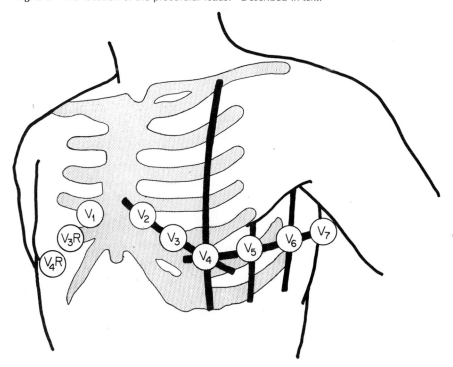

positive, or exploring, electrode is placed at various positions on the chest wall.

The standard precordial electrocardiogram consists of six unipolar leads V_1 through V_6. For descriptive purposes, leads V_1 and V_2 are called right-sided precordial leads; leads V_3 and V_4, midprecordial leads; and leads V_5 and V_6, left-sided precordial leads.

The location of these leads is as follows:

V_1 On the fourth intercostal space at the right sternal margin
V_2 On the fourth intercostal space at the left sternal margin
V_3 Midway between leads V_2 and V_4
V_4 On the fifth intercostal space at the midclavicular line
V_5 On the anterior axillary line at the horizontal level of lead V_4
V_6 On the midaxillary line at the horizontal level of lead V_4

Occasionally, additional leads are taken.   The nomenclature and location of these leads are as follows:

V_7	On the left posterior axillary line at the horizontal level of lead V_4
V_8	On the left midscapular line at the horizontal level of lead V_4
V_9	On the left paravertebral line at the horizontal level of lead V_4
V_E	At the tip of the ensiform process of the sternum
$V_{3R}, V_{4R}, V_{5R}, V_{6R}, V_{7R}, V_{8R}, V_{9R}$	At points on the right chest which are the counterparts of similarly numbered left-sided chest leads
HV or LV	Leads taken at higher or lower horizontal levels than the standard precordial leads, but in the same vertical planes; exact level should be indicated by a Roman numeral for the intercostal space, following the Arabic numeral of the position, for example, V_5III

As with the standard and unipolar extremity leads, a reference diagram may be constructed for the axes of the unipolar precordial leads (Fig. 3-6). Whereas the axes of the limb leads are located in the frontal plane, those of the precordial leads are located in the horizontal plane.   The axis of each unipolar precordial lead is on a line extending from the location of the exploring electrode to the dipole center of the heart.   In this horizontal reference figure the axes of the various precordial leads are approximately as follows: V_1, $+115°$; V_2, $+94°$; V_3, $+58°$; V_4, $+47°$; V_5, $+22°$; and V_6, $0°$.

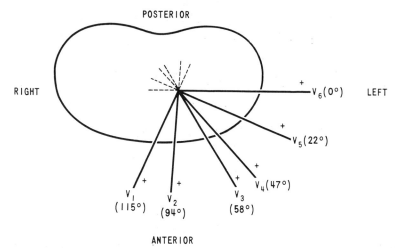

Fig. 3-6 The axes of the unipolar leads in the horizontal plane of the body (see Abildskov and Wilkinson).

ORTHOGONAL LEADS (FIG. 3-7)

An ideal lead system for electrocardiography and vectorcardiography would consist of three leads with the following characteristics: (1) The leads would be perpendicular to each other and to the horizontal, vertical, and sagittal axes of the body. (2) The amplitude of the three leads would be equal from a vectorial standpoint. (3) These leads would have the same strength and direction, not only for a single point within the heart, but for all points in the heart where electromotive forces are generated. Such leads are called corrected orthogonal leads. On theoretical grounds, such leads should contain all the information contained in the usual 12-lead electro-cardiogram. By convention, the horizontal lead is designated by the letter X; the vertical, by the letter Y; and the sagittal, by the letter Z.

Several corrected orthogonal lead systems have been devised. Because of its accuracy, simplicity, and convenience, the Frank lead system has been adopted by most workers in the field.

THE VECTOR CONCEPT

Any force having magnitude and direction can be considered a vector and represented by an arrow. Scalar quantities, although possessing magnitude, are not vectors because they lack direction.

Since electrical forces have magnitude and direction, they are vector quantities. In vector representation, the length of the arrow indicates the magnitude of the force; the inclination of the arrow, the direction in which

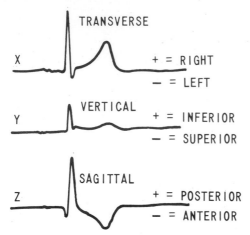

Fig. 3-7 Normal X, Y, and Z leads redrawn from an actual recording with the Frank lead system.

the force is acting; and the location of the arrowhead, the "sense," or polarity, of the force. By convention, for electrical forces, the arrow tip represents electrical positivity.

Vectors may be added by the use of parallelograms or triangles (Fig. 3-8). To add by the parallelogram method, the vectors are drawn from the same starting point, and a parallelogram is constructed with these vectors constituting two sides of the figure. The diagonal of the parallelogram is the resultant vector. To add by the triangle method, the vectors are drawn so that the tail of the second vector begins at the tip of the first. A line drawn from the tail of the first vector to the tip of the second vector is the resultant vector. When the resultant of several vectors is to be determined, the vectors are laid off head to tail. A line drawn from the tail of the first vector to the tip of the last vector is the resultant vector. To subtract two vectors, the vectors are drawn from a common starting point. A line connecting the tip of the second vector with the tip of the first represents the difference between these two vectors (the minus the second).

The vector concept (Fig. 3-9) assumes that the electromotive forces generated by the heart create a single electrical field in the tissue surrounding the heart. This electrical field extends to the surface of the body. Therefore, leads from the body surface can record the electrical events taking place in the heart. Since the electrical force produced by the heart at any given instant can be represented by a single equivalent dipole or vector, the deflections registered in any electrocardiographic lead are simply the projection of the instantaneous cardiac vector on the axis of that lead. The amplitude or voltage of the deflection is proportional to the projection of the vector on the axis of the lead. The deflection recorded in any lead, therefore, reflects the manner in which the lead "taps" the cardiac vector

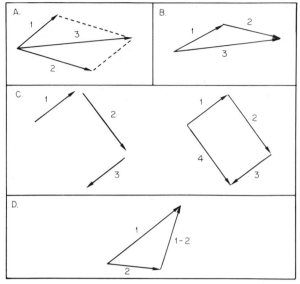

Fig. 3-8   Addition and subtraction of vectors.   (A) Addition of vectors 1 and 2 by the parallelogram method.   Vector 3 is the resultant vector.   (B) Addition of vectors 1 and 2 by the triangle method.   Vector 3 is the resultant vector.   (C) Addition of vectors 1, 2, and 3. Vector 4 is the resultant vector.   (D) Subtraction of vector 2 from vector 1.   The resultant vector is shown as 1 − 2.

and is essentially a record of the resultant electrical activity of all regions of the heart.

This point of view is in contrast to the local potentials, or semidirect lead, hypothesis.   The latter theory arose from the use of unipolar leads in electrocardiography.   It assumes that unipolar leads are semidirect leads and that the deflections recorded in a unipolar lead represent the potential variations in that region of the heart facing the exploring electrode.   Thus, for example, the right precordial leads are said to record primarily right ventricular surface potentials and the left precordial leads to record left ventricular surface potentials.

Although there is still controversy concerning these two theories, the weight of evidence supports the vector concept.   If the vector view is correct, it should be possible to derive scalar electrocardiograms from the spatial vectorcardiogram; contrariwise, if the local potentials theory is correct, this should not be possible.   Actually, scalar electrocardiograms can be drawn with great accuracy from the vector loop.   The unipolar lead approach cannot explain the fact that leads from opposite sides of the chest along an axis passing through the dipole center show patterns which are inverted images of each other and which actually cancel each other when fed into a comparator circuit.   Furthermore, the local potentials concept cannot explain the fact that in every individual, primarily negative deflections are recorded from one-half of the body surface and primary

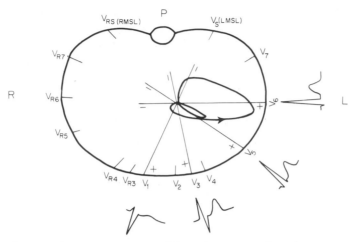

Fig. 3-9 The vector concept. Schematic representation of a cross section of the chest showing the relationship between the precordial leads and the horizontal plane projection of the spatial vectorcardiogram. The configuration of the precordial leads does not reflect right ventricular, transitional, or left ventricular potentials but is dependent upon the projection of the composite electrical forces of the heart on the axes of the leads. RMSL, right midscapular line; LMSL, left midscapular line. *(From A. Grishman and E. Donoso, Spatial Vectorcardiography, Mod. Concepts Cardiovasc. Dis., 30: 687, 1961. Used by permission of the American Heart Association, Inc.)*

positive waves are recorded from the other half. Finally, it cannot explain the frequent failure of the transitional precordial leads to overlie the interventricular septum, whose plane is more or less fixed anatomically in most individuals.

Some of the shortcomings of the vector concept were described in the discussion of the Einthoven triangle hypothesis. It seems appropriate also to mention that the heart is unquestionably a multipolar rather than a unipolar generator, that the dipoles may change position during the cardiac cycle, that there are high-frequency components produced by local potentials which are not revealed by conventional electrocardiographic leads, and that no set of body-surface leads is sufficiently remote from the heart to permit accurate vectorial summation of the cardiac dipoles. In spite of these deficiencies, various studies have indicated that between 80 and 90 percent of body-surface potentials may be attributed to the presence of a fixed single equivalent dipole.

CATHODE-TUBE VECTORCARDIOGRAPHY

In vectorcardiography the voltages recorded by the various leads are displayed on the screen of a cathode-ray tube. The oscilloscope has two sets of plates, which control the horizontal and vertical deflections of the electron beam.   To record the vectorcardiogram in the horizontal plane, the terminals of the X lead are connected to the horizontal plates and those of the Z lead to the vertical plates.   To display the vectorcardiogram in the frontal plane, the terminals of the Y lead are attached to the vertical plates and those of the X lead to the horizontal plates.   To show the vectorcardiogram in the sagittal plane, the terminals of the Z lead are connected to the horizontal plates and the terminals of the Y lead to the vertical plates.   Either the left or the right sagittal plane vectorcardiogram may be recorded.   The Committee on Electrocardiography of the American Heart Association has recommended that the sagittal plane should be viewed from the left.

Vectorcardiography in this book is based on the Frank system of electrode placement.   The vectorcardiograms recorded by this lead system are comparable to those recorded by other corrected lead systems.

The use of oscilloscopic vectorcardiography has increased in recent years.   Present evidence appears to indicate that the vectorcardiogram supplements the electrocardiogram but does not replace it.   The vector-cardiogram adds to the diagnostic accuracy of the electrocardiogram in approximately 15 percent of cases.

The vectorcardiogram aids in differentiating between normal variants, right ventricular enlargement, and right bundle branch block as causes of an RSR' configuration in the precordial leads.   The vectorcardiogram may prove to be more sensitive than the electrocardiogram in the early diagnosis of right and left ventricular enlargement and in the diagnosis of biventricular hypertrophy.   It may be superior to the standard electrocardiogram in the diagnosis of right, left, and biatrial hypertrophy.   It can help distinguish between ostium primum and ostium secundum defects.   It is likewise helpful in the diagnosis of myocardial infarction.   Patterns of myocardial infarction may be revealed more clearly in the vectorcardiogram than in the electrocardiogram.   This is particularly true in the case of inferior and posterobasal infarcts and when myocardial infarction and ventricular conduction defects are combined.   Moreover, when the electrocardi-ographic diagnosis of infarction is equivocal, the vectorcardiogram may establish the correct diagnosis.   Even though the vectorcardiogram is more sensitive than the electrocardiogram in the diagnosis of myocardial infarc-tion, it is probably not more specific. Timed vectorcardiograms have been reported to be useful in the analysis of cardiac arrhythmias.

VECTORELECTROCARDIOGRAPHY (VECTOR ANALYSIS OF THE ELECTROCARDIOGRAM, THE SPATIAL VECTOR METHOD)

The conventional scalar electrocardiogram may be interpreted according to the method of vector analysis originally proposed by Grant.   In this method, the vector is used to integrate, schematize, and present three-dimensionally the information contained in the various leads. Grant's method has been widely adopted because it not only increases the accuracy of electrocardiographic interpretation but also promotes a better understanding of electrocardiography. Accordingly, whenever deemed appropriate, the spatial vector method of analysis will be employed in this text, and criteria for diagnosis by this method will be described.

THE ELECTROCARDIOGRAM AND THE VECTORCARDIOGRAM

Both the electrocardiogram and vectorcardiogram record the electrical forces produced by the heart. They differ only in the methods by which these forces are displayed. The electrocardiogram depicts these forces as scalar deflections; the vectorcardiogram, as vector loops. Each electrocardiographic lead records the potential difference between two points on the body surface. The vectorcardiogram records the projection of the electromotive forces of the heart on a plane of the body. The vector loop does not contain any information not present in the two scalar leads that are combined to produce it. It is just a more convenient method for displaying this information.

Although based on electrophysiologic principles, both electrocardiography and vectorcardiography are fundamentally empiric sciences. Conventional electrocardiography stands on a solid basis of clinical experience supported by anatomic, physiologic, and radiologic evidence. Vectorcardiography is much newer. Despite the claims of the scientific purist, vectorcardiographic diagnosis cannot be based solely on a theoretical analysis of the vector loop.

REFERENCES

Abildskov, J. A., and R. S. Wilkinson, Jr.: The Relation of Precordial and Orthogonal Leads, *Circulation,* 27: 58, 1963.

Benchimol, A., and K. B. Dressler: Advances in Clinical Vectorcardiography, *Am. J. Cardiol.,* 36: 76, 1975.

Burger, H. C., and J. B. van Milaan: Heart Vector and Leads, *Brit. Heart J.,* 8: 157, 1946; 9: 154, 1947; and 10: 229, 1948.

Frank, E.: An Accurate, Clinically Practical System for Spatial Vectorcardiography, *Circulation,* 13: 737, 1956.

Goldberger, E.: A Simple Indifferent Electrocardiographic Electrode of Zero Potential and a Technique of Obtaining Augmented Unipolar Extremity Leads, *Am. Heart J.,* 23: 483, 1942.

Grant, R. P.: "Clinical Electrocardiography: The Spatial Vector Approach," McGraw-Hill, New York, 1957.

Grishman, A., and E. Donoso: Spatial Vectorcardiography, *Mod. Concepts Cardiovas. Dis.,* 30: 687, 693, 1961.

Johnston, F. D.: The Electrocardiogram, in W. A. Sodeman and W. A. Sodeman, Jr. (eds.), "Pathologic Physiology," 4th ed., W. B. Saunders, Philadelphia, 1967.

Langner, P.H., Jr.: An Octaxial Reference System Derived from a Nonequilateral Triangle for Frontal Plane Vectorcardiography, *Am. Heart J.,* 45: 835, 1953.

Wilson, F.N., F. D. Johnston, A. G. MacLeod, and P. S. Barker: Electrocardiograms That Represent the Potential Variations of a Single Electrode, *Am. Heart J.,* 9: 447, 1934.

CHAPTER 4

THE DERIVATION OF THE ELECTROCARDIOGRAM AND VECTORCARDIOGRAM

THE ATRIAL COMPLEX

Atrial Depolarization (Fig. 4-1)

As already stated, the excitatory process begins at the SA node and then spreads through both atria. Some evidence suggests that atrial depolarization is not entirely radial but is asymmetric, with the internodal tracts playing a significant role in the distribution of the atrial impulse. During the initial period of atrial activation, only the right atrium is depolarized. Shortly thereafter, excitation spreads to the interatrial septum and left atrium. During the final period of atrial activation, only the left atrium is depolarized.

For simplicity, atrial depolarization may be represented by three vectors, each of which may be regarded as originating at the SA node. The initial vector, representing right atrial forces, is directed inferiorly, anteriorly, and slightly leftward. The second vector, representing combined right and left atrial forces, is directed inferiorly, leftward, and usually slightly anteriorly or posteriorly. The terminal vector, representing left atrial forces, is directed leftward, inferiorly, and posteriorly.

The relationship of these vectors to the P wave of the electrocardiogram and the P loops of the vectorcardiogram is shown in Fig. 4-1.

From the diagram, it can be seen that the first half of the P wave is dominated by right atrial potentials; the last half, by left atrial potentials.

During the normal atrial depolarization of 90 ms, right atrial activation occurs from 0 to 70 ms, atrial septal excitation from 20 to 45 ms, and left

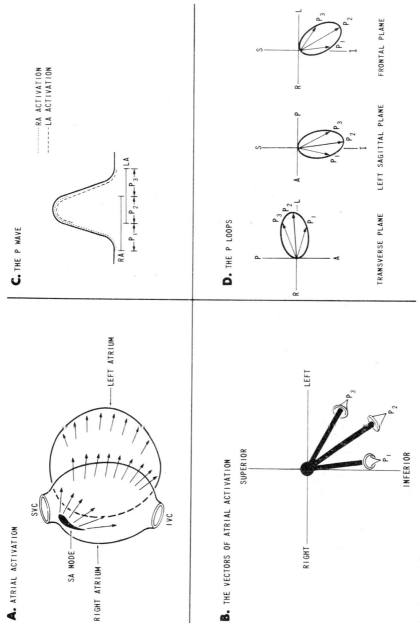

Fig. 4-1 Atrial activation. (A) Schematic representation of the vectors of atrial activation. (B) The three main vectors of atrial activation. P_1 represents right atrial forces; P_2, combined right and left atrial forces; and P_3, left atrial forces. (C) The derivation of the P wave, showing the contributions of the right and left atrial forces. (D) The relationship between the three vectors of atrial depolarization and the P loops in the transverse, left sagittal, and frontal planes.

atrial depolarization from 30 to 90 ms after the beginning of the surface P wave.

The mean P vector in the frontal plane lies near the $+60°$ axis on the hexaxial reference diagram. This means that the P wave is normally upright in leads I, II, and aVF; upright, diphasic, or inverted in leads III and aVL; and inverted in lead aVR. It is generally tallest in lead II. In the horizontal plane, the mean P vector generally lies between 0 and $+60°$. The vector of the right atrium is somewhat anteriorly directed; the vector of the left atrium, somewhat posteriorly oriented. The P wave is therefore often biphasic in leads V_1 and V_2, with the first part upright, representing right atrial activation, and the second part inverted, representing left atrial activation. Because the right precordial leads are closest to the atria, the P waves tend to be larger in these leads than in other precordial leads. In the left precordial leads (V_4 to V_6), the P wave is upright.

The planar P loops may be drawn by tracing the course of the three spatial vectors. The sequential changes in the direction of these vectors cause counterclockwise inscription of the P loop in the transverse, left sagittal, and frontal planes.

Atrial Repolarization (Fig. 4-2)

Atrial repolarization follows atrial depolarization. It produces a deflection called the *Tp* (or *Ta*) *wave*, which is ordinarily not seen because it is buried in the QRS complex. The direction of the Tp wave is generally opposite to the direction of the P wave. The Tp wave may cause pseudodepression of the junction (called *J*) between the QRS complex and the S-T segment.

Fig. 4-2   The time relationships between the electrical processes in the atria and ventricles. Note that the S-T$_p$ segment is superimposed on the P-R segment and the T$_p$ wave on a portion of the QRS complex and on the S-T complex. Changes in the magnitude and direction of the electrical forces during atrial repolarization may thus alter the configuration of the P-R and S-T segments. *(From J. Tranchesi, V. Adelardi, and J. M. de Oliveira, Atrial Repolarization— Its Importance in Clinical Electrocardiography, Circulation, 22: 635, 1960. Used by permission of the American Heart Association, Inc.)*

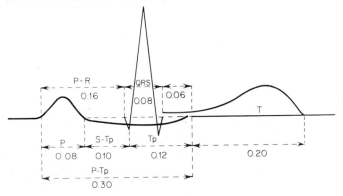

VENTRICULAR COMPLEX

The sequence of ventricular activation has been described in Chap. 2 on the anatomy and physiology of the conduction system.

Ventricular Depolarization (Figs. 4-3, 4-4)

Ventricular depolarization may be divided into four phases. Actually the process is continuous, so the division is purely arbitrary. It is done only for descriptive purposes.

It should be remembered that the deflections registered in any cardiac lead simply reflect the degree to which the cardiac vector is projected on the axis of that lead.

First Phase In this phase the left side of the interventricular septum is activated. Since the septum is more or less parallel to the frontal plane of the body, the vector of the electrical forces during this period is directed anteriorly, somewhat rightward, and either superiorly or inferiorly. The projection of this vector on the axes of the precordial leads causes the inscription of part of the upstroke of the R wave in the right-sided precordial leads, such as V_1 and V_2, and of a small Q wave in the left-sided leads, such as V_5 and V_6.

Second Phase In this phase septal activation proceeds from both the right and left sides of the interventricular septum. The electrical forces tend to counterbalance each other partially, but since a much larger region of the left septum is depolarized compared with that of the right, the net direction of septal activation is from left to right. In addition, septal activation also proceeds from apex to base and from front to back. While septal activation is proceeding, the activation spreads rapidly to both ventricles, but it occurs predominantly at the apex and lateral wall of the right ventricle and at the anterior apical portion of the left ventricle. Since the left ventricular potentials are larger, the resultant of the right and left ventricular vectors is directed anteriorly, slightly leftward, and somewhat inferiorly. The projection of this vector on the precordial lead axes causes these leads to register an upstroke.

Third Phase In this phase depolarization is largely completed in the septum and in the right ventricle, except for its posterobasal and conus portions. The bulk of the left ventricle, with the exception of its posterobasal region, is also activated. The left ventricular potentials are larger than those produced by the right; therefore they counterbalance the right, even though both are proceeding in opposite directions. The resultant vector during this phase has considerable magnitude and to a great extent determines the direction of the mean QRS vector. It is directed leftward, slightly posteriorly,

VENTRICULAR DEPOLARIZATION IN THE NORMAL HEART

SEQUENCE OF VENTRICULAR ACTIVATION

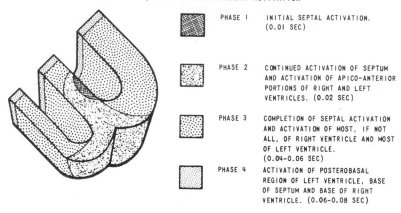

PHASE 1   INITIAL SEPTAL ACTIVATION. (0.01 SEC)

PHASE 2   CONTINUED ACTIVATION OF SEPTUM AND ACTIVATION OF APICO-ANTERIOR PORTIONS OF RIGHT AND LEFT VENTRICLES. (0.02 SEC)

PHASE 3   COMPLETION OF SEPTAL ACTIVATION AND ACTIVATION OF MOST, IF NOT ALL, OF RIGHT VENTRICLE AND MOST OF LEFT VENTRICLE. (0.04-0.06 SEC)

PHASE 4   ACTIVATION OF POSTEROBASAL REGION OF LEFT VENTRICLE, BASE OF SEPTUM AND BASE OF RIGHT VENTRICLE. (0.06-0.08 SEC)

VENTRICULAR ACTIVATION VECTORS IN THE TRANSVERSE PLANE

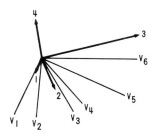

QRS COMPLEXES IN THE PRECORDIAL LEADS

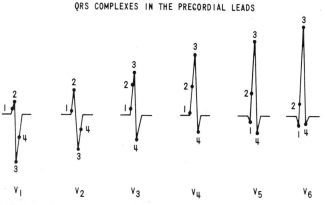

Fig. 4-3   Schematic representation of ventricular depolarization in the normal heart.   Described in text.

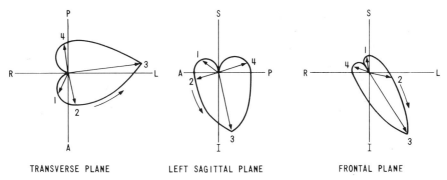

TRANSVERSE PLANE   LEFT SAGITTAL PLANE   FRONTAL PLANE

Fig. 4-4   The relationship between the four vectors of ventricular depolarization and the QRS vector loops in the transverse, left sagittal, and frontal planes.

and somewhat inferiorly.   The projection of this vector on the axes of the precordial leads causes the inscription of the nadir of the S wave in lead V_1 and the peak of the R wave in the left-sided leads.

Fourth Phase   In the final phase the basal portion of the interventricular septum and the posterobasal region of the left ventricle are activated. Depolarization of the pulmonary conus in the region of the crista supraventricularis also occurs about this time, but its overall contribution to the terminal forces is probably not significant.   The terminal vector is oriented posteriorly and either leftward or slightly to the right.   This vector is responsible for the inscription of the downstroke of the R wave and the final S wave in the left precordial leads.   Occasionally a final small R' wave is inscribed in lead V_1, which represents this terminal force.   The rSr' complex, which occurs as a normal variant in lead V_1, particularly in young people, is often referred to as the *crista pattern*. It has been so designated because some authorities believe that the small R' wave represents the forces produced by late depolarization of the crista supraventricularis.

In the standard or unipolar extremity leads, which are in the frontal plane of the body, the deflections recorded depend on the orientation of the axes of the leads with respect to the direction of the ventricular activation vectors.   There is considerable normal variation in the patterns produced; therefore these have not been described.

In summary, during ventricular depolarization, the right-sided precordial leads show predominantly negative complexes; the left-sided precordial leads, predominantly positive complexes; and the midprecordial leads at the transition zone, more or less equiphasic QRS complexes.   The findings in the standard and unipolar limb depend on the degree to which the cardiac vector is projected on the axes of these leads.   Since the cardiac vector normally shows a wide range of variation in magnitude and direction, the complexes recorded in these leads will reflect this variation.   For example, in adults the mean QRS vector normally may vary between -30

and $+90°$ or more in the frontal plane. Thus a lead like aVF (with an axis of $+90°$) normally may show either predominantly upright or predominantly downward QRS complexes, depending on whether the QRS vector is vertical or horizontal.

The planar QRS loops may be drawn by tracing the course of the four spatial vectors. In the transverse and the left sagittal planes, inscription of the QRS loop is counterclockwise. In the frontal plane, the direction of inscription is variable. Loops in this plane may show a clockwise, counterclockwise, or figure-of-eight configuration.

Ventricular Repolarization

Repolarization begins a short time after depolarization is completed. The sequence of events in ventricular repolarization is complex and not well understood. The overall direction of repolarization is opposite to that of depolarization. Thus the mean T vector in adults is relatively parallel to the mean QRS vector. This means that in the electrocardiogram, with the exception of lead V_1, the T waves are upright in the precordial leads and are almost invariably upright in leads I and II. In infants and children, the mean T vector normally may be directed leftward and posteriorly, which will result in negative T waves in leads V_1 to V_3. In the vectorcardiogram also, the spatial orientations of the T and QRS loops are similar. The direction of inscription of the T loop is usually the same as that of the QRS loop in each of the three planes.

REFERENCES

Durrer, D., R. T. van Dam, G. E. Freud et al.: Total Excitation of the Isolated Human Heart, *Circulation,* 41: 899, 1970.

Scher, A. M.: The Sequence of Ventricular Excitation, *Am. J. Cardiol.,* 14: 287, 1964.

————: Excitation of the Heart, in W. F. Hamilton (ed.), "Handbook of Physiology," vol. 1, sec. 2, The Circulation, American Physiological Society, Washington, D.C., 1962.

————: Excitation of the Heart: A Progress Report, in R. C. Schlant and J. W. Hurst (eds.), "Advances in Electrocardiography," Grune & Stratton, New York, 1972.

CHAPTER 5

THE NORMAL ELECTROCARDIOGRAM

GRID LINES (FIG. 5-2)

On the electrocardiogram, there is a series of horizontal and vertical lines which are used to measure the amplitude and duration of the various deflections, segments, and intervals. The former are 1 mm apart; the latter are also 1 mm apart, but each vertical line is a time line representing an interval of 0.04 s at the usual paper speed of 25 mm/s. Each fifth horizontal and vertical line is bolder than the others to facilitate measurement.

STANDARDIZATION (FIG. 5-2)

It is customary to standardize the electrocardiogram so that 1 mV (millivolt) will cause a deflection of 10 mm. The amplitude of the deflections can be recorded in terms of millimeters or millivolts. The standardization should be shown on every lead in the case of string galvanometer electrocardiographs. With direct-writing instruments, this need be done only once, preferably prior to recording the electrocardiogram.

VARIOUS COMPONENTS

The electrocardiographic record consists of a baseline and various deflections or waves. The letters P, Q, R, S, T, and U are used to designate the

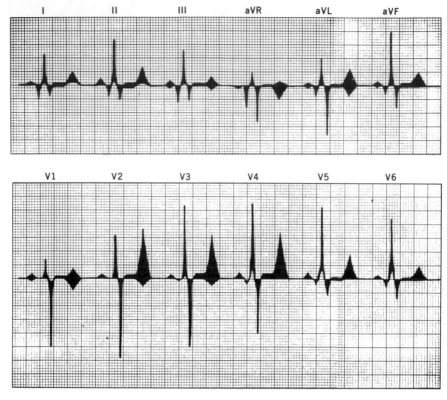

Fig. 5-1 The normal composite electrocardiogram. Prepared from the tables of normal values in the appendix from the "Electrocardiographic Test Book." The normal range of the P, Q, R, S, S-T, and T deflections is shown. The various time intervals and the intrinsicoid deflections are omitted. *(Redrawn from P. S. Ezra, The Normal Composite Electrocardiogram, Circulation, 24: 710, 1961. Used by permission of the American Heart Association, Inc.)*

six major waves or deflections of the normal electrocardiogram. The portions of the electrocardiogram between the deflections are called *segments*. The distances between waves are called *intervals*.

By convention, electrocardiographic connections are so arranged that positive forces record upward deflections; negative forces, downward deflections.

The duration of waves, complexes, intervals, and segments, expressed in seconds or fractions thereof, is always measured from their convex and not their concave curvatures.

The amplitude of deflections, as already stated, is recorded in millimeters or millivolts. Measurement of upward deflections is made from the upper edge of the baseline to the peak of the wave; downward deflections, from the lower edge of the baseline to the lowest point, or nadir, of the wave. This procedure corrects for the width of the baseline.

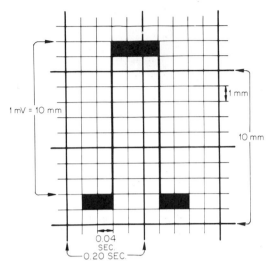

Fig. 5-2   The grid lines and standardization of the electrocardiogram.   In the drawing, 1 mV causes a deflection of 10 mm.   This is normal standardization.   See text.

P WAVE (FIG. 5-3)

The P wave represents depolarization of the atria.   Its duration indicates the time required for an impulse to pass from the SA node to the AV node (atrial conduction time).

Upward P waves are measured from the upper edge of the baseline to the summit of P.   Downward P waves are measured from the lower edge of the baseline to the lowest point of P.   Diphasic P waves are measured by adding the amplitudes above and below the baseline.

The width of the P wave is measured in hundredths of a second at its inner contours, where the forward and hind limbs of the deflection join the baseline.

Calculation of the P terminal force of a diphasic P wave in lead V_1 is illustrated in Fig. 5-4.   The P wave is divided into initial and terminal portions on the basis of morphology.   The duration (in seconds) and the amplitude (in millimeters) of the terminal component are measured.   The P terminal force is the algebraic product of these two values and is expressed in millimeter-seconds.   The P terminal force represents left atrial activation.

The duration of the intrinsicoid deflection of a biphasic P wave in lead V_1 is measured from the peak of the initial component to the nadir of the terminal component, as shown in Fig. 5-5.

The normal P wave has a rounded summit, but it may be slightly pointed or notched.

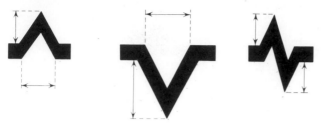

Fig. 5-3   Measurement of the P and T waves.   Described in text.

Normal Values

The following is a summary of the normal findings:

The amplitude of the P wave is normally 0.5 to 2.5 mm.

The maximum normal duration of the P wave is 0.07 s in infants under 1 year of age, 0.08 s in children between 1 and 12 years, 0.09 s in children between 12 and 16 years, and 0.10 s in older children and adults.

The P wave is usually largest in lead I or lead II.   It may be diphasic, flat, or inverted in lead III.   In sinus rhythms, the P wave is upright in leads I and II, inverted in lead aVR, upright in lead aVF, and upright, diphasic, or inverted in lead aVL.   It is usually diphasic in lead V_1 and sometimes in V_2.   However, it may be entirely inverted in these leads normally.   When the P wave is diphasic in lead V_1, the P terminal force is normally between

Fig. 5-4   Measurement of the P terminal force in lead V_1.   (A) The P wave is divided into initial and terminal portions.   The duration (in seconds) and the amplitude (in millimeters) of the terminal component are measured.   The P terminal force is the algebraic product of these two values and is expressed in millimeter-seconds.   (B) Examples: (1) Normal P terminal force.   (2) Abnormal P terminal force.   (Modified after J. J. Morris, E. H. Estes, Jr., R. F. Whalen et al., P-Wave Analysis in Valvular Heart Disease, Circulation, 29: 242, 1964.   Used by permission of the American Heart Association, Inc.)

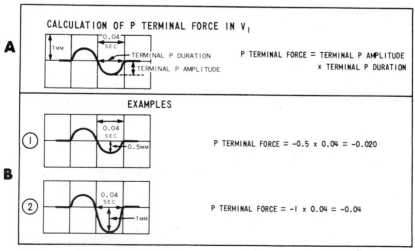

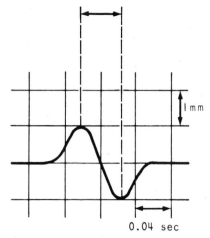

0.04 sec

Fig. 5-5 Measurement of the duration of the intrinsicoid deflection of a diphasic P wave in lead V_1. The duration is measured from the peak of the initial component to the nadir of the terminal component.

$+0.01$ and -0.03 mm-s. The duration of the intrinsicoid deflection of a diphasic P wave in lead V_1, is normally 0.03 s or less. In leads V_3 to V_6, the P wave is positive but may be of very low voltage.

The normal ratio of the duration of the P wave to that of the P-R segment is between 1.0 and 1.6.

Notching of the P wave per se is not abnormal unless the distance between the peaks exceeds 0.03 s and the P wave is abnormally wide.

Abnormality of the P Wave

Increased voltage or increased duration of the P wave is usually diagnostic of atrial abnormality. An increased P terminal force in lead V_1 or increased duration of the intrinsicoid deflection in this lead is usually indicative of left atrial abnormality. An abnormal P terminal force has been reported to occur in 7.1 percent of the resting electrocardiograms of healthy middle-aged men. An increased P terminal force may sometimes be seen in diffuse pulmonary disease in the absence of abnormality of the left atrium and, rarely, in some instances of right atrial enlargement.

An inverted P wave in lead I occurs in dextrocardia, in left atrial rhythm, and, rarely, in AV junctional rhythm or marked right atrial enlargement but most commonly results from reversal of the right and left arm leads.

Left axis deviation of the P wave (between 0 and $-30°$) in a sinus rhythm may be an early sign of left atrial enlargement in mitral stenosis or arterial hypertension but may also be seen in apparently healthy obese or elderly persons.

Right axis deviation of the P wave (beyond +75°) is commonly a sign of right atrial enlargement, seen most often in chronic obstructive pulmonary disease with or without cor pulmonale. However, it has been observed not infrequently in young, thin, asthenic but otherwise healthy persons.

The P wave is inverted in leads II, III, and aVF and is upright in lead aVR in AV junctional or low atrial rhythms.

Absence of P waves occurs in atrial standstill, during periods of sinus arrest, and in SA block. The P wave may not be recognizable in the conventional leads in some AV junctional rhythms. In atrial flutter and fibrillation, the P waves are replaced by other oscillations called F and f waves, respectively.

Atrial Repolarization

The Tp (or Ta) wave represents repolarization of the atria. Its direction is opposite to that of the P wave. The segment inscribed from the end of the P wave to the beginning of the Tp wave is called the S-Tp segments. It is recorded during the P-R segment and the beginning of the QRS complex, while the Tp wave is superimposed upon the final portion of the QRS complex and the S-T segment.

A downward S-Tp segment may normally cause depression of the P-R segment. When this occurs, there is also concordant depression (pseudo-depression) of the S-T segment, so that both the P-R and S-T segments behave as though they were arcs of a common circle or circumference.

Thus an S-T segment depression has no pathologic significance whenever it is preceded by a concordant and symmetric P-R segment depression. Abnormality is diagnosable only when the P-R and S-T segments are discordant, that is, when they correspond to arcs of different circles or circumferences (see Figs. 4-2 and 5-13).

P-R INTERVAL (FIG. 5-6)

The P-R interval represents the time required for a stimulus to travel from the SA node to the ventricles.

Fig. 5-6 Measurement of the P-R interval. Described in text.

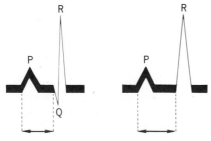

It is measured from the beginning of the P wave to the beginning of the QRS complex, regardless of whether the initial QRS deflection is a Q wave or an R wave.   Measurement is made in the standard or unipolar limb lead with the longest P-R interval.   The closest approximation to the true P-R interval is obtained by measuring the longest time interval between the beginning of the P wave and the end of the QRS complex in the bipolar and unipolar extremity leads and subtracting from this the longest QRS interval found in these leads.

Normal Values

The duration of the P-R interval is 0.12 to 0.20 s in adults, 0.10 to 0.18 s in adolescents between 14 and 17 years of age, and 0.10 to 0.17 s in children.   These values are valid for heart rates between 70 and 90 per minute.   For slower or more rapid heart rates, the maximum normal values for the P-R interval are listed in Table 1 in the Appendix.

Abnormality of the P-R Interval

Prolongation of the P-R interval is called first-degree AV block.   Atrioventricular block may develop as a result of drug action (e.g., digitalis or quinidine), myocardial disease (e.g., coronary artery disease), rheumatic fever, or infectious disease (e.g., diphtheria).

Although a short P-R interval may be a normal variant, it is more commonly associated with AV junctional or low atrial rhythms.   The Lown-Ganong-Levine syndrome and ventricular preexcitation are examples of other conditions that are associated with short P-R intervals.

QRS COMPLEX (FIGS. 5-7, 5-8)

The QRS complex represents depolarization of the ventricles.   The various components of the QRS complex are designated as follows:

Q wave   The initial downward deflection followed by an R wave
R wave   The first upward deflection whether preceded by a Q wave or not
S wave   The downward deflection following the R wave
R' wave   The second upward deflection
S' wave   The downward deflection following the R' wave
QS complex   A single negative deflection representing the entire QRS complex

Capital and small letters are often used to indicate approximately the amplitude of the various deflections.   A capital letter indicates a deflection of large amplitude; a small letter, one of low amplitude.

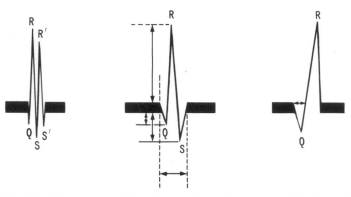

Fig. 5-7   Measurement of the QRS complex and its various deflections.   Described in text.

Although most deflections are smoothly inscribed, notching and slurring (Fig. 5-9) sometimes occur.   A *notch* is a slight distinct change in the direction of a deflection.   Localized thickening of a deflection is called a *slur*.

Measurement of the QRS interval (intraventricular conduction time) is always made in the standard or unipolar limb lead in which it is widest. It is measured from the beginning of the initial component to the end of the final component of the complex.

The height of the R wave is measured from the upper edge of the baseline to the peak of the R wave.   The depth of the Q, S, or QS components is measured from the lower edge of the baseline to the lowest point of the Q, S, or QS components, respectively.   The width of the Q wave is measured from the point where it begins to the point where the upstroke of the R wave crosses the baseline.   The reference level for determining the voltage of the QRS deflections is the point where the first component of the QRS begins.

Fig. 5-8   Nomenclature of the various QRS complexes.   Capital letters are employed to designate large deflections and letters in the lower case to indicate small deflections.

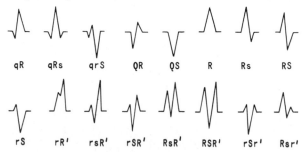

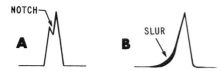

Fig. 5-9   Notching and slurring.

Q Wave

Abnormalities of the Q wave are of considerable importance in electrocardiographic diagnosis.   There is some disagreement among authorities on the criteria for the normal amplitude of the Q wave.   There is much less disagreement on the criteria for its width.   Since the width of the Q wave is of much greater importance than its amplitude, this is the more significant measurement.   Normal values for the Q wave are listed in Tables 2 to 4 in the Appendix.   The criteria for Q wave abnormality are summarized in Table 13-1.   The following is a summary of the normal findings in various leads.

Leads I and II   The Q wave is normally less than 0.04 s wide, less than 2 mm deep, and less than 25 percent of the succeeding R wave.

Lead III   The Q wave may be normally 0.04 s or more in width.   Its amplitude is variable, as is also the Q/R ratio.   It is normally 6 mm or less in depth.   The significance of a Q wave in lead III depends on the configuration of the QRS complex of lead aVF and lead II.   When there is a wide Q wave (0.04 s or more) in lead III, the association of wide Q waves in lead aVF and lead II as well almost always indicates that the wide Q wave is abnormal.   A Q wave in leads III and aVF in the presence of an initial R wave equal to or greater than 1.0 mm in lead aVR is usually abnormal and indicative of inferior or combined inferior and anterolateral myocardial infarction.   The occurrence of Q waves in leads III and aVF in association with a QR complex in lead aVR is not likely to be abnormal. A wide or deep Q_3 not associated with wide or deep Q waves in leads aVF and II is usually normal.   When Q waves are absent in leads aVF or aVL, an isolated Q_3, even if deep or wide, is normal.   This is commonly observed when the R wave in lead aVL is taller than that in aVF, since lead III = VF − VL.   The QS complexes that are sometimes seen in lead III may be abnormal or may occur as a normal variant.

Lead aVR   The Q wave may normally be 0.04 s or more in width.   The depth of the Q wave and the Q/R ratio are variable, but the Q/R ratio is normally greater than 1.0.   A QS deflection is seen commonly in both normal and abnormal subjects.   A QS complex in this lead may be observed with either normal or pathologic Q waves in leads III and aVF.   A QR pattern in lead aVR in association with an $S_1Q_3T_3$ pattern is consistent with acute cor pulmonale.   An rS complex in lead aVR with the R wave 1.0 mm or taller is usually abnormal and indicative of inferior or inferolateral myocardial infarction.

Lead aVL   The Q wave is normally less than 0.04 s wide, less than 2 mm deep, and less than 50 percent of the succeeding R wave.   When the voltage of the R wave is low (5 mm or less), Q/R ratios are unreliable from a diagnostic standpoint.   A wide Q wave (0.04 s or more) or QS complex may sometimes occur normally, particularly when the heart is vertical. The recognition of a wide Q wave as a normal variant is aided by its association with negative P and T waves in this lead and by the absence of abnormal Q waves in lead I and the lateral precordial leads, as well as by the absence of broad R waves in leads III and aVF.   Marked S-T segment elevation or abnormal T wave inversion in lead aVL is not seen in normal subjects with QR or QS patterns in this lead.

Lead aVF   The Q wave is normally less than 0.04 s wide, less than 2 mm deep, and less than 25 percent of the amplitude of the R wave.   When the voltage of the R wave is low (5 mm or less), Q/R ratios are unreliable from a diagnostic standpoint.   Occasionally, wide Q waves (0.04 s or more) or QS complexes can occur in some normal individuals.   Abnormal Q waves in lead aVF are usually indicative of inferior myocardial infarction, but may be seen in acute cor pulmonale and chronic lung disease with or without cor pulmonale.

Precordial Leads   A Q wave is normally found only in leads to the left of lead V_3.   When present, the Q wave is normally less than 0.04 s wide, less than 2 mm deep, and less than 15 percent of the succeeding R wave. A small Q wave may be normal in lead V_3 if it is less than 0.5 mm in depth, provided that the Q waves in leads to the left of lead V_3 are normal.

QS Complexes

QS complexes in leads aVF, III, and II are almost always normal.   This pattern is generally indicative of inferior infarction with or without left anterior fascicular block, but it is sometimes seen in emphysema (Fig. 18-5).   Usually the presence of other electrocardiographic abnormalities helps in the differential diagnosis between the two.   A QS complex in leads aVF and III associated with a qrS or an rS complex (in which the R wave is small and notched) in lead II suggests inferior infarction in the presence of left anterior fascicular block.   The pattern of QS complexes in leads aVF and III without Q waves in lead II is also suggestive of inferior infarction or emphysema, but it may be a normal variant.

   A QS complex may occur normally in lead aVL, particularly when the heart is vertical.   The recognition of a QS deflection as a normal variant is aided by its association with negative P and T waves in this lead and by the absence of abnormal Q waves in lead I, the lateral precordial leads, and broad R waves in leads III and aVF. `Moreover, the S-T segment is not abnormally elevated in lead aVL nor is there pathologic T wave inversion in this lead when the QS complex is a normal variant.

A QS deflection may occur normally in leads V_{3R} and V_1, and sometimes in lead V_2 as well, but very rarely in lead V_3. The most common causes of QS complexes in leads V_1 to V_3 are electrode misplacement, anteroseptal myocardial infarction, left ventricular enlargement, and emphysema with cor pulmonale.

Comments   Although abnormal Q waves are considered pathognomonic of myocardial infarction, there are exceptions. Abnormal Q waves and QS deflections simulating myocardial infarction have been noted in left ventricular hypertrophy, right ventricular hypertrophy, acute cor pulmonale, emphysema, ventricular preexcitation, idiopathic hypertrophic subaortic stenosis, diffuse myocardial disease (e.g., idiopathic cardiomyopathy), localized myocardial disease (e.g., tumor), left bundle branch block, Prinzmetal's angina, and conditions associated with shock and severe metabolic stress.

Transitory Q wave abnormalities have also been observed during bouts of tachycardia and during episodes of coronary insufficiency.

Reversal of the right and left arm electrodes may cause the appearance of a factitiously abnormal Q wave in lead I. Prominent Q waves may also appear in lead I in dextrocardia.

It has been held by many that respiratory or postural maneuvers may be helpful in deciding whether Q waves in leads III, aVF, and aVL are normal or abnormal. To the author's knowledge, no critical and systematic investigation has been made of the value of these maneuvers. It is claimed, for example, that deep inspiration will ordinarily cause an innocent Q_3 to disappear or decrease in size, whereas pathologic Q waves will be little affected. A recent study has shown that recording lead III in deep inspiration is not a reliable procedure for determining the significance of a Q_3 wave and can result in a false-negative diagnosis of inferior infarction. Presumably, the same reasoning can be applied to a QaVF deflection. It has also been stated, with respect to a Q wave in lead aVL, that the occurrence of changes in the relative amplitudes of the Q and R waves with assumption of an erect position implies that the deflection is normal.

Similarly, QS complexes in leads III and aVF are regarded as normal if bodily or respiratory movements change the QS deflection to an rS complex and as abnormal if the change is to a Qr complex. The reliability of these assumptions is open to question.

Duration of the QRS Complex

The maximum normal duration of the QRS interval is 0.08 s in children under 5 years of age, 0.09 s in children 5 to 14 years of age, and 0.10 s in older children and adults.

Voltage of the QRS Complex

Criteria for the normal amplitude of the various components of the QRS complex in the extremity and precordial leads are listed in Tables 2 to 6 in the Appendix. The following is a summary of the more pertinent normal findings. The criteria apply to children from 1 to 16 years of age and to adults over 16 years of age unless otherwise specified.

A more detailed discussion of the QRS complex may be found in the section on the conventional electrocardiogram including both the extremity and precordial leads, beginning on page 91.

Standard Limb Leads   The sum of the R wave in lead I and the S wave in lead III is normally 25 mm or less in adults and 30 mm in children. The amplitude of the R wave in lead I is less than 14 mm in adults. The sum of the R waves in leads II and III in children is less than 45 mm. When these values are exceeded, left ventricular enlargement may be present. Low voltage is said to be present when the largest QRS deflection in each lead is 5 mm or less.

Notching associated with low voltage of the QRS complex is abnormal in leads I and II but not in lead III. It is usually due to myocardial fibrosis or a ventricular conduction defect.

Unipolar Limb Leads   The height of the R wave in lead aVL is 11 mm or less; in aVF, 20 mm or less. The amplitude of the S wave in lead aVR is 14 mm or less. When these values are exceeded, left ventricular enlargement may be present. The amplitude of the initial R wave in lead aVR is less than 1 mm. Increased amplitude of the initial R wave in this lead is usually indicative of inferior or combined inferior and anterior myocardial infarction. When there is a late R wave in lead aVR, its amplitude is 5 mm or less. A tall, dominant late R wave in lead aVR is suggestive of right ventricular enlargement but may also be found in right bundle branch block, anterolateral or inferolateral myocardial infarction, left anterior hemiblock, and other conditions in which the mean QRS vector is directed superiorly.

Low voltage exists when the tallest deflection in each of the augmented unipolar limb leads is 5 mm or less.

Unipolar Precordial Leads   The amplitude of the R wave in lead V_1 is 6 mm or less in adults, 16 mm or less in children from 1 to 16 years of age, and less than 20 mm in infants under 1 year of age. In adults the R/S ratio is normally less than 1.0 in lead V_1 and greater than 1.0 in lead V_5 or V_6. The maximum normal R/S ratio in lead V_1 in children, according to age, is as follows: 0 to 3 months, 6.5; 3 to 6 months, 4.0; 6 months to 3 years, 2.4; 3 to 5 years, 1.6; and 6 to 15 years, 1.0. When these values are exceeded, the diagnosis of right ventricular enlargement should be suspected.

In adults, the height of the R wave in lead V_5 is 26 mm or less and in lead V_6 20 mm or less. The sum of the R wave in lead V_5 and the S wave in lead V_1 or V_2 is 35 mm or less.   The sum of the R wave in lead V_5 or V_6 and the S wave in lead V_1 is 30 mm or less.   The sum of the R wave in lead V_5 or V_6 and the S wave in lead V_1 or V_2 is 35 mm or less.   The sum of the R wave in lead V_4 or V_5 and the S wave in lead V_2 is 35 mm or less. The sum of the maximum R wave and the deepest S wave in the precordial leads is 45 mm or less.   The depth of the S wave in lead V_1 is 23 mm or less, and in lead V_2 it is 29 mm or less.   When these values are exceeded, the diagnosis of left ventricular enlargement should be considered.

In children, the amplitude of the R wave in lead V_5 or V_6 is less than 35 mm, and the sum of the R wave in lead V_5 and the S wave in lead V_2 is 60 mm or less in children under 11 years of age, and 55 mm in females and 65 mm in males between 11 and 16 years of age.   Voltages higher than these are suggestive of left ventricular enlargement.   The reader is also referred to Chap. 10, which covers ventricular enlargement.

When there is an R′ pattern with a normal QRS interval in lead V_1, the primary R wave is 8 mm or less, the secondary R wave is 6 mm or less, and the R′/S ratio is less than 1.0.

When the tallest QRS deflection in any of the precordial leads is less than 10 mm, low voltage is present.

Low Voltage (Fig. 5 10)   Low voltage of the QRS complexes occurs commonly as a normal variant but is not infrequently the result of such conditions as emphysema, coronary artery disease, anasarca, pleural and pericardial effusion, myxedema, obesity, and anemia.

INTRINSICOID DEFLECTION (FIG. 5-11)

While the intrinsicoid deflection has been thought to represent depolarization of that portion of the ventricular myocardium beneath the exploring electrode of a unipolar precordial lead, present opinion regards the intrinsicoid deflection as representing the turning point of the cardiac vector along the axis of derivation of the lead.

The time of onset of the intrinsicoid deflection is measured from the beginning of the QRS complex to the peak of the R wave.   It is usually measured only in the precordial leads.

Normal Values

In the right-sided precordial leads, such as V_1 or V_2, the time of onset of the intrinsicoid deflection is normally 0.03 s or less.   In the left-sided precordial leads, such as V_5 or V_6, it is normally 0.05 s or less in adults and 0.04 s or less in children under 16 years of age.

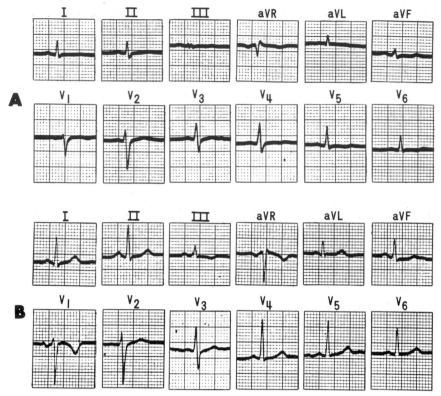

Fig. 5-10 Low voltage. (A) From a patient with classic myxedema. There is low voltage of all complexes in both the extremity and precordial leads. (B) After therapy with thyroid extract. The voltage of the various deflections is normal.

A delayed onset of the intrinsicoid deflection in the right precordial leads is found in right ventricular enlargement or right bundle branch block. In the left precordial leads, delayed onset of the intrinsicoid deflection occurs in left ventricular enlargement, in left bundle branch block, occasionally in myocardial fibrosis due to coronary arteriosclerosis, and rarely in other myocardial diseases.

S-T SEGMENT (FIGS. 5-12, 5-13)

The interval between the end of the QRS complex and the beginning of the T wave is the S-T segment. It represents the time during which the ventricles remain in the activated state and ventricular repolarization may begin. As previously noted, the junction between the QRS complex and the S-T segment is designated by the letter J.

In general, the contour of the S-T segment is of greater significance than the degree of its deviation above or below the baseline. A normal

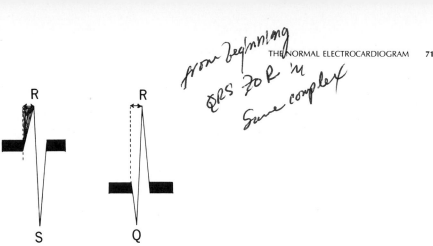

from beginning
QRS to R 'u
Gure complex

R R

S Q

Fig. 5-11 Measurement of the intrinsicoid deflection. Described in text.

S-T segment may show marked displacement, whereas an abnormal S-T segment may show little or no displacement from the baseline. When the T wave is normally upright, normally elevated S-T segments generally show slight upward concavity. When the T wave is normally inverted, normally depressed S-T segments show slight upward convexity.

The reference point for measurement of the degree of elevation or depression of the S-T segment is the T-P interval preceding or following the S-T segment in question, provided that it is isoelectric. When the T-P interval is not isoelectric or is absent, the P-R segment is used as the reference level. If the P-R segment is depressed, abnormal S-T segment elevation or depression is diagnosable only when the P-R and S-T segments are discordant and asymmetric, that is, when they correspond to arcs of a different circle or circumference. (See also section titled Atrial Repolarization earlier in this chapter.)

Elevation is measured from the upper edge of the isoelectric line to the upper edge of the S-T segment; depression is measured from the lower edge of the isoelectric line to the lower edge of the S-T segment.

Fig. 5-12 Measurement of elevation and depression of the S-T segment. Described in text.

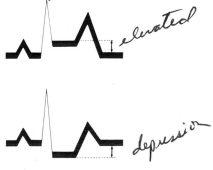

elevated

depression

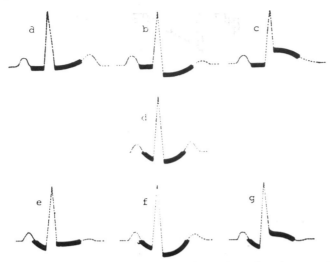

Fig. 5-13 Schematic representation of the relationships between displacements of the P-R and S-T segments: (a) normal; (b) subendocardial injury; (c) subepicardial injury; (d) sympathetic effect; (e) sympathetic effect of atrial injury plus slight subepicardial injury; (f) sympathetic effect plus subendocardial injury; (g) sympathetic effect plus subepicardial injury. (From J. Tranchesi, V. Adelardi, and J. M. de Oliveria, Atrial Repolarization: Its Importance in Clinical Electrocardiography, Circulation, 22: 635, 1960. Used by permission of the American Heart Association, Inc.)

Normal Values

The S-T segment is usually isoelectric, but it may normally deviate between -0.5 and $+1.0$ mm from the baseline in the standard and unipolar extremity leads. In the unipolar precordial leads and occasionally in the extremity leads, upward displacement of 2 or even 3 mm may be normal (Figs. 5-14, 5-15), provided the S-T segment, which often begins with a notch, is concave upward and the succeeding T wave is tall, broad-based, and upright. This normal variant has been attributed to "early repolarization." Downward displacement in excess of 0.5 mm is abnormal. In all instances, pseudodepression caused by a depressed P-R segment (Fig. 5-14) must be excluded. The average duration of the S-T segment is from 0.05 to 0.15 s.

Abnormality of the S-T Segment (Fig. 5-16)

Elevation of the S-T segment in epicardial leads may sometimes occur as a normal variant because of early repolarization. More often it is the result of myocardial infarction with subepicardial injury, acute pericarditis, or myocarditis. It may also be a reciprocal effect of a depressed S-T segment in an oppositely located lead. S-T segment elevation may rarely be caused by marked hyperpotassemia and also mitral valve prolapse.

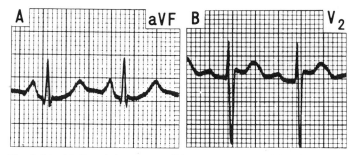

Fig. 5-14 (A) Pseudodepression of the S-T segment due to depression of the P-R segment. There is increased amplitude of the P wave (P pulmonale). (B) Normal upward S-T segment displacement. This type of S-T segment elevation is often erroneously regarded as abnormal and attributed to subepicardial injury.

The differential diagnosis between early repolarization and acute pericarditis, conditions which are commonly mistaken for each other, is discussed in Chap. 15.

Depression of the S-T segment in epicardial leads is often a nonspecific abnormality. It may be the result of digitalis effect or the administration of other drugs. It is a common finding in bundle branch block, left or right

Fig. 5-15 Upward S-T segment displacement in a normal subject without heart disease. Aside from the S-T segment elevations in leads I, II, aVF, and all the precordial leads, the electrocardiogram is within normal limits. The benign and fixed nature of the S-T segment changes was established by serial electrocardiograms.

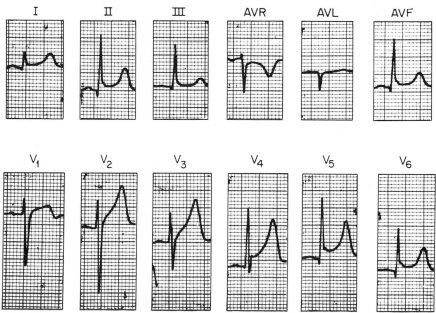

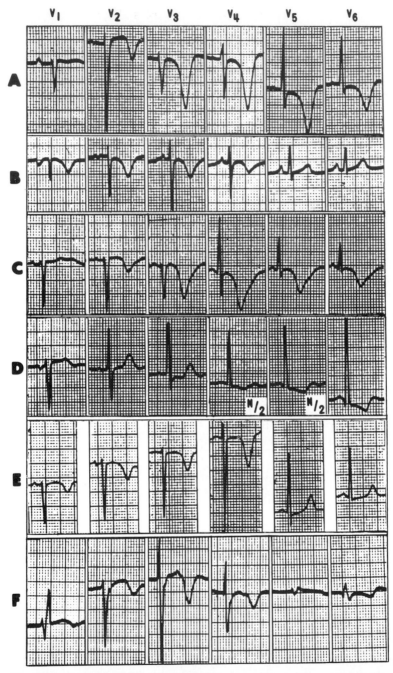

Fig. 5-16 Examples of S-T segment and T wave abnormalities. (*A*) Anterior myocardial ischemia due to coronary artery disease. (*B*) Right ventricular strain in a patient with mitral stenosis, left atrial hypertrophy, and pulmonary hypertension. (*C*) S-T-T changes in a patient with subarachnoid hemorrhage. (*D*) Left ventricular hypertrophy and strain. (*E*) Hypocalcemia with T wave inversion. (*F*) T wave inversion in a patient with complete heart block following a Stokes-Adams attack.

ventricular enlargement, electrolyte abnormalities, subendocardial anoxemia, and shock. S-T segment depression may also be a reciprocal effect
of an elevated S-T segment in an oppositely located lead. Transient S-T
segment and T wave changes are common during bouts of tachycardia
even in normal hearts and occasionally may persist for some time after the
attack (posttachycardia syndrome).

T WAVE (FIG. 5-3)

The T wave represents repolarization of the ventricles.
    Upright T waves are measured from the upper level of the baseline to
the summit of the T wave. Inverted T waves are measured from the lower
level of the baseline to the lowest point of the T wave. Diphasic T waves
are measured by adding the amplitudes above and below the baseline.
    The width of the T wave is measured in hundredths of a second at its
inner contours, where the forward and hind limbs join the baseline.
    The normal T wave has asymmetrical limbs and a rounded summit.
The slope of the forward limb is more gradual than that of the hind limb.

Normal Values

The range of normal values for the T wave in the various leads is given in
Tables 2, 3, and 7 in the Appendix.

Standard Limb Leads

The T wave measures 1.0 to 5.0 mm or more in the lead in which the T
wave is tallest. The T wave is upright in leads I and II. It is often flat,
diphasic, or inverted as much as 1.5 mm in lead III. In lead I, the T wave
is usually greater than 0.5 mm in amplitude. Inverted T waves in lead I
in the presence of clearly positive QRS complexes in this lead are always
abnormal. The normal duration of the T wave is from 0.10 to 0.25 s.

Unipolar Extremity Leads

Lead aVR   The T wave is normally always inverted in this lead.

Lead aVL   When the QRS complex shows an R, Rs, qR, or qRs pattern,
the T wave is upright and measures 1.0 to 5.0 mm. However, flattening
or inversion of the T wave up to 1.0 mm is normal, particularly when the
R wave is less than 5 mm in amplitude. When the QRS complex shows
an rS, QS, or Qr pattern, the T wave may be upright, flat, or diphasic. It
may even be inverted as much as 2.5 mm normally. When the T wave is
normally inverted in this lead, the P wave is usually inverted also.

Lead aVF   The T wave is usually upright and up to 5.0 mm in amplitude. It can, however, be normally flattened, diphasic, or inverted as much as 1.0 mm normally.

Precordial Leads

In adults, the T wave is usually inverted in lead V_1 but upright in the remainder of the standard precordial leads.   In some young adults under 30 years of age, the T wave may normally be inverted in leads V_1, V_2, and V_3.   However, in adults over 30 years of age, T wave inversion is usually normal only in lead V_1.   Isolated T wave negativity at the apex is a rare normal variant (Fig. 5-17).   The height of the T wave is usually not above 10 mm in any of the precordial leads, but this value may be exceeded in some normal individuals.

In children, the oldest age at which inverted or diphasic T waves occur normally is presented in the following table:

Lead	Inverted T Waves	Diphasic T Wave
V_1	16 years	16 years
V_2	12 years	16 years
V_3	10 years	15 years
V_4	5 years	11 years
V_5	15 hr	14 hr
V_6	8 hr	1 day

SOURCE: R. F. Ziegler, "Electrocardiographic Studies in Normal Infants and Children," Charles C Thomas, Publisher, Springfield, Ill., 1951.

Abnormality of the T Wave (Figs. 5-16, 5-18, 5-19)

Normally the T wave in lead V_6 is upright and taller than that in lead V_1. In the presence of an otherwise normal electrocardiogram and a positive T wave in lead V_1, the pattern of T_{V_1} taller than T_{V_6} is suggestive, but not diagnostic, of myocardial abnormality, particularly ischemic, hypertensive, or valvular heart disease.   The pattern is also a not uncommon normal variant, particularly in healthy men.

Most T wave abnormalities are of a nonspecific nature.   T wave abnormalities may indicate primary heart disease, especially coronary artery disease, or heart disease secondary to systemic disease.   However, abnormal T waves occur frequently in healthy persons as a variant pattern or as a result of physiologic stimuli.

Two normal variants have been discussed previously: the juvenile T wave pattern and isolated T wave negativity at the apex.   Two other variants occur in patients with normal hearts but with skeletal abnormalities.   Patients with funnel chest may show T wave inversion in leads V_1 to V_3 and

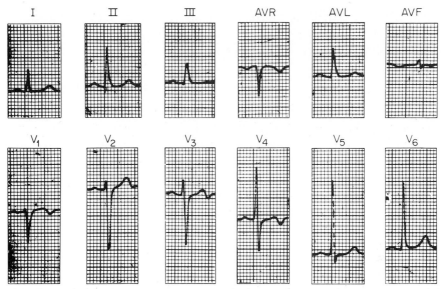

Fig. 5-17 Isolated T wave negativity in a normal subject. The inverted T waves are recorded in an area of T wave positivity. The T wave is upright in lead V_2, dips in leads V_3 and V_4, and is again upright in leads V_5 and V_6. The electrocardiogram is otherwise within normal limits.

occasionally in the left precordial leads. In the "straight back" syndrome, T wave inversion is common in leads II, III, and aVF and sometimes in leads V_5 and V_6 as well. T wave abnormalities are sometimes observed in otherwise healthy asthenic or neurotic individuals. Physiologic T wave changes may be the result of a change in body position, hyperventilation (Fig. 5-18), anxiety, drinking ice water, fever, high altitude, and other stimuli.

Functional T wave changes tend to show a great deal of lability under various conditions. When nonspecific T waves changes occur in the electrocardiogram and their etiology cannot be determined, repeat electro-cardiograms should be performed after hyperventilation, deep inspiration,

Fig. 5-18 T wave changes induced by hyperventilation.

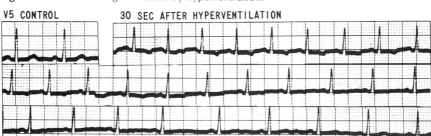

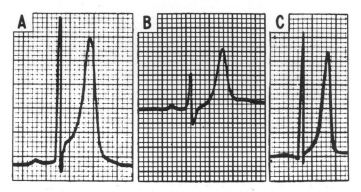

Fig. 5-19   Tall T waves.   (A) Lead V$_5$.   Acute subendocardial ischemia at the onset of anterior myocardial infarction.   (B) Lead V$_3$.   Reciprocal T wave elevation in strictly posterior myocardial infarction.   (C) Lead V$_4$.   Hyperkalemia.

standing, and fasting.   With these maneuvers, functional T wave changes will often disappear if they have been present or reappear if they have been temporarily absent.   The disappearance of T wave inversions after the administration of potassium salts or the appearance of T wave inversions following the oral ingestion of 100 g of glucose is strong evidence that the T wave abnormality is physiologic.   Functional T wave changes will also tend to disappear after sedation or after the administration of 0.5 mg atropine subcutaneously or intravenously.   Ordinarily, all the foregoing procedures will have little or no effect on organic T wave abnormalities.   Isoproterenol appears to reverse primary T wave abnormalities in patients with normal QRS durations but leaves them unaltered in patients with myocardial infarction or pericarditis.

Abnormally tall, upright T waves (Fig. 5-19) in the precordial leads occur in a small percentage of normal persons.   The voltage of the T waves is also increased in anterior and posterobasal myocardial infarction, angina pectoris, hyperpotassemia, anemia, left ventricular hypertrophy, and other conditions.   The normal tall T wave characteristically arises from an elevated S-T segment and is not narrow or symmetrical.   It is seen best in leads V$_3$ to V$_5$.   Usually the pattern is stable over a long period of time. Hyperpotassemic T waves are symmetrical, have a sharp peak, a narrow base, and a relatively short Q-T interval, and their amplitude may exceed that of the R wave.   The T waves tend to be wide in ischemic heart disease. In cases of anterior myocardial infarction, the tall T waves occur at the onset and are transitory.   They are presumably caused by acute subendo-cardial ischemia.   In posterobasal myocardial infarction, tall T waves in the precordial leads are a reciprocal effect of posterior T wave inversions. In left ventricular hypertrophy, tall T waves in leads V$_1$ to V$_3$ or V$_4$ occur in systolic overloading; in leads V$_4$ to V$_6$, in diastolic overloading; and from V$_2$ to V$_6$, in combined types of overloading.

Giant massive T wave inversion (see Fig. 5-16), especially in the precordial leads, may occur in several conditions. When the T wave inversion is symmetrical, deep, and narrow, coronary artery disease or severe right ventricular hypertrophy is the usual cause. Broad, bizarre, asymmetrical, deep T wave inversion, often associated with a prolonged Q-T interval, is most commonly the result of cerebral disease, notably subarachnoid hemorrhage. Similar changes may be noted in patients with complete heart block following Stokes-Adams attacks and in some individuals following vagotomy. In patients with heart disease, T wave inversions may sometimes become more prominent during bradycardia.

Short and Weir have reported that asymmetrical T wave inversion expressed by a T wave asymmetry ratio of 2.0 or greater (the so-called "strain" pattern), even in the absence of voltage criteria for left ventricular hypertrophy, has a strong association with ventricular enlargement in patients without bundle branch block and who are not receiving digoxin or a similar drug.

Symmetrical T wave inversion is more characteristic of ischemia.

U WAVE (FIG. 5-20)

The U wave is a small deflection sometimes seen following the T wave. Its true significance is unknown, but many believe it to be caused by afterpotentials at the beginning of diastole; others, to repolarization of the Purkinje system. The U wave is usually tallest in leads V_2 and V_3. Its maximum amplitude usually does not exceed 1.0 mm, but it sometimes may normally reach 2.0 mm in height. The U wave is generally 5 to 25 percent of the amplitude of the T wave. The polarity of the U wave is usually the same as that of the T wave. However, the U wave may be upright in the right precordial leads when the T wave is inverted (as in the

Fig. 5-20   The U wave. (A) Normal U wave. (B) Large U wave in hypopotassemia. (C) Large U wave in left ventricular hypertrophy. (D) Negative U wave.

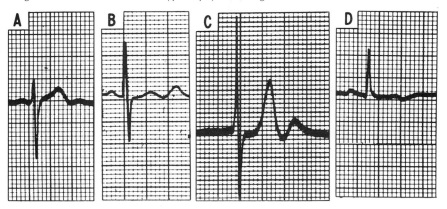

juvenile T wave pattern), and it may be upright in lead III when the T wave is inverted.   It is usually negative in lead aVR.

Abnormality of the U Wave (Fig. 5-20)

The amplitude of the U wave may be increased by bradycardia, forced inspiration, and exercise.   Other conditions that may heighten the U wave include hypopotassemia, hypothermia, drugs (e.g., digitalis, quinidine, procainamide, and isoproterenol), increased intracranial pressure, left ventricular hypertrophy, myocardial disease, complete heart block, and hypercalcemia.

A negative U wave is considered to be highly specific for the presence of heart disease and is usually associated with other electrocardiographic abnormalities.   The clinical conditions most commonly associated with negative U waves are systemic hypertension, aortic and mitral regurgitation, and ischemic heart disease.   Reversal of U wave inversion may be observed in patients with hypertension when the blood pressure is reduced.

Inversion of the U wave during exercise is considered indicative of coronary artery disease.

Q-T INTERVAL

The Q-T interval represents electrical systole.   It is the time required for depolarization and repolarization of the ventricles to take place.   It varies with age, sex, and heart rate.

The Q-T interval is measured from the beginning of the QRS complex to the end of the T wave.

The Q-T interval is difficult to determine accurately.   Although the longest interval found in any lead from the body surface is regarded as the one most nearly correct, it is important to select for measurement a lead in which the T wave is seen clearly and not deformed by a U wave. Otherwise, it is possible to erroneously measure the Q-U rather than the Q-T interval.

Normal Values

The usual normal range of the Q-T interval in adults is from 0.35 to 0.44 s.

The Q-T interval for various heart rates can be determined by Bazett's formula:

$$\text{Q-T corrected, or Q-T}_c = \frac{\text{Q-T (s)}}{\sqrt{\text{R-R interval (s)}}}$$

The Q-T interval is prolonged if the corrected Q-T interval exceeds 0.425 s.

The normal Q-T interval according to heart rate, age, and sex can be determined from Tables 8 to 10 in the Appendix.

Abnormality of the Q-T Interval

Prolongation of the Q-T interval may be primary (idiopathic) or secondary. The idiopathic variety includes the Jervell-Lange-Nielsen syndrome, the Romano-Ward syndrome, and sporadic types. These forms of Q-T interval prolongation are often associated with cardiac arrhythmias, syncopal spells, and sudden death due to ventricular fibrillation or asystole.

Secondary types of Q-T interval prolongation include: (1) drug-induced causes (e.g., antiarrhythmic agents, quinidine, phenothiazines, tricyclic antidepressants); (2) metabolic abnormalities (e.g., hypocalcemia, hypo-magnesemia, hepatic dysfunction); (3) myocardial disease (e.g., myocardial infarction, myocarditis, congestive heart failure); (4) lesions of the central nervous system (e.g., subarachnoid hemorrhage, cerebral thrombosis); (5) autonomic nervous system dysfunction (e.g., radical neck surgery); (6) mitral valve prolapse; and (7) miscellaneous disorders (e.g. congenital heart block).

Prolongation of the Q-T interval is indicative of delayed repolarization of the myocardium and is not infrequently associated with serious ventricular arrhythmias (e.g., torsades de pointes), syncope, and sudden death.

The Q-T interval may be shortened by digitalis, hypercalcemia, and sometimes by hyperpotassemia.

CALCULATION OF THE HEART RATE (FIG. 5-21)

In the electrocardiogram the number of 0.04-s time lines per minute is 1,500.

When the rhythm is regular, the heart rate can be calculated by either of the methods listed below. In each instance the figure obtained is the heart rate.

1   Divide the number of 0.04-s time lines in an R-R or P-P interval into 1,500.
2   Divide the cycle length or the time between the peaks of two successive R waves or P waves, expressed in seconds or fractions thereof, into 60.

When the rhythm is irregular, several R-R intervals and the number of 0.04-s time lines in the same interval are counted. The former figure divided by the latter and multiplied by 1,500 is the heart rate per minute.

The heart rate can be determined by the use of Tables 11 and 12 in the Appendix.

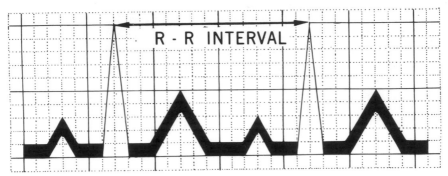

Fig. 5-21 Calculation of the heart rate.   In the example shown, there are fifteen 0.04-s time lines in an R-R interval.   Thus the R-R interval, or cycle length, is 0.6 s (15 × 0.04 = 0.6). The heart rate is 100 per minute (60 ÷ 0.6 = 100 or 1,500 ÷ 15 = 100).   See text.

ELECTRICAL AXIS AND SPATIAL VECTORS

The determination of the electrical axis of the atrial and ventricular complexes is of considerable importance in electrocardiographic diagnosis.

An instantaneous electrical axis represents the direction of the electrical forces at a given instant during the cardiac cycle.   The modal electrical axis refers to the average of the many directions taken by the action current during the cardiac cycle.   The mean electrical axis indicates the average direction of the activation process during the cardiac cycle. The instantaneous and modal electrical axes are determined by linear measurement of the amplitude and direction of the deflections in the standard limb leads; the mean electrical axis, by measurement of the area of the complexes. Instantaneous, modal, and mean electrical axes may be determined for the P wave, the QRS complex, and the T wave in both the frontal and the horizontal planes of the body. Statements concerning axis deviation in clinical electrocardiography usually refer to deviations of the modal electrical axis, although the term "mean electrical axis" is often erroneously used in its stead.

The direction of the electrical axis of the QRS complex in the frontal plane may be determined from standard leads I, II, and III by using either the Einthoven triangle or the triaxial reference figure of Bayley.

In the case of the Einthoven triangle (see Fig. 3-1), the net amplitude and direction of the QRS complexes in any two of the standard bipolar leads are plotted on the sides of the triangle, and the axis is determined by polar coordinates.   Basically the same procedure is used with the triaxial reference figure.   This method is too cumbersome for routine use.

The frontal-plane mean electrical axis of the QRS complex, P waves, or T waves can be determined by the use of Tables 14 and 15 in the Appendix.   These tables use leads I and III.   The values obtained are comparable to the results recorded by the use of other lead combinations.

However, for an individual patient, large axis differences (up to 35°) may occur occasionally. In a patient in whom the axis is considered to be of diagnostic importance, it is probably worth averaging axes determined by different lead combinations. For this purpose, Table 16, devised by Laiken and his coworkers, is suggested. However, for most clinical situations, the method described by Grant in the next section is adequate.

DETERMINING THE ELECTRICAL AXIS IN THE FRONTAL PLANE BY VECTOR ANALYSIS (FIGS. 5-22, 5-23, 5-24)

QRS Complex

1   Vector analysis for the determination of the mean electrical axis in the frontal plane is based on the principle that when a vector is parallel to a lead, the algebraic sum of the positive and negative components of the deflection is largest in that lead, and when a vector is perpendicular to a lead, the algebraic sum of the positive and negative components in that lead is zero.

2   The most accurate method for determining the mean electrical axis of the QRS complex utilizes the net area rather than the amplitude of the various components of the QRS complex. When the areas of these deflections are measured, they are added algebraically. The values obtained, whether positive, negative, or zero, are used to plot the axis. Unfortunately, determination of the net areas of the QRS complexes is a somewhat burdensome chore. Therefore, unless a ventricular conduction defect is present or the deflections vary considerably in width, measurement of the size of the deflections usually suffices for most clinical purposes.

3   The mean electrical axis can be estimated to the nearest 30° by sight inspection of the standard extremity leads (Fig. 5-22). The procedure involves determination of the algebraic sum of the components of the QRS complex in these leads. If the resultant deflection is conspicuously larger in one lead than in either of the other two, the mean vector must be relatively parallel with the axis for that lead. When the net deflection is positive, the mean vector is oriented along the positive side of the lead axis; if negative, along the negative side of the lead axis. On the other hand, if the resultant deflection is smaller in one of the standard leads than in either of the other two, the mean vector must be relatively perpendicular to the axis of that lead, but one of two directions are possible. The problem is solved by noting whether the net deflections in the other two leads are positive or negative and plotting the mean vector to satisfy their polarity. For example, if the algebraic sum of the deflections in lead II (axis +60°) is zero, the mean vector must be perpendicular to this lead axis. There are two possibilities: an axis of

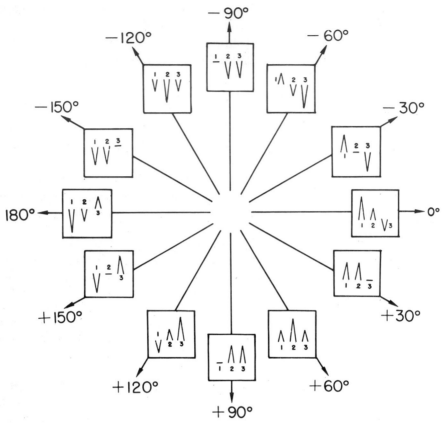

Fig. 5-22 Estimation of the electrical axis in the frontal plane to the nearest 30° by sight inspection of the standard leads. The net amplitudes of the deflections in leads I, II, and III for each axis are shown within the squares.

−30 or one of +150°. If the resultant deflection in lead I is positive and that in lead III negative, the axis is located at −30°. On the other hand, if the resultant deflection in lead I is negative and that in lead III positive, the axis is directed at +150°. This and other examples are graphically illustrated in Fig. 5-22. Estimation of the electrical axis to the nearest 30° is not sufficiently accurate for electrocardiographic interpretation unless the mean vector happens to fall well within the normal or abnormal range. Greater accuracy in the determination of the electrical axis is possible by following the procedure outlined in the succeeding paragraphs.

4 The hexaxial reference diagram (Figs. 3-1D, 5-25) is used. Errors are avoided by checking to see that the sum of leads I and III equals lead II (Einthoven's law) and that the sum of the unipolar limb leads is zero.

5 The extremity leads are inspected to see if any lead can be found in which the algebraic sum of the QRS deflections is zero. If such a lead

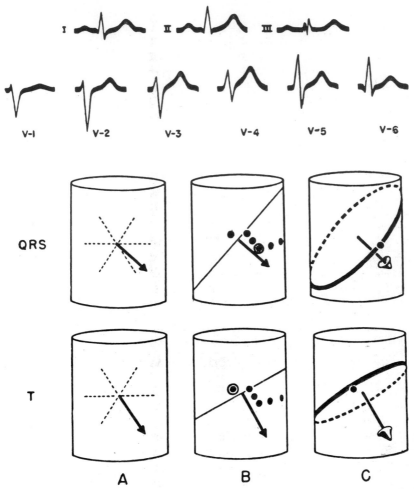

Fig. 5-23 Procedure for plotting the mean spatial QRS and T vectors from the standard limb leads and the six conventional precordial leads. (A) From the deflections in the limb leads, the QRS and T vectors are plotted on the triaxial reference diagram. (Their directions should be altered to conform also to the unipolar limb leads.) The plotting of a vector is based on the principle that when a vector is parallel to a lead the largest deflection appears on that lead, and when a vector is perpendicular to a lead it records its smallest deflection on that lead, or the net area of the deflection is zero. (B) Encircle the precordial lead in which the transitional complex is located. A line is drawn perpendicular to the vector at its origin, representing a diameter of the null or transitional plane. (C) Draw an ellipse symmetrically around the null-plane diameter and through the encircled precordial electrode position. The mean spatial vector is perpendicular to the plane which this ellipse defines, and its direction can be shown by drawing the arrowhead of the vector three-dimensionally. *(From R. P. Grant, "Clinical Electrocardiography,"* © *1957 by McGraw-Hill, Inc., New York. Used with permission of McGraw-Hill Book Company.)*

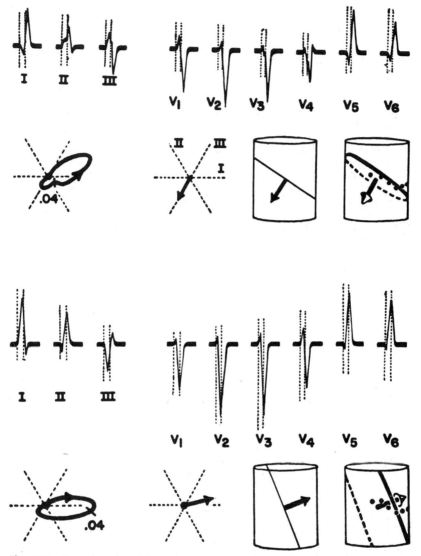

Fig. 5-24 Procedure for plotting the mean vector for the first 0.04 s of the QRS interval. Two electrocardiograms with different directions for the initial 0.04-s vector are shown. The vector loops were drawn from the limb leads. The same principles are employed as in Fig. 5-23, except that only the first 0.04 s of the QRS complex on each lead is used. This is the portion between the dotted lines. In the upper tracing, leads V_2, V_3, and V_4 have as much positive as negative area during this interval. Therefore all three are transitional, and the null pathway runs through all three electrode positions. The same principles may be used to determine the mean vector for the terminal 0.04 s of the QRS interval, except that only the final 0.04 s of the QRS complex is employed for this purpose. *(From R. P. Grant, "Clinical Electrocardiography," © 1957 by McGraw-Hill, Inc., New York. Used with permission of McGraw-Hill Book Company.)*

is present, it is immediately established that the mean vector is directed perpendicularly to the axis of this lead.   To determine which way the vector points, select a second lead whose axis is rotated 90° away from the lead which is at zero potential.   If the resultant QRS complex is positive in the second lead, the mean vector is oriented along the positive side of its lead axis.   On the other hand, if one resultant complex is negative, it is directed along the negative side of its lead axis.   For example, if the QRS complex in lead aVF is equiphasic, the mean electrical axis must be either at 0 or +180°.   Thus a predominantly positive QRS deflection in lead I indicates an axis of 0°, whereas a predominantly negative deflection in this lead reveals the axis to be +180°.

6   If there is no lead in which the positive and negative components are equal, choose the lead with the largest *net* QRS deflection, because the QRS vector must be relatively parallel with the axis of this lead.   If the net QRS deflection is upright, the mean vector is projected along the positive half of the lead axis; if downward, the mean vector is directed along the negative half of the lead axis.   By further alterations in the direction of the plotted vector to conform with the findings in the remaining limb leads, the mean QRS vector in the frontal plane can be localized fairly accurately.   If the net deflections in two adjacent leads are equal, the mean vector obviously lies between the two lead axes. It is well to remember that when comparing deflections in the bipolar leads with those in the augmented unipolar limb leads, the voltages in the latter should be multiplied by 1.15.

7   In right bundle branch block, it is usually necessary only to determine the mean QRS vector for the first half of the QRS complex (approximately the first 0.06 s), since this portion represents the unblocked forces.   The last half of the QRS complex is almost invariably rightward in this condition.   With respect to the left bundle branch block, the mean QRS vector should be determined for the entire QRS complex.

P, S-T Segment, and T Waves

The procedure outlined above is also applicable for determining the axis of the P waves, the S-T segment, and the T wave.

NORMAL VALUES FOR THE ELECTRICAL AXIS IN THE FRONTAL PLANE (FIG. 5-25)

P Wave

The mean electrical axis of the P wave (ÂP) is usually between +30 and +60°, with a range between 0 and +90°.   In normal adults, the maximum inferior P vector usually does not exceed +75°.

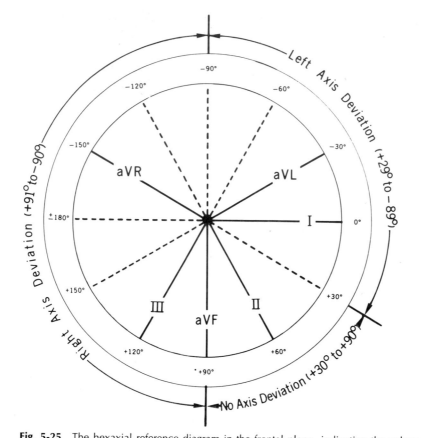

Fig. 5-25   The hexaxial reference diagram in the frontal plane, indicating the values for no axis deviation, left axis deviation, and right axis deviation.

QRS Complex

No Axis Deviation   The mean electrical axis of the QRS complex (ÂQRS) lies between +30 and +90°.

Left Axis Deviation   The mean electrical axis of the QRS complex lies between +29 and −89°.

Right Axis Deviation   The mean electrical axis of the QRS complex lies between +91 and −90°.
    The values for no axis deviation, left axis deviation, and right axis deviation are purely descriptive and do not imply normality or abnormality. The range of normal values is variable.   Age and body build are significant factors in determining the normality or abnormality of the degree of axis deviation in any individual.

Abnormal Left Axis Deviation   Abnormal left axis deviation is present in adults when the mean electrical axis lies between − 30 and − 89°.   Left axis deviation between + 29 and − 29° is usually normal in adults.

Abnormal left axis deviation is present in children when the mean electrical axis lies to the left of + 60° in the first week of life, to the left of + 20° from 1 week to 3 months of age, and to the left of 0° from 3 months to 16 years of age.

Abnormal Right Axis Deviation   Abnormal right axis deviation is present in adults when the mean electrical axis lies between + 110 and − 90°. Right axis deviation with a mean electrical axis between + 90 and + 110° may be abnormal but is frequently a normal variant, particularly in young adults or asthenic persons.

Abnormal right axis deviation is present in children when the mean electrical axis lies to the right of + 120° in children from 3 months to 16 years of age.   In infants under 1 month of age, marked right axis deviation may occur normally, and it is difficult to define standards of abnormality. In infants between 1 and 3 months of age, abnormal right axis deviation is probably present if the mean electrical axis lies to the right of + 140°.

T Wave

The mean electrical axis of the T wave (ÂT) lies between − 11° and + 76°.

QRS-T Angle

The angle between the mean spatial QRS vector and the mean spatial T vector is quite narrow normally.

Adults   The QRS-T angle in the frontal plane is usually less than 60° wide. As a general rule, the T vector tends to lag behind the QRS vector as the latter moves rightward or leftward.   A QRS-T angle over 90° is indicative of a primary T wave abnormality unless a ventricular conduction defect is present.   When ventricular conduction defects occur, the QRS-T angle tends to be abnormally wide (secondary T wave abnormality).   In such instances, the recognition of primary T wave abnormalities is based on criteria other than the width of the QRS-T angle.

In the transverse or horizontal plane, the QRS-T angle should not exceed 90° normally.   Angles above 60° are usually abnormal.

Children   The QRS-T angle may normally be 90° or more in either the frontal or transverse planes.

PROCEDURE FOR DETERMINING THE ELECTRICAL AXIS
AND SPATIAL VECTORS (FIGS. 5-23, 5-24)

1 From the findings in the standard limb leads and by using the triaxial or hexaxial reference system, determine and plot the frontal plane direction of the mean vector of the deflection being studied. This can be done for the P wave, the QRS complex, the initial and terminal 0.04-s portions of the QRS complex, the S-T segment, and the T wave. The method was outlined in the preceding section.

2 A line is drawn perpendicular to the vector at its origin. This is the null plane or pathway for the vector.

3 The mean vector is visualized within a cylinder. The frontal plane vector is retained, and its origin is located at the center of the cylinder.

4 The transitional or null deflection is identified in the unipolar precordial leads. The null pathway must pass through this electrode position.

5 An ellipse is drawn around the null-plane diameter.

6 The mean vector is then titled anteriorly or posteriorly, as the case may be, depending upon where the null pathway passes through the electrode position at which the transitional deflection is recorded.

7 The spatial direction of the vector can be shown by drawing the arrowhead of the vector three-dimensionally.

THE VENTRICULAR GRADIENT

The area enclosed by the QRS complex ($\hat{A}_{QRS}$) represents the electrical forces developed during ventricular depolarization. The area enclosed by the S-T segment and T wave ($\hat{A}_T$) represents the electrical forces developed during ventricular repolarization. If repolarization were simply the reverse of depolarization and occurred at the same rate, then the area of the S-T segment and T wave would equal the area of the QRS complex but would be opposite in sign. However, since there are local variations in the duration of the excited state of the normal heart, $\hat{A}_T$ does not equal $\hat{A}_{QRS}$, and the directions of both the QRS complex and T wave are similar. The relationship between the area of the QRS complex, on the one hand, and the area of the S-T segment and T wave, on the other, can be expressed in terms of the *ventricular gradient* ($\hat{A}_{QRST}$, or G). If a vector representing the area of the QRS ($\hat{A}_{QRS}$) is added by the parallelogram law to a vector representing the area of the S-T segment and T wave ($\hat{A}_T$), a mean vector is obtained ($\hat{A}_{QRST}$). This is the ventricular gradient. The normal heart has a ventricular gradient, and its normal range in the standard limb leads has been determined.

It is obvious that alterations in the T wave occurring without concomitant alteration of the QRS complex will change the ventricular gradient. It would seem, therefore, that the determination of the ventricular gradient would be helpful in distinguishing between primary and secondary T wave changes, especially when the former are superimposed upon the latter.   In actual practice, however, determination of the ventricular gradient is a tedious, time-consuming procedure and subject to inaccuracies.   Determination of the ventricular gradient is not a practical everyday tool in electrocardiography.

The mean length of the ventricular gradient in the frontal plane is approximately 46μV-s.   The normal ventricular gradient in the frontal plane does not deviate by more than 30° in either direction from the mean electrical axis.   When this value is exceeded, the ventricular gradient is abnormal.

THE NORMAL 12-LEAD ELECTROCARDIOGRAM[1]

Standard and Unipolar Extremity Leads

The normal values for the various complexes and intervals have been described in the preceding sections.   No attempt will be made to describe the various QRS patterns seen in the limb leads, since there is considerable normal variation.   The findings in each of the extremity leads depend on the extent to which each lead axis taps the cardiac vector.   When the mean QRS vector is horizontal, leads I, II, and aVL will show predominantly positive QRS deflections and leads aVF and III will show predominantly negative QRS deflections.   When the mean QRS vector is vertical, leads I and aVL will exhibit QRS deflections that are largely downward and leads II, III, and aVF will show QRS deflections that are upright.   As long as the mean electrical axis is within the normal range, lead aVR will always show predominantly negative deflections in the absence of disease.

Precordial Leads

The general configuration of the various complexes and their normal values have already been described in the sections dealing with the P wave, QRS complex, S-T segment, and T wave. However, further amplification is necessary with respect to the QRS complexes.

Right-sided precordial leads normally show small R waves followed by broad, deep S waves. The left-sided precordial leads usually show small Q waves followed by tall R waves and sometimes final small S waves. In the midprecordial leads, the R and S waves are usually about equal in size. Notching and slurring are common in these leads.

The ratio of R to S waves in the precordial electrocardiogram normally increases between any two consecutive leads to the right of the transition

---

[1] Figures 5-31 to 5-35 are examples of normal electrocardiograms showing varying degrees of axis deviation.

zone.   A retrogression of this ratio between any pair of pretransition leads may be an early sign of right ventricular enlargement.

A shallow S wave in lead V_1 associated with a small R wave in this lead and relative deep S waves in leads V_2 and V_3, especially in the presence of right axis deviation, is also suggestive of right ventricular enlargement.   However, a small S wave in lead V_1 is sometimes a normal variant.

The R wave increases in amplitude progressively from lead V_1 to lead V_4 or V_5 and then becomes smaller.   A QS deflection may occur normally in leads V_{3R} and V_1 and rarely in lead V_2 as well (Fig. 5-26).   It is not a normal finding in any other precordial lead.   In lead V_2 the R wave is usually taller than in lead V_1, but it may be the same size without necessarily indicating abnormality.   Once an R wave is present in a right precordial lead, it should not decrease in size or disappear in a lead immediately to the left.   Failure of this sequential increase in R wave amplitudes to occur in the precordial leads is often referred to as *poor progression of the R waves*.

Poor R wave progression (*assuming correct electrode placement*) is considered to be present if the absolute magnitude of the R wave is 3.0 mm or less in lead V_3 and the R wave in lead V_2 is equal to or smaller than the R wave in lead V_3.   Poor R wave progression is found in about 8 to 10 percent of routine tracings in hospitalized patients.   It is a common occurrence in normal young adults, particularly women.   However, it may be an expression of abnormality.   It may be found in anterior myocardial infarction, left ventricular enlargement, chronic pulmonary disease, right ventricular enlargement (particularly cor pulmonale), left bundle branch block, left anterior fascicular block, diffuse or localized myocardial disease, and idiopathic hypertrophic subaortic stenosis.

Reversed R wave progression is the presence of decreasing R wave amplitude in consecutive right precordial leads.   It is somewhat more

Fig. 5-26   QS deflection in leads V_1 and V_2 in a normal subject without heart disease.

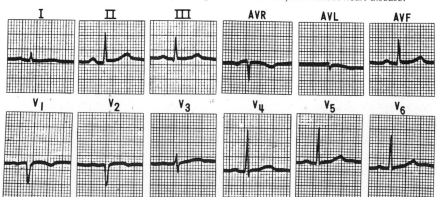

specific for anterior myocardial infarction than the other disorders listed in the preceding paragraph.

Poor R wave progression and its differential diagnosis is discussed in greater detail in Chap. 21.

The presence of qR, qrS, QR, or Qr patterns in the right-sided precordial leads is always abnormal. Such patterns may be indicative of right ventricular enlargement; acute cor pulmonale, myocardial infarction, myocardial infarction with right bundle branch block, left anterior fascicular block, or ventricular preexcitation.

Abnormal Q waves in the left precordial leads are usually diagnostic of myocardial infarction but may be the result of other conditions simulating myocardial infarction.

When QS or QR patterns occur in the midprecordial leads, differentiation between anterior infarction and other causes for these deflections may sometimes be accomplished by taking leads V_3 and V_4 at the level of the ensiform cartilage. In such low V leads, infarctional QS complexes generally persist unchanged, but noninfarctional QS complexes are often replaced by rS deflections. In doubtful cases, vectorcardiography may be decisive in establishing the correct diagnosis.

An R' wave may occur normally in the right precordial leads (Figs. 5-27, 5-28), particularly in children and young adults. The normal R' has been attributed to late depolarization of the cristal supraventricularis (hence the name *crista pattern*), but it may also be the result of normal late activation of the posterobasal region of the left ventricle and the interventricular septum and the projection of these forces on the lead V_1 axis.

When the RSR' pattern is normal, the QRS duration is normal, the primary R wave in leads V_{3R} and V_1 is 8 mm or less, the secondary R wave is 6 mm or less, and the R'/S ratio is less than 1.0 in any lead from the right side of the precordium. Normal R' waves tend to disappear when additional lower right chest leads are taken (Fig. 5-28). However, abnormal R' waves persist unchanged or are replaced by abnormally large, notched R waves in these additional leads (Figs. 5-27, 5-29). Moreover, when an RSR' pattern occurs in lead V_1 or V_2, or both, its absence in lead V_{3R} (Fig. 5-28) or the presence of an R' wave in lead V_2 that is 1.0 mm taller than the R' wave in lead V_{3R} suggests that the secondary R wave represents a normal variant.

RSR' patterns in lead V_1 with a normal QRS interval may also be found in the $S_1S_2S_3$ syndrome, right ventricular enlargement, left anterior hemiblock, strictly posterior myocardial infarction, acute cor pulmonale, emphysema with or without cor pulmonale, and incomplete right bundle branch block.

An RSR' complex in lead V_1 with a prolonged QRS duration is found in right bundle branch block, right bundle branch block with right ventricular both, may be normal variants but more often are indicative of right ventricular enlargement, strictly posterior myocardial infarction, right bundle branch

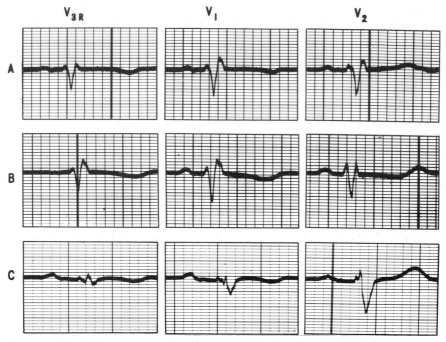

Fig. 5-27 The RSR' complex in the right precordial leads, showing the similarity between complexes produced by normal variants and heart disease: (A) normal variant; (B) congenital heart disease; (C) congenital heart disease. There is a small R' wave, but the R'/S ratio is greater than 1.0 which indicates that this RSR' complex is abnormal. See text. (From F. A. Tapia and W. L. Proudfit, Secondary R Waves in Right Precordial Leads in Normal Persons and in Patients with Cardiac Disease, Circulation, 21: 28, 1960. Used by permission of the American Heart Association, Inc.)

block, or ventricular preexcitation. Less frequent causes of prominent R waves in the right precordial leads include idiopathic hypertrophic subaortic stenosis, Duchenne muscular dystrophy, congenital dextroversion, and rare cases of chronic constrictive pericarditis.

Marked notching or slurring of the QRS complexes in the right or left precordial leads is usually indicative of a ventricular conduction defect, ventricular hypertrophy, or myocardial fibrosis. However, slight notching or slurring may be normal in these leads. In the midprecordial leads, notching or slurring of the transitional complexes is normal.

THE ELECTRICAL POSITION OF THE HEART

In the unipolar method of electrocardiographic interpretation, the electrical position of the heart is regarded as the result of its rotation about three axes: anteroposterior, longitudinal, and transverse. The anteroposterior axis runs horizontally through the center of the heart from front to back. The longitudinal axis runs through the center of the heart from apex to base. The transverse axis runs through the center of the heart from side to side.

The relative horizontal or vertical position of the heart is determined primarily by rotation about the longitudinal axis and, to a lesser extent, by its rotation about the anteroposterior axis.   Rotation about the antero-posterior axis causes the apex of the heart to point either horizontally or vertically.   Rotation about the longitudinal axis is determined by viewing the heart from an apex-to-base direction along the extension of the longitudinal axis.   When the heart is rotated clockwise on the longitudinal axis, the right ventricle comes to lie more superiorly and the left ventricle more inferiorly.   When there is counterclockwise rotation, the left ventricle moves superiorly and the right ventricle inferiorly.   Backward or forward rotation of the apex is governed by rotation about the transverse axis.

According to the semidirect lead hypothesis, the unipolar extremity leads record the potential variations of those surfaces of the heart which they face.   Because the base of the heart is fixed anatomically, the right arm lead (aVR), regardless of the position of the heart, almost always faces its cavities and therefore registers intracavitary potentials.   The left arm and

Fig. 5-28   Disappearance of R' waves in the lower precordial leads.   The R' wave is absent in lead V$_{3R}$.   The voltage of the R and R' waves is normal.   From a normal subject.   See text. *(From F. A. Tapia and W. L. Proudfit, Secondary R Waves in Right Precordial Leads in Normal Persons and in Patients with Cardiac Disease, Circulation, 21: 28, 1960.   Used by permission of the American Heart Association, Inc.)*

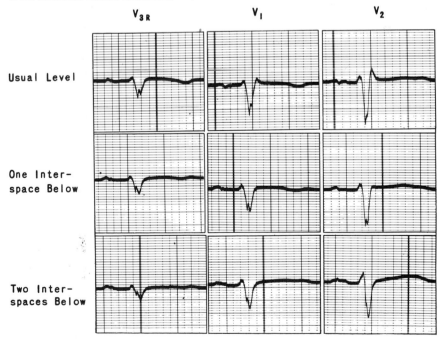

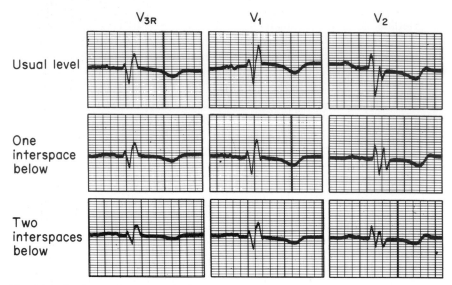

Fig. 5-29   Persistent R' waves in the lower precordial leads with an R' wave of 8 mm and an R'/S ratio greater than 1.0 in lead V_1.   From a patient with an interatrial septal defect. See text.   *(From F. A. Tapia and W. L. Proudfit, Secondary R Waves in Right Precordial Leads in Normal Persons and in Patients with Cardiac Disease, Circulation, 21: 28, 1960.   Used by permission of the American Heart Association, Inc.)*

left leg leads (aVL and aVF, respectively) usually face either the right ventricular epicardium or the left ventricular epicardium, or both, depending on the position of the heart.   The left arm lead may face the cavities when the heart is vertical.   The potentials recorded by these leads will therefore depend on the surface of the heart to which they are related.   In contrast, the precordial leads are not very much affected by the position of the heart. According to the unipolar method of interpretation, in most normal hearts the right-sided precordial leads register the potential variations of the epicardial surface of the right ventricle, the left-sided precordial leads register those of the corresponding surface of the left ventricle, and the midprecordial leads register the potential variations of the transitional zone between the two.

Wilson defined five electrical positions of the heart by correlating the findings in the unipolar extremity leads with those in the precordial leads. These positions are the vertical, semivertical, intermediate, semihorizontal, and horizontal.   They are illustrated in Fig. 5-30.   Representative examples are shown in Figs. 5-31 to 5-35.

Studies have demonstrated no significant correlation between the electrical and anatomic axes in the frontal plane, between the electrical axis and rotation of the heart about its longitudinal axis, or between the location of the interventricular septum and the transition zone of the precordial leads.   The electrical variations are greater than can possibly

PRECORDIAL LEADS	VERTICAL	SEMIVERTICAL	INTERMEDIATE	SEMIHORIZONTAL	HORIZONTAL
V1 & V2	aVL	aVL	aVL	aVL	aVL
V5 & V6	aVF	aVF	aVF	aVF	aVF
	AXIS ABOUT +90°	AXIS ABOUT +60°	AXIS ABOUT +30°	AXIS ABOUT 0°	AXIS ABOUT -30°

Fig. 5-30   The electrical position of the heart.   *Vertical position:* The ventricular complexes of lead aVL resemble those of leads V_1 and V_2; the ventricular complexes of lead aVF resemble those of leads V_5 and V_6.   *Semivertical position:* The ventricular complexes of lead aVF resemble those of leads V_5 and V_6; the ventricular complexes of lead aVL are small.   *Intermediate position:* The ventricular complexes of leads aVL and aVF are similar in size and form and like those of leads V_5 and V_6.   *Semihorizontal position:* The ventricular complexes of lead aVL resemble those of leads V_5 and V_6; the ventricular complexes of lead aVF are small.   *Horizontal position:* The ventricular complexes of lead aVL resemble those of leads V_5 and V_6; the ventricular complexes of lead aVF resemble those of leads V_1 and V_2.   The approximate electrical axis to which each of these positions corresponds is shown in the diagram.

be explained by known rotations of the heart about any anatomic axis. The electrical positions should be abandoned in favor of the description of the mean spatial vector of the QRS complex (Fig. 5-36) as indicated in the section on the electrical axis.

SPECIAL LEADS

Esophageal Leads (Fig. 5-37)

Esophageal leads are sometimes useful in the diagnosis of arrhythmias, because large atrial deflections may be recorded in these leads.

Fig. 5-31   A normal electrocardiogram in which the electrical position of the heart is vertical. The electrical axis is about +90°.

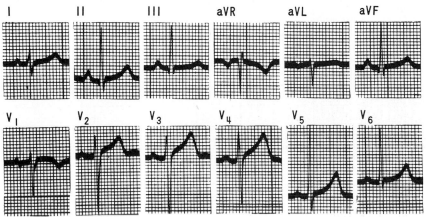

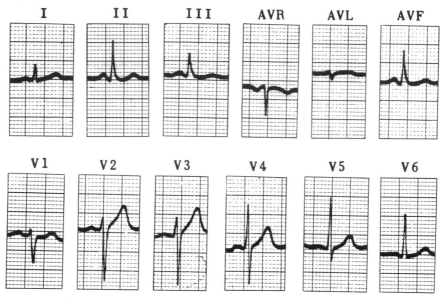

Fig. 5-32 A normal electrocardiogram in which the electrical position of the heart is semivertical. The electrical axis is about +60°.

Fig. 5-33 A normal electrocardiogram in which the electrical position of the heart is intermediate. The electrical axis is about +30°.

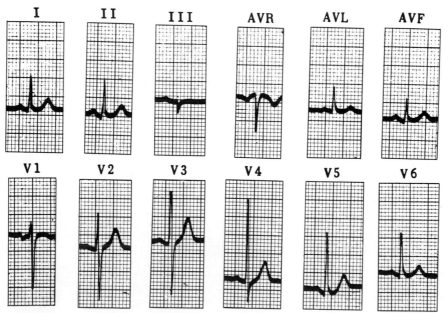

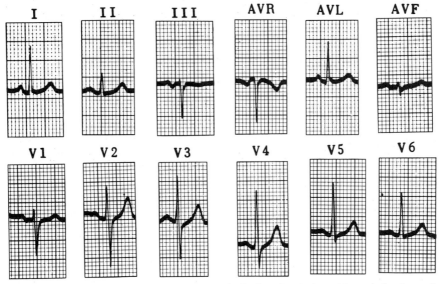

Fig. 5-34 A normal electrocardiogram in which the electrical position of the heart is semihorizontal. The electrical axis is about 0°.

Leads at the ventricular level, ordinarily located at a distance of 50 to 60 cm from the nares, show upright P waves and QRS complexes resembling those found in the left precordial leads, although S waves are frequently absent.

Leads at the atrial level, ordinarily located at a distance between 25 and 40 cm from the nares, show diphasic P waves with an initial positive component and a final negative component and QR ventricular complexes with inverted T waves

Fig. 5-35 A normal electrocardiogram from an elderly woman, in which the electrical position of the heart is horizontal. The electrical axis is about −30°.

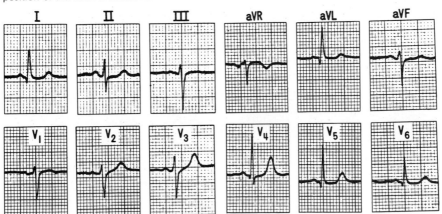

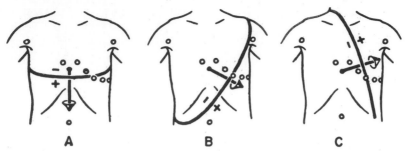

A   **B**   **C**

Fig. 5-36 The mean QRS vector for the vertical (*A*), intermediate (*B*), and horizontal (*C*) position of the heart. The distribution of positivity and negativity on the chest with these three directions of the mean QRS vector is shown. The resemblances between the QRS deflections in the unipolar extremity leads and the precordial leads, used by Wilson to determine the electrical positon of the heart, are seen to depend on whether these leads are located in areas of relative positivity or negativity. Thus, in the intermediate position, because leads aVL, aVF, V_5, and V_6 all lie in the area of relative positivity, their QRS complex must perforce resemble one another. *(From R. P. Grant, "Clinical Electrocardiography," © 1957 by McGraw-Hill, Inc., New York. Used with permission of McGraw-Hill Book Company.)*

Esophageal leads are designated by the letter E. The distance of the electrode tip from the nares is measured in centimeters expressed as a subscript, for example, E_{50}.

Atrial Leads (Fig. 5-38)

Right atrial leads, like esophageal leads, show atrial activity more clearly than conventional leads. They are particularly useful when atrial activity is not recognizable in the conventional electrocardiogram or when the

Fig. 5-37 The normal unipolar esophageal leads. Redrawn from an actual electrocardiogram.

NORMAL ESOPHAGEAL LEADS

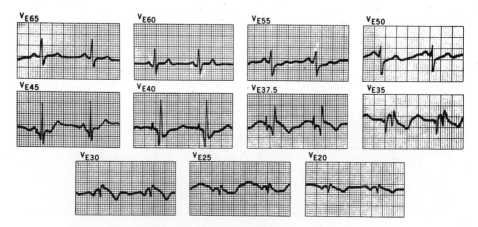

Intracardiac Electrocardiogram
With Platinum Electrode Wire

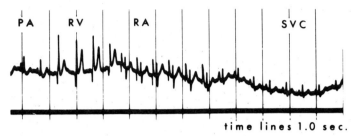

time lines 1.0 sec.

Fig. 5-38 Intracardiac electrocardiogram with platinum electrode wire, showing changes in configuration as the electrode is passed through the heart. Note the increase in size of the P wave as the electrode passes from the superior vena cava SVC into the right atrium RA. With the passage of the catheter into the right ventricle RV, the P waves become very small while the QRS complexes increase in size. In the pulmonary artery PA, the complexes are similar to those in the superior vena cava. In patients with large right atria, the complexes in the pulmonary artery may be similar to those in the right atrium. *(Courtesy of Dr. John H. K. Vogel.)*

atrial mechanism is in doubt. Atrial leads are easily obtained by using the technique described by Vogel and his associates, as well as by other methods (Dreifus and Najami). Atrial leads are preferable to esophageal leads because of their simplicity and because discomfort to the patient is minimized. Leads located high in the right atrium show negative P waves; those in the midatrium, diphasic P waves; and low atrial leads, upright P waves. Atrial leads are useful in the differential diagnosis of supraventricular arrhythmias and in determining the atrial mechanism in AV junctional, ventricular, or other complex arrhythmias.

Leads for Monitoring

A simple transsternal lead is often used for determining atrial activity. This lead is derived by recording lead I with the right arm electrode on the manubrium and the left arm electrode at the right sternal border in the fourth or fifth intercostal space. The lead is correctly placed when the QRS complex is diphasic and atrial activity is clearly defined. Minor adjustments in electrode placement may be necessary to secure the desired result.

Marriott and Fogg have shown that a modified V_1 lead (MCL_1) is superior to other transsternal leads for monitoring disturbances of rhythm and conduction. To obtain this lead, the positive electrode is placed at the usual V_1 position and the negative electrode near the left shoulder.

The ground electrode is positioned near the right shoulder.   The hookup is illustrated in Fig. 5-39.   The diagnostic advantages of this lead system (aside from leaving the precordium free for examination or for the application of paddles for cardioversion) are as follows (Figs. 5-40 to 5-42): (1) It permits distinction between right and left ventricular ectopic beats.   (2) It is useful in differentiating between right and left bundle branch block.   (3) It is of help in the recognition of the RBB-Q_{V1} pattern which is sometimes a precursor of complete AV block.   (4) It is helpful in differentiating between the right bundle branch type of aberrant ventricular conduction and left ventricular ectopy.   (5) The P waves are usually well-defined.   (6) Finally, it is easy to switch to a modified lead III (MCL_3) to determine P wave polarity or to a modified CL_6 (MCL_6) as an aid in the differential diagnosis between aberrant ventricular conduction and ventricular ectopic activity.

It is worth emphasizing that no single lead is always adequate for monitoring.   Whenever warranted by circumstances, a standard 12-lead electrocardiogram should be recorded, preferably with a multichannel machine.

Holter Monitoring

Holter monitoring has become a widely used and helpful aid in cardiac diagnosis.   It is of great value in the documentation of arrhythmias and

Fig. 5-39   The hookup for constant monitoring with MCL_1 (unbroken lines) with alternative temporary placement of the positive electrode to obtain MCL_6 and M_3 (dashed lines).   (*From H. J. L. Marriott and E. Fogg, Constant Monitoring for Cardiac Dysrhythmias and Blocks, Mod. Concepts Cardiovasc. Dis., 39: 103, 1970.   Used by permission of the American Heart Association, Inc.*)

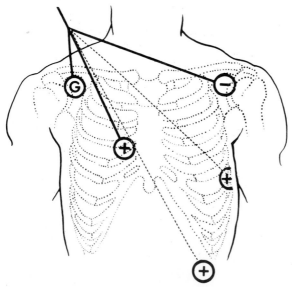

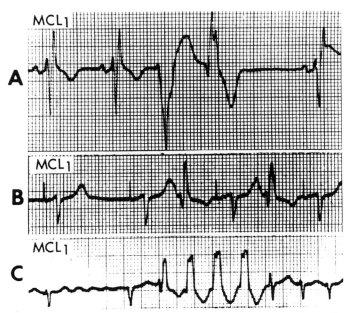

Fig. 5-40 Typical QRS configuration in lead MCL₁. (A) Normal sinus beats with right bundle branch block (RBBB) interrupted by successive right ventricular (rS) and left ventricular (qRR') premature systoles. (B) Atrial pacing with atrial premature beats with RBBB type of aberration. The P' waves are superimposed on the T waves of the paced beats. (C) Atrial fibrillation with a run of anomalous beats. The first beat shows an rsR' pattern, indicating that the run consists of aberrant and not ventricular ectopic beats. (From H. J. L. Marriott and E. Fogg, Constant Monitoring for Cardiac Dysrhythmias and Blocks, Mod. Concepts Cardiovasc. Dis., 39: 103, 1970. Used by permission of the American Heart Association, Inc.)

conduction disturbances. Correlating the patient's symptoms and activity with the electrocardiographic findings may provide the explanation for such symptoms as dizziness, syncope, and palpitation. Holter monitoring may establish electrocardiographic confirmation of classical angina, atypical angina, and Prinzmetal's angina. It has proven to be of value in the evaluation of drug therapy and in the assessment of pacemaker function.

HIS BUNDLE ELECTROGRAMS

The transmission of impulses through the AV node, the bundle of His, the bundle branches, their subdivisions, and the Purkinje network is not recorded in surface electrocardiographic leads. Until recent years, the nature of impulse transmission through the conduction system could only be surmised from the deductions of many notable investigators

His bundle recordings have not only confirmed many of the conclusions reached by earlier investigators but have added much new information about impulse formation and conduction in the heart. The current upsurge

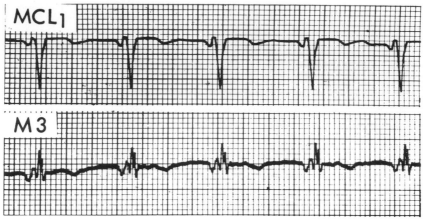

Fig. 5-41   The M_3 lead confirms the retrograde polarity of the P waves in an AV junctional rhythm when MCL_1 is not diagnostic. *(From H. J. L. Marriott and E. Fogg, Constant Monitoring for Cardiac Dysrhythmias and Blocks, Mod. Concepts Cardiovasc. Dis., 39: 103, 1970. Used by permission of the American Heart Association, Inc.)*

of interest in the study of extracellular recordings of the human AV conduction system received its impetus from animal studies conducted by Alanis and his coworkers in 1958.   The technique for recording the His bundle electrogram in humans was devised by Scherlag and his associates in 1969.

Value of His Bundle Recordings

His bundle recordings have proved to be invaluable investigative and research tools for the following purposes:

1   Study of the electrophysiology of the heart
2   Learning the effects of drugs on the AV conduction system
3   Precise localization of the site of AV conduction defects in all degrees of AV block
4   Evaluation of unilateral and bilateral bundle branch block, bifascicular block, and trifascicular block
5   Investigation of the mechanism of cardiac arrhythmias
6   Diagnosis and differential diagnosis of arrhythmias
a   Differentiation between ventricular and supraventricular arrhythmias (e.g., ventricular tachycardia vs. supraventricular tachycardia with abnormal QRS complexes, ventricular ectopy vs. aberrant ventricular conduction)
b   Elucidation of arrhythmias involving the AV junction
c   Evaluation of complex arrhythmias such as concealed conduction, supernormal conduction, pseudo AV block secondary to nonpropagated

His bundle depolarizations, concealed reentry in the AV node, and AV nodal entrance block

d   Study of the mechanism involved in ventricular preexcitation (W-P-W syndrome) and the Lown-Ganong-Levine syndrome (short P-R interval, normal QRS complex, and paroxysmal tachycardia)

e   In conjunction with other techniques, such as atrial pacing and pharmacologic interventions, to obtain information concerning the prognosis and management of AV conduction defects and dysrhythmias

Obviously the final word has not been said about the ultimate place

Fig. 5-42   (A) The second and fourth beats in both strips show RBBB type of aberration (rSR′, in MCL₁, qRs in MCL₆).   The sixth beat in both strips is characteristic of left ventricular ectopy (qR in MCL₁, rS in MCL₆).   (B) The upper strip (MCL₁) shows a tachycardia at a rate of 200, consistent with either a supraventricular tachycardia with aberrant ventricular conduction or left ventricular tachycardia.   The qRs contour in lead MCL₆ favors aberrancy.   This is confirmed in the bottom strip of MCL₁, where the beat initiating each run of abnormal beats is triphasic (rsR′).   *(From H. J. L. Marriott and E. Fogg, Constant Monitoring for Cardiac Dysrhythmias and Blocks, Mod. Concepts Cardiovasc. Dis., 39: 103, 1970.   Used by permission of the American Heart Association, Inc.)*

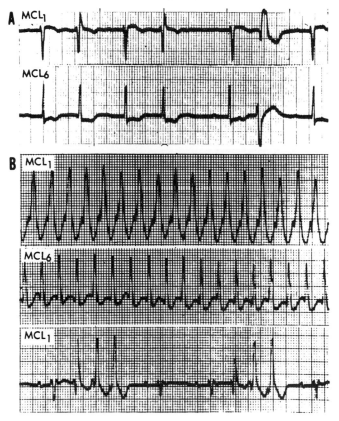

of the His bundle electrogram. Additional correlations between His bundle recordings and the clinical and pathologic findings are necessary to define more precisely the role of this technique in clinical medicine.

Technique

The electrode catheter technique for recording the electrical activity of the ventricular conduction system consists of the percutaneous introduction of a bipolar, tripolar, or multipolar electrode catheter into a femoral vein and its advancement fluoroscopically across the tricuspid value into the right ventricular cavity. The catheter is then withdrawn across the tricuspid valve until a sharp biphasic or triphasic spike appears between the atrial and ventricular electrogram. This spike is the His deflection. Usually surface leads are recorded simultaneously (e.g., I, II, III, V_1).

Definition of Terms and Normal Values

By means of simultaneous recordings of the His bundle electrogram and appropriate surface leads, it is possible to subdivide the P-R interval into several segments or components (Fig. 5-43).

The *P wave* represents atrial activity as recorded in the surface electrocardiogram.

The *A wave* is the low right atrial electrogram recorded with the His bundle catheter.

The *H* or *BH* (bundle of His) *potential* is a biphasic or triphasic wave, 15 to 20 ms in duration, located between the atrial and ventricular electrograms. In the presence of sinus rhythms at a constant rate, it is found at the same time (± 3 ms) in the P-R interval during successive cardiac cycles.

The *RB* (right bundle) *potential* is a fast biphasic or triphasic wave, 10 to 12 ms in duration, between the H potential and the onset of ventricular depolarization.

The *LB* (left bundle) *potential*, demonstrable only in left ventricular recordings, is a rapid biphasic or triphasic deflection, ranging from 10 to 15 ms in duration, between the H potential and the onset of ventricular activation. The LB potential usually precedes the RB potential by 3 ms or less in normal subjects.

The *V wave or complex* is the ventricular electrogram recorded from the vicinity of the AV junction.

The *P-H time* is the interval from the onset of the P wave to the first rapid deflection of the H potential. The normal P-H time is 119 $\pm$ 38 ms. The P-H interval reflects the sum of intraatrial and AV nodal conduction time. During atrial pacing, the P-H time is measured from the pacing impulse to the H deflection.

The *P-A time* is the interval from the onset of the P wave to the first

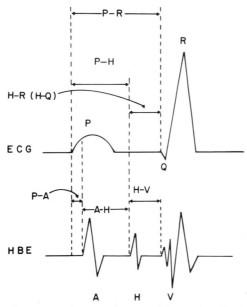

Fig. 5-43   Schematic diagram of the His bundle electrogram (HBE) and its relationship to the electrocardiogram (ECG).   Described in text.   The code is as follows: *P* = P wave; *P-R* = P-R interval; *P-H* = P-H interval; *A-H* = A-H interval; *H-V* = H-V interval; *A* − atrial electrogram; *H* = His bundle potential; *V* = ventricular electrogram.

high-frequency component of the low right atrial electrogram. It represents intraatrial conduction time, and its normal value is 27 ± 18 ms.   During atrial pacing, the P-A time is measured from the pacing impulse to the onset of the A wave.

The *A-H time* is the interval from the onset of the A wave to the H deflection.   It represents primarily AV nodal conduction time but probably also includes conduction in the proximal portion of the bundle of His.   Its normal value is 92 ± 38 ms.

The *H-V time* is the interval between the His deflection and the onset of ventricular activation in any lead.   It represents primarily conduction in the bundle branches and the Purkinje network, but probably also includes conduction in the distal portion of the bundle of His.   The normal H-V time is 43 ± 12 ms.

Effect of Atrial Pacing

In humans, spontaneous increases in heart rate induced by physiologic stimuli such as exercise, or by pharmacologic means such as sympatho-mimetic drugs or atropine, are associated with a decrease in the P-R interval.   The enhancement of conduction is attributed to neurohumoral effects.   However, when the heart rate is increased by atrial pacing, there is a progressive increase in the AV conduction time, indicating that neurohumoral mechanisms are not affected.

His bundle electrograms recorded in normal subjects during right atrial pacing have shown that as the heart rate is increased, there is progressive prolongation of the P-H and A-H intervals without any change in the H-V time. The site of conduction delay is thus within the AV node. At the more rapid-paced atrial rates, the Wenckebach phenomenon and more advanced degrees of block may occur. In these instances also, the delay in AV conduction is located proximal to the bundle of His.

The usefulness of His bundle recordings in the evaluation of suspected conduction system disease is enhanced by the use of atrial pacing at varied rates. Atrial pacing stresses the conduction system, often allowing demonstration of block not apparent during normal sinus rhythm. The development of second-degree block proximal to the His bundle at paced rates below 130 per minute probably reflects AV nodal dysfunction. The occurrence of second-degree block distal to the bundle of His at any heart rate (up to 200 per minute) probably (but not invariably) represents intraventricular conduction disease.

Timed premature atrial depolarization during His bundle recording allows measurement of the refractory periods of the AV conduction system. A wide range of normal values for refractory periods has been reported in the literature. The data published by Josephson and Seides may be regarded as representative: effective refractory period (ERF) of the atrium, 170 to 300 ms; ERF of the AV node, 330 to 525 ms; ERF of the His-Purkinje system, 330 to 450 ms; and ERF of the ventricles, 170 to 290 ms.

Clinical Applications

The clinical applications of His bundle recordings in the study of drug effects, atrial fibrillation or flutter, aberrant ventricular conduction, AV junctional rhythms, differential diagnosis of ventricular and supraventricular arrhythmias, AV block, bundle branch block, bifascicular block, trifascicular block, ventricular preexcitation, and complex arrhythmias will be considered under the appropriate headings later in the text.

REFERENCES

Criteria Committee of the New York Heart Association: "Diseases of the Heart and Blood Vessels: Nomenclature and Criteria for Diagnosis," 6th ed. and 7th ed., Little, Brown, Boston, 1964 and 1973.
Barker, J. M.: "The Unipolar Electrocardiogram: A Clinical Interpretation," Appleton-Century-Crofts, New York, 1952.
Damato, A. N., and S. H. Lau: Clinical Value of the Electrogram of the Conducting System, *Progr. Cardiovasc. Dis.*, 13: 119, 1970.

Daoud, F. S., B. Surawicz, and L. S. Gettes: Effect of Isuprel on the Abnormal T Wave, *Am. J. Cardiol.*, 30:810, 1972.

Denes, P., and K. M. Rosen: His Bundle Electrograms: Clinical Applications, *Cardiovasc. Clin.*, 6 (1): 68, 1974.

DePasquale, N. P., and G. E. Burch: Analysis of the RSR' Complex in Lead V_1, *Circulation*, 28: 362, 1963.

Dreifus, L. S., and M. Najami: Right Atrial Electrocardiography, *J.A.M.A.*, 195: 678, 1965.

Evans, W.: The Effect of Deep Breathing on Lead III of the Electrocardiogram, *Brit. Heart J.*, 13: 457, 1951.

Forfang, K., and J. Eriksen: Significance of P Wave Terminal Force in Presumably Healthy Middle-Aged Men, *Am. Heart J.*, 96: 739, 1978.

Gerson, M. C., and G. J. Insenmeyer, III: Diagnostic Significance of U Wave Inversion, *Practical Cardiology*, 8: 132, 1982.

Grant, R. P.: "Clinical Electrocardiography: The Spatial Vector Approach," McGraw-Hill, New York, 1957.

———: The Relationship between the Anatomic Position of the Heart and the Electrocardiogram: A Criticism of "Unipolar" Electrocardiography, *Circulation*, 7: 890, 1953.

Guntheroth, W. G., C. O. Ovenfors, and D. Ikkos: Relationship between the Electrocardiogram and the Position of the Heart as Determined by Biplane Angiocardiography, *Circulation*, 23: 69, 1961.

Helfant, R. H., and B. J. Scherlag: "His Bundle Electrocardiography," Medcom Press, New York, 1974.

Jacobson, D., and V. Schrire: Giant T Wave Inversion, *Brit. Heart J.*, 28: 768, 1966.

James, T. N.: QT Prolongation and Sudden Death, *Mod. Concepts Cardiovasc. Dis.*, 38: 35, 1969.

Josephson, M. E., and S. F. Seides: "Clinical Cardiac Electrophysiology," Lea & Febiger, Philadelphia, 1979.

Kishida, H., Cole, J. S., and B. Surawicz: Negative U Wave: A Highly Specific but Poorly Understood Sign of Heart Disease, *Am. J. Cardiol.*, 49: 2030, 1982.

Kossman, C. E.: The Normal Electrocardiogram, *Circulation*, 8: 920, 1953.

Laiken, S., N. Laiken, R. A. O'Rourke, and J. S. Karliner: A Rapid Method for Frontal Plane Axis Determination Scalar Electrocardiograms, *Am. Heart J.*, 85: 620, 1973

Lepeschkin, E.: "Modern Electrocardiography: The P-Q-R-S-T-U Complex," vol. 1, Williams & Wilkins, Baltimore, 1951.

———: The U Wave of the Electrocardiogram, *Mod. Concepts Cardiovasc. Dis.*, 38: 39, 1969.

———: Physiologic Basis of the U Wave, in R. C. Schlant and J. W. Hurst (eds.), "Advances in Electrocardiography," Grune & Stratton, New York, 1972.

Marriott, H. J. L. and E. Fogg: Constant Monitoring for Cardiac Dysrhythmias and Blocks, *Mod. Concepts Cardiovasc. Dis.*, 39: 103, 1970.

Narula, O. S. (ed.): "His Bundle Electrocardiography and Clinical Electrophysiology," F. A. Davis, Philadelphia, 1975.

Okamoto, N., E. Simonson, and H. Blackburn: The $T-V_1 > T-V_6$ Pattern for Electrocardiographic Diagnosis of Left Ventricular Hypertrophy and Ischemia, *Circulation*, 31: 719, 1965.

————, K. Kaneko, E. Simonson, and O. H. Schmitt: Reliability of Individual Frontal Plane Axis Determination, *Circulation*, 44: 213, 1971.

Pinto I. J., N. C. Nanda, A. K. Biswas, and V. G. Parulkar: Tall Upright T Waves in the Precordial Leads, *Circulation*, 36: 708, 1967.

Rosen, K. M.: Catheter Recording of His Bundle Electrograms, *Mod. Concepts Cardiovasc. Dis.*, 42: 23, 1973.

Shettigar, U. R., H. N. Hultgren, J. F. Pfeifer, and M. J. Lipton: Diagnostic Value of Q Waves in Inferior Myocardial Infarction, *Am. Heart J.*, 88: 170, 1974.

Short, D. and J. Weir: Significance of Asymmetrically Inverted T Wave, *Br. Heart J.*, 49: 564, 1983.

Simonson, E.: "Differentiation between Normal and Abnormal in Electrocardiography," Mosby, St. Louis, 1961.

Spodick, D. H.: Differential Characteristics of the Electrocardiogram in Early Repolarization and Acute Pericarditis, *New Engl. J. Med.*, 295: 523, 1976.

Surawicz, B., R. G. Van Horne, J. R. Urbach, and S. Bellet: QS- and QR-Pattern in Leads V_3 and V_4 in Absence of Myocardial Infarction: Electrocardiographic and Vectorcardiographic Study, *Circulation*, 12: 391, 1955.

Tapia, F. A., and W. I. Proudfit: Secondary R Waves in Right Precordial Leads in Normal Persons and in Persons with Cardiac Disease, *Circulation*, 21: 28, 1960.

Tranchesi, J., V. Adelardi, and J. M. de Oliveira: Atrial Repolarization: Its Importance in Clinical Electrocardiography, *Circulation*, 22: 635, 1960.

Vincent, G. M., J. A. Abildskov, and M. J. Burgess: Q-T Interval Syndromes, *Progr. Cardiovasc. Dis.*, 16: 523, 1974.

Vogel, J. H. K., H. Averill, K. Tabari, and S. G. Blount, Jr.: Detection of Intracardiac Shunts with the Platinum Electrode, Using a Simplified Percutaneous Approach. *Am. Heart J.*, 67: 610, 1964.

Wasserburger, R. H., W. J. Alt, and C. J. Lloyd: The Normal RS-T Elevation Variant, *Am. J. Cardiol.*, 8: 184, 1961.

Watanabe, Y.: Purkinje Repolarization as a Possible Cause of the U Wave in the Electrocardiogram, *Circulation*, 51: 1030, 1975.

Weisbart, M. H., and E. Simonson: The Diagnostic Accuracy of Q3 and Related Electrocardiographic Items for the Detection of Patients with Posterior Wall Myocardial Infarction, *Am. Heart J.*, 50: 62, 1955.

Wilson, F. N., F. D. Johnston, F. F. Rosenbaum, H. Erlanger, C. E. Kossman, H. Hecht, N. Costen, R. Menzes de Olivera, R. Scarsi, and P. S. Barker: Precordial Electrocardiogram, *Am. Heart J.*, 27: 19, 1944.

————, ————, ————, and P. S. Barker: On Einthoven's Triangle, the Theory of Unipolar Electrocardiographic Leads, and the Interpretation of the Precordial Electrocardiogram, *Am. Heart J.*, 32: 277, 1946.

Winsor, T. (ed.): "Electrocardiographic Test Book," American Heart Association, New York, 1956.

Zema, M. J., and P. Kligfield: ECG Poor R-Wave Progression—Review and Synthesis, *Arch. Intern. Med.*, 142: 1145, 1982.

CHAPTER 6

THE NORMAL VECTORCARDIOGRAM

TERMINOLOGY

The vectorcardiogram is recorded in the transverse (horizontal), sagittal, and frontal planes of the body.

The E point is the zero point on the vectorcardiogram. The X, Y, and Z axes as well as the three planes of the body intersect at the E point.

The letter E stands for the equivalent cardiac dipole. The symbol $\hat{E}$ is often used to represent E as a vector quantity and $s\hat{E}$ as a spatial vector quantity. The letter A is recommended for this purpose by the Committee on Electrocardiography of the American Heart Association.

The P loop is the loop of atrial activation; the QRS loop, the loop of ventricular depolarization; and the T loop, the loop of ventricular repolarization.

The O point is the point at which the QRS vector loop begins; the J point, the point at which it ends. The QRS loop is divided into an initial deflection, a body composed of efferent and afferent limbs, and a terminal deflection.

The maximum QRS vector is a line drawn from the O point to the farthest point of the loop.

The magnitude of a spatial vector can be determined by using the formula

$$s\hat{E} = \sqrt{E_x^2 + E_y^2 + E_z^2}$$

in which $s\hat{E}$ is the magnitude of the spatial vector and E_x, E_y, and E_z are the magnitudes of the projection of the spatial vector on the X, Y, and Z leads.

The half-area vector is the vector, drawn from the O point, which divides the QRS loop into two equal areas.

The maximum QRS width is the greatest width of the QRS loop as measured on a line perpendicular to the maximum QRS vector.

Timing of the loop is obtained by interrupting the electron beam of the oscilloscope at fixed intervals. The loop thus appears as a set of dashes. Usually the timing is arranged so that dashes occur at intervals of either 2.0 or 2.5 ms. Since all the loops shown in this text are schematic, the dash lines are omitted.

The S-T vector is the vector joining the O and J points.

The T loop begins at the J point and ends at the E point.

Because of the difficulty in determining the mean QRS and T vectors, the QRS-T angle is usually calculated from the maximum QRS and T vectors.

ABBREVIATIONS

The following abbreviations are used customarily:

$$
\begin{aligned}
\text{CW} &= \text{clockwise} \\
\text{CCW} &= \text{counterclockwise} \\
\text{TP} &= \text{transverse plane} \\
\text{SP} &= \text{sagittal plane} \\
\text{LSP} &= \text{left sagittal plane} \\
\text{FP} &= \text{frontal plane} \\
\text{xy} &= \text{frontal plane} \\
\text{zy} &= \text{sagittal plane} \\
\text{xz} &= \text{transverse (horizontal) plane} \\
\text{A} &= \text{integrated value (or area) of a force, including its duration as} \\
&\quad \text{well as magnitude} \\
\text{H}° &= \text{the angle between a vector and the X axis in the transverse} \\
&\quad \text{plane} \\
\text{S}° &= \text{the angle between a vector and the Z axis in the left sagittal} \\
&\quad \text{plane} \\
\text{F}° &= \text{the angle between a vector and the X axis in the frontal plane} \\
\text{max} &= \text{maximum} \\
\text{mV} &= \text{millivolt} \\
\text{ms} &= \text{millisecond}
\end{aligned}
$$

Examples

0.04QRSxz = the 0.04-s vector of the QRS in the transverse plane.
maxQRS vector F° + 60° = the maximum QRS vector in the frontal plane is at +60°.

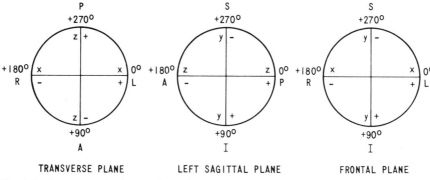

Fig. 6-1   Conventional reference frame for angular measurements of planar vectors.

NOMENCLATURE OF ANGLES

It has been customary to use the reference frame as shown in Fig. 6-1 for angular measurements of planar vectors.   The American Heart Association Committee on Electrocardiography has recommended use of the reference frames in Fig. 6-2 for these measurements.   Since the new system of notation is strange to some persons, in this text the angles of vectors are recorded in the traditional manner, but the value according to the recommended system follows in parentheses.

NORMAL VALUES

Normal values for the various components of the P, QRS, and T loops are listed in Tables 17 and 18 in the Appendix.

Fig. 6-2   Reference frame for angular measurements of planar vectors recommended by the American Heart Association Committee on Electrocardiography.   (*From Circulation,* 35: 585, 1967.)

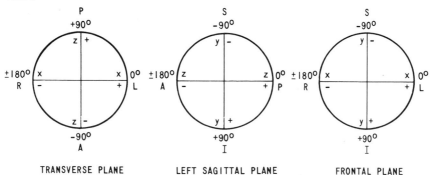

THE P LOOP (FIG. 9-7)

The P loop begins at the E point and ends at the O point. The loop is open because the Tp vector, representing atrial repolarization, is directed oppositely to the P loop. The O point is usually superior, posterior, and to the right of the E point.

In the TP, the P loop is usually inscribed in a CCW manner with the initial portion directed anteriorly and the terminal portion posteriorly. Sometimes the loop shows a figure-of-eight pattern. The maximum P vector does not exceed 0.1 mV. The magnitude of the anteriorly directed forces does not exceed 0.06 mV in adults and 0.08 mV in children. The maximum posterior P vector is 0.04 mV or less in both children and adults. The maximum leftward P vector is 0.09 mV in adults and 0.13 mV in children.

In the LSP, the P loop rotates CCW with the initial portion directed anteriorly and the terminal portion posteriorly. Its overall direction is inferior. The maximum P vector is 0.18 mV or less.

In the FP, inscription of the P loop is CCW. The loop is directed inferiorly and leftward. The maximum P vector is 0.2 mV or less.

THE QRS LOOP (FIG.6-3)

The initial portion of the loop, representing septal activation, is always directed anteriorly and, usually, rightward and superiorly.

The body of the loop, representing ventricular depolarization, is directed leftward, inferiorly, and posteriorly.

The terminal portion of the loop, representing late activation of the posterobasal region of the left ventricle and the base of the interventricular septum, is directed posteriorly, either slightly leftward or rightward, and superiorly or inferiorly.

The initial and terminal portions of the loop are often inscribed slowly, but slowing does not normally exceed 20 ms for the initial deflection or 30 ms for the terminal vector.

Transverse Plane

The QRS loop in the TP is usually oval in shape. Inscription of the loop is invariably CCW. The initial forces are directed anteriorly and usually rightward. The 20-ms vector is always directed anteriorly. The main body of the loop is located posteriorly. The average maxQRS vector is at 327° (H° + 33°), and its magnitude is usually less than 2.2 mV. The terminal deflection is directed posteriorly. However, less than 20 percent of the loop area is located in the right posterior quadrant.

THE NORMAL VECTORCARDIOGRAM

TRANSVERSE PLANE

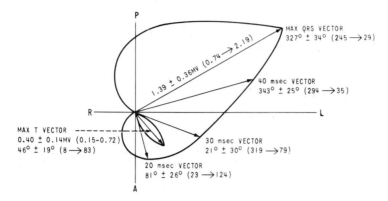

LEFT SAGITTAL PLANE

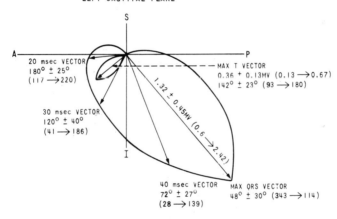

FRONTAL PLANE

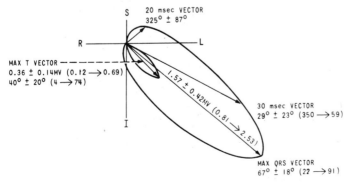

Fig. 6-3 The normal vectorcardiogram. The values shown are based on the data of H. W. Draper et al. (*From Circulation*, 30: 853, 1964.)

Left Sagittal Plane

The QRS loop in the LSP is usually oval-shaped. Inscription of the loop is invariably CCW. The initial forces are directed anteriorly and usually superiorly, but sometimes inferiorly. The 25-ms vector is always directed inferiorly. The main body of the loop is located inferiorly. The average maxQRS vector is at 48° (S° + 48°), and its magnitude is usually less than 1.8 mV.

Frontal Plane

The QRS loop in the FP tends to be long and narrow. Inscription of the loop is CW in 65 percent of cases, figure-of-eight in 25 percent, and CCW in 10 percent. As a general rule, horizontal loops rotate CCW and vertical loops CW. The CCW inscription of a vertical loop is rare, but CW inscription of a horizontal loop sometimes occurs. The initial forces are usually directed rightward and superiorly, but the findings are variable. The average maxQRS vector is at 41° (F° + 41°), and its magnitude is less than 2 mV. The direction of the terminal forces is variable.

THE S-T VECTOR

The S-T vector is normally small and does not exceed 0.1 mV in any plane.

THE T LOOP

The T loop tends to be elliptical in shape. The efferent limb is inscribed more slowly than the afferent limb. The T loop usually has a leftward, posterior, and inferior direction. Inscription of the T loop is usually CCW in both the TP and LSP; in the FP, it may be CW or CCW. As a rule, CW rotation of the T loop in the TP is indicative of heart disease.

THE QRS-T ANGLE

According to Benchimol, the angle between the maxQRS and the maxT vector in any plane should not exceed 75° in normal subjects. The QRS-T angle is usually narrowest in the FP and widest in the LSP.

DERIVATION OF THE SCALAR ELECTROCARDIOGRAM FROM THE VECTORCARDIOGRAM

The standard and unipolar limb leads can be derived with reasonable accuracy from the FP loop by use of the hexaxial reference diagram devised by Langner (Fig.6-4).

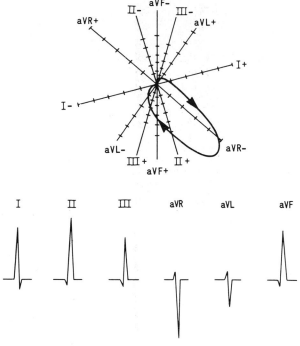

Fig. 6-4 Derivation of the QRS complexes of the limb leads from the frontal plane QRS loop by using the hexaxial reference diagram of Langner. (*From Am. Heart J.*, 45: 835, 1953.)

Fig. 6-5 Derivation of the QRS complexes of the precordial leads from the transverse plane QRS loop by using the reference system of Abildskov and Wilkinson. (*From Circulation*, 27: 58, 1963.)

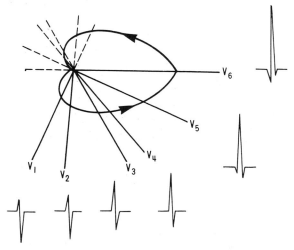

The precordial leads can similarly be derived from the TP loop by use of the reference diagram suggested by Abildskov and Wilkinson (Fig. 6-5).

REFERENCES

Benchimol, A,.: "Vectorcardiography," Williams & Wilkins, Baltimore, 1973.

Bristow, J. D.: A Study of the Normal Frank Vectorcardiogram, *Am. Heart J.,* 61:242, 1961.

Chou, T-C., R. A. Helm, and S. Kaplan: "Clinical Vectorcardiography," 2d ed., Grune & Stratton, New York, 1974.

Draper, H. W., C. J. Peffer, F. W. Stallman, D. Littman, and H. V. Pipberger: The Corrected Orthogonal Electrocardiogram and Vectorcardiogram in 510 Normal Men (Frank Lead System), *Circulation,* 20: 853, 1964.

Forkner, C. E., Jr., P. G. Hugenholtz, and H. D. Levine: The Vectorcardiogram in Normal Young Adults. Frank Lead System, *Am. Heart J.,* 62: 237, 1961.

Hoffman, I. (ed.): "Vectorcardiography—1965," North-Holland, Amsterdam, 1966.

———(ed.), R. I. Hamby and E. Glassman (co-eds.): "Vectorcardiography 2," North-Holland, Amsterdam, 1971.

Hugenholtz, P. G., and J. Liebman: The Orthogonal Vectorcardiogram in 100 Normal Children (Frank System), *Circulation,* 26: 891, 1962.

McCall, B. W., A. G. Wallace, and E. H. Estes, Jr.: Characteristics of the Normal Vectorcardiogram Recorded with the Frank Lead System, *Am. J. Cardiol,* 10: 514, 1962.

CHAPTER 7

ABNORMALITIES OF THE T WAVE OR VECTOR

There are two general types of T wave abnormalities: (1) primary T wave abnormalities, in which repolarization is altered independently of depolarization, and (2) secondary T wave abnormalities, in which an alteration in repolarization is directly dependent upon a change in the sequence of depolarization.

PRIMARY ABNORMALITIES (FIG. 7-1)

Metabolic Abnormalities

These occur in such disorders as hypothyroidism, anemia, shock, and nutritional disorders.

1 The T waves are decreased in amplitude but are otherwise unchanged. The QRS complexes are normal.
2 The T vector is reduced in size but is not changed in direction. The QRS-T angle is usually normal.

Abnormalities Due to Ischemia

The term *ischemia* is used here in an electrical sense only. Anatomic ischemia may or may not be present.

PRIMARY T WAVE OR VECTOR ABNORMALITIES

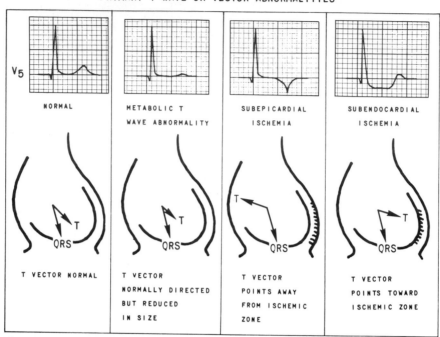

Fig. 7-1 Schematic representation of the primary abnormalities of the T wave or vector. (Modified from R. P. Grant, "Clinical Electrocardiography," © 1957 by McGraw-Hill, Inc., New York. Used with permission of McGraw-Hill Book Company.)

1 In subepicardial ischemia, the T waves overlying the ischemic zone are symmetrically inverted. In subendocardial ischemia, the T waves overlying the ischemic zone are symmetrically upright and tall.

2 In subepicardial ischemia, the T vector points away from the ischemic zone; in subendocardial ischemia, it points toward the ischemic zone. The particular direction which the T vector takes depends on the direction of the mean QRS vector and on the location of the ischemic region.

3 The QRS-T angle and the ventricular gradient are abnormal.

SECONDARY ABNORMALITIES (FIG. 7-2)

1 The presence of an intraventricular conduction defect, such as bundle branch block, identifies this type of abnormal T wave or vector.

2 The ventricular gradient is normal although the QRS-T angle may be abnormally wide.

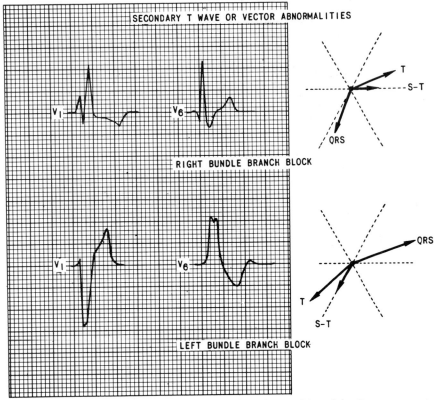

Fig. 7-2 Schematic representation of the secondary abnormalities of the T wave or vector which occur in bundle branch block.

FUNCTIONAL ABNORMALITIES

Functional T wave abnormalities, similar to those seen in organic heart disease, may occur in response to various physiologic stimuli. Sometimes they are also observed in otherwise healthy asthenic or neurotic individuals.

SUMMARY

The relationship between the mean QRS, S-T, and T vectors in various conditions is illustrated schematically in Fig. 8-3.

REFERENCE

Grant, R. P.: "Clinical Electrocardiography: The Spatial Vector Approach," McGraw-Hill, New York, 1957.

CHAPTER 8

ABNORMALITIES OF THE S-T SEGMENT OR VECTOR

DISPLACEMENT AS A NORMAL VARIANT (FIG. 8-1)

1 In the precordial leads or even in the limb leads, upward displacement exceeding accepted standards may nevertheless be normal, provided the S-T segment is concave upward and the T wave is tall, broad-based, and upright.

2 The QRS-T angle is narrow. The S-T vector is relatively parallel to the T vector, which is increased in magnitude.

DIGITALIS (FIG. 8-1)

1 The QRS complex is unaltered. The S-T segment is depressed and sagging. Its contour is concave upward or sloped downward in a straight line. Initially, the T wave is decreased in amplitude. Later, there is inversion of its proximal portion although the final portion is upright. The Q-T interval is shortened.

2 The QRS vector is unchanged. The T vector is reduced in magnitude but is little changed in direction. The S-T vector is in the opposite direction of the mean QRS vector.

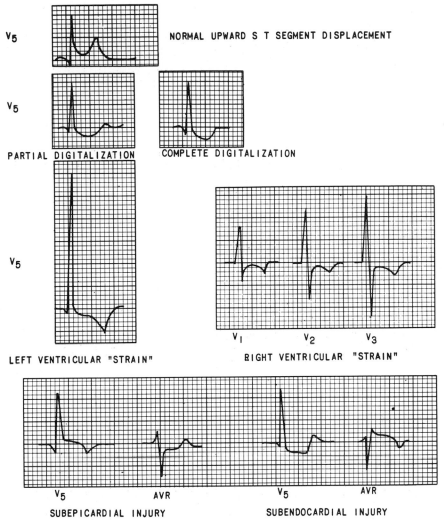

Fig. 8-1 Abnormalities of the S-T segment produced by normal variants, digitalization, left ventricular strain, right ventricular strain, subepicardial injury, and subendocardial injury. See text.

LEFT VENTRICULAR "STRAIN" (FIG. 8-1)

1   In the left precordial leads, the S-T segment is depressed, convex upward, and associated with asymmetrical T wave inversion. When the mean QRS vector is horizontal, similar changes occur in lead aVL and lead I. When the mean QRS vector is vertical, similar changes occur in lead aVF and lead III. The above changes are associated with a normal or very slightly prolonged QRS interval and with voltage changes indicative of left ventricular enlargement.

2   The mean QRS vector is normally directed but increased in magnitude. The S-T segment and T wave vectors have the same direction, and both are nearly 180° from the mean QRS vector. The S-T vector is smaller in magnitude than the mean T vector.

RIGHT VENTRICULAR "STRAIN" (FIG. 8-1)

1   In the right precordial leads, the S-T segment is depressed and the T wave inverted in association with QRS changes of right ventricular enlargement. In the limb leads, similar S-T and T wave changes often occur in leads aVF, III, and II. The QRS interval is normal.
2   The mean QRS vector shows right axis deviation. The S-T and T vectors are opposite in direction to the mean QRS vector and therefore point leftward and posteriorly.

SUBEPICARDIAL INJURY (FIG. 8-1)

1   In epicardial leads overlying the injured zone, the S-T segment is elevated and convex upward and the T wave is inverted. In endocardial leads beneath the injured zone, the S-T segment is depressed and concave upward and the T wave is upright.
2   The S-T vector points toward the injured zone and the T vector away from it.

SUBENDOCARDIAL INJURY (FIG. 8-1)

1   The S-T segment is depressed, horizontal, or downward-sagging and the T wave is upright in epicardial leads overlying the injured region. In endocardial leads beneath the injured region, the S-T segment is elevated and convex upward and the T wave is inverted.
2   The S-T vector points away from the injured region and the T vector toward it.

PERICARDITIS (FIG. 8-2)

Early Stage

1   In leads overlying the involved pericardium, usually aVL, aVF, and the left precordial leads, the S-T segments are elevated and often concave upward. Lead aVR usually shows a depressed S-T segment. The T wave generally shows no changes at this stage. The QRS complexes are unchanged, except perhaps for a decrease in voltage.

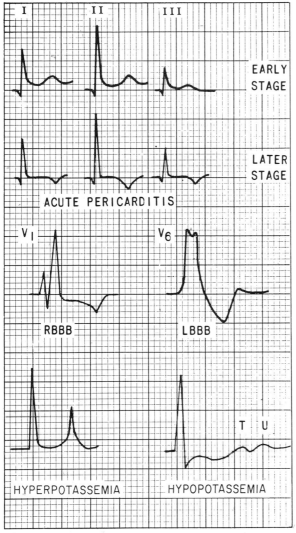

Fig. 8-2 Abnormalities of the S-T segment produced by acute pericarditis, right bundle branch block, left bundle branch block, hyperpotassemia, and hypopotassemia.   See text.

2   The S-T vector points toward the center of the involved pericardium. The T vector is unchanged.

Later Stage

1   The S-T segments become isoelectric, but the T waves become inverted in leads overlying the involved pericardium.   In lead aVR, the T wave may be upright.

MEAN QRS, S-T, and T VECTORS IN VARIOUS ENTITIES

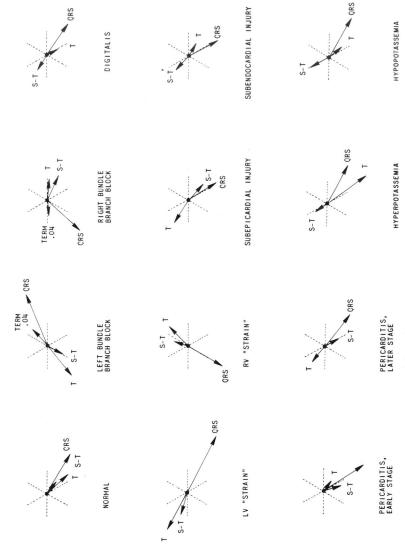

Fig. 8-3   Schematic representation of the relationship between the mean QRS, S-T, and T vectors in various entities.

2   The T vector points away from the center of the ventricular pericardium in a direction that is rightward and superior.

BUNDLE BRANCH BLOCK (FIG. 8-2)

1   The S-T segment and the T wave are displaced in a direction opposite to the main ventricular deflection.   The QRS interval is prolonged.
2   The S-T and T vectors are more or less parallel to each other but are opposite in direction to the mean QRS vector direction.

HYPERPOTASSEMIA (FIG. 8-2)

1   In the early stages of potassium intoxication, the T waves may be tall and peaked.   The S-T segment may be depressed.
2   The S-T vector may be opposite to the mean QRS vector.   The T vector is not altered in direction but is increased in magnitude.

HYPOPOTASSEMIA (FIG. 8-2)

1   The T wave is commonly reduced in size, and the U waves are prominent.   The S-T segment is depressed.
2   The S-T vector is opposite to the mean QRS vector.   The T vector is reduced in magnitude but not altered in direction.

SUMMARY

The relationship between the mean QRS, S-T, and T vectors in various conditions is illustrated schematically in Fig. 8-3.

REFERENCE

Grant, R. P.: "Clinical Electrocardiography: The Spatial Vector Approach," McGraw-Hill, New York, 1957.

CHAPTER 9

ATRIAL ABNORMALITIES

ATRIAL ABNORMALITY, ENLARGEMENT, OR HYPERTROPHY

Theoretical Considerations

The normal mean P vector is the resultant of the vectors generated by both atria. The initial portion of the P wave is produced primarily by the right atrium; the midportion, by both atria; and the terminal portion, by the left atrium. The right atrial P vector is anteriorly directed, whereas the left atrial P vector is posteriorly oriented. The mean P vector is directed leftward, inferiorly, and either slightly anteriorly or posteriorly.

In right atrial enlargment, the mean P vector is increased in magnitude and is rotated more rightward, inferiorly, and anteriorly, which results in P waves of increased amplitude in leads II, III, and aVF and in diphasic P waves of increased amplitude in the right precordial leads with large, positive initial components—the "so-called P pulmonale pattern." In left atrial enlargement, the mean P vector is shifted somewhat posteriorly and is of increased duration, not only because the left atrium is activated last, but probably because of an intra- or interatrial conduction defect, which results in broad P waves in leads I and II and diphasic P waves with broad, negative terminal components in the right precordial leads—the "so-called P mitrale pattern."

The direction of atrial repolarization is not altered in atrial enlargement. The only change that may be seen is displacement of the P-R and S-T segments in a direction opposite to that of the P wave, resulting from the increased magnitude of the S-Tp and Tp vectors. The P-R and S-T segment deviations are concordant.

From the foregoing, it would appear that the diagnosis of atrial hypertrophy or enlargement should be fairly simple. Actually, this is not true. One reason is that there is considerable normal variation in the voltage, duration, morphology, and direction of the P wave. Another is that the configuration of the P wave may change in the same person from time to time under the influence of physiologic stimuli. Abnormal P waves occur in perfectly healthy subjects, and, conversely, normal P waves may be found in the presence of atrial disease. Moreover, the P wave is notoriously sensitive to autonomic influences. Acceleration of the heart rate alone may cause peaking and increased voltage of the P wave. And even when the electrocardiogram shows "unequivocal" evidence of right or left atrial enlargement, neither may be present. Furthermore, overlapping of patterns is not unusual, so that sometimes right atrial enlargement is simulated by left atrial enlargement or other conditions.

Because conditions other than hypertrophy or enlargement cause P wave changes, the term *abnormality*, rather than either of the foregoing terms, is commonly used to designate alterations in P wave morphology. This term is probably more correct, but the terms *hypertrophy* and *enlargement* have gained acceptance by common usage.

RIGHT ATRIAL ABNORMALITY, ENLARGEMENT, OR HYPERTROPHY (FIGS. 9-1, 9-2, 18-4, 21-1, 23-4)

Diagnosis

Conventional Criteria

1   The P wave is 2.5 mm or more in amplitude in leads II, III, and aVF. In some cases of congenital heart disease (P congenitale), the P wave may be taller in leads I and II than in leads II and III. The P wave is usually tall, thin, and peaked (P pulmonale). Sometimes it is "gothic" in appearance.
2   The P wave is 0.11 s or less in duration.
3   The mean electrical axis of the P wave is shifted rightward to $+75°$ or more.
4   The right precordial leads show diphasic P waves, often with increased voltage of the initial component (1.5 mm or more), except in emphysema, where the terminal component or the entire P wave may be inverted.

Comments

Right atrial enlargement is actually demonstrable in only one-half of patients exhibiting the P pulmonale pattern. Thus this pattern is not specific for

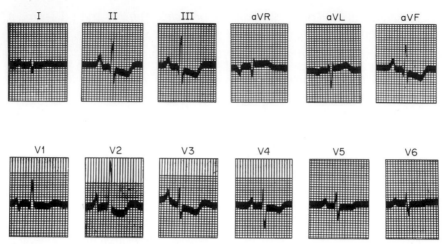

Fig. 9-1 Right atrial and right ventricular enlargement, right ventricular strain, and digitalis effect in a patient with chronic cor pulmonale. There is right axis deviation (+100°). The P waves are abnormally tall and peaked, with the P vector directed inferiorly (P pulmonale). A qR pattern is present in lead V_1 and a tall R wave in lead V_2. The R/S ratio in leads V_5 and V_6 is less than 1.0. Digitalis effect is best seen in leads II, III, and aVF; the strain pattern, in the precordial leads.

right atrial enlargement. Not infrequently, the P pulmonale pattern represents left atrial enlargement or another condition altogether. The P wave may increase in amplitude with an increase in heart rate, even in normal subjects, and so simulate P pulmonale. The P pulmonale pattern may occur in emphysema with or without right atrial hypertrophy, and it may be found in coronary artery disease, acute left ventricular failure, and hypoxemia. In tricuspid atresia, the P wave is usually tall and notched in leads I and II, with the first peak taller than the second (P tricuspidale).

The recognition of left atrial enlargement rather than right as the cause of the P pulmonale pattern is favored by an abnormal P terminal force in lead V_1 in the presence of left ventricular enlargement. Conversely, the diagnosis of right atrial enlargement is favored by the absence of these findings and the presence of changes consistent with right ventricular enlargement or pulmonary disease. In doubtful cases, the vectorcardiogram may be helpful in arriving at the correct diagnosis.

LEFT ATRIAL ABNORMALITY, ENLARGEMENT, OR
HYPERTROPHY (FIGS. 9-3, 10-4)

Diagnosis

Conventional Criteria

1 The duration of the P waves exceeds normal values (0.07 s in infants under 1 year of age, 0.08 s from 1 to 12 years, 0.09 s from 12 to 16

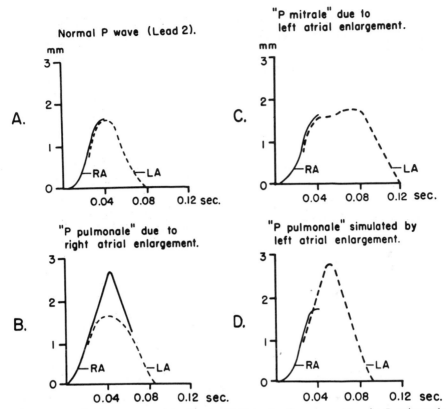

Fig. 9-2 Mechanisms proposed by Chou and Helm for the appearance of a P pulmonale pattern in left atrial enlargement. *(From I-C. Chou and R. A. Helm, The Pseudo P Pulmonale, Circulation, 32: 96, 1965. Used by permission of the American Heart Association, Inc.)*

years, and 0.10 s above the age of 16 years). The P wave is typically notched and slurred in leads I and II (P mitrale). Notching of itself is not abnormal unless the P wave shows high voltage or increased duration, or both, or the summits are more than 0.03 s apart.

2 The mean axis of the terminal component of the P wave in the FP is shifted leftward to +30° or beyond. This is recognized by a positive terminal P deflection in leads I and aVL or a negative terminal P deflection in leads III and aVF. The initial P forces are usually unchanged in direction, but in some instances the mean electrical axis of the entire P wave is also shifted leftward to between +45 and −30°.

3 The right precordial leads show diphasic P waves with wide and deep terminal components. The P terminal force is −0.04 mm · s or more. An increased P terminal force is a common finding in rheumatic mitral valvular disease. An abnormal P terminal force has been reported to occur in 7.1 percent of middle-aged men without cardiovascular disease. It may also be seen in some patients with chronic pulmonary disease

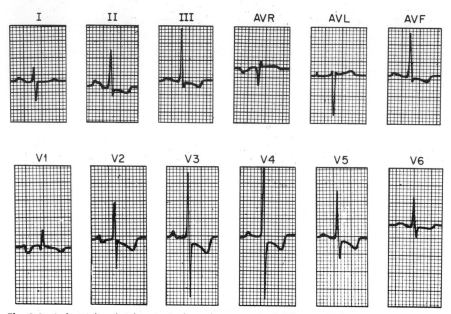

Fig. 9-3   Left atrial and right ventricular enlargement and right ventricular strain in a patient with mitral stenosis.   The P waves are broad and notched.   There is a qR pattern with an inverted T wave in lead V$_1$.   The S-T segments are depressed and the T waves inverted in the precordial leads.

in the absence of left atrial enlargement and, rarely, in right atrial enlargement.

4   The duration of the intrinsicoid deflection of a diphasic P wave in lead V$_1$, measured from the peak of the initial component to the nadir of the final component, exceeds 0.03 s.

Comments

The pattern of left atrial enlargement was evaluated by Josephson and his coworkers.   Left atrial size and pressure as well as interatrial conduction were correlated with electrocardiographic left atrial enlargement using echocardiography, mean pulmonary capillary wedge pressure, and the activation time from the P wave to the coronary sinus.   The Josephson team concluded that the electrocardiographic pattern of left atrial enlargement is produced by an interatrial conduction defect that, in turn, may have multiple causes.   The pattern manifested no consistent relationship to elevation of the pulmonary capillary wedge pressure or the dimension of the left atrium determined echocardiographically.   An increased left atrial size correlated only in patients with rheumatic mitral valve disease. Elevated pulmonary capillary wedge pressure correlated with electrocardiographic left atrial enlargement only in patients with cardiomyopathy. In patients with coronary artery disease, neither echocardiographic left atrial enlargement nor elevated pulmonary capillary wedge pressure correlated with the electrocardiographic left atrial enlargement. Josephson and coworkers therefore suggested that the term *left atrial enlargement* was inappropriate for this pattern and should be replaced by *interatrial conduction defect*. The author of this text prefers the term *intraatrial block* to *interatrial conduction delay*.

Left atrial abnormality is a common finding in mitral and aortic valvular disease but may occur in coronary artery disease, acute myocardial infarction, acute pulmonary edema, constrictive pericarditis, idiopathic hypertrophic subaortic stenosis, cardiomyopathy, coarctation of the aorta, diastolic overloading of the left ventricle, and endocardial cushion defects. Left atrial abnormality is a frequent finding in systemic hypertension even when the heart size is normal. Left atrial abnormality does not occur in pulmonary embolism.

COMBINED ATRIAL ABNORMALITY, ENLARGEMENT, OR HYPERTROPHY (FIGS. 9-4, 23-8)

There is both increased amplitude and duration of the P waves.

CRITERIA OF MACRUZ ET AL. FOR THE DIAGNOSIS OF ATRIAL ENLARGEMENT

The durations of the P wave and of the P-R segment are measured. The normal ratio of the duration of the P wave to that of the P-R segment is from 1.0 to 1.6.

Right Atrial Enlargement   The P/P-R segment ratio is less than 1.0.

Left Atrial Enlargement   The P/P-R segment ratio is greater than 1.6.

Fig. 9-4 Biatrial enlargement and right ventricular strain in a patient with mitral and tricuspid stenosis. The waves are both abnormally broad and tall. Right ventricular strain is manifested by the inverted T waves in the precordial leads and can be considered evidence of right ventricular enlargement.

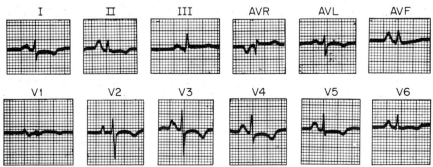

Comments

The index of Macruz is based on the following theoretical considerations:

When the right atrium is enlarged, the voltage of the P wave, but not its duration, is increased. However, because of the increased size of the right atrium, transmission of the impulse from the SA to the AV node is slightly delayed. Accordingly, the ratio of the duration of the P wave to that of the P-R segment will decrease as the P-R interval lengthens.

When the left atrium is enlarged, the P wave is of increased duration. The P-R interval, however, is normal, because transmission of the impulse from the SA to the AV node via the right atrium is not delayed. Accordingly, the ratio of the duration of the P wave to that of the P-R segment will increase as the P wave broadens.

Biatrial enlargement will increase both the numerator and denominator of the ratio, and thus the P/P-R segment ratio may remain normal. However, in such cases there should be distinct prolongation of both the P wave and the P-R segment.

Although based on physiologic principles, the Macruz index is of limited value in the diagnosis and differential diagnosis of atrial enlargement. It is frequently normal when atrial enlargement is present, particularly in the case of right atrial enlargement. The Macruz index often fails to distinguish between right and left atrial enlargement and appears to be of little value in the diagnosis of combined atrial enlargement.

UNUSUAL AXIS OF THE P WAVE

Left axis deviation of the P wave (between 0 and $-30°$) in a sinus rhythm may be an early sign of left atrial enlargement in mitral stenosis or arterial hypertension but may also be seen in apparently healthy obese or elderly persons.

Right axis deviation of the P wave ($+75°$ or more) is commonly a sign of right atrial enlargement, seen most often in chronic obstructive pulmonary disease with or without cor pulmonale. However, it may be observed not infrequently in young, asthenic, but otherwise healthy individuals.

A negative P wave in lead I may be found in the following conditions: most commonly, as a result of reversal of the right and left arm leads, but also in dextrocardia, left atrial and AV junctional rhythms, and severe right atrial enlargement.

ATRIAL INJURY AND INFARCTION (FIG. 9-5)

Normally, the S-Tp and Tp vectors have a direction opposite to that of the P vector. In atrial injury due to infarction or trauma, the S-Tp and Tp vectors tend to point in the same direction as the P vector. The S-Tp and

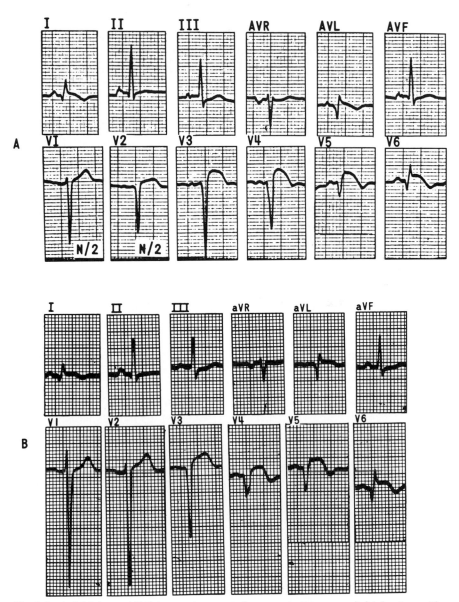

Fig. 9-5 Atrial injury. (A) Taken at the onset of acute anterior myocardial infarction. The P waves are splintered and notched. The P-R segment is elevated in leads II, III, aVF, V_5, and V_6 but is depressed in leads aVR, V_1, and V_2. (B) Taken a few days later. Signs of atrial injury have disappeared, but signs of ventricular infarction persist.

Tp vectors in atrial injury due to acute pericarditis are directed opposite to the mean P vector (see Chap. 15). These changes in the S-Tp and Tp vectors produce the P-Tp segment displacements.

Atrial infarction is almost invariably associated with infarction of the ventricles and is frequently accompanied by atrial arrhythmias.

Major Criteria for Diagnosis (Liu et al.)

1 Elevation of the P-Tp segment greater than 0.5 mm in leads V_5 and V_6 with reciprocal depression of the P-Tp segment in leads V_1 and V_2.
2 Elevation of the P-Tp segment over 0.5 mm in lead I, with its depression in leads II or III.
3 Depression of the P-Tp segment more than 1.5 mm in the precordial leads and more than 1.2 mm in leads I, II, and III in the presence of any form of atrial arrhythmia.

Minor Criteria for Diagnosis (Liu et al.)

1 Abnormal P waves that are M-shaped, W-shaped, irregular, or notched.
2 Depression of the P-Tp segment of small amplitude without elevation of this segment in other leads cannot be regarded by itself as positive evidence of atrial infarction.

INTRAATRIAL BLOCK (FIG. 9-6), INTERATRIAL CONDUCTION DELAY

A P wave with a duration of 0.12 s or with other electrocardiographic patterns of left atrial enlargement is regarded by some authorities as evidence of an interatrial conduction defect or intraatrial block. (See section on Left Atrial Abnormality earlier in the chapter.)

Fig. 9-6 Intraatrial block. The P wave is 0.16 s wide. Its terminal component is deviated leftward. The patient had radiologic evidence of left atrial enlargement.

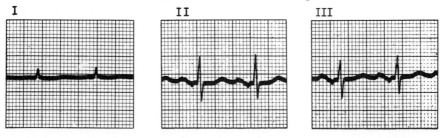

I   II   III

THE VECTORCARDIOGRAM IN ATRIAL ENLARGEMENT (FIG. 9-7)

Right Atrial Enlargement

1   Inscription of the P loop is usually CCW in all three planes.
2   In the TP, most of the P loop is directed anteriorly. The magnitude of the anteriorly directed forces is 0.07 mV or more in adults and 0.09 mV or greater in children under 15 years of age. The maximum P vector may exceed 0.10 mV.
3   In the LSP, most of the P loop is located anteriorly and inferiorly. The maximum P vector may exceed 0.18 mV.
4   In the FP, orientation of the P loop is more vertical than usual. The maximum P vector may exceed 0.20 mV.

Left Atrial Enlargement

1   The duration of the P loop is usually increased.
2   In the TP, most of the P loop is directed leftward and posteriorly. Inscription of the P loop is CCW or figure of eight, with the initial portion CCW and the terminal portion CW. The maximum posterior P vector commonly exceeds 0.05 mV. The maximum leftward P vector is 0.10 mV or more in adults and 0.14 mV or greater in children under 15 years of age.
3   The findings in the LSP and FP are not usually helpful diagnostically.

Biatrial Enlargement

In biatrial enlargement there is increased voltage of the anterior and posterior components of the loop. Normal values for both these vectors are exceeded. The characteristic changes are seen best in the TP and in the LSP, which typically shows a broad triangular loop.

REFERENCES

Arevalo, A. C., M. Spagnuolo, and A. R. Feinstein: A Simple Electrocardiographic Indication of Left Atrial Enlargement, *J.A.M.A.*, 185: 96, 1963.
Benchimol, A.: "Vectorcardiography," Williams & Wilkins, Baltimore, 1973.
Chou, T. C., and R. A. Helm: The Pseudo P Pulmonale, *Circulation*, 32: 96, 1965.
———— and S. Kaplan: "Clinical Vectorcardiography," 2d ed., Grune & Stratton, New York, 1974.
Forfang, K., and J. Erikssen: Significance of P Wave Terminal Force in Presumably Healthy Middle-Aged Men, *Am. Heart J.*, 96: 739, 1978.
Gamboa, R., W. Gersony, and A. S. Nadas: The Electrocardiogram in Tricuspid Atresia and Pulmonary Atresia with Intact Ventricular Septum, *Circulation*, 34: 24, 1966.
Gooch, A. S., J. B. Calatayud, P. A. Gorman, J. L. Saunders, and C. A. Caceres:

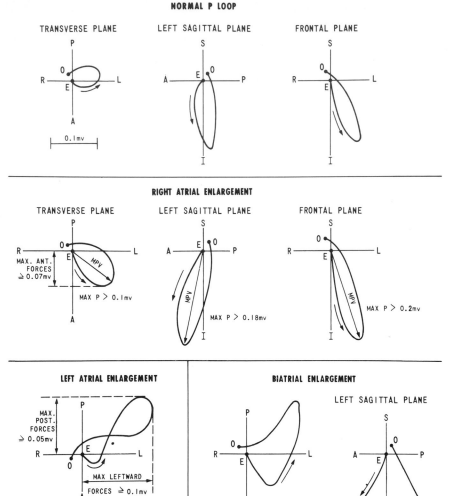

Fig. 9-7 Schematic representation of the normal P loop and of the P loops in right, left, and biatrial enlargement.

Leftward Shift of the Terminal P Forces in the ECG Associated with Left Atrial Enlargement, *Am. Heart J.*, 71: 727, 1966.

Gross, D.: Electrocardiographic Characteristics of P Pulmonale Waves of Coronary Origin, *Am. Heart J.*, 73: 453, 1967.

Human, G. P., and H. W. Snyman: The Value of the Macruz Index in the Diagnosis of Atrial Enlargement, *Circulation*, 27: 935, 1963.

Josephson, M. E., J. A. Kastor, and J. Morganroth: Electrocardiographic Left Atrial Enlargement, *Am. J. Cardiol.*, 39: 967, 1977.

Kahn, M., J. Scheuer, F. Wachtel, A. Grishman, and E. Donoso: An Evaluation of the Ratio of P-Wave Duration to P-R Segment in the Diagnosis of Atrial Enlargement, *Am. Heart J.*, 60: 23, 1960.

Liu, C. K., G. Greenspaw, and R. T. Peccirillo: Atrial Infarction of the Heart, *Circulation*, 23: 331, 1961.

Macruz, R., J. K. Perloff, and R. B. Case: A Method for the Electrocardiographic Recognition of Atrial Enlargement, *Circulation*, 17: 882, 1958.

Morris, J. J., E. H. Estes, Jr., R. A. Whalen, H. K. Thompson, Jr., and H. D. McIntosh: P-Wave Analysis in Valvular Heart Disease, *Circulation*, 21: 242, 1964.

Puech, P.: The P Wave: Correlation of Surface and Intra-Atrial Electrocardiograms, *Cardiovasc. Clin.*, 6 (1): 43, 1974.

Selvester, R. H., and L. J. Haywood: High Gain, High Frequency Atrial Vectorcardiograms in Normal Subjects and in Patients with Atrial Enlargement, *Am. J. Cardiol.*, 24: 8, 1969.

Tarazi, R. C., A. Miller, E. Frolich, and H. P. Dustan: Electrocardiographic Changes Reflecting Left Atrial Abnormality in Hypertension, *Circulation*, 34: 818, 1966.

Thomas, P., and D. Dejong: The P Wave in the Electrocardiogram in the Diagnosis of Heart Disease, *Brit. Heart J.*, 16: 241, 1954.

CHAPTER 10

VENTRICULAR HYPERTROPHY, OR ENLARGEMENT

Although it is usually not possible in the electrocardiogram to distinguish between ventricular hypertrophy and dilatation, the term *hypertrophy* has gained acceptance by common usage. Actually the term *enlargement* is preferable, since it includes both hypertrophy and dilatation.

LEFT VENTRICULAR HYPERTROPHY, OR ENLARGEMENT
(FIGS. 10-1 to 10-5, 11-9, 11-10, 11-16, 11-21, 13-35)

Theoretical Considerations

In left ventricular hypertrophy there is increased voltage of those QRS deflections which represent left ventricular potentials. The voltage changes are probably brought about by several factors, but two seem most important: (1) An enlarged ventricle with thickened walls and increased surface area produces greater potentials than does a normal ventricle; (2) enlargement brings the heart closer to the chest wall, so that the voltages recorded by the precordial leads are greater.

In left ventricular hypertrophy the mean QRS vector tends to be rotated leftward, posteriorly, and often somewhat superiorly and has increased magnitude. The general sequence of ventricular activation is unaltered. The changes in the mean QRS vector tend to produce large upright deflections in the left precordial leads and deep negative deflections in the right precordial leads. This is primarily an accentuation of normal findings.

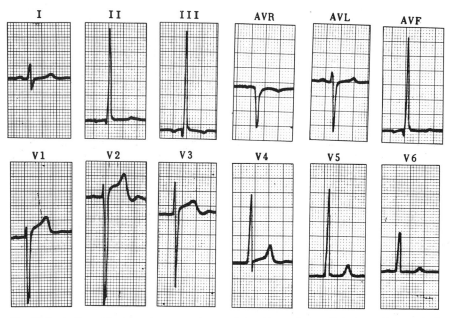

Fig. 10-1 Left ventricular enlargement in an adult with aortic insufficiency. There is high voltage of the R wave in leads aVF and V_5. The sum of the R_{V5} and S_{V1} waves exceeds normal values, as does the sum of the R_2 and R_3 waves. The QRS-T angle in the frontal plane is abnormally wide. This is indicative of a T vector abnormality, even though the T waves are upright in the precordial leads.

The findings in the limb leads depend on the extent of the projection of the cardiac vector on the axes of the leads. Horizontal (leftward) direction of the vector, which is most frequent, will cause tall, upright deflections to appear in leads I and aVL and large negative deflections to be inscribed in lead III. If the vector is directed vertically (rightward), as occasionally happens, leads aVF, II, and III will show the largest deflections. When the vector is markedly posteriorly directed, it will not project significantly in any of the limb lead axes, since these are in the frontal plane, and the limb leads may thus appear normal. However, if the mean QRS vector is primarily directed leftward in a direction parallel to the frontal plane, the precordial complexes will appear normal, but large deflections will be recorded in the limb leads.

Left ventricular hypertrophy is often accompanied by slight prolongation of the QRS interval. This results from the longer time required for the completion of the activation process in a thickened, compared with a normal, left ventricle.

In some instances of left ventricular hypertrophy, the time of onset of the intrinsicoid deflection in the left precordial leads is delayed. In unipolar electrocardiography this has been attributed to the longer time required for the impulse to travel from endocardium to epicardium through a thickened

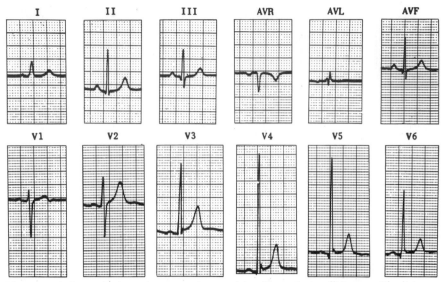

Fig. 10-2 Left ventricular enlargement in an adult with aortic insufficiency. There is no deviation of the electrical axis. There is high voltage of the R wave in lead V_5. The sum of the maximum R wave (in lead V_4) and the maximum S wave (in lead V_1) in the precordial leads exceeds 45 mm. The S-T segments and the T waves are normal. This is an example of diastolic overloading of the left ventricle.

Fig. 10-3 Left ventricular enlargement and strain. There is high voltage of the R wave in leads aVL and V_5. The R_{V5} wave plus the S_{V1} wave exceeds normal values, as does the sum of the R_1 and S_3 waves. There is left axis deviation $(+15°)$. The S-T segments and T waves show changes characteristic of the strain pattern. This is an example of systolic overloading of the left ventricle in a patient with hypertensive heart disease.

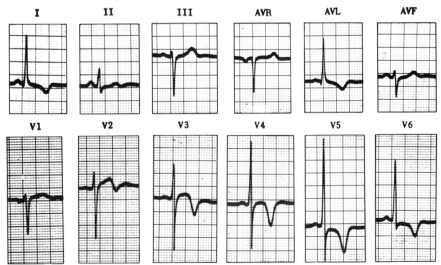

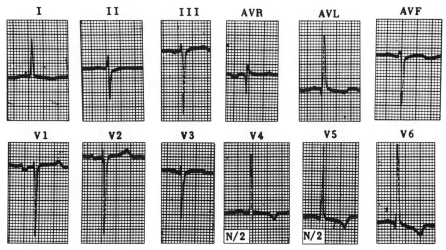

Fig. 10-4 Left ventricular enlargement and strain with left anterior fascicular block. There is abnormal left axis deviation ($-60°$). There is high voltage of the R wave in leads aVL and V_5. The R_1 wave plus the S_3 wave exceeds normal values, as does the sum of the R_{V5} and S_{V1} waves. This is an example of systolic overloading of the left ventricle in a patient with hypertensive heart disease. There is also left atrial abnormality.

musculature. This belief is predicated on the radial transmission of the impulse from endocardium to epicardium. Actually, there is significant tangential as well as radial spread of the impulse through the free wall of the left ventricle, so that this concept cannot be accepted. It is simpler and more accurate to regard the intrinsicoid deflection as representing the turning point of the cardiac vector along the axis of derivation of the lead.

Left ventricular hypertrophy is often accompanied by change in the direction of the S-T and T vectors. These vectors then point in a direction opposite to that of the mean QRS vector. This is the left ventricular strain pattern. The left precordial leads show depressed S-T segments and inverted T waves. In the limb leads, when the mean QRS vector is horizontal, similar changes occur in leads I and aVL. However, when the mean QRS vector is vertical, these changes occur in leads III and aVF and sometimes in lead II. The mechanism of these S-T and T wave alterations is unknown. Some authorities believe that the altered repolarization is caused by relative coronary insufficiency.

Diagnosis

The electrocardiogram in left ventricular enlargement may be normal, may show nonspecific abnormalities, or may present specific diagnostic alterations.

Conventional Criteria The diagnosis of left ventricular enlargement is based primarily on increased voltage of those QRS deflections which represent left ventricular potentials. Also important diagnostically are S-T segment and T wave changes in left ventricular epicardial leads, left atrial abnormality, abnormal left axis deviation, and a delayed onset of the intrinsicoid deflection in the left precordial leads. Criteria for the diagnosis of left ventricular enlargement are usually valid only when the QRS interval is less than 0.12 s.

Voltage of the QRS

Adults

Precordial Leads

1   The sum of the R wave in lead V_5 or V_6 and the S wave in lead V_1 or V_2 is greater than 35 mm in adults above the age of 30 years (40 mm in those between 20 and 30 years and 60 mm in the 16- to 20-year age group), or
2   The sum of the maximum R and the deepest S waves in the precordial leads is greater than 45 mm, or
3   The amplitude of the R wave in lead V_5 is greater than 26 mm, or
4   The amplitude of the R wave in lead V_6 is greater than 20 mm, or
5   The R wave in lead V_6 is taller than the R wave in lead V_5, provided there are dominant R waves in both these leads.

Extremity Leads

1   The sum of the R wave in lead I and the S wave in lead II is 26 mm or more, or
2   The amplitude of the R wave in lead I is 14 mm or more, or
3   The amplitude of the S wave in lead aVR is 15 mm or more, or
4   The amplitude of the R wave in lead aVF is 21 mm or more, or
5   The amplitude of the R wave in lead aVL is 12 mm or more.

The precordial lead criteria give high sensitivity with a reasonably acceptable degree of specificity. The point score system of Romhilt and Estes has comparable sensitivity but greater specificity. The limb lead criteria are less sensitive but highly specific.

Children (under 16 Years of Age)

1   The amplitude of the R wave in lead V_5 or V_6 is 35 mm or more, or
2   The sum of the R wave in lead V_5 and the S wave in lead V_2 is greater than 60 mm in children under 11 years of age or greater than 55 mm in females and 65 mm in males between 11 and 16 years, or

3   The sum of the R wave in lead I and the S wave in lead III is 30 mm or more, or

4   The sum of the R waves in leads II and III is 45 mm or more, or

5   The amplitude of the R wave in lead aVL is 12 mm or more, or

6   The amplitude of the R wave in lead aVF is 21 mm or more, or

7   The R/S ratio in lead V_1 is less than the maximum normal for the age: under 1 year, 0.8; 1 to 5 years, 0.2; and 6 to 15 years, 0.1 or less.

8   Deep Q waves in leads V_5 and V_6 or in leads II, III, and aVF are suggestive of left ventricular enlargement (septal hypertrophy), especially if accompanied by tall R and T waves in these leads.

9   In infants and children there is normally right ventricular preponderance. The amplitude of the R wave in lead V_1 exceeds the R wave of lead V_6 from birth to 6 months of age.   The amplitudes of the R wave in leads V_1 and V_6 are approximately equal from 6 months to 1 year.   After 1 year of age, the amplitude of the R wave in lead V_6 exceeds the R wave of lead V_1.   Any significant change in these ratios, with dominance of the R wave in lead V_6 compared with the R wave of lead V_1, is suggestive of left ventricular preponderance and of the probable diagnosis of left ventricular enlargement.

Intrinsicoid Deflection

The time of onset of the intrinsicoid deflection in lead V_5 or V_6 exceeds 0.05 s in adults and 0.04 s in children.   This finding assumes greater significance in the presence of a tall R wave in the corresponding lead. The intrinsicoid deflection in lead V_1 or V_2 is normal.

   Measurement of the time of onset of the intrinsicoid deflection in the left precordial leads is of limited value in the diagnosis of left ventricular enlargement because it is so frequently normal in this condition, but when it is delayed, it adds to the specificity of the diagnosis.   The intrinsicoid deflection may also be delayed in ventricular conduction defects.

S-T Segment and T Wave Changes

The S-T segment is depressed and convex upward with asymmetrical inversion of the T wave in leads showing high voltage of the QRS complex (tall R waves).   This is commonly noted in leads V_4 to V_6, in leads I, II, and aVL when the mean QRS vector is horizontal and in leads II, III, and aVF when the mean QRS vector is vertical.   This combination of S-T segment and T wave alteration is commonly referred to as the *left ventricular strain pattern*.   However, this pattern is not specific for enlargement.   It may be caused by digitalis, coronary artery disease, electrolyte disturbances, myocarditis, etc.   It is best regarded as a nonspecific abnormality, but it does support the diagnosis of left ventricular enlargement if the magnitude of the QRS deflections is increased.   The left ventricular strain pattern is often associated with positive S-T segment displacement in the right precordial leads.

As indicated in Chap. 5 under the heading Abnormality of the T Wave, asymmetric T wave inversion expressed by a T wave asymmetry ratio of 2.0 or greater, even in the absence of voltage criteria for hypertrophy, is strongly associated with left ventricular enlargement.

Summary

Possible or *probable left ventricular enlargement* (often called *left ventricular enlargement by voltage criteria*) is diagnosed when the electrocardiogram shows voltage abnormalities as described above. The greater the number of such abnormalities in any tracing, the greater the likelihood that left ventricular enlargement is present.

Definite left ventricular enlargement is diagnosed in the presence of indisputable and preferably multiple voltage abnormalities if they are accompanied by S-T segment and T wave changes typical of left ventricular strain, left atrial abnormality, or abnormal left axis deviation. The diagnosis is further supported by the presence of a delayed onset of the intrinsicoid deflection in the left precordial leads, although this requirement is by no means essential for the definitive diagnosis of left ventricular enlargement.

Point Score System for the Diagnosis of Left Ventricular Hypertrophy

Romhilt and Estes have introduced the following point score system for the diagnosis of left ventricular hypertrophy:

1 *Amplitude of the QRS complex*: Positive if any one of the following is present: 3
a Largest R or S in the limb leads $\geq$ 20 mm
b S_{V1} or $S_{V2} \geq$ 30 mm
c R_{V5} or $R_{V6} \geq$ 30 mm
2 *ST-T segment*: Positive if the left ventricular strain pattern with an ST-T vector oppostie to the mean QRS vector is present:
   Without digitalis   3
   With digitalis   1
3 *Left atrial involvement*: Positive if the P terminal force in lead V_1 is abnormal.   3
4 *Abnormal left axis deviation*: Positive if the electrical axis of the QRS complex is $-30°$ or more   2
5 *QRS duration*: Positive if the QRS duration is $\geq$ 0.09 s   1
6 *Intrinsicoid deflection*: Positive if the intrinsicoid deflection in lead V_5 or $V_6 \geq$ 0.05 s   1

Definite left ventricular hypertrophy is present if the point score is 5 or more.

Probable left ventricular hypertrophy is diagnosed if the point score is 4.

This is probably one of the best sets of criteria that have been proposed. The point score system has a high degree of specificity. However, improved sensitivity would be desirable. Users of this system should not ignore the customary criteria for voltage abnormality. The criterion of $R_{V6} > R_{V5}$ may be added to the voltage criteria of the point score system with a value of 3 points. The author does not use the point score system.

Comments on the Electrocardiographic Diagnosis

Voltage Criteria   The electrocardiographic diagnosis of left ventricular enlargement is based primarily on increased voltage of those deflections which represent left ventricular potentials. It should be pointed out that voltage criteria are somewhat inaccurate: (1) There are some normal persons, particularly thin, elderly, emaciated persons, adolescents, and young adults, whose electrocardiograms will show excessive voltage in the absence of left ventricular enlargement; (2) in some people with left ventricular enlargement, the electrocardiogram may fail to record voltages exceeding maximum normal values. This occurs not only because of bodily habitus but also because complicating conditions, such as coronary artery disease, emphysema, and serous effusions, may reduce the amplitude of the QRS deflections recorded at body surface. The voltage criteria listed above will include a small percentage of both false-positive and false-negative diagnoses. In making the electrocardiographic diagnosis of left ventricular enlargement, it is well to be circumspect and to evaluate carefully such factors as body build, the thickness of the chest wall, and the presence of complicating disease.

Left Axis Deviation   Abnormal left axis is frequently listed as a criterion for the diagnosis of left ventricular enlargement. While left axis deviation may complicate left ventricular enlargement, left axis deviation per se is not diagnostic of left ventricular enlargement. When left axis deviation occurs in association with left ventricular enlargement, it is generally indicative of left anterior hemiblock, but even then it may be due to other causes. Abnormal left axis deviation supports the diagnosis of left ventricular enlargement only when the voltage criteria are fulfilled. It should also be noted that left ventricular enlargement may be present without concomitant left axis deviation. For example, the electrical axis may be normal or deviated to the right in the presence of left ventricular enlargement. Even in children, left axis deviation does not necessarily mean left ventricular enlargement, because it is often due to other conditions, such as tricuspid atresia, an ostium primum defect, or a single ventricle.   The reader is referred to Chap. 20 for more information on left axis deviation.

Left Atrial Abnormality   The electrocardiographic findings compatible with left atrial abnormality are common to all diseases involving the left side of the heart.   Left atrial enlargement caused by mitral stenosis is not associated with left ventricular enlargement unless there is mitral insufficiency or concomitant aortic valvular disease.   However, left atrial abnormality occurs so frequently in left ventricular enlargement, regardless of cause, that the presence of electrocardiographic signs of left atrial abnormality may offer indirect evidence of the presence of left ventricular enlargement or of a left-sided lesion potentially capable of causing it (e.g., systemic hypertension).

Pseudoinfarction Patterns   Poor progression of the R waves or even reversal of normal R wave progression in the right precordial leads, with or without the appearance of Q waves or QS complexes in these leads, may occur in left ventricular hypertrophy in the absence of associated anteroseptal myocardial infarction or fibrosis (see Figs. 13-15 to 13-19).   The reduction in size of the initial R wave over the right precordium is explained by the leftward displacement of the initial vectors of depolarization, a frequent occurrence in left ventricular enlargement.

When QS or QR patterns occur in the midprecordial leads, anterior infarction may sometimes be differentiated from left ventricular hypertrophy by taking leads V_3 and V_4 at the level of the ensiform cartilage.   In such low V leads, QS complexes due to infarction generally persist unchanged, but those due to hypertrophy are replaced by rS deflections.   In doubtful cases the vectorcardiogram may be decisive in establishing the correct diagnosis.   Other causes for these abnormalities are discussed in the section on the differential diagnosis of myocardial infarction.

Left Ventricular Enlargement and Incomplete Left Bundle Branch Block (Fig. 11-16)

Left ventricular enlargement may be diagnosed by the usual voltage criteria in the presence of incomplete left bundle branch block (QRS duration less than 0.12 s, absent Q waves in leads I, aVL, V_5, and V_6, and notching or slurring of the uptstroke of the R wave in these leads).

Left Ventricular Enlargement and Complete Left Bundle Branch Block

The diagnosis of left ventricular enlargement in the presence of complete left bundle branch block is suggested if the sum of the voltages of S_{V2} and R_{V5} is 45 mm or more.   Increased QRS duration ($\geqq 0.14$ s), and electrocardiographic left atrial enlargement also strongly support the diagnosis of left ventricular enlargement in the presence of complete bundle branch block.

Left Ventricular Enlargement and Right Bundle Branch Block (Figs. 11-9, 11-10)

Coexistence of left ventricular enlargement should be suspected in right bundle block when the amplitude of the R wave in lead V_5 or V_6 is 20 mm or more or other voltage criteria for left ventricular enlargement are fulfilled.

Left Ventricular Enlargement and Myocardial Infarction (Fig. 13-35)

If the conventional voltage criteria are met, left ventricular enlargement may be diagnosed in the presence of myocardial infarction.

Left Ventricular Enlargement and Primary ST-T Abnormalities

Primary T wave abnormalities in the presence of left ventricular enlargement are suggested by the occurrence of T wave inversions in the right precordial leads or in leads II, III, and aVF (when there is left axis deviation).   Such findings are usually indicative of ischemia, as are deep, symmetrically inverted T waves in leads I, aVL, and V_4 to V_6.

Primary ST-T abnormalities resulting from drug effects, (e.g., digitalis, quinidine), electrolyte disturbances, or injury can ordinarily be recognized in the presence of left ventricular enlargement.

Vectorelectrocardiographic Criteria

1   The mean QRS vector is normally directed but is increased in magnitude. The conventional criteria for voltage abnormalities previously described are employed to determine whether the vector is increased in magnitude.
2   The S-T and T vectors may be normal or may show the characteristics of left ventricular strain.

THE VECTORCARDIOGRAM IN LEFT VENTRICULAR HYPERTROPHY (FIG. 10-5)

In left ventricular hypertrophy, the initial QRS vectors, while remaining anteriorly directed, tend to shift leftward from their usual rightward and anterior orientation.   The cause for this phenomenon is not understood. The leftward displacement of the initial forces accounts for the reduction

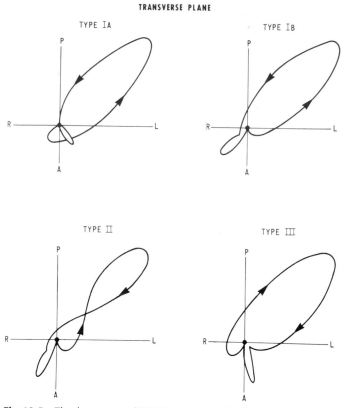

Fig. 10-5   The three types of QRS loop patterns found in the TP in left ventricular hypertrophy. In Type IA, the initial vector is directed rightward and anteriorly, whereas in type IB, it is directed leftward and anteriorly.   Described in text.

in the size of the R waves in the right precordial leads, a common finding in left ventricular hypertrophy.   It also explains the decrease in the size of the Q waves, or their disappearance, in the left precordial leads in some cases of left ventricular hypertrophy.   Because of the increased muscle mass of the left ventricle, the magnitude of the QRS loop is increased and its direction is displaced to a more posterior and leftward position.   The S-T vector and T loop are generally directed oppositely to the mean QRS vector.

QRS Loop

Transverse Plane   In left ventricular hypertrophy three types of QRS loop patterns may be found in the TP (Varriale et al.).

1 *Type I (most common):* The loop is ovoid or elongated and is inscribed in a CCW manner. The 0.02QRS vector is directed anteriorly, either to the right (Type 1*A*), or more frequently, to the left (Type I*B*).

2 *Type II (less common):* There is a figure-of-eight loop in which there is CCW inscription of the proximal portion and CW inscription of the distal portion. The relative size of the proximal and distal loops is variable. The 0.02QRS vector is directed anteriorly and to the left. This figure-of-eight loop probably represents a form of incomplete left bundle branch block.

3 *Type III (rare):* There is a narrow CW loop with the 0.02QRS vector directed rightward and anteriorly. Although the loop pattern resembles that of complete left bundle branch block, it is distinguished from the latter by its lesser duration and the absence of slowing in the mid and terminal portions of the loop. This pattern also resembles that found in anterolateral myocardial infarction.

In all three types of loop pattern, the 0.03QRS and 0.04QRS vectors are directed more posteriorly than normal.

The magnitude of the maxQRS vector is usually greater than 2.0 mV below the age of 40 years and 1.9 mV above this age. Its direction is usually posterior 330° (H° + 30°).

Type II and Type III loops usually represent more advanced degrees of left ventricular hypertrophy than does Type I.

Left Sagittal Plane   Inscription of the loop is variable but is most often CCW.

The magnitude of the maxQRS vector is usually increased to 2.0 mV or more, and its direction is posterior and often superior to +30° (S° + 30°).

Frontal Plane   Inscription of the loop is variable but is usually CCW. The magnitude of the maxQRS vector is usually increased to 20.0 mV or more. The direction of the maxQRS vector is located between +60 and −20°. Superior displacement of the vector above −30° suggests the coexistence of left anterior fascicular block.

S-T Vector

The S-T vector is usually displaced rightward, superiorly, and anteriorly.

T Loop

The T loop is usually displaced rightward, superiorly, and anteriorly. In the TP, the T loop vector is greater than +70° (H° − 70°).

QRST Angle

The angle subtended by the maximum QRS and T vectors in the planar projection is variable but is frequently wide and may approach 180°.

Criteria of Varriale et al. for the Vectorcardiographic Diagnosis of Left Ventricular Hypertrophy

The diagnosis is based on five vectorcardiographic findings:

1   The magnitude of the maxQRS vector in the TP is 2.0 mV or more.
2   The magnitude of the maxQRS vector in the FP is 2.0 mV or more.
3   The magnitude of the maxQRS in the LSP is 1.6 mV or more.
4   The angle of the maxQRS vector in the TP is displaced posteriorly to +330° (H° + 30°) or more.
5   The angle of the maxQRS vector in the LSP is displaced superiorly to +30 (S° + 30°) or more.

Definite left ventricular hypertrophy is diagnosed when at least four of the criteria are fulfilled.

Probable left ventricular hypertrophy is diagnosed when three of the criteria are fulfilled.

Possible left ventricular hypertrophy is diagnosed when two of the criteria are fulfilled.

Criteria of Romhilt et al. for the Vectorcardiographic Diagnosis of Left Ventricular Hypertrophy

1   The maxQRS vector in the TP is greater than 2.2 mV below the age of 50 years and 1.8 above this age.
2   The maxT vector in the TP is greater than 70° (H° − 70°).

RIGHT VENTRICULAR HYPERTROPHY, OR ENLARGEMENT (FIGS. 9-1, 9-3, 10-6 TO 10-12, 11-7, 11-8, 18-3 TO 18-6, 21-1, 21-2, 21-4, 23-4, 23-6)

Theoretical Considerations

The normal adult electrocardiogram is essentially a levocardiogram, because the ventricular mass is composed largely of left ventricle. To offset this left ventricular predominance so that the specific diagnostic alterations of right ventricular hypertrophy become apparent in the electrocardiogram, the right ventricle must enlarge considerably. Even then diagnostic signs may fail to appear. This accounts for the relative frequency with which the electrocardiogram is normal in the presence of right ventricular hypertrophy.

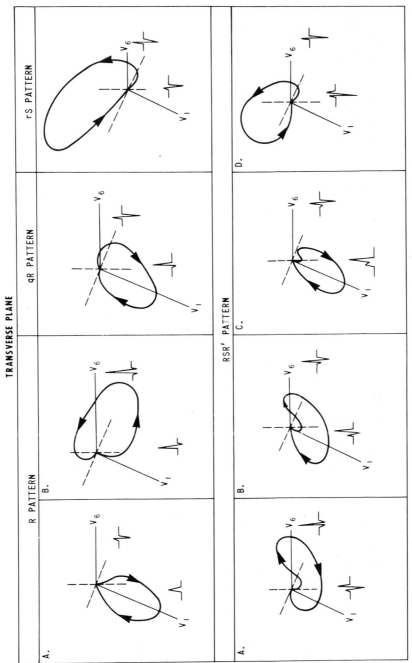

Fig. 10-6 Genesis of the precordial electrocardiogram in right ventricular hypertrophy. Described in text.

The electrocardiogram of normal infants and children, on the other hand, is characterized by right ventricular preponderance. Right ventricular hypertrophy in children increases the normal tendency to right axis deviation and produces a further increase in right ventricular potentials. However, the differentiation between physiologic and pathologic right ventricular preponderance in young children is often difficult or impossible because of the similarities and overlap in the electrocardiographic patterns.

Prolongation of the QRS interval does not occur in right ventricular hypertrophy unless an intraventricular conduction defect is also present. This is because activation of even a considerably enlarged right ventricle takes no longer than normal left ventricular activation.

The time of onset of the intrinsicoid deflection is delayed in the right precordial leads in right ventricular hypertrophy, because the vectors representing activation of the right ventricle usually occur later in the QRS interval than they do normally and are of increased magnitude.

Three basic ventricular patterns are seen in the right precordial leads in the ventricular hypertrophy: (1) a tall R wave and its variants, Rs or RS deflections; (2) an RSR' pattern and its variants, rsR', rSR', and rsr' complexes; and (3) a qR complex. A fourth pattern consisting of rS deflections in all the precordial leads is seen occasionally.

The derivation of these patterns is more easily understood when they can be visualized. In the Fig. 10-6 diagram, the genesis of each particular pattern is explained in terms of its relationship to a particular type of QRS vector loop. Only the findings in the transverse plane are illustrated.

Fig. 10-7 Early right ventricular enlargement due to congenital heart disease. There is slightly increased voltage of the R wave in lead V_1, with an R/S ratio greater than 1.0.

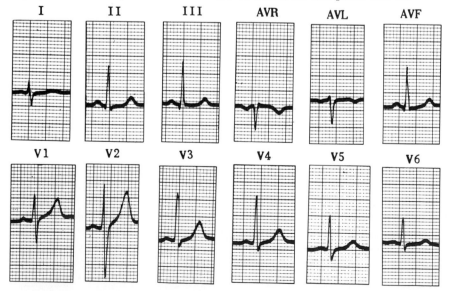

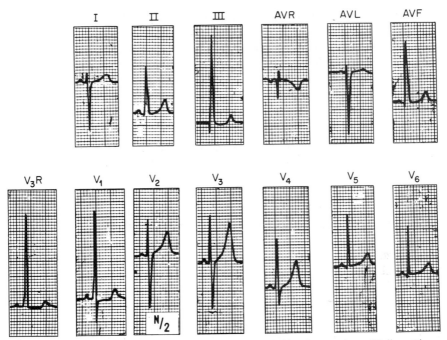

Fig. 10-8 Right ventricular enlargement in a 7-year-old child with a tetralogy of Fallot. There is abnormal right axis deviation ($+120°$). There is a tall R wave in lead V_1, with an R/S ratio of 4.0. Lead aVR shows a QR complex. The T waves are upright in the right precordial leads, which indicates that the degree of hypertrophy is as yet not severe enough to cause T wave inversion.

In the R pattern of right ventricular hypertrophy, the initial and also the remaining QRS vectors are directed rightward anteriorly. The right precordial leads will then show tall R waves and the left precordial leads rS complexes. Occasionally the R pattern results when most of the QRS vectors are directed anteriorly and the terminal forces point posteriorly. All the precordial leads will then show dominant R waves.

In the usual RSR' pattern, the initial QRS vectors are normally directed and are not increased in magnitude. This results in the inscription of an initial r wave in lead V_1. The depth of the S wave depends on the degree to which the succeeding vectors, representing left ventricular potentials, are rotated leftward. The terminal QRS vector, however, is directed rightward, anteriorly, and often inferiorly and may be of increased magnitude. This will cause a final R' to be recorded in lead V_1 and an S wave in leads V_5 and V_6. The right precordial leads will thus show rsR' patterns, the left precordial leads will show qRS complexes, and an $S_1R_2R_3$ pattern will be observed in the standard leads. If the terminal vector is directed rightward and anteriorly, but also superiorly, the standard leads will record an $S_1S_2S_3$ pattern. An rsr' pattern may also be produced by a combination of a normal initial vector, succeeding vectors that are displaced posteriorly, and a final vector which is located sufficiently rightward and anteriorly to project on the positive side of the lead V_1 axis. In this case, rsr' complexes will appear in the right precordial leads and rS complexes in the remaining precordial leads.

In the qR pattern of right ventricular hypertrophy, the initial septal vector, instead of being directed rightward and anteriorly, is displaced leftward so that it falls on the negative portion of the lead V_1 axis. Why this should occur has never been explained. The remaining QRS vectors are directed rightward and anteriorly, which results in a qR pattern in lead V_1 and RS or rS deflections in the left precordial leads.

The pattern of rS complexes in all the precordial leads occurs when there is marked posterior and rightward displacement of the QRS forces, and it results in rS deflections in all the precordial leads.

Usually there is little change in the direction of the S-T and T vectors in right ventricular hypertrophy. However, when hypertrophy is marked, the S-T and T vectors may point leftward and posteriorly away from the lie of the right ventricle and opposite to the direction of the mean QRS vector. This is the right ventricular strain pattern. The right precordial leads and sometimes leads II, III, and aVF show depressed S-T segments and inverted T waves. The mechanism of these S-T segment and T wave changes is unknown.

Diagnosis

The electrocardiogram is frequently normal in the presence of right ventricular enlargement. Abnormalities, when present, may be specific or nonspecific.

Conventional Criteria   The diagnosis of right ventricular enlargement is usually based on the presence of four types of changes in the electrocardiogram: (1) high voltage of those QRS deflections which represent right ventricular potentials, (2) delay in the onset of the intrinsicoid deflection in leads overlying the epicardial surface of the right ventricle, (3) S-T segment and T wave changes in these leads, and (4) abnormal right axis deviation. Criteria for the diagnosis of right ventricular enlargement are usually valid only when the QRS interval is less than 0.12 s.

Voltage of the QRS

Adults

qR or qRs Pattern in Leads V_1 and/or V_{3R}   This pattern is diagnostic of right ventricular enlargement regardless of the amplitude of the deflections, provided preexcitation, myocardial infarction, or the combination of myocardial infarction and right bundle branch block are ruled out.

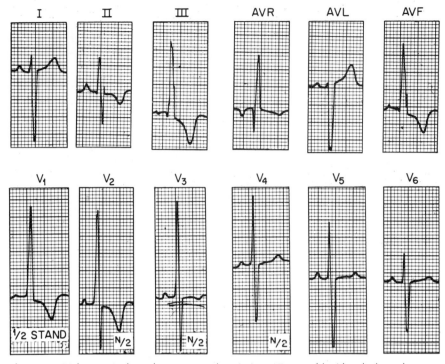

Fig. 10-9 Right ventricular enlargement and strain in a 17-year-old with valvular pulmonary stenosis. There is abnormal right axis deviation ($+140°$). There is an R pattern in lead V_1 and a qR complex in lead aVR. The R/S ratio in lead V_5 is less than 1.0. The T waves are inverted in leads V_1 through V_3. This is an example of systolic overloading of the right ventricle.

R, Rs, or RS Pattern in Leads V_1 and/or V_{3R}   The predominant deflection is a tall and/or broad (0.04 s or more) R wave.

1   The R wave in lead V_1 is 7 mm or more
2   The R/S ratio in lead V_1 is 1.0 or more
3   The R/S ratio in lead V_5 or V_6 is 1.0 or less

R' Pattern (rSr', rsR', rSR', RsR') in Leads V_1 and/or V_{3R} with a Normal QRS Interval   When the primary R wave is more than 8 mm, the secondary R wave exceeds 6 mm, or the R'/S ratio is greater than 1.0 in any of the right-sided precordial leads, right ventricular enlargement is probably present.

In right ventricular enlargement, the R' waves generally persist unchanged or are replaced by abnormally large, notched R waves in leads taken two interspaces below leads V_{3R}, V_1, and V_2. On the other hand, when with an R' pattern in lead V_1 or V_2, or both, the R' wave is absent in V_{3R} or the R' wave in lead V_2 exceeds the R' wave in lead V_{3R} by 1 mm or more, it is probable that the R' wave represents a normal variant. An R'

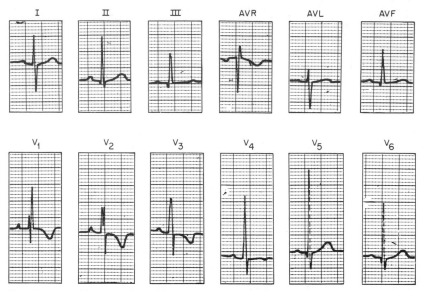

Fig. 10-10   Right ventricular enlargement in a child with an ostium secundum type of atrial septal defect.   The electrical axis is about +90°.   There is an rSR' complex in lead V_1.   The secondary R wave measures 12 mm.   This is an example of diastolic overloading of the right ventricle.

wave of low amplitude in lead V_1 together with a markedly delayed intrinsicoid deflection (0.07 s or more) is more indicative of right bundle branch block than of right ventricular enlargement.

The taller the R' wave and the narrower the associated QRS interval, the greater the likelihood that right ventricular enlargement is the cause of the R' wave.

The rsR' complex found in lead V_1 in patients with atrial septal defect has been shown to represent right ventricular outflow tract hypertrophy.

Incomplete right bundle branch block should be diagnosed in the presence of a QRS duration of 0.09–0.11 s if the R' wave in lead V_1 and the S waves in leads I and V_6 measure 0.04 s or more in width.

rS Pattern in All the Precordial Leads   This pattern is suggestive, but not diagnostic, of right ventricular enlargement.   It may be found in emphysema with or without cor pulmonale.

Children (under 16 Years of Age)

qR or qRs Pattern in Leads V_1 and/or V_{3R}   This pattern is diagnostic of right ventricular enlargement regardless of the amplitude of the deflections, provided preexcitation is ruled out.

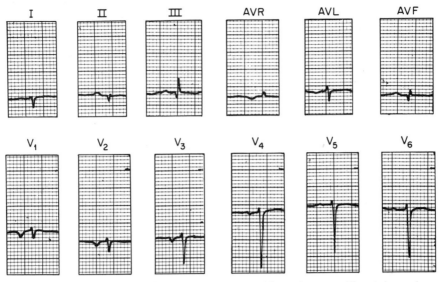

Fig. 10-11   Right ventricular enlargement in a patient with emphysema.   There is low voltage in the extremity leads, with abnormal right axis deviation (+140°).   The P vector is directed inferiorly, and rS complexes are present in all the precordial leads.

R, rR, Rs, or RS Pattern in Leads V_1 and/or V_{3R}

1   The R wave in lead V_1 is 20 mm or more in infants under 1 year of age and is greater than 16 mm in children over this age, or

2   The R/S ratio in lead V_1 exceeds the following values:

Age	Values
0–3 months	6.5
3–6 months	4.0
6 months–3 years	2.4
3–5 years	1.6
6–15 years	1.0

or

3   The R/S ratio in lead V_5 or V_6 is 1.0 or less.

R' Pattern (rSr', rsR', rSR', RsR') in Leads V_1 and/or V_{3R} with a Normal QRS Interval   See the second paragraph under Voltage of the QRS, Adults on page 157.

Intrinsicoid Deflection

The time of onset of the intrinsicoid deflection in lead V_1 or V_2 exceeds 0.03 s in children and is delayed to 0.04 to 0.06 s in adults.   The intrinsicoid deflection in leads V_5 and V_6 is normal.   Measurement of the time of onset

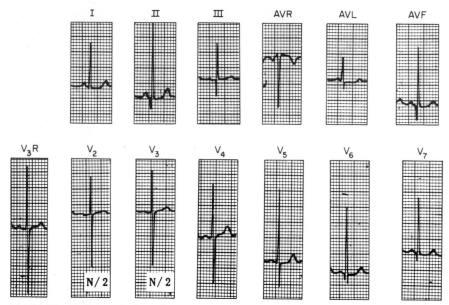

Fig. 10-12   Right ventricular enlargement in a 1-year-old baby.   The only abnormality is a positive T wave in leads V_{3R} and V_1.   A positive T wave in these leads in a child after the second or third day of life is indicative of right ventricular enlargement.

of the intrinsicoid deflection has limited value in the diagnosis of right ventricular enlargement, because when it is delayed, the electrocardiogram usually shows other abnormalities which permit the diagnosis to be made.

S-T Segment and T Wave Changes

The S-T segment is depressed and the T wave is inverted in the right-sided precordial leads and often in leads II, III, and aVF as well.   This is the right ventricular strain pattern, and like the left ventricular strain pattern, it is a nonspecific abnormality.

Abnormal Right Axis Deviation

Abnormal right axis deviation is the commonest sign of right ventricular enlargement.

Right axis deviation of $+100$ or greater in adults is strongly suggestive of right ventricular enlargement in the absence of anterolateral or inferior myocardial infarction, left posterior fascicular block, or right bundle branch block.   Right axis deviation of $+110$ or more in the absence of anterolateral or inferior infarction, left posterior fascicular block or right bundle branch block is usually diagnostic of right ventricular enlargement.   However, right ventricular enlargement may occur without abnormal right axis deviation.

Right axis deviation to the right of $+120°$ in children from 3 months to 16 years of age is strongly suggestive of right ventricular enlargement. In infants under 1 month of age, marked right axis deviation is probably present if the mean electrical axis lies to the right of $+140°$.

When the R_3 and S_1 waves have high voltage, the probability that the right axis deviation is caused by right ventricular enlargement is increased.

Other Patterns

Atrial Enlargement

Right atrial enlargement is often an indirect sign of right ventricular enlargement. In older children and adults, in the absence of left ventricular enlargement, the presence of left atrial enlargement (e.g., in mitral stenosis) should lead to a careful search for electrocardiographic evidence of right ventricular enlargement.

Right Bundle Branch Block

Right bundle branch block may be a manifestation of right ventricular enlargement but is more often due to other causes.

Positive T Wave in Lead V_1

A positive T wave in lead V_1 from the third or fourth day of life to the twelfth year, particularly when associated with an R/S ratio greater than 1.0 in this lead, is strongly suggestive of right ventricular enlargement.

qR Pattern in Lead aVR

A qR pattern with an R wave of 5 mm or more and with a Q/R ratio less than 1.0 is suggestive of right ventricular enlargement (especially in children), but it may also occur in other conditions associated with marked superior deviation of the mean QRS vector.

Deep S Wave Syndrome

Deep S waves in the right- and mid-precordial leads are usually associated with left ventricular enlargement. However, such deep S waves are sometimes the result of right ventricular enlargement. Clues to the right-sided origin of such deflections are right axis deviation and the presence of a dominant R wave in lead V_{3R}, V_{4R}, or both.

Shallow S Wave Syndrome

A shallow S wave in lead V_1 (particularly if it is 2.0 mm or less) associated with a small R wave in this lead and relatively deep S waves in leads V_2

and V_3, especially in the presence of right axis deviation, is suggestive of right ventricular enlargement. However, a small S wave in lead V_1 is sometimes a normal variant. The presence of a shallow S wave in lead V_1 in association with signs of left ventricular enlargement suggests the diagnosis of biventricular hypertrophy.

R/S Ratio in the Right Precordial Leads

A drop in the R/S ratio between any two consecutive leads to the right of the transition zone may be an early sign of right ventricular enlargement.

Summary

Probable right ventricular enlargement may be diagnosed when the electrocardiogram shows increased voltage of those deflections representing right ventricular potentials, R'/S or R/S ratio abnormalities in lead V_1 and/ or the left precordial leads as listed above, or right axis deviation greater than 100° in older adults in the absence of other possible causes for this condition. The greater the number of such abnormalities in any tracing, the greater the likelihood that right ventricular enlargement is present.

Definite right ventricular enlargement may be diagnosed when leads V_1 and/or V_{3R} show a dominant R wave (Rs, R, rR', qR, qRs, QR) with R exceeding normal values and with an R/S ratio greater than 1.0, in the absence of other causes for this abnormality. When there is an R' pattern (rsr', rSR', RSR') in leads V_1 and/or V_{3R} with a QRS interval less than 0.12 s, right ventricular enlargement may be diagnosed if there is increased voltage of the R or R' waves and the R'/S or R/S ratio is greater than 1.0 in V_1 or the R/S ratio in V_5 or V_6 is less than 1.0. Abnormal right axis deviation of +110° or more in adults is diagnostic of right ventricular enlargement in the absence of myocardial infarction or right bundle branch block. In children from 3 months to 16 years, right axis deviation of +120° or more is virtually diagnostic of right ventricular enlargement. The diagnosis of right ventricular enlargement is further supported by the presence of the right ventricular strain pattern and by a delayed onset of the intrinsicoid deflection in lead V_1 or V_2.

Another approach to the diagnosis of right ventricular enlargement is the use of a point score system as shown in Table 10-1.

Comments on the Electrocardiographic Diagnosis

Conventional Criteria   The electrocardiographic diagnosis of right ventricular enlargement is even less accurate than that of left ventricular enlargement. The value of the criteria listed above, as well as those proposed by others, is limited by the inclusion of a significant number of false-positive and false-negative diagnoses. The use of less rigid criteria results in fewer

TABLE 10-1   ELECTROCARDIOGRAPHIC CRITERIA OF RIGHT VENTRICULAR ENLARGEMENT IN ADULTS WITHOUT CONDUCTION DEFECTS KNOWN NOT TO HAVE INFARCTION

Sign	Points
Ratio reversal (R/S V_5: R/S $V_1 \leqq 0.4$)	5
qR in V_1	5
R/S ratio in $V_1 > 1$	4
S in $V_1 < 2$mm	4
R in V_1 + S in V_5 or $V_6 > 10.5$ mm	4
Right axis deviation $> 110°$	4
S in V_5 or $V_6 \geqq 7$ mm and each $\geqq 2$ mm	3
R/S in V_5 or $V_6 \leqq 1$	3
R in $V_1 \geqq 7$ mm	3
$S_1, S_2,$ and S_3 each $\geqq 1$ mm	2
S_1 and Q_3 each $\geqq 1$ mm	2
R' in V_1 earlier than 0.08 s and $\geqq 2$ mm	2
R peak in V_1 or V_2 between 0.04 and 0.07 s	1
S in V_5 or $V_6 \geqq 2$ mm but < 7 mm	1
Reduction in V lead R/S ratio between V_1 and V_4	1
R in V_5 or $v_6 < 5$ mm	1

Interpretation of point score:
   10 points: Right ventricular enlargement
   7 to 9 points: Probable right ventricular enlargement or hemodynamic overload
   5 to 6 points: Possible right ventricular enlargement or hemodynamic overload
These criteria do not take into account serial electrocardiographic comparisons. Such additional data may alter the interpreter's impression of the likelihood of fixed enlargement or dynamic overload.
SOURCE: Horan, L. G. and N. C. Flowers, page 226, in E. Braunwald (ed): "Heart Disease: A Textbook of Cardiovascular Medicine," W. B. Saunders Co., Philadelphia, 1980. Used by permission.

false-negative diagnoses but in a greater number of false-positive diagnoses. The reverse is true if more stringent criteria are employed. Another limiting factor with respect to most of the criteria in the literature is their lack of applicability to the electrocardiograms of both children and adults. Separate criteria have been listed, therefore, for the diagnosis of right ventricular enlargement in children and adults.

Right Axis Deviation   The diagnosis of right ventricular enlargement should not be based on this finding alone unless it is clearly abnormal and other causes for right axis deviation are ruled out. Aside from its occurrence as a normal variant, right axis deviation may be seen in emphysema with or without cor pulmonale, anterolateral myocardial infarction, left posterior hemiblock, and inferior myocardial infarction with left posterior hemiblock.

Tall and/or Broad R Waves in Leads V_1 and/or V_{3R} Abnormally tall and/or broad initial R waves in lead V_1 or V_{3R} are not pathognomonic of right ventricular enlargement, since they may also occur in strictly posterior myocardial infarction, right bundle branch block, and preexcitation and as a reciprocal effect of deep Q waves in the left precordial leads or as a normal variant. The differential diagnosis of these conditions is discussed below and in the section on the differential diagnosis of strictly posterior myocardial infarction in Chap. 13.

R' Waves in Leads V_1 and/or V_{3R} with a Normal QRS Interval   This finding is not pathognomonic of right ventricular enlargement. It may occur in normal persons, the $S_1S_2S_3$ syndrome, left anterior hemiblock, strictly posterior myocardial infarction, acute cor pulmonale, pulmonary emphysema with or without cor pulmonale, and incomplete right bundle branch block. The differential diagnosis of these entities is discussed later in this chapter.

Pseudoinfarction Patterns in Right Ventricular Enlargement   Right ventricular enlargement may mimic anteroseptal infarction when there is a loss of the initial R wave or the presence of small Q waves in the right- and mid-precordial leads. Acute cor pulmonale commonly produces a pseudoinfarction pattern with Q waves in leads III, aVF, and sometimes II.

Left Posterior Fascicular Block   This condition may mimic right ventricular enlargement because it produces right axis deviation, an S_1Q_3 pattern, and tall R waves in leads II, III, and aVF. Left posterior fascicular block occurs much less frequently than right ventricular enlargement and is often associated with right bundle branch block. In order to diagnose left posterior fascicular block, a vertical heart, emphysema, right ventricular enlargement, and anterolateral infarction must be excluded on clinical grounds.

Differential Diagnosis of an RSR' Complex in Lead V_1 with a Normal QRS Interval

Normal   An RSR' complex may occur normally in lead V_1. The normal RSR' complex is usually not more than 0.08 s wide. When the RSR' complex is normal, the primary R wave is 8 mm or less, the secondary R wave is 6 mm or less, and the R'/S ratio is less than 1.0 in any lead from the right side of the precordium. Normal R' waves tend to disappear when additional right lower-chest leads are taken. However, abnormal R' waves persist unchanged or are replaced by an abnormally large, notched R wave in these additional leads. Furthermore, when an R' wave occurs in lead V_1 or V_2, or in both, its absence in lead V_{3R} or the presence of an R' wave in lead V_2 that is 1.0 mm taller than the R' deflection in lead V_{3R} suggests that the secondary R wave represents a normal variant.

$S_1S_2S_3$ Syndrome   This is characterized by deep S waves in the three standard limb leads. The $S_1S_2S_3$ syndrome may occur as a normal variant but is also seen in congenital or acquired right ventricular enlargement, emphysema with or without cor pulmonale, and myocardial infarction. In the $S_1S_2S_3$ syndrome, the terminal QRS vector is primarily directed rightward and superiorly, but if it is anteriorly directed as well, R' waves will appear in the right precordial leads.

Right Ventricular Enlargement   In this condition, the voltages of the primary and/or secondary R waves exceed the normal values given under Normal (above) and/or the R'/S ratio is greater than 1.0 in at least one of the right precordial leads. Furthermore, if additional right lower-chest leads are taken, the R' wave usually persists unchanged or is replaced by an abnormally large, notched R deflection. The terminal QRS vector is directed rightward, anteriorly, and usually inferiorly, so that right axis deviation is present.

Left Anterior Fascicular Block   This condition is characterized by mean and terminal QRS vectors that are primarily directed leftward and superiorly and produce abnormal left axis deviation. Should the vector be directed sufficiently anteriorly, an R' wave may be inscribed in a right precordial lead. However, since the initial QRS vector is of normal duration, abnormal Q waves do not occur. Leads aVL and I show qR patterns and leads II, III, and aVF show rS deflections. Concomitant signs of left ventricular enlargement may or may not be present.

Anterior Infarction with Left Anterior Fascicular Block   This condition is characterized by a terminal QRS vector that is directed leftward and superiorly, which results in abnormal left axis deviation. An R' wave may be present in the right precordial leads if the vector is also anteriorly directed. However, the initial QRS vector is abnormally wide, which results in the presence of 0.04-s Q waves in leads aVL and I and broad R waves in the inferior extremity leads when the infarct is lateral. Abnormal Q waves may also be present in the left precordial leads.

Strictly Posterior Myocardial Infarction   The ventricular complex in the right precordial leads in strictly posterior myocardial infarction consists either of a broad and/or tall R wave or of an RSR' or rR complex. The initial QRS vector points anteriorly. The clinical picture and the vector-cardiogram, which shows CCW rotation and anterior displacement of the QRS vector loop, may be of further aid in the diagnosis of this entity.

Acute Cor Pulmonale   An RSR' complex in lead V_1 may occur transiently in acute cor pulmonale. The rapidly changing electrocardiographic pattern, the presence of other abnormalities seen in acute cor pulmonale, and the clinical history are helpful diagnostically.

Emphysema with or without Cor Pulmonale   The clinical features and the presence of other electrocardiographic abnormalities seen in this condition are useful in establishing emphysema as the cause of an RSR' pattern in lead V_1.

Incomplete Right Bundle Branch Block   Right bundle branch block is difficult to diagnose and differentiate from right ventricular enlargement in the absence of prolongation of the QRS interval.   There is still controversy as to whether the RSR' pattern with a QRS interval of less than 0.12 s is a true incomplete right bundle branch block or whether it is related to a focal hypertrophy of the right ventricle.   According to Scott, when the R' in lead V_1 is 0.04 s or longer in duration, in association with S waves of similar duration in lead I, incomplete right bundle branch block should be diagnosed.   If, in addition, the criteria for right ventricular hypertrophy are fulfilled, this diagnosis should be added.   The diagnosis of right ventricular hypertrophy in the presence of incomplete right bundle branch block based on the voltage of the secondary R wave in lead V_1 is not secure but is more reliable in children than in adults.

Comment   It is not always possible to differentiate between the various causes of an RSR' pattern in lead V_1.   In doubtful cases, the vectorcardiogram may be helpful in establishing the correct diagnosis (Fig. 10-13).

Vectorelectrocardiographic Criteria

Right ventricular enlargement may take any or a combination of three forms:

1   Right axis deviation
2   Marked rightward and anterior direction of the initial QRS vector, resulting in an initial R wave in lead V_1 that is taller or broader, or both, than normal
3   Marked rightward, anterior, and inferior direction of the terminal QRS vector, resulting in an R' wave of increased amplitude in lead V_1

Right Ventricular Dilatation

Right ventricular dilatation may occur conjointly with right ventricular hypertrophy, or it may occur acutely in the absence of right ventricular hypertrophy.

The following electrocardiographic findings, especially if reversible, are suggestive of right ventricular dilatation:

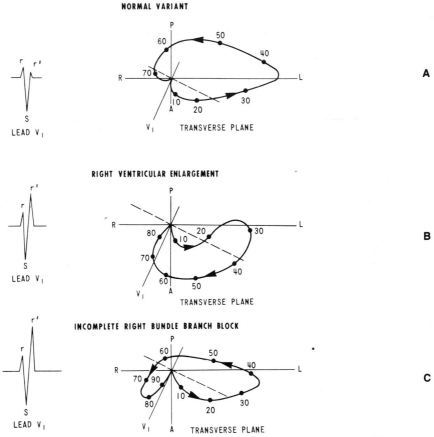

Fig. 10-13 The value of the vectorcardiogram in the differential diagnosis of an RSR' complex in lead V₁ with a QRS duration of less than 0.12 s. The relationship between the TP vector loop and lead V₁ is shown. An RSR' complex in lead V₁ may result from different causes: (A) normal variant, in which a *CCW* loop is written whose initial and terminal deflection are directed rightward and anteriorly but in which there is *no terminal conduction delay;* (B) right ventricular enlargement, in which the initial and terminal portions of the *CW-inscribed* loop are directed rightward and anteriorly; and (C) incomplete right bundle branch block, in which the normal initial and *slowly inscribed terminal portions* of the loop are also directed rightward and anteriorly but in which the inscription of the loop is *CCW*.

1   The right ventricular strain pattern
2   An rS pattern in the right and sometimes also in the left precordial leads with a shift in the transition zone to the left
3   Rarely, a QR pattern in lead V₃ᵣ or V₁, or both, in connection with 1 and 2 above
4   Complete or incomplete right bundle branch block

Right Ventricular Enlargement and Bundle Branch Block

The diagnosis of right ventricular enlargement in the presence of bundle branch block is discussed in Chap. 11.

Right Ventricular Enlargement and Primary ST-T Abnormalities

The presence of T wave inversion in the left precordial leads is suggestive of ischemia unless right ventricular enlargement is extreme.   T wave inversion in leads I and aVL is also probably ischemic in the presence of right ventricular hypertrophy.   On the other hand T wave inversion in the right precordial or inferior limb leads may be part of the electrocardiographic pattern of right ventricular enlargement, so that ischemia in these regions is difficult to diagnose in the presence of right ventricular hypertrophy.

THE VECTORCARDIOGRAM IN RIGHT VENTRICULAR HYPERTROPHY (FIG. 10-14)

Anterior displacement of the TP QRS loop and reversal of rotation from CCW to CW are the characteristic findings of right ventricular hypertrophy. In some instances of right ventricular hypertrophy, however, although there is anterior displacement of the QRS loop in this plane, CCW rotation is preserved.   In still others, the QRS loop in the TP is oriented posteriorly and inscribed in CCW fashion.   There is thus a great deal of variation in the configuration, inscription, and orientation of the QRS loop in right ventricular hypertrophy.

The findings in the TP are the most significant from a diagnostic standpoint.

The QRS loops in right ventricular hypertrophy may be classified into three groups (Chou, Helm, and Kaplan): Type I, Type II, and Type III.

Type I QRS Loop   In the TP, the QRS loop is displaced anteriorly and rightward so that most of the loop is located in the right anterior quadrant.

Rotation of the QRS loop is characteristically CW, or if the loop presents a figure-of-eight configuration, inscription of the initial portion is CCW and that of the distal portion CW.

The 0.03QRS and 0.04QRS vectors are directed more rightward and anteriorly than in the normal.

The terminal vectors are directed rightward and anteriorly.

In the FP, inscription of the loop is almost always CW. In the LSP, it is usually CW.

The S-T vector is generally small.   The T loop is usually directed posteriorly and leftward, and its inscription is usually CW.

The Type I QRS loop is often encountered in congenital heart disease. It may also occur in mitral stenosis and in cor pulmonale due to emphysema.

TRANSVERSE PLANE

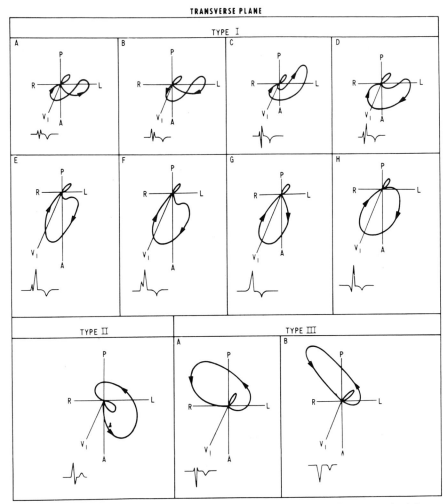

Fig. 10-14   The vectorcardiogram in right ventricular enlargement.   The seemingly different configurations of the right-sided precordial leads in Type I right ventricular enlargement are actually very closely related, as seen from an inspection of the QRS vector loops.   The differences lie chiefly in the extent to which the CW-inscribed vector loops are deviated anteriorly and rightward.   In Type II, the QRS loop is displaced anteriorly but is rotated CCW. In Type III, rotation of the loop is CCW, but much of the loop is displaced posteriorly and rightward.

Type II QRS Loop   In the TP, the QRS loop shows forward displacement. One-half or more of the loop area is located anteriorly.   Usually the loop is large and broad.   Rotation of the loop is CCW.

The 0.03QRS and 0.04QRS vectors are directed more anteriorly and rightward than in the normal.

Inscription of the loop is usually CCW in the LSP and CW in the FP.

The S-T vector and T loop show little change.

The Type II loop is usually associated with mild to moderate degrees of right ventricular hypertrophy.

Type III QRS Loop   In the TP, the QRS loop, which may be broad or narrow, shows backward and rightward displacement so that 20 percent or more of the loop area is located in the right posterior quadrant.

Inscription of the QRS loop is usually CCW, although sometimes the loop presents a figure-of-eight appearance.

Inscription of the loop in the LSP is variable; in the FP, it is usually CW.

The S-T vector and T loop are usually unremarkable.

The Type III QRS loop is usually associated with cor pulmonale due to emphysema, mitral stenosis, and occasionally ostium primum defects.

COMBINED VENTRICULAR HYPERTROPHY, OR ENLARGEMENT
(FIGS. 10-15, 10-16)

Combine ventricular enlargement is a diagnosis that is very difficult to establish with certainty, particularly in adults.   Oftentimes the electrocardiogram will show evidence of enlargement of only one of the hypertrophied ventricles.   At other times the potentials from the two hypertrophied

Fig. 10-15 Biventricular enlargement and digitalis effect.   There is right axis deviation (+120°), and qRS patterns with inverted T waves are seen in leads V_{3R} and V_1, which indicate right ventricular enlargement.   However, the sum of the R_{V5} and S_{V2} waves and the depth of the S wave in lead V_2 exceed normal values, so that left ventricular enlargement is also present.   The contour of the S-T segments, particularly in the left precordial leads, together with the relatively short Q-T interval, is indicative of digitalis effect.

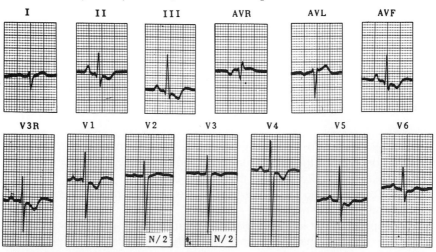

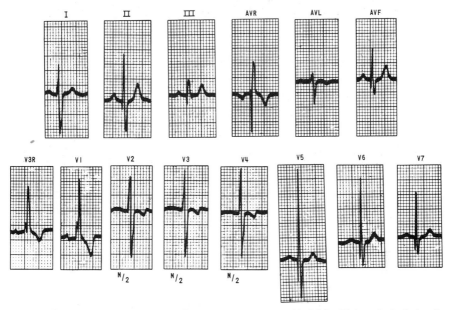

Fig. 10-16 Combined ventricular enlargement in a 6-year-old child.   Right axis deviation is present.   There is an abnormally tall rR' complex in lead V_1, which indicates right ventricular enlargement.   The Q waves are unusually deep in the left precordial leads, owing to septal hypertrophy.   The sum of the R_{V_5} and S_{V_2} waves exceeds 60 mm.   The last finding is diagnostic of left ventricular enlargement.

ventricles may counterbalance each other so that the electrocardiogram may appear normal.

Diagnosis

Biventricular enlargement may be suspected under the following circumstances:

1 The precordial leads show voltage changes diagnostic of both right and left ventricular enlargement.

2 The electrocardiogram shows definite evidence of right ventricular enlargement plus one or more of the following signs:

a High voltage of the R wave in lead V_5 or V_6, especially if the intrinsicoid deflection is delayed, the S-T segment is depressed, and the T wave is inverted in these leads or the sum of the R wave in lead V_5 or V_6 and of the S wave in lead V_1 or V_2 exceeds the normal range for the age of the individual

b Deep Q waves in the left precordial leads and/or in leads II, III, and aVF

c Large equiphasic QRS complexes in the midprecordial leads and/or in two or more limb leads (Katz-Wachtel sign)

3 The electrocardiogram shows definite evidence of left ventricular enlargement plus one or more of the following signs:
a Right axis deviation
b A significant R or R' wave in lead V_1 and/or an R/S or an R'/S ratio greater than 1.0 in this lead
c A tall R wave, 5 mm or more, in lead aVR with a Q/R ratio less than 1.0
d A deep S wave in lead V_5 or V_6, or both
4 The electrocardiogram shows the shallow S wave syndrome described by Scott, consisting of a very shallow S wave in lead V_1 in association with a deep S wave in lead V_2, small R waves in these leads, relatively tall R waves over the left precordium, and displacement of the transition zone to the left.
5 A normal electrocardiogram in the presence of marked cardiac enlargement demonstrable by other means should suggest diagnosis of biventricular enlargement.

The Vectorcardiogram in Combined Ventricular Hypertrophy

No satisfactory criteria are available for the vectorcardiographic diagnosis of biventricular hypertrophy.

The increased electric potentials from the hypertrophied ventricles may counterbalance each other, resulting in an essentially normal QRS loop. In some instances the preponderance of one ventricle (usually the left) produces a vectorcardiogram suggestive of hypertrophy of that ventricle alone.

Chou, Helm, and Kaplan have found the following changes helpful in the diagnosis: (1) the presence of large anterior forces in the QRS loop with the maximum voltage greater than 0.6 mV when the loop is otherwise typical of left ventricular enlargement, (2) large right posterior forces with the QRS loop area in the right posterior quadrant greater than 20 percent of the total in a vectorcardiogram otherwise typical of left ventricular hypertrophy, and (3) CW or CCW rotation of the QRS loop in the TP suggesting right ventricular hypertrophy in association with a CCW loop in the FP.

Benchimol's criteria for the diagnosis of biventricular hypertrophy are as follows: (1) the presence of large posterior forces in the SP and TP, a maxQRS vector exceeding 2.2 mV, and CW rotation of the FP QRS loop; (2) a maxQRS vector in the FP between $+70°$ and $+140°$ with CW rotation and predominantly posteriorly directed forces in the TP with the maxQRS vector exceeding 2.2 mV; and (3) a maxQRS anterior vector in the TP greater than 0.08 mV associated with a maximum posterior vector in this plane more than 2.2 mV.

Varriale et al. have reported that in approximately two-thirds of cases with known biventricular hypertrophy there was abnormal posterior displacement of a CCW QRS loop in the TP, associated usually with right axis deviation and CW inscription of the loop in the FP.

SYSTOLIC AND DIASTOLIC OVERLOADING OF THE VENTRICLES

The concept of systolic and diastolic overloading of the right and left ventricles proposed by Cabrera and Monroy is an attempt to correlate electrocardiographic patterns of enlargement with the associated hemo-dynamic alterations. Experience has shown that although the correlation is frequently useful, it is not always accurate or reliable. The electrocar-diogram, therefore, cannot substitute for definitive hemodynamic studies.

The concept is predicated on the assumption that the ventricular response to pressure work in systole is different from response to flow work in diastole and that this difference is recognizable in the electrocardiogram. The term *systolic overloading* indicates that the ventricle is contracting against abnormally high resistance during systole. The ventricle responds by increased contraction forces during systolic ejection, which ultimately leads to the development of concentric hypertrophy. The term *diastolic overloading* indicates that the ventricle is contracting against an increased residual blood volume in diastole, which results from either increased flow or valvular insufficiency. The greater the diastolic filling, the greater the initial length of the fibers and hence the more powerful the cardiac contraction. The basic compensation is ventricular dilatation and increased stroke volume.

Systolic Overloading of the Right Ventricle (Figs. 10-9, 23-4)

Systolic overloading of the right ventricle occurs primarily in such congenital lesions as isolated pulmonary stenosis and the tetralogy of Fallot and in such acquired lesions as mitral stenosis, cor pulmonale, and pulmonary hypertension.

Electrocardiographic Findings

1 Right axis deviation.
2 High voltage of the R wave in lead V_1 or V_{3R} with an RS, Rs, qR, qRs,R, or rR complex. The R wave is often tall in lead aVR as well.
3 The right ventricular strain pattern with depression of the S-T segment and T wave inversion in leads V_1, V_2, and V_3, and often in leads II, III, and aVF as well.

Diastolic Overloading of the Right Ventricle (Fig. 10-10)

Diastolic overloading of the right ventricle occurs chiefly in uncomplicated ostium secundum defects, anomalous pulmonary venous drainage, and tricuspid insufficiency.

Electrocardiographic Findings

1   An R' complex in lead V_1 or V_{3R} associated with right axis deviation, a delayed intrinsicoid deflection, and a QRS complex which is of either normal or increased duration.
2   The association of an R' complex in lead V_1 or V_{3R} with left axis deviation is strongly suggestive of an ostium primum defect or atrio-ventricularis communis, or both, although there are other causes for this pattern.

Systolic Overloading of the Left Ventricle (Figs. 10-3, 10-4)

Systolic overloading of the left ventricle occurs most frequently in essential hypertension, aortic stenosis, and coarctation of the aorta.

Electrocardiographic Findings

1   The Q wave in lead V_6 is usually less than 2 mm in depth.
2   There is high voltage of the R waves in leads V_5 and V_6 and of the S waves in leads V_1 and V_2.
3   The left ventricular strain pattern is present, with depressed S-T segments and inverted T waves in the left precordial leads and usually in leads I and aVL as well.

Diastolic Overloading of the Left Ventricle (Figs. 10-1, 10-2)

Diastolic overloading of the left ventricle occurs in such conditions as ventricular septal defect, patent ductus arteriosus with left-to-right shunt, peripheral arteriovenous fistula, and aortic and mitral insufficiency.

Electrocardiographic Findings

1   The Q wave in lead V_6 is usually 2 mm or more in depth.
2   There is high voltage of the R waves in leads V_5 and V_6 and of the S waves in leads V_1 and V_2.
3   The T waves are tall and peaked in leads V_5 and V_6.

Comments

While the concept of systolic and diastolic overloading of the right and left ventricles is attractive on theoretical grounds, its clinical usefulness is limited.   For example, systolic overloading of the right ventricle in some cases of valvular pulmonary stenosis and the tetralogy of Fallot may be manifested by the appearance of R' complexes in the right precordial leads. Conversely, some ostium secundum defects may show electrocardiographic evidence of systolic overloading instead of diastolic overloading.   Further-more, high voltage of the R waves in the left precordial leads, with or without S-T segment and T wave changes, may occur in both systolic and diastolic overloading of the left ventricle and even in their absence.

REFERENCES

Allenstein, B. J., and H. Mori: Evaluation of Electrocardiographic Diagnosis of Ventricular Hypertrophy Based on Autopsy Comparison, *Circulation*, 21: 401, 1960.

Benchimol, A.: "Vectorcardiography," Williams & Wilkins, Baltimore, 1973.

Cabrera, E. C., and A. Gaxiola: A Critical Re-evaluation of Systolic and Diastolic Overloading Patterns, *Progr. Cardiovasc. Dis.*, 2: 219, 1959–1960.

―――― and J. R. Monroy: Systolic and Diastolic Overloading of the Heart. I. Physiologic and Clinical Data, *Am. Heart J.*, 43: 661, 1952.

―――― and ――――: Systolic and Diastolic Overloading of the Heart. II. Electrocardiographic Data, *Am. Heart J.*, 43: 669, 1952.

Chou, T-C., R. A. Helm, and S. Kaplan: "Spatial Vectorcardiography," 2d ed., Grune & Stratton, New York, 1974.

Cueto, J., H. Toshima, G. Armijo, N. Tuna, and C. W. Lillehei: Vectorcardiographic Studies in Acquired Valvular Disease with Reference to the Diagnosis of Right Ventricular Hypertrophy, *Circulation*, 33: 588, 1966.

Gamboa, R., P. G. Hugenholtz, and A. S. Nadas: Corrected (Frank), Uncorrected (Cube), and Standard Electrocardiographic Lead Systems in Recording Augmented Right Ventricular Forces in Right Ventricular Hypertension, *Brit. Heart J.*, 28: 62, 1966.

Griep, A. H.: Pitfalls in the Electrocardiographic Diagnosis of Left Ventricular Hypertrophy, *Circulation*, 20: 30, 1959.

Holt, D. H., and D. H. Spodick: The R_{V6}: R_{V5} Voltage Ratio in Left Ventricular Hypertrophy, *Am. Heart J.*, 63: 1962.

Klein, R. C., Z. Vera, A. Neumann, A. N. DeMaria, and D. T. Mason: Electrocardiographic Diagnosis of Left Ventricular Enlargement in the Presence of Left Bundle Branch Block, *Circulation*, Part II, 58: 766, 1978.

Kossman, C. E., H. B. Burchell, R. D. Pruitt, and R. C. Scott: The Electrocardiogram in Ventricular Hypertrophy and Bundle-branch Block, *Circulation*, 26: 1337, 1962.

Lasser, R. P.: Diagnostic Application of the Electrocardiogram: Systolic and Diastolic Overload Patterns of Right and Left Ventricular Enlargement, in A. M. Master and E. Donoso (eds.), "Visual Aids in Cardiological Diagnosis," chap 6, Grune & Stratton, New York, 1960.

Liu, C. K., and D. De Cristofaro: Sensitivity and Specificity of Electrocardiographic Evaluation of LVH in 364 Unselected Autopsy Cases, *Am. Heart J.*, 76: 596, 1968.

McPhie, J.: Left Ventricular Hypertrophy: Electrocardiographic Diagnosis, *Australasian Ann. Med.*, 7: 317, 1958.

Milnor, W. R.: Electrocardiogram and Vectorcardiogram in Right Ventricular Hypertrophy and Right Bundle-branch Block, *Circulation*, 16: 348, 1957.

Ray, C. T., L. G. Horan, and N. C. Flowers: An Early Sign of Right Ventricular Enlargement, *J. Electrocardiol.*, 3: 57, 1970.

Roman, G. T., T. J. Walsh, and E. Massie: Right Ventricular Hypertrophy: Correlation of Electrocardiographic and Anatomic Findings, *Am. J. Cardiol.,* 7: 481, 1961.

Romhilt, D. W., and E. H. Estes, Jr.: A Point-score System for the EGG Diagnosis of Left Ventricular Hypertrophy, *Am. Heart J.,* 75: 752, 1968.

————, K. E. Bove, R. J. Norris, E. Conyers, S. Conradi, D. T. Rowlands, and R. C. Scott: A Clinical Appraisal of the Electrocardiographic Criteria for the Diagnosis of Left Ventricular Hypertrophy, *Circulation,* 40: 185, 1969.

————, J. C. Greenfield, Jr., and E. H. Estes, Jr.: Vectorcardiographic Diagnosis of Left Ventricular Hypertrophy, *Circulation,* 37: 15, 1968.

Scott, R. C.: The Electrocardiographic Diagnosis of Right Ventricular Hypertrophy in the Adult, *Heart Bull.,* 16:65, 1967.

————: The Correlation between the Electrocardiographic Patterns of Ventricular Hypertrophy and the Anatomic Findings, *Circulation,* 21:256, 1960.

————: Ventricular Hypertrophy, *Cardiovasc. Clin.,* 5(3): 219, 1973.

Shubin, H., and D. C. Levinson: The Deep S Wave in Leads V_1, V_2, and V_3 in Right Ventricular Hypertrophy, *Circulation,* 18: 410, 1958.

Sokolow, M., and T. P. Lyon: The Ventricular Complex in Left Ventricular Hypertrophy as Obtained by Unipolar Precordial and Limbs Leads, *Am. Heart J.,* 37:16 1949.

———— and ————: The Ventricular Complex in Right Ventricular Hypertrophy as Obtained by Unipolar Precordial and Limb Leads, *Am. Heart J.,* 38: 273, 1949.

Varriale, P., J. C. Alfenito, and R. J. Kennedy: The Vectorcardiogram of Left Ventricular Hypertrophy, *Circulation,* 33: 569, 1966.

———— and R. J. Kennedy: The Vectorcardiogram of Combined Ventricular Hypertrophy: Posterior Counterclockwise Loops (Frank System), *Brit. Heart J.,* 31: 457, 1969.

Walker, C. H. M., and R. L. Rose: Importance of Age, Sex and Body Habitus in the Diagnosis of Left Ventricular Hypertrophy from the Precordial Electrocardiogram in Childhood and Adolescence, *Pediatrics,* 28: 705, 1961.

CHAPTER 11

VENTRICULAR
CONDUCTION DEFECTS

In clinical electrocardiography, bundle branch block patterns with a QRS duration of 0.12 s or more are arbitrarily designated as *complete* and those with a QRS duration less than 0.12 s as *incomplete*.

The separation is arbitrary, but it is useful. Ordinarily, when the QRS interval is prolonged to 0.12 s or more in bundle branch block, ventricular depolarization is so altered that it is difficult or impossible to make the additional diagnosis of right or left ventricular hypertrophy. This is particularly true in the case of left bundle branch block. However, when the block is incomplete, the usual criteria for hypertrophy are applicable.

CLASSIFICATION

Ventricular conduction defects may be classified as follows:

1 Right bundle branch block
2 Left bundle branch block
a Predivisional, or block in the main left bundle branch
b Divisional, or simultaneous block in both divisions of the left bundle branch
3 Diffuse intraventricular block
4 Nonspecific intraventricular block (intramyocardial or intramural block)
5 Left anterior fascicular block
6 Left posterior fascicular block

7   Right bundle branch block with left anterior fascicular block
8   Right bundle branch block with left posterior fascicular block
9   Left bundle branch block with left anterior fascicular block
10 Left bundle branch block with left posterior fascicular block
11 Bilateral bundle branch block, or simultaneous block in the two main bundle branches.
12 Trifascicular block, or simultaneous block in the right bundle branch and the two fascicles of the left bundle branch.

ANATOMIC BASIS OF VENTRICULAR CONDUCTION DEFECTS

The same diseases which produce complete AV block can also cause bundle branch block. However, bundle branch block is found most frequently in coronary heart disease, hypertension, and aortic valve disease. Although complete heart block is commonly idiopathic in origin, this is not true of bundle branch block. The only exception is bifascicular block.

Anatomic lesions in the conduction system are demonstrable in most cases of bundle branch block except for incomplete right bundle branch block. In the latter condition, no pathologic changes can be found. However, in complete right bundle branch block and in both complete and incomplete left bundle branch block, fibroelastic replacement of cells can be found in most cases. In unilateral bundle branch block, lesions are often seen in the contralateral bundle branch as well, but these are apt to be less pronounced.

It should be emphasized that occasional cases of bundle branch block show no lesions in the conduction system and that severe disease of the conduction system may sometimes exist without electrocardiographic evidence of bundle branch block.

The pathologic findings in bilateral and "masquerading" bundle branch block consist of lesions of both bundle branches.

In left anterior fascicular block with or without concomitant right bundle branch block, there is poor correlation with specific involvement of the anterior fascicle. More often, the fascicular block appears related to more generalized lesions of the left bundle branch. On the other hand, the lesions underlying the pattern of left posterior fascicular block are less disseminated and are generally limited to the posterior fascicle.

RIGHT BUNDLE BRANCH BLOCK

Theoretical Considerations (Fig. 11-1)

It is generally agreed by authorities that in right bundle branch block, the cardiac vector is not significantly altered during the first 0.06 to 0.08 s of

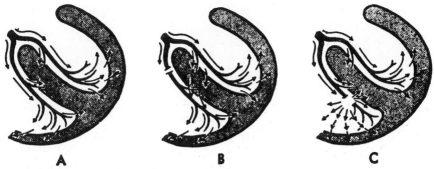

Fig. 11-1 Theories of the mechanism of right bundle branch block. The common bundle and the right and left bundle branches are shown. (*A*) Normal ventricular conduction. (*B*) Classical theory of right bundle branch block with the block located early in the course of the right bundle branch. Excitation crosses the septum from the left bundle and regains entrance into the right bundle below the site of the block. (*C*) Grant's theory, with excitation leaking from the site of the block to stimulate the blocked region of the right ventricle by direct intramyocardial spread. The site of the block is more distal along the course of the right bundle branch. Other explanations of the mechanism of right bundle branch block are mentioned in the text. *(From R. P. Grant, "Clinical Electrocardiography," © 1957 by McGraw-Hill, Inc., New York. Used with permission of McGraw-Hill Book Company.)*

the QRS interval but is abnormal during the final 0.04 to 0.08 (average 0.06) s of the QRS interval. This abnormal terminal QRS vector is directed rightward and anteriorly and is responsible for the inscription of an R′ wave in the right precordial leads and of a final wide S wave in lead I and the left precordial leads.

Authorities agree that the left ventricle is activated normally and that septal activation takes place entirely in a left-to-right direction. The site of the block is disputed. Some authorities believe that the block is located in the proximal portion of the right bundle branch. Two alternative explanations are offered for the mechanism of right ventricular activation in this theory: (1) There is direct fiber-to-fiber spread of the activation process, beginning at the right side of the interventricular septum with the arrival of the impulse at this point, and (2) excitation takes place by resumption of conduction in the right bundle branch below the site of the block after some delay by an "electrical barrier" in the septum. Other authorities believe that the block is more peripheral in the right bundle branch and that not all the right ventricle is affected by the block. Two possible explanations are offered for the mechanism of right ventricular activation in this hypothesis: (1) The localized blocked region of the right ventricle is activated late in the QRS interval by direct myocardial spread of the stimulus rather than by the Purkinje plexus, and (2) there is "escape," or "leakage," of excitation at the site of the block, so that activation of the blocked portion of the right ventricle takes place by direct fiber-to-fiber spread of the stimulus from the point of leakage. The variable but definite prolongation of the QRS interval is ascribed to the longer duration of excitation by intramyocardial spread compared with the more rapid conduction through the Purkinje system.

Clinical Significance

Right bundle branch block is usually associated with organic heart disease but is sometimes found in healthy persons. Ischemic, rheumatic, and hypertensive heart disease and also cor pulonale are the usual types of heart disease encountered in this condition.

Ventricular Depolarization (Fig. 11-2)

The sequence of ventricular activation in right bundle branch block may be divided into four phases. Actually the process is continuous, so the division is purely arbitrary; it is made only for simplicity.

First Phase In the initial phase, since the left bundle branch is intact, the septum is activated normally from left to right. The septal vector is directed rightward and anteriorly and causes the inscription of part of the upstroke of the R wave in the right precordial leads and of a small Q wave in the left precordial leads and sometimes in lead I.

Second Phase During the second phase, since the right bundle branch is blocked, activation continues in the septum in a left-to-right direction and begins in the apical and anterior portion of the left ventricle. Since the left ventricular potentials are larger than those produced in the septum, the resultant of the left ventricular and septal vectors is still directed anteriorly, but somewhat leftward. This vector is responsible for the completion of the initial R wave in the right precordial leads and the registration of part of the upstroke of the R wave in the left precordial leads and lead I.

Third Phase During the third phase, left-to-right septal activation continues and activation proceeds through the anterolateral and basal regions of the left ventricle until it is finally completed in this chamber. Again the left ventricular potentials are dominant, so that the vector is directed leftward, more or less posteriorly, and inferiorly. During this phase, an S wave is inscribed in the right precordial leads and the peak of the R wave is recorded in the left precordial leads and in lead I.

Fourth Phase During the fourth phase, which is of relatively long duration, there is completion of left-to-right septal activation, activation of the apical and anterior portion of the right ventricle, and finally, activation of the free wall and the remainder of the right ventricle. This vector is directed rightward, anteriorly, and superiorly or horizontally or inferiorly. During this phase the final R' wave, which is larger and wider than the initial R wave, is written in the right precordial leads, and a wide, terminal S wave is recorded in the left precordial leads and lead I.

VENTRICULAR DEPOLARIZATION IN RIGHT BUNDLE BRANCH BLOCK

SEQUENCE OF VENTRICULAR ACTIVATION

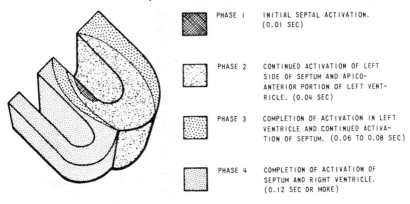

PHASE 1   INITIAL SEPTAL ACTIVATION.
(0.01 SEC)

PHASE 2   CONTINUED ACTIVATION OF LEFT
SIDE OF SEPTUM AND APICO-
ANTERIOR PORTION OF LEFT VENT-
RICLE. (0.04 SEC)

PHASE 3   COMPLETION OF ACTIVATION IN LEFT
VENTRICLE AND CONTINUED ACTIVA-
TION OF SEPTUM. (0.06 TO 0.08 SEC)

PHASE 4   COMPLETION OF ACTIVATION OF
SEPTUM AND RIGHT VENTRICLE.
(0.12 SEC OR MORE)

VENTRICULAR ACTIVATION VECTORS IN THE TRANSVERSE PLANE

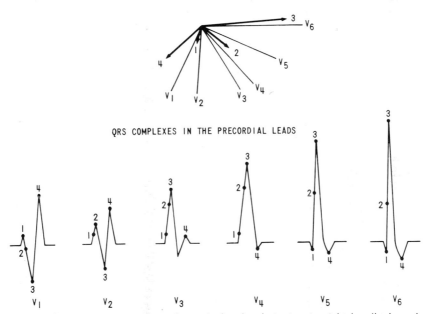

Fig. 11-2 Schematic representation of ventricular depolarization in right bundle branch block. Described in text.

Ventricular Repolarization

In right bundle branch block there is a change in the direction of repolarization secondary to the altered sequence of ventricular depolarization. The S-T and T vectors tend to rotate away from the mean QRS vector, which produces S-T segment depression and T wave inversion in the right precordial leads. Although the QRS-T angle is therefore widened, the ventricular gradient remains normal unless primary S-T and T vector abnormalities are superimposed.

Diagnosis of Complete Right Bundle Branch Block (Figs. 11-3, 11-4)

Conventional Criteria

1 The QRS complex is 0.12 s or more wide in the extremity leads.
2 Right-sided precordial leads, such as leads V_{3R}, V_1, and V_2, show wide RSR′ patterns. The secondary R wave ordinarily has greater amplitude than the primary R wave. The S-T segment is depressed and the T wave is downward in these leads.
3 Left-sided precordial leads, such as leads V_5 and V_6, show wide QRS patterns with a wide final S wave. The T wave is upright in these leads.
4 The time of onset of the intrinsicoid deflection in lead V_1 or V_2 is often delayed to 0.07 s or more, whereas in lead V_5 or V_6 it is normal.
5 Lead I shows a broad QRS complex with a wide final S wave.

Vectorelectrocardiographic Criteria

1 The QRS interval is prolonged.
2 The terminal, slowly inscribed QRS vector is directed rightward, anteriorly, and inferiorly or horizontally or superiorly and produces a broad, slurred S wave in lead I and a wide prominent R′ wave in lead V_1.

Fig. 11-3 Right bundle branch block. The QRS interval measures 0.12 s. There are wide S waves in leads I, V_5, and V_6. An RSR′ complex with a delayed intrinsicoid deflection is present in lead V_1. The T wave changes are secondary to the block.

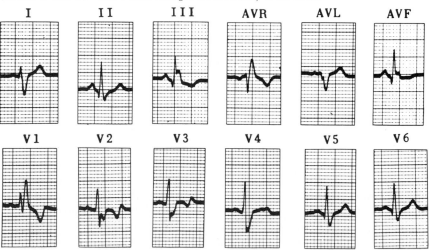

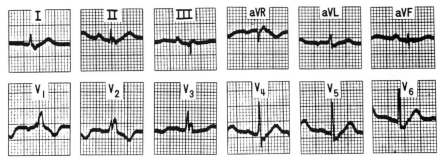

Fig. 11-4 Right bundle branch block. The QRS interval measures 0.12 s. There are wide S waves in leads I, aVL, V$_5$, and V$_6$. There is an rsR' complex in lead V$_1$, with a delayed onset of the intrinsicoid deflection. The T wave changes are secondary to the block.

Differential Diagnosis of an RSR' Complex in Lead V$_1$ with a Prolonged QRS Interval

Uncomplicated Right Bundle Branch Block   Aside from the prolongation of the QRS interval and the presence of an RSR' pattern in lead V$_1$, there is almost always a broad S wave in lead I and the left precordial leads. The intrinsicoid deflection in lead V$_1$ is markedly delayed. The orientation of the terminal QRS vector is rightward, anterior, and inferior or horizontal or superior. The mean frontal plane vector for the first 0.06 to 0.08 s of the QRS complex is in the normal range.

Right Bundle Branch Block with Left Anterior Fascicular Block   Signs of right bundle branch block are present in both the extremity and precordial leads. In addition, there is abnormal left axis deviation of the first 0.06 to 0.08 s of the QRS complex in the limb leads. (See also the section on right bundle branch block with left anterior fascicular block later in this chapter.)

Right Bundle Branch Block with Left Posterior Fascicular Block   Signs of right bundle branch block are present in both the extremity and precordial leads. In addition, there is right axis deviation of the first 0.06 to 0.08 s of the QRS complex in the limb leads. Other possible causes for the right axis deviation of the unblocked forces must be excluded. (See also the section on right bundle branch block with left posterior fascicular block later in this chapter.)

Right Bundle Branch Block with Right Ventricular Enlargement   Diagnostic signs of right bundle branch block are noted in the electrocardiogram. In addition, the amplitude of the R' wave is 15 mm or more or there is abnormal right axis deviation of the *unblocked* forces. However, the diagnosis of right ventricular enlargement in the presence of right bundle branch block is rarely secure. When there is right axis deviation of the first 0.06 to 0.08 s of the QRS complexes in the frontal plane, left posterior fascicular block must be excluded.

Right Bundle Branch Block with Myocardial Infarction   In addition to the signs of right bundle branch block, abnormal Q waves indicative of myocardial infarction are present.   The anatomic location of the infarct determines the leads in which the abnormal Q waves are found.   When anteroseptal infarction and right bundle branch block are combined, the initial R wave of the RSR' complex in the right precordial leads is replaced by an abnormal Q wave.   The right precordial leads then show wide QR complexes in which the time of onset of the R wave is delayed.

Right Bundle Branch Block with Strictly Posterior Myocardial Infarction   The coexistence of right bundle branch block and strictly posterior myocardial infarction is difficult to diagnose in the scalar electrocardiogram.   It may be suspected when there are tall, notched R waves (RR' complexes) in leads V_{3R} and V_1 (if the frontal plane QRS axis is within normal limits), particularly when associated with tall upright T waves in the right precordial leads.   The vectorcardiogram is a superior method for the diagnosis of these combined abnormalities.

Incomplete Right Bundle Branch Block (Fig. 11-5)

1   Incomplete right bundle branch block is the condition in which the electrocardiographic criteria of right bundle branch block are fulfilled but in which the QRS interval is between 0.09 and 0.11 s in duration.

2   The differentiation of incomplete right bundle branch block from right ventricular enlargement when there is an R' pattern in lead V_1 with a duration less than 0.12 s may present a difficult problem.   When a broad (0.04 s or more) R' wave in lead V_1 is associated with a similarly wide S wave in lead I, the diagnosis of incomplete right bundle branch block should be made.   If the criteria for right ventricular hypertrophy are also fulfilled, this diagnosis should be added.

3   Other causes for an RSR' pattern in lead V_1 or V_{3R}, or both, with a QRS interval less than 0.12 s must also be differentiated from incomplete right bundle branch block.   These include the normal crista pattern, the $S_1S_2S_3$ syndrome, left anterior hemiblock, anterior infarction with left anterior hemiblock, posterobasal myocardial infarction, acute right ventricular dilatation (as in acute cor pulmonale), and emphysema with or without cor pulmonale.   The reader is referred to the previous chapter for further details.

4   In doubtful cases, the vectorcardiogram may help to differentiate between the various causes of an RSR' pattern in lead V_1 (see Fig. 10-13).

5   It has been suggested (Moore et al.) that incomplete right bundle branch block may be due to a focal hypertrophy of the right ventricle rather than to delayed conduction within the right bundle branch.

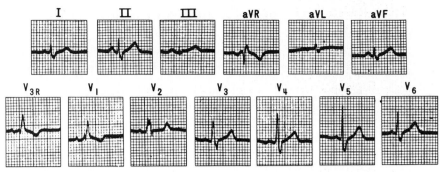

Fig. 11-5 Incomplete right bundle branch block. The QRS interval is 0.10 s. There is a wide S wave in leads I, aVL, and the left precordial leads. An rsR' complex is present in leads V_{3R} and V_1.

VECTORCARDIOGRAM IN RIGHT BUNDLE BRANCH BLOCK

Complete Right Bundle Branch Block (Fig. 11-6)

The duration of the QRS loop is prolonged to 0.12 s or more, but its overall magnitude is normal.

The specific diagnostic alterations are seen best in the TP.

The QRS loop in complete right bundle branch block consists of two portions: the main body of the loop and the terminal appendage.

In the TP, the initial vectors and the efferent limb retain their normal orientation. The afferent limb, however, is displaced anteriorly. The slowly inscribed terminal appendage is always directed rightward and anteriorly. The duration of the terminal conduction delay averages 60 ms, with a range between 30 and 80 ms. Terminal slowing should be visible in at least two planar loops. As a rule there is CCW inscription of the efferent limb. The loop then turns sharply, forming the afferent limb. The afferent limb and terminal appendage are then inscribed in a CCW, figure-of-eight, or CW fashion.

Inscription of the QRS loop is variable in the LSP and FP.

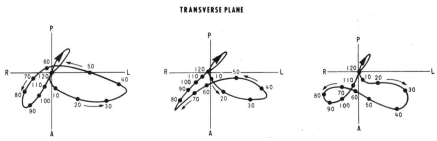

Fig. 11-6 Representative examples of the TP QRS loop in complete right bundle branch block. The numbers indicate the time in milliseconds after the beginning of the QRS loop. Described in text.

The S-T vector and the T loop are directed oppositely to the long axis of the QRS loop.

Incomplete Right Bundle Branch Block

In incomplete right bundle branch block, the QRS loop, the S-T vector, and the T loop are similar to those in complete right bundle branch block. The QRS duration, of course, is shorter.

RIGHT BUNDLE BRANCH BLOCK WITH RIGHT VENTRICULAR ENLARGEMENT (FIGS. 11-7, 11-8)

The diagnosis of right ventricular enlargement in the presence of right bundle branch block is rarely secure but may be suspected under the following circumstances:

1   The electrocardiogram shows the usual findings of right bundle branch block.
2   There is abnormal right axis deviation of the initial 0.06 to 0.08-s QRS vector, representing the unblocked portion of the QRS complex. However, a vertical heart, left posterior hemiblock, and other conditions must be ruled out as causes of the right axis deviation.

Fig. 11-7   Right bundle branch block and right ventricular enlargement in a patient with chronic cor pulmonale.   The QRS interval is 0.12 s wide.   There is a wide S wave in lead I and an RSR' complex in lead V_1, in which the secondary R wave measures 20 mm.   In right bundle branch block, a secondary R wave exceeding 15 mm in the right precordial leads is often, but not invariably, indicative of concomitant right ventricular enlargement.

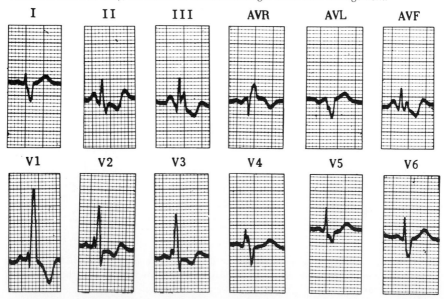

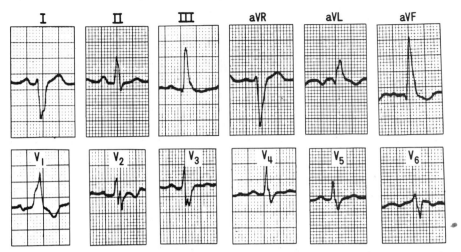

Fig. 11-8 Right bundle branch block with right ventricular enlargement. The QRS interval is 0.14 s. There is marked right axis deviation of the unblocked forces, a wide S wave in lead I and the left precordial leads, and a slurred, broad R wave in lead V_1. From a patient with cor pulmonale secondary to recurrent pulmonary embolization.

3 The amplitude of the R' wave in lead V_1 is 15 mm or greater. However, there are frequent instances of right bundle branch block in which the R' wave exceeds this value in the absence of right ventricular hypertrophy.

4 Tall secondary R waves are more reliable indicators of concomitant right ventricular enlargement in children than in adults.

RIGHT BUNDLE BRANCH BLOCK WITH LEFT VENTRICULAR ENLARGEMENT (FIGS. 11-9, 11-10)

The diagnosis of left ventricular enlargement in the presence of right bundle branch block is difficult but may be suspected under the following circumstances:

1 The electrocardiogram shows the usual findings of right bundle branch block.

2 The voltage criteria for the diagnosis of left ventricular hypertrophy are fulfilled. (An R wave in lead V_5 or V_6 that is 20 mm or more is considered adequate for this purpose by Scott.)

VECTORCARDIOGRAM IN RIGHT BUNDLE BRANCH BLOCK WITH VENTRICULAR HYPERTROPHY (FIG.11-11)

There are no completely satisfactory criteria for the diagnosis of ventricular hypertrophy in the presence of right bundle branch block.

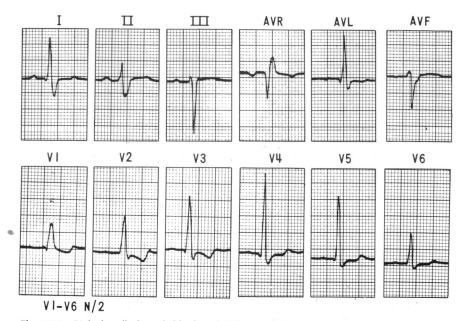

Fig. 11-9 Right bundle branch block with left ventricular enlargement. In addition to the typical features of right bundle branch block, the voltage criteria for left ventricular hypertrophy are fulfilled. Standardization is half-normal in all the precordial leads.

Fig. 11-10 Right bundle branch block, left ventricular enlargement, and abnormal left axis deviation. The QRS interval measures 0.12 s. There is a wide S wave in lead I and RSR' complexes in leads V_{3R} to V_4. There is high voltage of the R wave in lead aVL, and the sum of the R_1 and S_3 waves exceeds normal values, which indicates left ventricular enlargement. The electrical axis is at about $-60°$. The combination of right bundle branch block and abnormal left axis deviation is due to right bundle branch block with left anterior fascicular block.

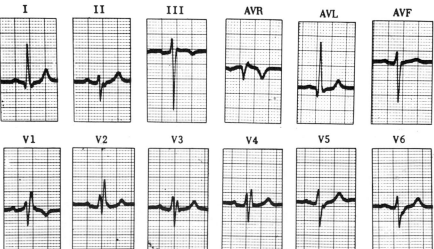

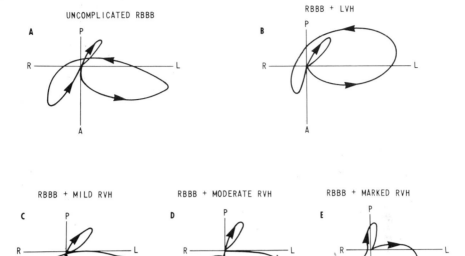

Fig. 11-11   The vectorcardiogram in right bundle branch block with ventricular enlargement. Described in text.   RBBB = right bundle branch block; RVH = right ventricular hypertrophy; LVH = left ventricular hypertrophy.

Baydar and his group concluded on the basis of their studies that only the findings in the TP are useful in this regard.   They found that in this plane, in uncomplicated right bundle branch block, the midtemporal portion of the QRS loop is slightly posterior to the null, or E, point.   They also found that ventricular hypertrophy does not alter the rightward and anterior location of the characteristic terminal appendage of right bundle branch block nor does it affect the conduction delay.   With coexisting left ventricular enlargement and right bundle branch block, there is marked posterior displacement of the midtemporal portion of the loop.   When right ventricular hypertrophy and right bundle branch block coexist, the characteristic feature is anterior displacement of the QRS loop.   With mild right ventricular hypertrophy the midtemporal portion of the loop is located anterior to the null point, but its initial portion continues to be inscribed in a CCW direction.   With moderate right ventricular hypertrophy there is further anterior displacement of the QRS loop, but the initial portion of the loop shows CW rotation.   In severe right ventricular hypertrophy there is marked anterior displacement of the QRS loop and the entire loop is rotated CW.

LEFT BUNDLE BRANCH BLOCK

Theoretical Considerations

In left bundle branch block the entire sequence of ventricular activation is altered. The primary abnormality is a change in the direction of the initial 0.04-s vector, which points leftward and posteriorly and is more or less parallel to the mean QRS vector.

It is generally accepted that the block is located proximally in the left bundle branch. It is also believed that the first portion of the interventricular septum to be activated is the lower third of the right septal surface in the region of the anterior papillary muscle. The reminder of the right septal surface and the right ventricular wall are activated normally.

With respect to the mechanism of left ventricular activation, there are four schools of thought (Fig. 11-12). One school (Sodi-Pallares and associates) holds that there is an "electrical barrier" between the right and left septal masses which causes a delay in the passage of the impulse from right to left. However, once the stimulus reaches the left septal surface by direct fiber-to-fiber conduction, activation of this surface and the free left ventricular wall proceeds through the Purkinje network at a normal rate and in a normal direction. A second group (Becker and associates) believes that the interventricular septum is activated smoothly, but slowly, by muscle conduction from right to left. By the time this is complete, however, activation of the right ventricle proceeds to the epicardium, and in the anterior septal region there is epicardial-to-endocardial spread by muscle conduction. After septal activation is completed, the impulse enters the subendocardial Purkinje network and is then distributed to the free wall of the left ventricle. A third group (Grant and Dodge) holds that there is "escape" of excitation from the conduction system into the myocardium at the site of the block. Thereafter, the spread of activation to the remainder of the left ventricle is by intramyocardial spread along the myocardial syncytium instead of along the normal conduction pathways. A fourth school (Barker) believes that there is slow uniform activation across the septum from right to left. Once the impulse reaches the left side of the septum, excitation of the left ventricle takes place by the resumption of conduction in the left bundle branch below the site of the block.

Left bundle branch block may be predivisional or divisional. In the former instance, the lesion is located in the main left bundle branch; in the latter, there is simultaneous block in the anterior and posterior fascicles. Divisional and predivisional left bundle branch block are indistinguishable electrocardiographically.

Clinical Significance

Left bundle branch block is usually caused by arteriosclerotic, hypertensive, or rheumatic heart disease, but it may be due to other causes. Very rarely,

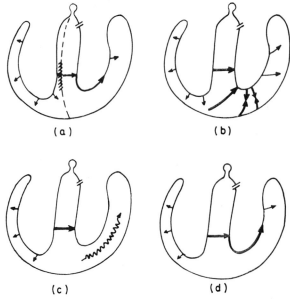

(a)   (b)

(c)   (d)

Fig. 11-12 Proposed mechanisms of ventricular activation in left bundle branch block. Described in text. (a) Mechanism proposed by Sodi-Pallares et al. (b) Mechanism proposed by Becker et al. (c) Mechanism proposed by Grant and Dodge. (d) Mechanism proposed by Barker. *(From R. C. Scott, Left Bundle Branch Block—A Clinical Assessment: Part I, Am. Heart J., 70: 535, 1965. Used by permission.)*

it occurs in otherwise healthy individuals. In the overwhelming majority of cases, left bundle branch block is associated with anatomic hypertrophy of the left ventricle.

Ventricular Depolarization (Fig. 11-13)

The sequence of ventricular activation in left bundle branch block may be divided into four phases. Again, this division is arbitrary and is made for descriptive purposes only.

First Phase   In the initial phase, since the left bundle branch is blocked, activation is initiated on the right side of the septum and proceeds in a right-to-left and apex-to-base direction across the septum. Simultaneously, activation spreads to the apical and anterior portion of the right ventricle. The septal vector is directed leftward, posteriorly, and inferiorly; the right ventricular vector is directed rightward, anteriorly, and inferiorly. The resultant vector depends on the magnitude and direction of the two component vectors. If septal potentials dominate significantly, the vector is directed leftward, posteriorly, and inferiorly, which results in the inscription of the downstroke of a QS complex in lead V_1 and of the upstroke of an R wave in leads V_6 and I. If right ventricular potentials are significant,

VENTRICULAR DEPOLARIZATION IN LEFT BUNDLE BRANCH BLOCK

SEQUENCE OF VENTRICULAR ACTIVATION

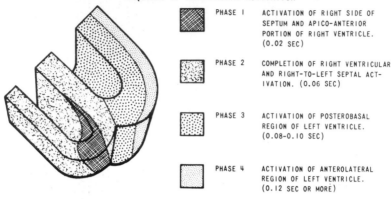

PHASE 1   ACTIVATION OF RIGHT SIDE OF
SEPTUM AND APICO-ANTERIOR
PORTION OF RIGHT VENTRICLE.
(0.02 SEC)

PHASE 2   COMPLETION OF RIGHT VENTRICULAR
AND RIGHT-TO-LEFT SEPTAL ACT-
IVATION. (0.06 SEC)

PHASE 3   ACTIVATION OF POSTEROBASAL
REGION OF LEFT VENTRICLE.
(0.08-0.10 SEC)

PHASE 4   ACTIVATION OF ANTEROLATERAL
REGION OF LEFT VENTRICLE.
(0.12 SEC OR MORE)

VENTRICULAR ACTIVATION VECTORS IN THE TRANSVERSE PLANE

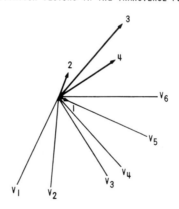

QRS COMPLEXES IN THE PRECORDIAL LEADS

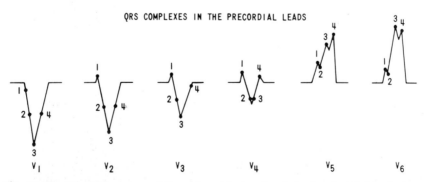

Fig. 11-13 Schematic representation of ventricular depolarization in left bundle branch block. Described in text.

the vector, although still directed leftward and inferiorly, is rotated anteriorly, which results in the registration of a small R wave in lead V_1 and of the upstroke of an R wave in leads V_6 and I.

Second Phase During this phase, activation of the right ventricle is completed, but depolarization continues in the septum in a right-to-left direction and is eventually completed. The septal potentials dominate so that the vector is directed quite leftward and posteriorly and more or less horizontally. It is responsible for the registration of the downstroke of the QS or rS deflection in lead V_1 and for the upstroke of the R wave in leads V_6 and I.

Third Phase In this phase, left ventricular activation takes place, but the direction is somewhat abnormal, so that activation is completed within the posterior and basal region but continues in the anterior and lateral portions of the left ventricle. The vector points markedly leftward and posteriorly. The nadir of the S wave in lead V_1 and the peak of the initial R wave in leads V_6 and I are recorded during this phase.

Fourth Phase In the final phase, left ventricular activation is completed in the anterior and lateral walls of the left ventricle. This vector is directed leftward but more anteriorly than in the preceding phase. It is responsible for the peak of the R' wave and its subsequent downstroke in leads V_6 and I and for the hind limb of the S wave in lead V_1.

Ventricular Repolarization

In left bundle branch block there is a change in the direction of repolarization secondary to the altered sequence of ventricular depolarization. The S-T and T vectors tend to rotate away from the mean QRS vector and so produce S-T segment depression and T wave inversion in the left precordial leads and in lead I. Although the QRS-T angle is widened, the ventricular gradient remains normal unless primary S-T and T vector abnormalities are superimposed.

Diagnosis of Complete Left Bundle Branch Block (Figs. 11-14, 11-15)

Conventional Criteria

1 The QRS complex is 0.12 s or more wide in the extremity leads.
2 In the majority of cases, initial R waves followed by wide, deep S waves are present in the right and midprecordial leads. However, wide QS deflections may sometimes be seen in lead V_1 or even in leads V_2 and V_3. Once an R wave appears in a right-sided precordial lead, its amplitude usually increases progressively in leads to the left. The transitional zone is shifted to the left.

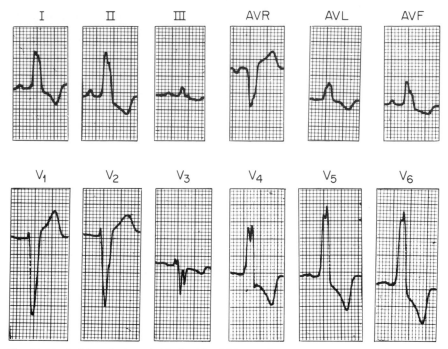

Fig. 11-14 Left bundle branch block. The QRS complex measures 0.14 s. A broad, bifid R wave with a delayed intrinsicoid deflection is present in leads V_5 and V_6, and also in lead I. Significant, too, is the absence of Q waves in leads I and aVL and the left precordial leads, and the absence of an S wave in lead I.

3 Left-sided precordial leads, such as V_6, show broad, notched, or slurred R waves or RsR′ patterns. Q waves are usually absent. When present, they are rarely more than 0.02 s in duration. The S-T segments are depressed, and the T waves are inverted in these leads.

4 The time of onset of the intrinsicoid deflection in lead V_6 is often delayed to 0.07 s or more. In lead V_1 or V_2 it is normal.

5 The findings in the standard and unipolar limb leads are somewhat variable. In leads I and aVL there are usually broad, slurred, or notched R waves with absent Q and S waves. If Q waves are present in lead I, they are less than 0.03 s wide. In lead aVL, however, wide Q waves are often found even in uncomplicated left bundle branch block. In leads II, III, and aVF there are RS complexes, although occasionally a QS complex or Q wave may be seen in leads III and aVF. According to some authorities, QS complexes or Q waves do not occur in lead II in uncomplicated left bundle branch block.

Vectorelectrocardiographic Criteria

1 The QRS interval is 0.12 s or more in duration.
2 The mean QRS vector points leftward and posteriorly.

3   When left bundle branch block develops, the initial QRS vector is always changed in direction to point leftward and posteriorly.
4   The angle between the initial and mean QRS vectors is narrow and rarely exceeds 45°.

Incomplete Left Bundle Branch Block (Fig. 11-16)

The term *incomplete* left bundle branch block has been applied to the condition in which criteria for the diagnosis of left bundle branch block are met but the QRS interval is less than 0.12 s wide.

Criteria for Diagnosis

1   The QRS complex is from 0.10 to 0.12 s wide in the extremity leads.
2   In the left precordial leads and lead I, there is notching or slurring of the upstroke of the R wave.
3   Q waves are absent in leads I and aVL and the left precordial leads.
4   The time of onset of the intrinsicoid deflection is delayed to 0.06 s or more in the left precordial leads.

Left Bundle Branch Block with Ventricular Enlargement

The overwhelming majority of patients with complete left bundle branch block have anatomic evidence of left ventricular hypertrophy. The diag-

Fig. 11-15 Left bundle branch block with abnormal left axis deviation. The QRS interval is prolonged to 0.14 s. The electrical axis is at about −50°. The poor R wave progression noted in the right precordial leads is a common finding in uncomplicated left bundle branch block and is not necessarily indicative of anterior infarction.

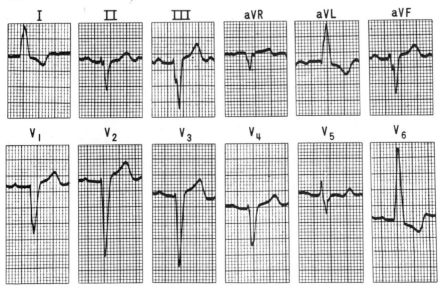

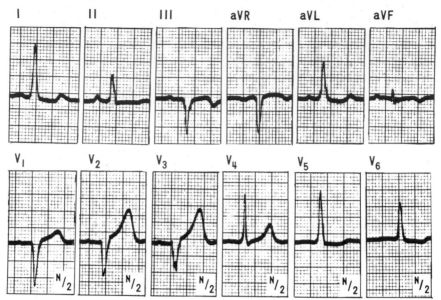

Fig. 11-16 Incomplete left bundle branch block. The electrocardiogram is typical of left bundle branch block. The QRS interval is 0.11 s. The sum of the R_{V_6} and S_{V_2} waves exceeds normal values, which indicates coexisting left ventricular hypertrophy. 1965. *Used by permission.)*

nosis of left ventricular enlargement in the presence of left bundle branch block is suggested electrocardiographically if the sum of the S wave in lead V_2 and the R wave in lead V_5 is 45 mm or more. The diagnosis is also strongly supported if the QRS duration is 0.14 s or greater, or if signs of left atrial enlargement are present.

Left ventricular enlargement may be diagnosed by the usual voltage criteria in the presence of incomplete left bundle branch block.

When right axis deviation with a prominent S wave in lead I occurs in complete left bundle branch block, the diagnosis of right ventricular enlargement should be entertained. However, a similar pattern may be produced by a combination of left bundle branch block and left posterior fascicular block or by infarction of the free wall of the left ventricle in association with left bundle branch block.

VECTORCARDIOGRAM IN LEFT BUNDLE BRANCH BLOCK

Complete Left Bundle Branch Block (Fig. 11-17)

The duration of the QRS loop is prolonged to 0.12 s or more.

The specific diagnostic alterations are observed best in the TP. In this plane, the QRS loop typically is found to be elongated and narrow. The initial vector, although displaced leftward, retains its anterior orientation.

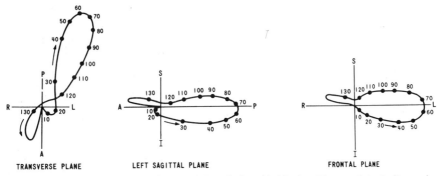

TRANSVERSE PLANE   LEFT SAGITTAL PLANE   FRONTAL PLANE

Fig. 11-17 The vectorcardiogram in left bundle branch block. The numbers indicate the
time in milliseconds after the beginning of the QRS loop. Described in text.

The main body of the loop is inscribed posteriorly and to the left in a CW
direction. A distinctive feature is the conduction delay noted in the mid
and terminal portions of the QRS loop. The magnitude of the maxQRS
vector is increased above normal. The S-T vector and T loop are directed
rightward and anteriorly, oppositely to the long axis of the QRS loop.

INTERMITTENT BUNDLE BRANCH BLOCK (FIG. 11-18)

Intermittent bundle branch block is usually attributed to a prolongation of
recovery in one of the bundle branches. Intermittent bundle branch block
is commonly rate-related. Above a particular critical rate, impulses reach
the affected bundle during the prolonged refractory period, causing slow
conduction or block. Below the critical rate, impulses reach the damaged
fascicle after recovery is completed, so that intraventricular conduction
becomes normal. Thus the conduction defect become apparent only when
the heart rate is sufficiently rapid and disappears when it slows.

Fig. 11-18 (A) Intermittent right bundle branch block (lead V_1); (B) intermittent left bundle
branch block (lead I).

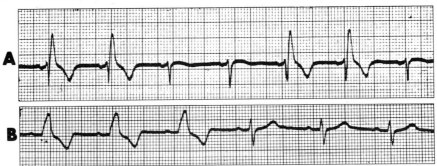

Cases also occur in which bundle branch block appears only after long diastolic intervals, so that the bundle branch block is bradycardia-dependent. Many different mechanisms have been suggested for this phenomenon, such as vagal effects, concealed conduction, and supernormality. Rosenbaum and his coworkers believe that it is related to hypopolarization of the involved fascicle in the presence of spontaneous diastolic depolarization.

Cases of bradycardia-dependent bundle branch block are almost invariably associated with tachycardia-dependent bundle branch block. When the cycle lengths are intermediate in duration, ventricular conduction becomes normal.

According to Rosenbaum, most cases of intermittent left bundle branch block are predivisional and ischemic in origin.

DIFFUSE INTRAVENTRICULAR BLOCK

The QRS interval is widened with but little change in the contour of the QRS complex. The initial, mean, and terminal QRS vectors are unchanged in direction, but their duration is increased. This type of block may be produced by quinidine, hyperpotassemia, and other conditions.

NONSPECIFIC INTRAVENTRICULAR BLOCK

This refers to an intraventricular conduction defect (abnormally wide or notched QRS complexes, or both) which cannot be placed in any specific category. Synonyms are intramyocardial or intramural block.

THE MONOFASCICULAR, BIFASCICULAR, AND TRIFASCICULAR BLOCKS AND BILATERAL BUNDLE BRANCH BLOCK

The Monofascicular Blocks

The anatomy of the conduction system was discussed in detail in Chap. 2. It will be recalled that the bundle of His divides into right and left bundle branches. Shortly after its origin, the left bundle branch block divides into two main groups of fibers (Fig. 11-19): one group, called the *anterior fascicle or division of the left bundle*, radiates superiorly and anteriorly to reach the anterolateral wall of the left ventricle; the other group, called the *posterior fascicle or division of the left bundle* is distributed to the inferoposterior wall of the left ventricle. A third group, called the *septal, central, or medial fascicle of the left bundle branch*, supplies the midseptal area. The three divisions anastomose peripherally in the subendocardial layers of the ventricle via the Purkinje network. Since the function of the septal fascicle has not been determined, it will not be discussed further. Consideration will be given only to the bundle of His, the bundle branches, and their subdivisions.

Normally, excitation spreads down the AV node, the bundle of His, the bundle branches, and simultaneously through the anterior and posterior fascicles. If, however, one of the divisions is blocked, the sequence of excitation is altered. Thus, if the anterior fascicle is blocked, excitation will travel through the fibers of the inferior fascicle and then spread superiorly. Accordingly, the initial 0.02-s QRS vector will be directed inferiorly and somewhat rightward, producing, as in the normal, a small 0.02-s Q wave in leads aVL and I and a small 0.02-s R wave in leads II, III, and aVF. The mean and terminal QRS vectors will be directed leftward and superiorly, resulting in a tall R wave in leads aVL and I and deep S waves in leads II, III, and aVF. Hence the QRS loop will rotate CCW, the terminal QRS vectors will be directed leftward and superiorly, the left axis deviation will occur, with or without slight prolongation of the QRS interval. According to the presently recommended nomenclature, this type of conduction defect is called *left anterior fascicular block.* Other names for this conduction defect are *left anterior hemiblock, left superior intraventricular block, left anterior division block,* and *superior parietal block.* If the lesion involving the anterior division is fibrosis or a similar process but is not an infarct, the initial QRS vector will remain normal. If the lesion is infarction, the initial 0.04-s vector will point rightward and inferiorly away from the infarcted area, resulting in a 0.04-s Q wave in leads aVL and I and often also in leads V_4 to V_6. This entity is called *anterior*

Fig. 11-19   Diagram of the left bundle branch and its anterior and posterior divisions. (*From R. C. Scott, Left Bundle Branch Block—A Clinical Assessment: Part I, Am. Heart J., 70: 535, 1965. Used by permission.*)

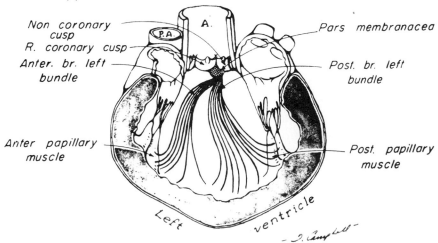

infarction with left anterior fascicular block. In the older literature, it was called anterior or superior peri-infarction block.

The same type of reasoning may be applied to block of the posterior fascicle or division of the left bundle branch. If this fascicle is blocked, excitation will travel through the anterior fascicle and then spread inferiorly. The initial QRS vector will be directed leftward and slightly superiorly. Thus a small initial 0.02-s R wave will appear in leads aVL and I and a small 0.02-s Q wave will be noted in leads II, III, and aVF. The mean and terminal QRS vectors will be directed inferiorly and often slightly rightward, resulting in large R waves in leads II, III, and aVF and S waves in leads I and aVL. Hence the QRS loop will rotate CW, with terminal forces directed inferiorly and slightly rightward, with or without slight prolongation of the QRS interval. This type of conduction defect is called *left posterior fascicular block.* Synonyms are *left posterior hemiblock, left inferior intraventricular block,* and *left inferior parietal block.* The findings in posterior fascicular block are similar, if not identical, to those observed in some normal individuals with vertical hearts, emphysema, right ventricular enlargement, and anterolateral infarction. If the lesion causing block of the inferior fascicle is an infarct, a 0.04-s Q wave will appear in leads aVF, III, and II. This entity is called *inferior infarction with left posterior fascicular block.* In the older literature, it bore the name of inferior peri-infarction block.

Left anterior fascicular block almost invariably indicates left ventricular disease. Myocardial fibrosis due to coronary artery disease is probably its most common cause. Myocardial infarction is the second most frequent cause. Other causes include diabetes and hypertension (probably due to subclinical coronary artery disease in these conditions), aortic valvular lesions, cardiomyopathy, myocarditis, and possibly some types of congenital heart disease (e.g., endocardial cushion defects, tricuspid atresia, corrected transposition, and single ventricle).

Left posterior fascicular block occurs much less frequently than left anterior fascicular block. It is often associated with right bundle branch block and AV conduction disturbances. It may be caused by coronary artery disease, cardiomyopathy, myocarditis, and Lenegre's disease.

The high frequency of block of the anterior fascicle compared to the rarity of block of the posterior fascicle has raised questions concerning the vulnerability of the two divisions. Rosenbaum has attributed the greater vulnerability of the anterior fascicle to the following factors: (1) a single blood supply derived from the perforating arteries of the left anterior descending coronary vessel; (2) its greater length and thinness compared to the posterior fascicle; (3) its location in the hemodynamically turbulent outflow tract of the left ventricle. He has reasoned that the posterior fascicle is better protected because (1) its fibers are the first to leave the bundle of His, with a short crossing from the septum to the inferior wall; (2) it is shorter and thicker than the anterior fascicle; (3) it belongs to the inflow tract of the left ventricle, which is a less turbulent region; and (4) it has a dual blood supply from branches of both the anterior and posterior descending arteries.

Diagnosis of Left Anterior Fascicular Block
(Left Anterior Hemiblock) (Figs. 11-20, 11-21)

1 The initial 0.02-s QRS vector is directed inferiorly and rightward, producing 0.02-s Q waves in leads aVL and I and 0.02-s R waves in leads II, III, and aVF. If superior infarction is present, abnormal 0.04-s Q waves will appear in leads aVL and I. When the infarct is anterolateral, abnormal Q waves will be noted in leads V_5, V_6, and I and aVL. In anteroseptal infarction, diagnostic Q or QS abnormalities are seen in leads V_1 to V_3 or V_4, and in localized anterior infarctions, these occur in the midprecordial leads.

2 The mean and terminal QRS forces in the frontal plane are directed leftward and superiorly to $-45°$ or more.

3 There are deep S waves in leads II, III, and aVF. The amplitude of the S wave in lead II exceeds that of the R wave in this lead, and S_3 is deeper than S_2.

4 There is a positive terminal deflection in leads aVL and aVR and a negative terminal deflection in lead II.

5 The QRS loop rotates CCW in the FP.

6 Usually the QRS interval is within normal limits. Widening, if it occurs, is ordinarily no greater than 0.02.

Fig. 11-20 Abnormal left axis deviation ($-45°$) due to left anterior fascicular block in a patient with chronic coronary artery disease. The electrocardiogram is otherwise normal. There is an R' wave in leads V_1 and V_2, which indicates that the terminal QRS vector, in addition to being directed leftward and superiorly, also points anteriorly.

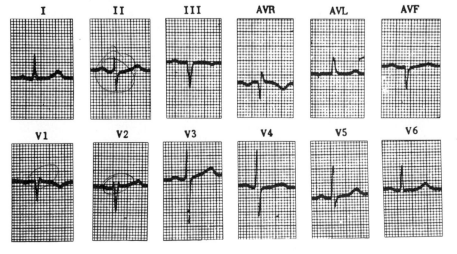

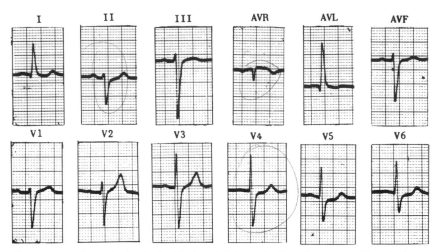

Fig. 11-21   Left anterior fascicular block with left ventricular enlargement.   There is abnormal left axis deviation (about $-55°$) with a qR pattern in leads aVL and I, and rS patterns in leads II, III, and aVF.   Voltage criteria for left ventricular enlargement are fulfilled: $R_1 + S_3$ is greater than 25 mm, and R_{aVL} exceeds 11 mm.

7 The following findings may occur in the precordial leads but are not necessary for the diagnosis of left anterior fascicular block:

a An R′ deflection in the right precordial leads (V_2 and V_3), especially in those recorded at a higher level, if the terminal QRS vector is directed anteriorly as well as superiorly.

b Relatively deep S waves in leads V_5 and V_6 which disappear in higher V leads, attributed to downward displacement of the electrical center of ventricular depolarization.

c Frequent absence of the Q wave in leads V_5 and V_6.

d The appearance of Q waves in leads V_1 to V_3, simulating anteroseptal infarction.   Differentiation is possible by recording low V leads, in which Q waves due to infarction persist and those caused by left anterior fascicular block disappear.

Comments

To make the diagnosis of left anterior fascicular block secure, other causes of abnormal left axis deviation such as emphysema, ventricular preexcitation, hyperkalemia, acute pulmonary embolism, inferior myocardial infarction, normal variants, etc., should be excluded.   If the mean QRS axis is about $-60°$ with a Q_1S_3 pattern, the diagnosis of left anterior fascicular block is quite certain.

Some authorities feel that an axis beyond $-30°$ is adequate for the diagnosis of left anterior fascicular block, provided the other criteria for the diagnosis are met.   Cases with a mean QRS axis between -30 and

−45° may in fact represent incomplete forms of left anterior fascicular block. However, in epidemiologic studies and in clinical practice, many persons with this degree of left axis deviation seem to be healthy, without evidence of heart disease. Whether such persons may have latent coronary artery disease is unknown.

Horwitz and associates have suggested that the diagnosis of left anterior fascicular block requires *both* abnormal left axis deviation and evidence of asynchronous activation of the left ventricle. According to them, a delay in conduction in the region of the affected fascicle can be considered present if the time of inscription of the intrinsicoid deflection in lead aVL exceeds 0.05 s and it is at least 0.01 s greater than in lead V_6. They found that the two criteria were satisfied in only 62 percent of cases with left axis deviation of −30° or more. However, the greater the leftward axis shift, the more likely was the possibility of a delayed intrinsicoid deflection in lead aVL. With an axis of −75° or more, the intrinsicoid deflection in lead aVL was invariably delayed. In contrast, only 2 percent of cases with a 0° axis and 9 percent with a −15° axis had significantly delayed intrinsicoid deflections in lead aVL compared to lead V_6 and would not have been recognized as possible instances of left anterior fascicular block if the axis criterion alone had been utilized. The authors suggested that since a significant number of tracings with marked left axis deviation did not have a regional delay in conduction, another explanation for the left axis deviation should be sought in these cases (e.g., horizontal heart, obesity, masked interior infarction), or regional delay might not be manifest in lead aVL. It should be recognized, however, that the validity of the proposed criteria, as admitted by these authors, has not yet been demonstrated in the human heart.

The occurrence of abnormal left axis deviation in the presence of pulmonary emphysema (Figs. 18-5, 20-2) raises a difficult diagnostic problem. Pryor and Blount, as well as others, believe that emphysema alone may cause abnormal left axis deviation (pseudo left axis deviation), which may be distinguished from the true left axis deviation of left anterior fascicular block by the following characteristics: (1) the P vector is directed relatively inferiorly, with prominent P waves in leads II, III, and aVF. (2) Low voltage QRS complexes are present in both the limb and precordial leads. (3) The terminal QRS vector is superior and sometimes rightward, producing a small terminal R wave in lead aVR that may equal or even exceed the terminal R wave in lead aVL. Since patients with emphysema not infrequently also have left ventricular disease, it is possible that the abnormal left axis deviation found in at least some of these patients may be due to concomitant left anterior fascicular block.

The $S_1S_2S_3$ pattern is characterized by R and S waves of approximately equal voltage in the three standard leads (and aVF). Usually the S wave is somewhat greater than the R wave in leads II and III, but S_1 is usually smaller than R_1. It may mimic left anterior fascicular block. Characteristically, S_3 is greater than S_2 in left anterior fascicular block, whereas in the $S_1S_2S_3$ pattern the voltage of S_2 exceeds that of S_3.

Left Ventricular Enlargement with Left Anterior Fascicular Block (Fig. 11-21)

When voltage changes of left ventricular enlargement occur in association with left anterior fascicular block, this diagnosis should be added.

Right Ventricular Enlargement with Left Anterior Fascicular Block

Right ventricular enlargement in association with left anterior fascicular block is a rare combination sometimes seen in ostium primum atrial septal defects and other congenital anomalies. However, it is not established that the abnormal left axis deviation seen in these conditions is actually due to left anterior fascicular block.

1 When left anterior fascicular block is marked and right ventricular enlargement is slight, or when left ventricular enlargement is also present, the electrocardiogram is typical of left anterior fascicular block, although signs of right ventricular enlargement may be seen in the right precordial leads.
2 As the degree of right ventricular enlargement increases, the mean QRS vector rotates CCW first to $-90°$ then to $-120°$, then to $-150°$, the presence of small Q waves in leads I and aVL and relatively prominent S_2 and S_3 deflections is indicative of the left anterior fascicular block.
3 When right ventricular enlargement is more marked, or when the degree of left anterior fascicular block is mild, the latter condition may be difficult or impossible to recognize. Conversely, when left anterior fascicular block is severe, even marked right ventricular enlargement may be unable to shift the QRS axis inferiorly.

Myocardial Infarction with Left Anterior Fascicular Block

This condition is discussed in Chap. 13.

Diagnosis of Left Posterior Fascicular Block (Left Posterior Hemiblock) (Figs. 11-22, 11-23, 13-32, 13-36)

1 The initial 0.02-s QRS vector is directed leftward and superiorly, producing a 0.02-s R wave in leads aVL and I and 0.02-s Q waves in leads II, III, and aVF. If inferior infarction is present, abnormal 0.04-s Q waves will appear in leads aVF, III, and II.
2 The main and terminal QRS forces are oriented inferiorly and to the

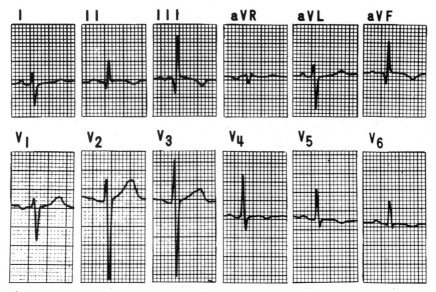

Fig. 11-22   Left posterior fascicular block in a patient with recent inferior myocardial infarction.   There is abnormal right axis deviation (about +120°) with an rS pattern in leads I and aVL, and qR patterns with relatively tall R waves in leads II, III, and aVF.   The abnormal Q waves and inverted T waves in the inferior leads are indicative of recent inferior myocardial infarction.   The patient had diffuse, severe, occlusive disease of all major coronary vessels demonstrable on arteriography.

right (beyond +90 and usually close to +120°) producing an S wave in leads aVL and I and rather tall R waves in leads II, III, and aVF.   The voltage of R_3 should equal or exceed that of R_2.

3   Usually the QRS interval is within normal limits.   Widening, if it occurs, ordinarily does not exceed 0.02 s.

4   The QRS loop is rotated CW in the frontal plane.

5   The following findings are commonly observed in the precordial leads but are not required for diagnosis:

a   The QRS complexes are predominantly positive in the lower V leads and predominantly negative in the higher V leads due to upward displacement of the electrical center of ventricular depolarization.

b   Q waves are often absent in leads V_5 and V_6, but small Q waves may appear in these leads recorded at a lower level.

6   The diagnosis of left posterior fascicular block is clinical as well as electrocardiographic.   It is necessary to exclude a vertical heart, chronic obstructive pulmonary disease (Fig. 18-6), right ventricular enlargement, and lateral infarction as causes of the right axis deviation.   In the appropriate clinical setting, i.e., in adults with medium or heavy body builds with the aforementioned causes excluded, and in the presence of predisposing diseases (e.g., coronary artery disease, hypertension), the diagnosis of left posterior fascicular block is likely.

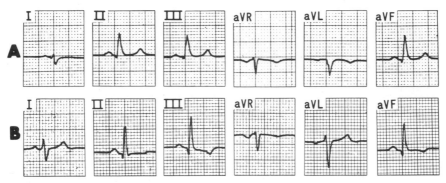

Fig. 11-23   (A) Left posterior fascicular block, in this case the residual of previous inferior myocardial infarction.   There is right axis deviation of the terminal 0.04-s QRS vector.   Small normal Q waves are present in leads II, III, and aVF.   The initial 0.04-s QRS vector is normally directed.   These findings are suggestive of left posterior fascicular block but are not diagnostic. That they are actually due to left posterior fascicular block, however, is shown by comparing A with B.   (B) A tracing taken on the same patient 2 years previously during an episode of acute inferior infarction.   Abnormal Q waves diagnostic of infarction are associated with the terminal 0.04-s QRS vector deformity of left posterior fascicular block.   By the time the electrocardiogram in A was recorded, the Q wave abnormality had disappeared, but the intraventricular block pattern persisted.

7   Left posterior fascicular block is not often an isolated lesion.   It is more commonly associated with right bundle branch block, inferior infarction, or both.

Myocardial Infarction with
Left Posterior Fascicular Block

This condition is discussed in Chap. 13.

The Bifascicular Blocks

Technically, the term *bifascicular block* refers to a block of any two fascicles of the ventricular conduction system.   In its common usage, however, the term refers to a combination of right bundle branch block with either left anterior fascicular block or left posterior fascicular block.   However, to avoid semantic errors, it is more meaningful to describe the specific conduction abnormalities in each case.

Right bundle branch block with left anterior fascicular block is commonly related to coronary artery disease in patients who are middle-aged. Below the age of 40 years, this bifascicular block may be caused by a cardiomyopathy or by aortic valve disease.   There is also a group of patients in whom this abnormality does not appear to be associated with any type of heart disease.   However, when these patients are followed, they frequently develop complete heart block.   The apparent cause is Lenegre's disease, a sclerodegenerative process specifically affecting the conduction system.   In elderly patients (usually above the age of 70 years), right bundle branch block with left anterior fascicular block may occur in the absence of other evidence of heart disease. These cases are caused by sclerosis of the left side of the cardiac skeleton, an entity called *Lev's disease*. These rather rarely develop complete AV block. Lev's disease may also cause right bundle branch block, left anterior fascicular block, left bundle branch block, and, less commonly, complete heart block by injuring the penetrating portion of the bundle of His. Surgical repair of ventricular septal defects, including the tetralogy of Fallot, aortic valve replacement, and tricuspid valve replacement, may also result in intraventricular blocks.

Right bundle branch block with left posterior fascicular block is caused chiefly by cardiomyopathy or myocarditis in patients below the age of 40 years. Above this age, this type of bifascicular block is sometimes due to coronary artery disease, but most frequently its etiology is unknown. It is likely that most of these cases are due to Lenegre's disease.

Right bundle branch block with left anterior fascicular block is the most common electrocardiographic pattern preceding the development of complete heart block. The incidence of progression to complete heart block is reported to be from 2 to 6 percent per year. The risk is believed to be considerably higher for patients with right bundle branch block and left posterior fascicular block.

Right Bundle Branch Block with Left Anterior
Fascicular Block (Figs. 11-24, 11-25, 11-26)

In the presence of left anterior fascicular block, right bundle branch block shifts the mean QRS axis in a CCW manner, first superiorly, then rightward and superiorly, and finally rightward and inferiorly. When the axis shift is moderate (ÂQRS between −60 and −75°) because of the predominance of left ventricular forces, the electrocardiogram becomes atypical, resulting in the pattern of "masquerading" bundle branch block. The electrocardiogram may also become atypical if the shift is large (ÂQRS between −150 and +150°) because of a predominance of right ventricular forces arising from an hypertrophied right ventricle.

When right bundle branch block and left anterior fascicular block are combined, there are three main directions of the QRS forces in the frontal plane. During the first 0.02 s of the QRS complexes, the forces point inferiorly and rightward to about +120°, resulting in a small Q wave in leads aVL and I and small R waves in leads II, III, and aVF. During the next 0.04 to 0.06 s of the QRS complexes, the forces are directed leftward and superiorly to −45° or more. The two initial vectors are due to the left anterior fascicular block. The terminal 0.04- to 0.06-s QRS vector, produced by right bundle branch forces, is directed rightward toward the +180° axis.

1   The initial 0.02-s QRS vector is directed rightward and inferiorly,

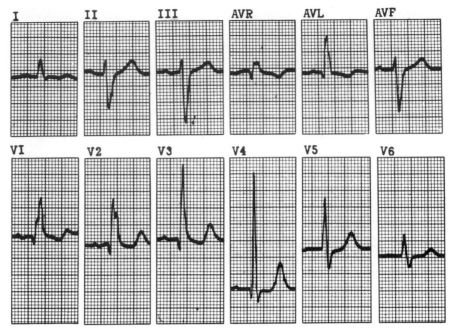

Fig. 11-24   Right bundle branch block with abnormal left axis deviation.   In addition, there are prominent Q waves in the right precordial leads due to old anteroseptal myocardial infarction.   The combination of right bundle branch block and abnormal left axis deviation of the unblocked forces is diagnostic of right bundle branch block with left anterior fascicular block.

    producing Q waves in leads aVL and I and small R waves in leads II, III, and aVF.

2   The mean vector for the first 0.06 to 0.08 s of the QRS complex is oriented leftward and superiorly above the $-45°$ axis (abnormal left axis deviation).

3   The terminal 0.04- to 0.06-s QRS vector is directed rightward and anteriorly and either inferiorly, horizontally, or superiorly.

4   Thus the limb leads typically show a qRS pattern in leads I and an initial rS pattern in leads III and aVF.

5   The precordial leads show the pattern of right bundle branch block, with an RSR' complex in lead V_1 and wide S waves in leads V_5 and V_6

Masquerading Bundle Branch Block

Masquerading bundle branch block is a term used to describe atypical electrocardiographic patterns associated with complete right bundle branch block.   Two types are recognized: (1) standard masquerading bundle branch block, in which the QRS pattern in the limb leads resembles that of left bundle branch block although the precordial electrocardiogram remains diagnostic of right bundle branch block; and (2) precordial masquerading bundle branch block, in which the right precordial pattern is that of right bundle branch block and the left precordial pattern that of left bundle branch block.

Masquerading bundle branch block is not a specific entity but is the result of right bundle branch block with varying combinations of left anterior fascicular block, intramural left ventricular block, left ventricular enlargement, and anterior myocardial infarction.

Standard Masquerading Bundle Branch Block (Figs. 11-26, 11-27, 11-28)

Atypical forms of right bundle branch block with left anterior fascicular block may occur. When the S wave in lead I becomes very small or disappears, the limb leads may resemble left bundle branch block although the precordial electrocardiogram remains typical for right bundle branch block. This is called *standard masquerading bundle branch block* by Rosenbaum. The sine qua non for this condition is a high degree of left anterior fascicular block superimposed on right bundle branch block, often associated with left ventricular hypertrophy and a localized block in the left ventricle.

Fig. 11-25 Complete right bundle branch block with left anterior fascicular block, a bifascicular block. The QRS interal is 0.16 s. Wide S waves are present in leads I and aVL, and the left precordial leads. RSR' complexes are seen in the right precordial leads. These findings are characteristic of right bundle branch block. There is abnormal left axis deviation (about −50°) of the first 0.06 s of the QRS complex in the frontal plane, with qR patterns in leads I and aVL, and rS deflections in leads II, III, and aVF. These findings are diagnostic of left anterior fascicular block.

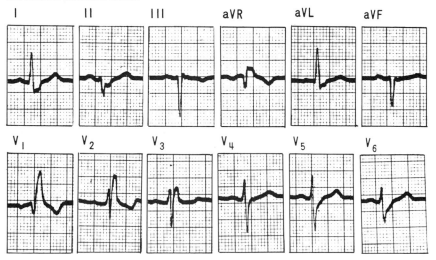

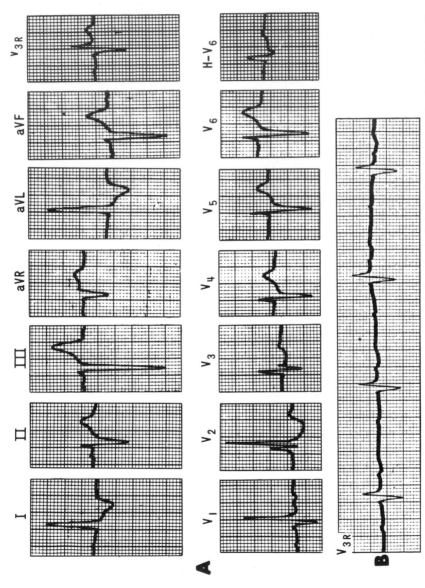

Fig. 11-26 (A) Standard masquerading bundle branch block. The limb leads show a pattern simulating left bundle branch block, but the precordial leads show the pattern of right bundle branch block. There is abnormal left axis deviation (about −60°) due to left anterior fascicular block. (B) Same patient as in (A), during complete AV block.

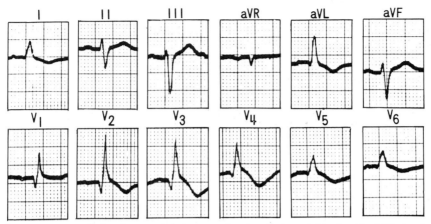

Fig. 11-27 Standard and precordial masquerading bundle branch block. The QRS duration is 0.12 s. The limb leads show an apparent pattern of left bundle branch block with abnormal left axis deviation. The precordial electrocardiograms exhibit the pattern of right bundle branch block in the right chest leads and the pattern of left bundle branch block on the left. Abnormal Q waves diagnostic of anterior myocardial infarction are also present.

1 Signs of right bundle branch block are noted in the precordial leads.
2 Signs of left anterior fascicular block consisting of deep S_2 and S_3 deflections, absence of an R′ wave in lead III, and an absent or very small S_1 are seen in the extremity leads. Q_1 may or may not be present.
3 The mean QRS axis is usually oriented between -60 and $-75°$.

Precordial Masquerading Bundle Branch Block
(Figs. 11-27, 11-28)

Some ventricular conduction defects show the pattern of right bundle branch block in the right precordial leads and left bundle branch block in

Fig. 11-28 Standard and precordial masquerading bundle branch block in a patient with old anterior and inferior myocardial infarction. First-degree AV block is present. The QRS interval is 0.12 s. The extremity leads show a pattern of what appears to be left bundle branch block. There is abnormal left axis deviation due to inferior infarction with left anterior fascicular block, but in lead V_6 left bundle branch block is simulated. Abnormal Q waves are seen in the precordial leads.

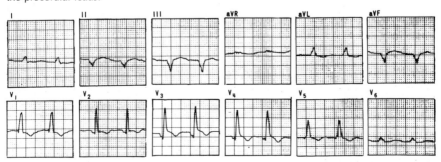

the left-sided leads.   This pattern has been termed *precordial masquerading bundle branch block.*

Precordial masquerading bundle branch block results from right bundle branch block associated with severe left ventricular hypertrophy, a localized block in the anterolateral wall of the left ventricle (often due to myocardial infarction), and usually left anterior fascicular block.   Presumably, the intramural left ventricular block, together with the left ventricular hypertrophy or the left anterior fascicular block, or both, produce predominant leftward forces which tend to cancel out the late rightward forces of the right bundle branch block in the left precordial leads and lead I.

Standard and precordial masquerading bundle branch block may occur in the same tracing (Figs. 11-26 and 11-27).   When precordial masquerading bundle branch block occurs in the absence of left anterior fascicular block, abnormal left axis deviation will not be seen in the limb leads.

Right Bundle Branch Block with Left Posterior
Fascicular Block (Fig. 11-29)

1   When right bundle branch block and left posterior fascicular block are combined, there are three main directions of the QRS forces in the FP. During the first 0.02 s of the QRS complex, the forces point superiorly and leftward to about −45°, resulting in small Q waves in leads II, III, and aVF and small R waves in leads I and aVL.   During the next 0.04 to 0.06 s, the forces are directed inferiorly and rightward to about +120°.   These initial vectors are due to the left posterior fascicular

Fig. 11-29 Right bundle branch block with left posterior fascicular block in a patient with old anterior and inferior myocardial infarction.   The tracing is typical of right bundle branch block, but there is also right axis deviation of the unblocked forces.

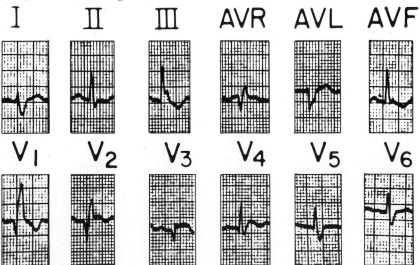

block. The terminal 0.04- to 0.06-s QRS vector, produced by right bundle branch block forces, is directed rightward toward the $+150$ to the $+180°$ axis.

2   The combination of right bundle branch block and left posterior fascicular block may be diagnosed when in right bundle branch block the vector for the first half of the QRS complex is directed at about $+120°$ with an S_1Q_3 pattern in the standard leads, provided a vertical heart, emphysema, right ventricular enlargement, and lateral wall infarction can be excluded.   The diagnosis is further supported by the presence of tall R waves in leads II, III, and aVF and of AV conduction disturbances.

3   The findings in the precordial leads in right bundle branch block with left posterior fascicular block are generally as follows:

a   The normal Q wave found in leads V_4 to V_6 is generally absent. However, small Q waves may be present in leads V_4 to V_6 recorded at a lower level.

b   A Q wave is commonly recorded in lead V_1, even in the absence of anteroseptal infarction.

c   There is a tendency for large R/S ratios to occur in the left precordial leads.

d   The QRS complexes are predominantly negative in high V leads and largely positive in low V leads.

Bilateral Bundle Branch Block
(Figs. 11-30, 11-31)

Block in the His-Purkinje system, rather than block in the AV node or bundle of His, is the most common cause of complete AV block.   There are no adequate criteria for determining the precise location of the site of complete heart block from the surface electrocardiogram alone.   However, it is often possible to diagnose bilateral bundle branch block electrocardiographically prior to the development of complete heart block or during periods when AV conduction returns.

1   A definite diagnosis of bilateral bundle branch block can be made if the patterns of right and left bundle branch block, accompanied by changes in the P-R interval, occur alternately or intermittently in the same patient (Fig. 11-30).   The mechanism of this phenomenon is explained in Fig. 11-31.

2   If the patterns of right bundle branch block and left bundle branch block appear at different times in the same patient but the P-R interval remains constant, the diagnosis of bilateral bundle branch block is reasonably secure.

3   The combination of first- and second-degree AV block with bundle branch block may represent bilateral bundle branch block (i.e, complete block in one bundle branch with incomplete block in the contralateral

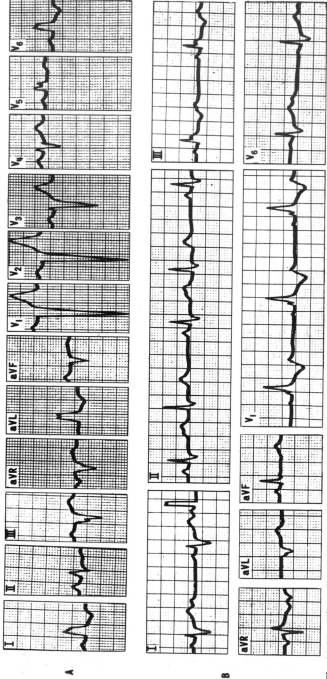

Fig. 11-30 Bilateral bundle branch block manifested by intermittent left and right bundle branch block accompanied by changes in AV conduction. In A, there is normal sinus rhythm with left bundle block and a P-R interval of 0.22 s. In B, recorded at another time from the same patient, there is right bundle branch block, a P-R interval of 0.16 s in the conducted beats, and 2:1 AV block in all leads except lead II. This lead shows a Wenchkebach phenomenon with 3:2 AV condition. The patient ultimately developed complete AV block.

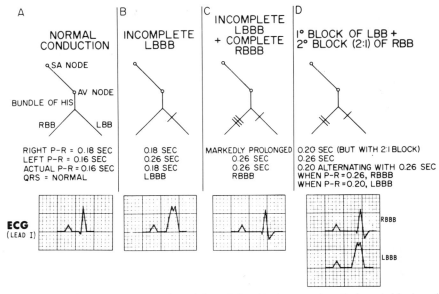

Fig. 11-31 Schematic representation of the relationship between bundle branch block and AV conduction. In A, normal conduction is portrayed. The left P-R interval is assumed to be 0.16 s, the right, 0.18 s. The shorter left P-R interval is accounted for by the earlier arrival of the impulse on the left side of the interventricular septum. The actual P-R interval is 0.16 s, and the QRS complex is normal. In B, first-degree block is assumed to be present in the left bundle branch with normal conduction preserved on the right. The left P-R interval measures 0.26 s and the right 0.18 s. The actual P-R interval is 0.18 s, because excitation reaches the ventricles from the right side. The QRS complex shows left bundle branch block. In C, third-degree block is present on the right. The right P-R interval is markedly prolonged; the left is delayed to 0.26 s. The actual P-R interval is 0.26 s, because activation reaches the ventricles via the left bundle branch. The QRS complex shows right bundle branch block. In D, first-degree block of the left bundle branch is associated with a 2:1 second-degree block on the right. When an impulse is conducted through the right bundle branch, the P-R interval is 0.20 s and the QRS complex shows left bundle branch block. However, when the impulse to the right bundle branch is blocked, it will be transmitted to the left bundle branch at a P-R interval of 0.26 s with a QRS pattern of right bundle branch block. Thus the electrocardiogram shows alternating right and left bundle branch block accompanied by changes in the P-R interval. *(After Rosenbaum and Lepeschkin.)*

bundle branch). However, when bundle branch block is accompanied by incomplete AV block, the latter may be sited in the AV node, the bundle of His, or the other bundle branch. The exact location of the block can only be determined by the use of His bundle recordings. Thus, the finding of bundle branch block together with incomplete AV block in surface leads can only suggest the possibility or probability of bilateral bundle branch block.

The Trifascicular Blocks (Figs. 11-32, 11-33)

The term *trifascicular block* refers to a combination of right bundle branch block with intermittent left anterior *and* left posterior fascicular block.

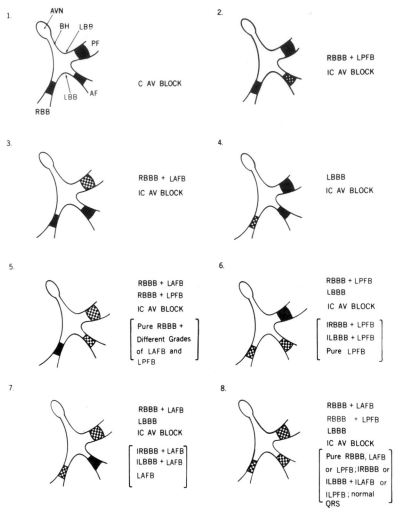

Fig. 11-32 The trifascicular blocks. The drawings represent the eight possible trifascicular blocks described in the text. In the diagrams, the bracketed symbols show the less common manifestations of the trifascicular blocks. The blacked-out areas indicate complete block in the involved bundle(s) or fascicle(s). The stippled areas represent unstable or intermittent conduction. The abbreviations used are as follows: AVN = AV node; BH = bundle of His; LBB = left bundle branch; PF = posterior fascicle; AF = anterior fascicle; RBB = right bundle branch; C = complete; IC = incomplete; ILBBB = incomplete left bundle branch block; IRBBB = incomplete right bundle branch block; LAFB = left anterior fascicular block; LPFB = left posterior fascicular block. (Modified from M. B. Rosenbaum, M. C. Elizari, and J. O. Lazarri, "The Hemiblocks," Tampa Tracings, Oldsmar, Fla. 1970. Used by permission.)

Trifascicular block is a possibility only when right bundle branch block is associated with *either* left anterior or left posterior fascicular block and incomplete AV block (because the AV block may be sited in the AV node, the bundle of His, or the left bundle proximally, rather than in the remaining fascicle).

There are eight possible trifascicular blocks (Rosenbaum et al.): (1) Block is present in the right bundle branch as well as in the two divisions of the left bundle, resulting in complete AV block. (2) Block is permanent in the right bundle branch and the posterior fascicle of the left bundle branch and intermittent in the anterior fascicle. The electrocardiogram

Fig. 11-33 Trifascicular block, first-degree AV block, and Mobitz Type II second-degree AV block. Two different types of QRS complexes are seen. Those marked by an asterisk show the pattern of right bundle branch block with left anterior fascicular block. The other QRS complexes show right bundle branch block with left posterior fascicular block. The occurrence of right bundle branch block with both left anterior and left posterior fascicular block in the same tracing establishes the diagnosis of trifascicular block. The P-R interval of the conducted beats is constant at 0.36 s. Occasional P waves are blocked. The diagnosis of Mobitz Type II second-degree AV block is based on the findings of intermittently blocked P waves in the presence of a constant, prolonged P-R interval. In the illustration, the arrows point to the P waves.

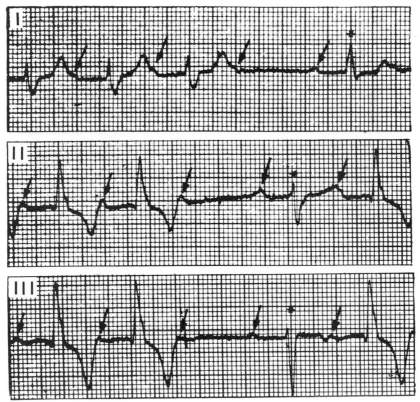

will show right bundle branch block with left posterior fascicular block and varying degrees of incomplete AV block.   (3) Block is permanent in the right bundle branch and the anterior fascicle of the left bundle branch and intermittent in the posterior fascicle.   The electrocardiogram will show right bundle branch block with left anterior fascicular block and varying degrees of incomplete AV block.   (4) Block is permanent in both divisions of the left bundle branch and intermittent in the right bundle branch.   The electrocardiogram will show left bundle branch block and incomplete AV block.   (5) Block is permanent in the right bundle branch and intermittent in both divisions of the left bundle branch.   The electrocardiogram may show right bundle branch block with either left anterior or left posterior fascicular block and incomplete AV block.   (6) Block is permanent in the posterior fascicle of the left bundle branch and intermittent in the anterior fascicle and right bundle branch.   The electrocardiogram will usually show right bundle branch block (with left posterior fascicular block) or left bundle branch block, and incomplete AV block.   Less likely possibilities are incomplete right bundle branch block with left posterior fascicular block, incomplete left bundle branch block with left posterior fascicular block, and pure left posterior fascicular block.   (7) Block is permanent in the anterior fascicle and intermittent in the posterior fascicle and right bundle branch.   The electrocardiogram will usually show right bundle branch block (with left anterior fascicular block) or left bundle branch block, and incomplete AV block.   Less likely possibilities are incomplete right bundle branch block with left anterior fascicular block, incomplete left bundle branch block with anterior fascicular block, and pure left anterior fascicular block.   (8) Block is unstable or intermittent in all three fascicles.   The electrocardiogram most likely will show right bundle branch block (with either left anterior or left posterior fascicular block) or left bundle branch block, left anterior fascicular block, or left posterior fascicular block; incomplete right or left bundle branch block with either left anterior or posterior fascicular block or a normal QRS complex.

Bilateral Bundle Branch Block
and Trifascicular Block

1   The term *bilateral bundle branch block* should be reserved for cases in which the patterns of both right and left bundle branch block are observed in the same patient.   The diagnosis of incomplete bilateral bundle branch block may be suggested in cases of unilateral bundle branch block (either right bundle branch block with a normal QRS axis or left bundle branch block) combined with incomplete AV block. Confirmation of the diagnosis requires demonstration of a prolonged H-V interval in His bundle recordings.

2   The term *trifascicular block* should be employed to designate cases in which right bundle branch block with left anterior and left posterior

fascicular block are observed in the same patient.   The diagnosis of possible trifascicular block may be suggested in patients with bifascicular block and incomplete AV block, in which the His bundle electrogram shows prolongation of the H-V interval.   It may also be considered under the circumstances outlined under the heading, The Trifascicular Blocks, earlier in this chapter.

3   In actual practice, it is preferable to use the specific names of the conduction disturbances observed in the electrocardiograms rather than to designate the abnormalities as bilateral bundle branch block or trifascicular block.   For example, when right bundle branch block with either left anterior or left posterior fascicular block is accompanied by incomplete AV block, a description suggesting all the likely possibilities is preferable to the use of the term trifascicular block.

BUNDLE BRANCH BLOCK AND AXIS DEVIATION

A combination of right bundle branch block and right axis deviation of the first half of the QRS complex is indicative of concomitant left posterior fascicular block, provided the other criteria for the diagnosis are met and other possibile causes of right axis deviation are excluded.

A combination of right bundle branch block and abnormal left axis deviation of the first half of the QRS complex is indicative of concomitant left anterior fascicular block, provided the other criteria for the diagnosis are met.

The combination of left bundle branch block and right axis deviation is rare and suggests coexistent right ventricular enlargement, left posterior fascicular block, or infarction of the free wall of the left ventricle.

The combination of left bundle branch block and abnormal left axis deviation occurs frequently.   However, its significance is difficult to evaluate.   It is first necessary to consider the effect of left bundle branch block per se on the QRS axis.   Rosenbaum et al. have studied the problem in detail.   In about two-thirds of cases, left bundle branch block shifts the original mean QRS axis direction about 40° leftward.   In about one-fifth of cases, left bundle branch block shifts the prior mean QRS axis about 20° rightward.   In the remaining cases, left bundle branch block shows an axis superior to −45°.   In approximately 30 percent of these cases, left anterior fascicular block is found in the electrocardiogram during the absence of left bundle branch block, but in the remaining 70 percent, left bundle branch block alone is responsible for the abnormally directed QRS axis. In left bundle branch block, therefore, a mean QRS axis superior to −45° may suggest that left anterior fascicular block is present, but it must then be assumed that the left bundle branch block is not "complete," regardless of the duration of the QRS complexes.   This is because when left bundle branch block is truly complete, the mean QRS direction is shifted relatively to the right and will thus conceal the existence of left anterior fascicular block.

Lichstein and his associates, in a study of patients with complete left bundle branch block and left axis deviation, found that the majority develop left axis deviation (due to left anterior fascicular block) separately, either before or after the appearance of the left bundle branch block. They concluded that, at least in these patients, the combination of left bundle branch block and left axis deviation represents a combination of predivisional and divisional block of the left bundle branch.

THE HIS BUNDLE ELECTROGRAM IN VENTRICULAR CONDUCTION DEFECTS

It will be recalled from Chap. 5 that the P-H time represents the sum of the intraatrial and AV nodal conduction time; the A-H interval, conduction through the AV node and probably the proximal portion of the bundle of His; and the H-V time, conduction through the bundle branches, the Purkinje network, and probably the distal portion of the bundle of His.

Narula and others have performed detailed studies on His bundle recordings in ventricular conduction defects. The statistical data in the succeeding paragraphs are those reported by Narula.

It is estimated that 70 percent of patients with isolated left anterior fascicular block and a narrow QRS complex have normal H-V times. An abnormal H-V time in such cases is probably indicative of conduction delay in the bundle of His proximal to its bifurcation into the bundle branches.

Cases with left posterior fascicular block and a narrow QRS complex are rare and theoretically should show normal H-V times. The incidence of abnormal H-V time was 40 percent in five patients studied by Narula.

The majority of patients (68 percent) with right bundle branch and a normal QRS axis have a normal H-V time. Even those with first-degree AV block generally have a normal H-V time, indicating that even when the P-R interval is prolonged, the major delay is the result of block in the AV node.

Virtually all patients (87 percent) with right bundle branch and right posterior fascicular block and a normal P-R interval have abnormal H-V times but normal A-H times, indicating additional damage in the remaining fascicles of the His-Purkinje system. When first-degree block coexists, the major delay responsible for the long P-R interval occurs in either the AV node or the His-Purkinje system.

The vast majority (72 percent) of patients with right bundle branch block and left anterior fascicular block, with or without myocardial infarction, have an abnormal H-V time, indicating additional disease in the His-Purkinje system. When right bundle branch block with left anterior fascicular block is associated with a normal P-R interval, the A-V time is usually normal even when the H-V time is prolonged. When this type of bifascicular block is combined with first-degree AV block, the H-V interval is almost invariably prolonged. However, the major delay responsible for the prolongation of the P-R interval is usually found in the A-H interval. Less often, it may occur during the H-V interval or during both the A-H and H-V intervals.

The H-V time is abnormal in 79 percent of patients with left bundle branch block and a normal P-R interval and in 80 percent of those with a prolonged P-R interval, indicating damage in the contralateral bundle branch. In patients with first-degree AV block and left bundle branch block, the principal delay in the P-R interval is produced by an abnormal A-H time (disease of the AV node) in addition to a comparatively slight prolongation of the H-V time.

SOME THERAPEUTIC IMPLICATIONS IN VENTRICULAR CONDUCTION DEFECTS

The decision whether or not to institute permanent transvenous-demand pacemakers in patients with ventricular conduction defects such as bifascicular, trifascicular, or bilateral bundle branch block is based largely on the physician's subjective judgment. In the presence of cardiac symptoms related to paroxysmal second-degree or advanced AV block, a permanent pacemaker is usually recommended. Bilateral bundle branch block (alternating bundle branch block) is also an indication for permanent pacing. When the clinical symptomatology is imprecise, Holter monitoring and electrophysiologic studies including determination of the basal H-V interval, atrial pacing, programmed atrial depolarizations, and the evaluation of drug effects are probably indicated. Based on the results of testing, a decision can be made whether or not to implant a permanent cardiac pacemaker. (See Table 11-1.)

TABLE 11-1 INTRAVENTRICULAR CONDUCTION DISTURBANCES: RECOMMENDATIONS FOR CLINICAL CARDIAC PACING

	H-V ≦ 55 ms	H-V = 60 to 99 ms	H-V ≧ 100 ms
LBBB, RBBB, IVCD	No	Yes, with symptoms†	Yes
RBBB + LAHB or LPHB	No*	Yes, with symptoms†	Yes
Alternating BBB	‡	Yes	Yes

NOTE: LBBB = left bundle branch block; RBBB = right bundle branch block; LAHB = left anterior hemiblock; LPHB = left posterior hemiblock; BBB = bundle branch block.
* Except in cases of clearly documented cardiac syncope
† Noncardiac causes of symptoms excluded
‡ Rarely occurs
SOURCE: M. E. Josephson and S. F. Seides, "Clinical Cardiac Electrophysiology," Lea & Febiger, Philadelphia, 1979, p. 117. Used by permission.

VECTORCARDIOGRAM IN THE FASCICULAR AND BIFASCICULAR BLOCKS

Left Anterior Fascicular Block (Fig. 11-34A)

The characteristic pattern is best described in the FP and LSP.

1   In the absence of other abnormalities, the magnitude of the spatial QRS loop is in the normal range. The duration of the QRS loop is no greater than 100 ms or does not exceed by more than 20 ms its duration during normal conduction. Slight terminal conduction delay may be observed.
2   Rotation of the loop in the FP is CCW in the overwhelming majority of cases. The CCW rotation of the initial 30-ms QRS vector is helpful in differentiating this condition from inferior infarction, which generally shows CW rotation of this vector. The initial 10- and 20-ms QRS vectors are directed inferiorly, and the maximum QRS deflection vectors are displaced superiorly. Most of the QRS loop area is located in the left superior quadrant.
3   In the LSP, the QRS loop rotates CCW in the majority of cases, but figure-of-eight and CW rotation may also occur. The maximum QRS deflection is directed superiorly and posteriorly. Most of the QRS loop area is located in the posterosuperior quadrant.
4   In the TP, the QRS loop usually presents no diagnostic features. Rotation is CCW and sometimes figure of eight. CW rotation does not occur unless anterior myocardial infarction is associated.

Fig. 11-34 The frontal plane vectorcardiogram in left anterior (A) and left posterior (B) fascicular block.

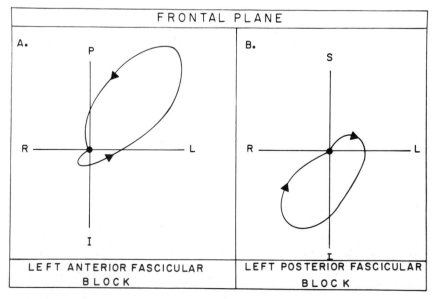

FRONTAL PLANE

A.

B.

LEFT ANTERIOR FASCICULAR BLOCK   LEFT POSTERIOR FASCICULAR BLOCK

5   The ST-T vectors and T loop are normal in the absence of associated disease.

Left Posterior Fascicular Block (Fig. 11-34B)

The characteristic pattern is seen best in the FP and LSP.

1   The duration of the QRS loop is no greater than 100 ms or does not exceed by more than 20 ms its duration during normal conduction. Slight terminal conduction may be observed. The magnitude of the QRS loop is in the normal range.
2   Rotation of the loop in the FP is CW. The 10- and 20-ms vectors are directed leftward and superiorly. The maximum QRS deflection is directed inferiorly and rightward to about +110°. Most of the loop area is located in the right inferior quadrant.
3   In the LSP, the QRS loop rotates CCW. Most of the QRS loop area is located in the inferoposterior quadrant.
4   In the TP, inscription of the QRS loop is CCW, with the main QRS vectors directed posteriorly and rightward. At least 20 percent of the loop area is located in the right posterior quadrant.
5   The ST-T vectors and T loop are normal in the absence of associated disease.
6   The vectorcardiographic differential diagnosis between right ventricular hypertrophy and left posterior fascicular block may be difficult or impossible. Left posterior fascicular block should not be diagnosed unless a vertical heart, emphysema, right ventricular enlargement, and lateral-wall myocardial infarction can be excluded on clinical grounds.

Left Anterior Fascicular Block with Right Bundle Branch Block

The vectorcardiogram shows the characteristic features of left anterior fascicular block in the FP and the findings of right bundle branch block in the TP.

Left Posterior Fascicular Block with Right Bundle Branch Block

The vectorcardiogram shows the characteristic features of left posterior fascicular block in the FP and the findings of right bundle branch block in the TP.

REFERENCES

Baydar, I. D., T. J. Walsh, and E. Massie: A Vectorcardiographic Study of Right Bundle Branch Block with the Frank Lead System. Clinical Correlation in

Ventricular Hypertrophy and Chronic Pulmonary Disease, *Am. J. Cardiol.*, 15: 185, 1965.

Benchimol, A.: "Vectorcardiography," Williams & Wilkins, Baltimore, 1973.

Chou, T-C., R. A. Helm, and S. Kaplan: "Clinical Vectorcardiography," 2d ed., Grune & Stratton, New York, 1974.

Demoulin, J. C., and H. E. Kulbertus: Pathologic Basis of Left Posterior Hemiblock, *Am. J. Cardiol.*, 37: 131, 1976.

Denes, P., R. C. Dhingra, D. Wu et al.: H-V Interval in Patients with Bifascicular Block (Right Bundle Branch Block and Left Anterior Hemiblock), *Am. J. Cardiol.*, 35: 23, 1975.

Dodge, H. T., and R. P. Grant: Mechanism of QRS Complex Prolongation in Man: Right Ventricular Conduction Defects, *Am. J. Med.*, 21: 534, 1956.

Grant, R. P.: Mechanisms of QRS Prolongation in Left Ventricular Conduction Disturbances, *Am. J. Med.*, 20: 834, 1956.

Hecht, H. H. et al.: Atrioventricular and Intraventricular Conduction—Revised Nomenclature and Concepts, *Am. J. Cardiol.*, 31: 232, 1973.

Helfant, R. H., and B. J. Scherlag: "His Bundle Electrocardiography," Medcom Press, New York, 1974.

Horwitz, S., E. Lupi, J. Hayes et al.: Electrocardiographic Criteria for the Diagnosis of Left Anterior Fascicular Block, *Chest*, 68: 317, 1975.

Lenegre, J.: Etiology and Pathology of Bilateral Branch Block in Relation to Complete Heart Block, *Progr. Cardiovasc. Dis.*, 6: 409, 1964.

Lepeschkin, E.: Electrocardiographic Diagnosis of Bilateral Bundle Branch Block in Relation to Heart Block, *Progr. Cardiovasc. Dis.*, 6: 445, 1964.

Lev, M., and S. Bharali: Atrioventricular and Intraventricular Conduction Disease, *Arch. Intern. Med.*, 135: 405, 1975.

Lichstein, E., R. Mahaptra, P. R. Gupta, and K. D. Chadda: Significance of Complete Left Bundle Branch Block with Left Axis Deviation, *Circulation*, 58 (Suppl II): 766, 1978.

Moore, E. N., J. P. Boineau, and D. F. Patterson: Incomplete Right Bundle Branch Block: An Electrocardiographic Enigma and Possible Misnomer, *Circulation*, 44: 678, 1971.

Narula, O. S. (ed.): "His Bundle Electrocardiography and Clinical Electrophysiology," F. A. Davis, Philadelphia, 1975.

———: Intraventricular Conduction Defects, in O. S. Narula (ed.), "His Bundle Electrocardiography and Clinical Electrophysiology," F. A. Davis, Philadelphia, 1975.

Pryor, R.: The Clinical Significance of Left Ventricular Blocks, *Bull. N. Y. Academy of Medicine*, 47: 973, 1971.

———: Fascicular Blocks and the Bilateral Bundle Branch Block Syndrome, *Am. Heart J.*, 83: 441, 1972.

——— and S. G. Blount, Jr.: The Clinical Significance of True Left Axis Deviation: Left Intraventricular Blocks, *Am. Heart J.*, 72: 391, 1966.

Rosenbaum, M.: Types of Right Bundle Branch Block and Their Clinical Significance, *J. Electrocardiol.*, 1: 221, 1968.

———: Types of Left Bundle Branch Block and Their Clinical Significance, *J. Electrocardiol.*, 2: 197, 1969.

———: The Hemiblocks: Diagnostic Criteria and Clinical Significance, *Mod. Concepts Cardiovasc. Dis.*, 39: 141, 1970.

————, M. V. Elizari, and J. O. Lazzari: "The Hemiblocks," Tampa Tracings, Oldsmar, Fla.,1970.

———— et al.: The Differential Electrocardiographic Manifestations of Hemiblocks, Bilateral Bundle Branch Block, and Trifascicular Blocks, in R. C. Schlant and J. W. Hurst (eds.), "Advances in Electrocardiography," Grune & Stratton, New York, 1972.

———— et al.: The Clinical Causes and Mechanisms of Intraventricular Conduction Disturbances, in R. C. Schlant and J. W. Hurst (eds.), "Advances in Electrocardiography," Grune & Stratton, New York, 1972.

———— et al.: "The Mechanism of Intermittent Bundle Branch Block: Relationship to Prolonged Recovery, Hypopolarization and Spontaneous Diastolic Depolarization, *Chest,* 63: 666, 1973.

———— and E. Lepeschkin: Bilateral Bundle Branch Block, *Am. Heart J.,* 50: 38, 1955.

Scanlon, P. J.: Right Bundle-Branch Block Associated with Left Superior or Inferior Intraventricular Block—Associated with Acute Myocardial Infarction, *Circulation,* 42: 1135, 1970.

————, R. Pryor, and S. G. Blount, Jr.: Right Bundle-Branch Block Associated with Left Superior or Inferior Intraventricular Block—Clinical Setting, Prognosis, and Relation to Complete Heart Block, *Circulation,* 42: 1123, 1970.

Schloff, L. D., L. Adler, E. Donoso, and C. K. Friedberg: Bilateral Bundle Branch Block, *Circulation,* 35: 790, 1965.

Scott, R. C.: Left Bundle Branch Block—A Clinical Assessment, *Am. Heart J.,* 70: 535, 691, 813, 1965.

Unger, P. N., M. E. Lesser, U. H. Kugel, and M. Lev: Concept of "Masquerading" Bundle Branch Block: An Electrocardiographic-Pathological Correlation, *Circulation,* 17: 397, 1958.

Wallace, A. G., E. H. Estes, Jr., and B. W. McCall: The Vectorcardiographic Findings in Left Bundle Branch Block: A Study Using the Frank Lead System, *Am. Heart J.,* 63: 508, 1962.

CHAPTER 12

THE PREEXCITATION, OR WOLFF-PARKINSON-WHITE (W-P-W), SYNDROME

THEORETICAL CONSIDERATIONS

Ventricular preexcitation is said to be present when, in relation to atrial events, the whole or part of the ventricular myocardium is activated by the atrial impulse sooner than would be expected if the impulse reached the ventricles only by way of the normal AV conduction system.

It is currently accepted that there are one or more accessory pathways which permit a supraventricular impulse to partially or completely bypass the AV node and activate part of the ventricle prematurely. The atrial impulse may be conducted to the ventricles through either the accessory pathway or the normal AV conduction pathway or both. An accessory bundle has been demonstrated histologically in about one-half of the patients with ventricular preexcitation who have been studied carefully at postmortem examination.

Studies of the possible anatomic pathways for conduction from the atria to the ventricles, cited in Chap. 2, provide the anatomic background for the explanation of the various forms of anomalous AV conduction (Fig. 12-1). According to Ferrer, in the *classic form of W-P-W syndrome*, the impulse is transmitted through the bundle of Kent (producing the short P-R interval), to the ipsilateral ventricle (initiating preexcitation), and later to the contralateral ventricle (which results in a prolonged QRS interval). Alternatively, excitation may travel over the bypass tract of James, with attendant shortening of the P-R interval, and then over the Mahaim fibers to the ventricles (which produces the delta wave and wide QRS complex). When there is a *short P-R interval and a normal QRS complex,* it is assumed that only the bypass tract of James is utilized. This mechanism could explain the short P-R interval and normal QRS complex of at least some cases of the Lown-Ganong-Levine syndrome. In cases with a *normal P-R interval but with a delta wave and a wide QRS complex,* Ferrer believes that the impulse is conducted normally through the AV junction after its entrance at the crest of the AV node. The P-R interval is thus not shortened. However, because transmission to the ventricles takes place in the Mahaim tract, a delta wave and a broad QRS deflection are inscribed.

Since the bypass tracts presumably conduct bidirectionally, reentry may explain the frequency of supraventricular arrhythmias in this syndrome.

Fig. 12-1 Summary of anatomic tracts probably responsible for anomalous AV conduction of classic W-P-W (top left and top right), anomalous AV conduction with a short P-R interval but normal QRS duration (bottom left), and anomalous AV conduction with normal or prolonged P-R interval, delta wave, and wide QRS complex. *(From M. I. Ferrer, New Concepts Relating to the Preexcitation Syndrome, J.A.M.A., 201: 1038, 1967. Used by permission.)*

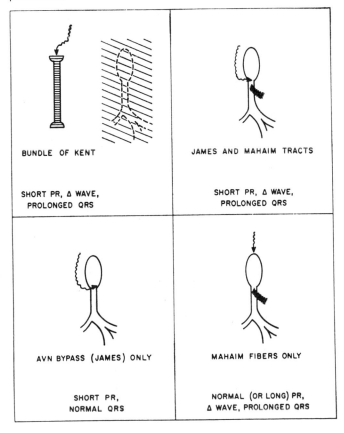

BUNDLE OF KENT

SHORT PR, Δ WAVE,
PROLONGED QRS

JAMES AND MAHAIM TRACTS

SHORT PR, Δ WAVE,
PROLONGED QRS

AVN BYPASS (JAMES) ONLY

SHORT PR,
NORMAL QRS

MAHAIM FIBERS ONLY

NORMAL (OR LONG) PR,
Δ WAVE, PROLONGED QRS

Thus an impulse descending to the ventricles through the AV junction may turn around and reenter the atria through the accessory pathway, or less often it may travel down the accessory pathway, turn around, and then return to the atria by way of the AV node. In either case, reentry and reexcitation of the atria may induce an arrhythmia, particularly if the atrial tissues are in the vulnerable phase of recovery. Some investigators believe that the supraventricular tachycardias in this syndrome may be due to functional longitudinal dissociation of the AV node alone.

It has been suggested that the term *anomalous atrioventricular excitation* be used to describe the electrocardiographic abnormality of ventricular preexcitation irrespective of its clinical correlation with tachycardia. Under this circumstance, the term *Wolff-Parkinson-White, or preexcitation syndrome,* would be reserved for the combination of anomalous atrioventricular excitation with episodes of paroxysmal tachyarrhythmia.

The preceding classification of the anatomic connections described by the terms Kent fibers, James fibers and Mahaim fibers, has been objected to by various authorities because it is imprecise and does not permit sufficient flexibility in the explanation of electrophysiologic and pathologic observations. The European Study Group for preexcitation has devised a new classification of the preexcitation syndromes based on their proposed anatomic connections. These connections are as follows, with the previous terminology listed in parentheses: (1) accessory AV connection (Kent bundle, also called the Paladine tract in the septum); (2) atriofascicular bypass tract (atrio-Hisian fiber); (3) intranodal bypass tract (James fiber); (4) nodoventricular connection (Mahaim fiber); and (5) fasciculoventricular connection (Mahaim fiber).

Multiple bypass tracts have been demonstrated in some individuals. Concealed accessory pathways conducting only in retrograde fashion are involved in the genesis of many cases of paroxysmal supraventricular tachycardia.

CLASSIFICATION

Depending on the direction of inscription of the delta wave, the W-P-W syndrome may be divided into two major groups:

1   Type A (Fig. 12-2), in which the delta wave and the remainder of the QRS complex are upright in both the right and left precordial leads. Lead V_1 shows a dominant R wave with R, RS, Rs, RSr', or Rsr' patterns, and lead V_6 shows Rs or R deflections.
2   Type B (Fig. 12-3), in which the delta wave is predominantly downward in lead V_1, and upright in the left precordial leads. Thus the left precordial leads show tall R waves, and lead V_1 shows an rS, QS, or qrS pattern.
3   In addition, there are rare cases of preexcitation which cannot be classified into either of the foregoing categories.

a Type C, in which the delta wave is negative or isoelectric in leads V_5 and V_6 and positive in leads V_1 to V_4.

b Other variants, in which the delta waves are seen at locations different from those listed above.

4 As a general rule, in Type A cases, preexcitation occurs in the posterobasal region of the left ventricle; in Type B cases, in the posterobasal region of the right ventricle. In both instances, the spread of depolarization proceeds from epicardium to endocardium at the site of preexcitation.

Many authorities have recommended that the classification of AV bypass tracts into types A and B based on the major QRS forces in leads V_1 and V_2 should be abandoned because intracardiac and epicardial mapping as well as vectorcardiography have demonstrated a poor correlation between the location of bypass tracts and these electrocardiographic patterns.

CLINICAL SIGNIFICANCE

The W-P-W syndrome, which is probably congenital in origin, occurs at all ages but is seen most frequently in persons below the age of 30 years and predominantly in males. Although most cases occur in healthy persons,

Fig. 12-2 Ventricular preexcitation, Type A. The P waves are normal, the P-R interval is short, the QRS complex is broad, and delta waves are present. The prominent Q waves in leads II, III, and aVF may lead to the erroneous diagnosis of inferior myocardial infarction. The upright QRS complexes in both right and left precordial leads are characteristic of the Type A preexcitation syndrome.

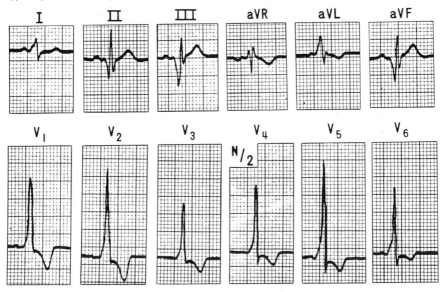

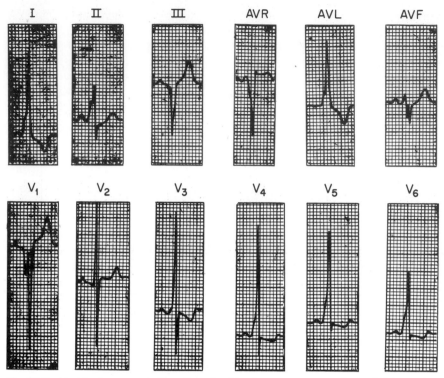

Fig. 12-3 Ventricular preexcitation, Type B. The P waves are normal, the P-R interval is short, the QRS deflection is broad, and delta waves are present. The downward-directed QRS complex in lead V_1 and the upright QRS complexes in the other precordial leads are characteristic of the Type B preexcitation syndrome.

organic heart disease is found in 30 to 40 percent of adults and 42 to 68 percent of children. A variety of congenital and acquired cardiac defects have been reported in patients with the preexcitation syndrome: Ebstein's anomaly, corrected transposition, idiopathic hypertrophic subaortic stenosis, septal defects, the tetralogy of Fallot, thyrotoxicosis, cardiomyopathies, and mitral valve prolapse.

Although surface electrocardiograms in some patients with idiopathic hypertrophic subaortic stenosis may suggest ventricular preexcitation, Josephson and Seides have failed to demonstrate electrophysiologic evidence of AV bypass tracts in two dozen cases.

CRITERIA FOR DIAGNOSIS (FIGS. 12-2, 12-3)

1 A short P-R interval, 0.12 s or less, in 85 percent of cases (and usually 0.10 s or less) in the presence of normal P waves.
2 A wide QRS interval, which exceeds 0.10 s in 70 percent of cases.

3 The presence of a *delta wave,* which is the diagnostic feature.   There is deformity and widening of the QRS complex by a heavily slurred or notched initial component, called the delta wave.   When the QRS deflection is upright, notching or slurring occurs on the ascending limb of the deflection; when downward, on the descending limb.

4 The P-J interval is 0.26 s or less whether conduction occurs via a normal or an anomalous pathway.   The widening of the QRS complex occurs at the expense of the P-R interval, which accounts for the constancy of the P-J interval during both types of conduction.

VARIATIONS

1 The concertina effect (Fig. 12-4) consists in progressive shortening of the P-R interval and a concomitant increase in the size of the delta wave and the duration of the QRS complex.   The reverse phenomenon may also occur, viz., the preexcitation complexes may show an increase in the P-R interval and narrowing of the QRS duration in successive beats until both return to normal values.   The concertina phenomenon has been attributed to variations in the amount of ventricular muscle undergoing premature activation.

2 The P-J interval may be shorter in anomalous beats than in normal beats.

3 The QRS complexes may change from an anomalous to a normal configuration during episodes of paroxysmal tachycardia.

OTHER FEATURES OF THE SYNDROME (FIGS. 12-5, 12-6)

1 Supraventricular arrhythmias occur in 40 to 80 percent of cases.   The approximate frequency and types of arrhythmias encountered in the W-P-W syndrome are as follows: atrial paroxysmal tachycardia, 70 percent; atrial fibrillation, 16 percent; supraventricular tachycardia, 10 percent; and atrial flutter, 4 percent.   Ventricular paroxysmal tachycardia is rare.   Premature systoles of atrial, AV functional, ventricular, or "bypass" tract origin my occur.   Atrioventricular dissociation, escape beats, and atrial and AV nodal parasystole may sometimes be seen.

Fig. 12-4   Concertina effect.   There is progressive shortening of the P-R intervals in successive beats, together with a corresponding increase in the size of the delta wave and in the duration of the QRS complexes.

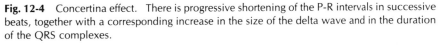
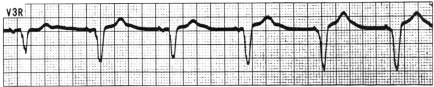

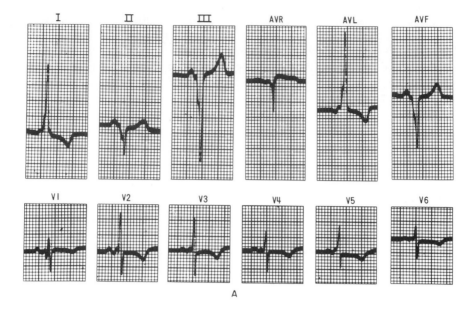

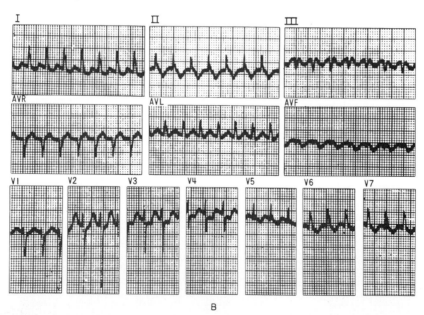

Fig. 12-5 (A) The W-P-W syndrome, Type B. There is normal sinus rhythm with anomalous AV conduction. From an elderly woman with frequent bouts of paroxysmal tachycardia. (B) Same patient as in (A), during a bout of supraventricular (probably atrial) tachycardia at a rate of 200 per minute. The QRS complexes are normal. The preexcitation complexes noted in (A) are no longer present.

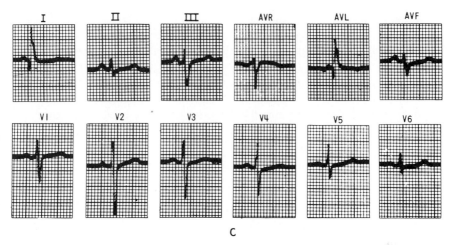

C

Fig. 12-5 (*Continued*)   (C) Same patient as in *A* and *B*, during sinus rhythm and normal AV conduction.   Signs of old superior myocardial infarction, manifested by deep Q waves in leads I and aVL, are now evident but were not present in records *A* or *B*.

The configuration of the QRS complexes is usually normal during paroxysms of tachycardia, but anomalous and aberrant ventricular conduction are observed frequently.   Aberrant ventricular conduction occurs in about 30 percent of supraventricular arrhythmias.

When atrial fibrillation occurs in the W-P-W syndrome, the ventricular response is usually quite rapid, often exceeding 200 beats per minute.   Aberration of the ventricular complexes is also common, so that ventricular tachycardia may be simulated.

Tachycardias with wide QRS complexes in the W-P-W syndrome may be due to reentry: (1) reentrant circuits may involve retrograde conduction over the accessory pathway and antegrade conduction over the normal pathway but with right or left bundle branch block; (2) retrograde conduction may take place over the normal pathway but with antegrade conduction over the accessory pathway; and (3) antegrade conduction may occur via one accessory pathway and retrograde conduction over another.   Supraventricular tachycardias not due to reentry may utilize only one accessory pathway for antegrade conduction.   Any wide QRS complex tachycardia observed in the absence of ventricular preexcitation may also occur in the W-P-W syndrome (e.g., ventricular tachycardia).

2   Atrioventricular block is uncommon in preexcitation.   However, all degrees of block have been reported in association with the syndrome.

3   A remarkable feature is the shift back and forth, even in the same tracing, between normal and anomalous conduction.

4   Q waves usually do not occur in leads I and aVL and in the left precordial leads because the delta vector is almost always directed leftward.   However, Q waves or QS deflections occur commonly in

leads II, III, and aVF (see Fig. 12-2) and in the right precordial leads (see Fig. 12-3). These Q waves or QS deflections may lead to the erroneous diagnosis of myocardial infarction. Similarly, the tall, broad R waves in the right precordial leads may suggest the diagnosis of right ventricular enlargement or strictly posterior myocardial infarction rather than preexcitation.

5   Secondary S-T segment and T wave changes occur but are variable and quite unstable.

6   The altered ventricular activation in the preexcitation syndrome obscures the electrocardiographic diagnosis of other entities (e.g., myocardial infarction and hypertrophy). These conditions can be diagnosed only when AV conduction is normal (Fig. 12-5), not when it is anomalous. However, left or right bundle branch block may sometimes be diagnosable during anomalous conduction.

Fig. 12-6   In *A* is shown paroxysmal atrial fibrillation with a ventricular response of about 220 per minute in a patient with the W-P-W syndrome. The QRST complexes during the tachycardia are unchanged from the preexcitation complexes during sinus rhythm, as shown in *B*. The rapid, irregular rhythm with wide QRS complexes may easily be mistaken for ventricular tachycardia.

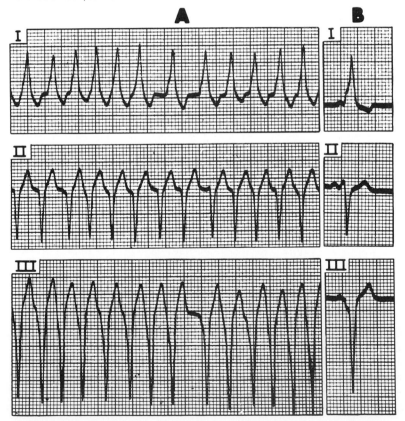

7 Exercise may reestablish normal AV conduction, but its effects are variable.

8 Drugs and vagal stimulation affect normal and anomalous conduction differently in the preexcitation syndrome. Digitalis, carotid sinus pressure, and vagal stimulation act to block normal AV conduction but have an insignificant effect on the accessory pathway. Their use tends to produce preexcitation. Quinidine and procainamide have a greater depressant effort on anomalous conduction than on AV conduction and hence will tend to terminate preexcitation. Atropine and isoproterenol also tend to abolish preexcitation, because they enhance conduction through the AV node. Recent studies suggest that lidocaine depresses anomalous .pathway conduction while propranolol depresses normal pathway conduction.

9 In atrial flutter, and especially atrial fibrillation, slowing of the AV nodal conduction by digitalis may serve to enhance conduction by the accessory pathway. Under such circumstances, the ventricles may be exposed to a deluge of atrial impulses, resulting in very fast and hemodynamically dangerous ventricular rates culminating in ventricular fibrillation and even death.

ELECTROPHYSIOLOGIC CONSIDERATIONS

Epicardial mapping, as well as electrophysiologic and anatomic studies in animals and humans, indicate that both the anomalous excitation and arrhythmias result from persistence of accessory atrioventricular pathways. Although there are three major postulated anatomic mechanisms for the W-P-W syndrome, more data are needed to confirm the functional importance of the various accessory pathways.

His bundle recordings and atrial pacing have proved useful in evaluating the electrophysiologic behavior of the normal and accessory AV pathways in patients with preexcitation.

In the His bundle electrogram, the P-delta interval is a measure of the conduction time through the anomalous pathway. The A-H time, on the other hand, reflects conduction through the normal AV pathway. In classic preexcitation, the A-H interval is usually normal and the H-V time short. Sometimes the H deflection may be recorded at the onset or even within the QRS complex.

The QRS complex in the W-P-W syndrome is considered by most authorities to be the result of fusion in ventricular activation between the impulse conducted through the accessory pathway and the AV node. If the P-delta and A-H times are close, the QRS complex is relatively narrow, whereas if the A-H interval is significantly longer than the P-delta time, the QRS tends to be wider and more aberrant.

Atrial pacing in conjunction with His bundle recordings may help to differentiate among the various types of preexcitation. Pacing at progressively faster atrial rates increases the delay at the AV node but has little or no effect on conduction through an accessory AV connection (Kent bundle). Hence, in this type of preexcitation, atrial pacing at progressively more rapid rates will gradually prolong the A-H interval but leave the P-delta time unaltered. The end result is an essentially unchanged P-R interval but a wider and more aberrant QRS complex. Since the nodoventricular and fasciculoventricular connections arise distal to the main body of the AV node, atrial pacing in this type of preexcitation will prolong both the A-H and P-delta times, resulting in longer P-R intervals but no change in the QRS complexes. When preexcitation results from conduction via an AV nodal bypass tract (James fiber), because the AV node is bypassed, atrial pacing will have little or no effect on either the P-R interval or the QRS complex.

DIFFERENTIAL DIAGNOSIS

Bundle Branch Block, Ventricular Hypertrophy, and Myocardial Infarction

The presence of wide QRS complexes in ventricular preexcitation may lead to the erroneous diagnosis of bundle branch block or other ventricular conduction defects. Similarly, because the voltages of the QRS deflections are often increased during anomalous conduction, ventricular hypertrophy may be diagnosed. Abnormal Q waves or QS deflections occur commonly during preexcitation in leads II, III, and aVF and in the right precordial leads. They may also occur in leads I and aVL, but this is rare. The presence of these Q waves or QS deflections may mislead into a diagnosis of myocardial infarction. Also, the tall, broad R waves seen so often in the right precordial leads may suggest the diagnosis of posterobasal myocardial infarction or right bundle block rather than preexcitation. In all these cases, the clues to correct diagnosis are the short P-R interval, the wide QRS complex, and most important, the presence of a delta wave.

Lown-Ganong-Levine Syndrome (Short P-R, Normal QRS, and Bouts of Tachycardia)

The classic W-P-W syndrome should be differentiated from the Lown-Ganong-Levine (L-G-L) syndrome. The diagnostic features of the latter are (1) a short P-R interval (0.12 s or less), (2) a QRS complex of normal configuration and duration (0.08 s or less), (3) extrasystoles, as well as frequent bouts of paroxysmal tachycardia. It occurs predominantly in middle-aged females in the absence of organic heart disease. Some authorities have considered this syndrome a variant form of ventricular preexcitation. In the majority of patients with the L-G-L syndrome, His bundle electrograms show a short A-H interval.

The presence of functionally operative accessory pathways (James fibers) which partially or completely bypass the AV node and reenter the conduction system in the lower portion of the node or the bundle of His has been held by some to be the most likely explanation for the short P-R interval and the normal QRS complexes. This undoubtedly is the most reasonable theory for the relatively small number of patients with this syndrome in whom the A-H interval remains constant during atrial pacing. However, other possibilities must be considered for those patients in whom the A-H interval increases during atrial pacing or in whom an initial increase in the A-H time is followed sequentially by a plateau response and further prolongation of the A-H time. An anatomically small AV node, a short or rapidly conducting intranodal pathway, isorhythmic AV dissociation, and sinoventricular rhythm have been suggested as alternative hypotheses.

The term *coronary nodal* rhythm has been used to describe rhythms characterized by normal P waves with short P-R intervals but without delta waves. This condition is discussed in Chap. 24.

It has been assumed that the underlying mechanism of the paroxysmal supraventricular tachycardias in the syndrome is reentry utilizing AV nodal bypass tracts or functional longitudinal dissociation of the AV node itself. However, in the group of patients studied by Monahan and his coworkers, all episodes of paroxysmal supraventricular tachycardia reflected either unifocal or multifocal atrial ectopic firing.

VECTORCARDIOGRAM IN THE W-P-W SYNDROME (FIG. 12-7)

The vectorcardiogram characteristically shows slow inscription of the initial portion of the QRS loop. The slowly inscribed portion is the delta deflection. Its duration varies between 0.02 and 0.08 s and is usually longer in Type A than in Type B.

Type A

In the TP, the delta deflection is directed anteriorly, either leftward or slightly rightward. The entire QRS loop is displaced anteriorly. There is usually CCW inscription of the loop, but a figure-of-eight pattern may occur.

In the FP, the orientation of the delta deflection is variable, but it is usually directed leftward and either superiorly or inferiorly. Inscription of the loop may be CW, CCW, or figure of eight.

Because the delta wave and the body of the QRS loop are directed anteriorly, the QRS complexes will be upright in all the precordial leads.

Since the delta vector is usually directed leftward, Q waves do not appear in leads I and aVL. However, if its orientation is rightward, Q waves may be present in these leads. When the delta wave is directed superiorly, Q waves or QS complexes appear in leads II, III, and aVF.

The initial slowing of the QRS loop is also visible in the LSP.

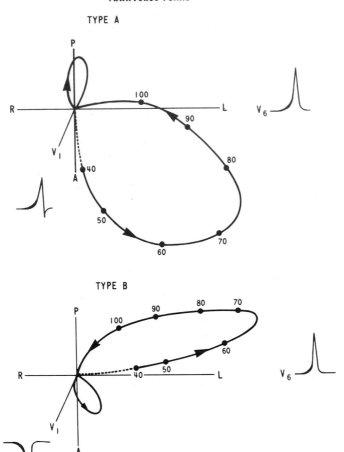

Fig. 12-7 Schematic representation of the vectorcardiogram in ventricular preexcitation, Types A and B. The QRS complexes in leads V_1 and V_6 are also diagramed. The numbers indicate the time in milliseconds after the beginning of the QRS loop. The dotted portions of the loop represent the delta vector. Described in text.

The orientation of the T loop is variable, but it is often discordant to the mean QRS vector.

Type B

In the TP, the delta deflection is directed leftward, usually posteriorly but sometimes anteriorly. The body of the loop is oriented to the left. Inscription of the loop is usually CCW, but a figure-of-eight pattern may occur.

In the FP, the delta deflection is directed leftward and either superiorly or inferiorly.

The leftward orientation of the delta vector in the TP causes downward inscription of the delta wave in lead V_1. However, it is upright in the other precordial leads.

Because of the leftward direction of the delta deflection in the FP, the delta wave is upright in leads I and aVL. If the delta vector is oriented superiorly, Q waves or QS complexes are recorded in leads II, III, and aVF.

The initial slowing of the QRS loop may also be seen in the LSP.

The orientation of the T loop is variable, but it is often discordant to the mean QRS vector.

REFERENCES

Anderson, R. H., A. E. Becher, C. Brechenmacker, M. J. Davies, and L. Rossi: Ventricular Preexcitation: A Proposed Nomenclature for Its Substrates, *European J. Card.*, 3: 27, 1975.

Boineau, J. P., E. N. Moore, W. C. Sealy, and J. K. Kasell: Epicardial Mapping in Wolff-Parkinson-White Syndrome, *Arch. Int. Med.*, 135: 422, 1975.

Caracta, A. R., A. N. Damato, J. J. Gallagher et al.: Electrophysiologic Studies in the Syndrome of Short P-R Interval, Normal QRS Complex, *Am. J. Cardiol.*, 31: 245, 1973.

Castellanos, A., Jr., C. A. Castillo, and A. S. Agha: Contribution of His Bundle Recordings to the Understanding of Clinical Arrhythmias, *Am. J. Cardiol.*, 28: 499, 1971.

————, ————, ————, and M. Tessler: His Bundle Electrograms in Patients with Short P-R Intervals, Narrow QRS Complexes, and Paroxysmal Tachycardia, *Circulation*, 43: 667, 1971.

————, E. Chapunoff, O. Maytin et al.: His Bundle Electrograms in Two Cases of Wolff-Parkinson-White (Preexcitation) Syndrome, *Circulation*, 41: 399, 1970.

Castillo, C. A., and A. Castellanos, Jr.: His Bundle Recordings in Patients with Reciprocating Tachycardias and Wolff-Parkinson-White Syndrome, *Circulation*, 42: 271, 1970.

Chung, K. Y., T. J. Walsh, and E. Massie: Wolff-Parkinson-White Syndrome, *Am. Heart J.*, 69: 116, 1965.

Denes, P., and K. M. Rosen: His Bundle Electrograms: Clinical Applications, *Cardiovasc. Clin.*, 6 (1): 69, 1974.

Durrer, D., L. Schoo, R. M. Schuilenburg, and H. J. J. Wellens: The Role of Premature Beats in the Initiation and Termination of Supraventricular Tachycardia in the Wolff-Parkinson-White Syndrome, *Circulation*, 36: 644, 1967.

Ferrer, M. I.: New Concepts Relating to the Preexcitation Syndrome, *J.A.M.A.*, 201: 1038, 1967.

Gallagher, E., E. L. C. Pritchett, W. C. Sealy, J. Kasell, and A. G. Wallace: The Preexcitation Syndromes, *Prog. Cardiovasc. Dis.*, 20: 285, 1978.

Hecht, H. H., R. Kennamer, M. Prinzmetal, F. F. Rosenbaum, D. Sodi-Pallares, L.

Wolff, C. Brooks, A. Pick, P. Rijlant, and J. C. Robb: Anomalous Atrioventricular Excitation: Panel Discussion, *Ann. N.Y. Acad. Sci.,* 65: 826, 1957.

Josephson, M. E., and S. F. Seides: "Clinical Cardiac Electrophysiology," Lea & Febiger, Philadelphia, 1979.

Lev, M.: Anatomic Considerations of Anomalous A. V. Pathways, in L. S. Dreifus and W. Likoff (eds.), "Mechanisms and Therapy of Cardiac Arrhythmias," Grune & Stratton, New York, 1966.

Lown, B., W. F. Ganong, and S. A. Levine: The Syndrome of Short P-R Interval, Normal QRS Complexes, and Paroxysmal Rapid Heart Action, *Circulation,* 5: 693, 1952.

Marriott, H. J. L., and H. M. Rogers: Mimics of Ventricular Tachycardia Associated with the W-P-W Syndrome, *J. Electrocardiol.,* 2: 77, 1969.

Massumi, R. A., Z. Vera, and D. T. Mason: The Wolff-Parkinson-White Syndrome: A New Look at an Old Problem, *Mod. Concepts Cardiovasc. Dis.,* 42: 41, 1973.

Monahan, J. P., P. Denes, and K. R. Rosen: Portable Electrocardiographic Monitoring: Performance in Patients with Short P-R Intervals Without Delta Waves, *Arch. Intern. Med.,* 135: 1188, 1975.

Narula, O.: Wolff-Parkinson-White Syndrome: A Review, *Circulation,* 47: 872, 1973.

Newman, B. J., E. Donoso, and C. K. Friedberg: Arrhythmias in the Wolff-Parkinson-White Syndrome, *Progr. Cardiovasc. Dis.,* 9: 14, 1966.

Oehnell, R. F.: Pre-excitation, A Cardiac Abnormality, *Acta Med. Scand., Suppl.,* 152: 1, 1944.

Pick, A., and L. N. Katz: Disturbances of Impulse Formation and Conduction in the Pre-excitation (WPW) Syndrome: Their Bearing on Its Mechanism, *Am. J. Med.,* 19: 759, 1955.

Scherf, D.: Mechanisms of Arrhythmias Associated with the WPW Syndrome, in L. S. Dreifus and W. Likoff (eds.), "Mechanisms and Therapy of Cardiac Arrhythmias," Grune & Stratton, New York, 1966.

Sherf, L., and T. N. James: A New Look at Some Old Questions in Clinical Electrocardiography, *Henry Ford Hosp. Med. Bull.,* 14: 265, 1966.

Wolff, L.: Wolff-Parkinson-White Syndrome: Historical and Clinical Features, *Progr. Cardiovasc. Dis.,* 2: 677, 1960.

Zipes, D. P., D. A. Rothbaum, and R. L. De Joseph: Pre-excitation Syndrome, *Cardiovasc. Clin.,* 6 (1): 209, 1974.

CHAPTER 13

MYOCARDIAL INFARCTION

THEORETICAL CONSIDERATIONS (FIGS. 13-1, 13-2)

A typical transmural myocardial infarct consists of three zones: (1) a central *zone of necrosis*, or dead tissue; (2) a *zone of injury* which surrounds the dead zone; and (3) a *zone of ischemia* which surrounds the injured region.

The zone of ischemia accounts for the T wave or T vector abnormalities. In ischemia the direction of repolarization is reversed, so that the T wave points opposite to its usual direction. Stated otherwise, the T vector points away from the ischemic region. The zone of injury produces the S-T vector abnormalities. In transmural or subepicardial injury, the S-T vector points toward the injured zone. Thus epicardial leads show elevated S-T segments, and endocardial leads show depressed S-T segments. The reverse is true in subendocardial injury, in which the S-T vector points away from the site of injury and results in S-T segment depression in epicardial leads and S-T segment elevation in endocardial leads. The zone of necrosis, or the dead zone, is responsible for the change in the direction of the initial 0.04-s vector. Normally during the first 0.04 s of ventricular depolarization, electrical forces are generated in the subendocardial regions of the left ventricle. The resultant of these vectors, the 0.04-s vector, is more or less parallel to the mean QRS vector, pointing leftward, inferiorly, and posteriorly. Since dead tissue is electrically inert, when infarction develops, no electrical forces are produced by the infarcted region during the first 0.04 s of the QRS interval. The initial 0.04-s vector thus tends to

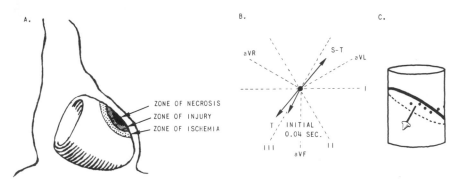

Fig. 13-1 Myocardial infarction. *A* is a schematic representation of an acute anterolateral myocardial infarct with a central zone of necrosis surrounded by zones of injury and ischemia. The three zones account for, respectively, the mean initial 0.04-s QRS vector, the S-T vector, and the T vector abnormalities that take place in myocardial infarction. In *B*, these vectors are plotted on the triaxial figure, and in *C*, the initial QRS vector is drawn three-dimensionally. From an inspection of the diagrams, it can be seen that wide Q waves together with elevated S-T segments and inverted T waves will be present in leads I, aVL, V₅, and V₆.

point away from the site of the infarct. Since, for practical purposes, most cases of myocardial infarction involve the left ventricle, the initial 0.04-s vector will point away from the infarcted region of the left ventricle. The projection of this initial 0.04-s vector in the frontal plane on the negative half of any of the limb lead axes will result in the appearance of deep, wide Q waves in that lead, but may likewise result in the inscription of broad R waves when projected on the positive half of any of the limb lead axes. Similarly, abnormal Q or R waves may occur in the precordial leads, which are located in the horizontal plane of the body, depending upon the projection of the initial 0.04-s vector on the axes of these leads. When an infarct is large and transmural, the dead zone will not generate any electrical forces throughout ventricular depolarization. The vector generated during the entire QRS interval will point away from the infarct, so that leads overlying the infarct will show QS deflections.

DIAGNOSIS

Conventional Criteria

The electrocardiographic diagnosis of myocardial infarction can be established with certainty only when abnormality of the initial 0.04 s of the QRS complex (abnormal Q, QS, or R waves) is combined with typical T wave abnormalities or characteristic S-T segment alterations, or both.

Q Wave Abnormalities

Q waves are abnormal in leads I, II, and aVF if they are 0.04 s or more wide, greater than 2 mm in depth, and more than 25 percent of the following R wave. In lead aVL, these values are 0.04 s or more in width, greater than 2 mm in depth, and more than 50 percent of the succeeding R wave in the presence of an upright P wave. When the voltage of the R wave is low (5 mm or less), Q/R ratios are unreliable from a diagnostic standpoint. A wide Q wave or QS complex may sometimes occur normally. The recognition of a wide Q wave in lead aVL as a normal variant is aided by its association with negative P and T waves in this lead and by the absence of abnormal Q waves in lead I and broad R waves in leads III and aVF. The significance of a Q_3 depends on whether Q waves are also present in leads aVF and II. When there is a wide Q_3 (0.04 s or greater), the association of abnormal Q waves in leads aVF and II indicates that the wide Q_3 is abnormal. A Q wave in leads aVF and III in the presence of an initial R wave in lead aVR that is 1.0 mm or more is indicative of inferior or inferolateral myocardial infarction. A wide or deep Q_3 not associated with wide or deep Q waves in leads aVF and II is usually normal. When Q waves are absent in lead aVF or aVL, an isolated Q_3, even if deep or wide, is normal. This is commonly observed when the R wave in lead aVL is taller than that in aVF, since lead III = $V_F - V_L$.

In the precordial leads, a Q wave is normally found only in leads to the left of lead V_2. In the left precordial leads, the criteria for Q wave abnormality include a width of 0.04 s or more, a depth exceeding 2 mm, and an amplitude greater than 15 percent of the succeeding R wave.

Fig. 13-2 Mechanism of the initial 0.04-s QRS vector deformity in myocardial infarction. A is normal. During the first 0.04 s of the QRS interval, vectors are generated simultaneously from all regions of the subendocardial layers of the ventricles and produce a resultant mean vector for the first 0.04 s shown in B. C shows myocardial infarction. No electrical forces are produced by the infarcted region during the first 0.04 s of the QRS interval. The resultant mean vector for the first 0.04 s thus tends to point away from the site of the infarct, as shown in D. (From R. P. Grant, "Clinical Electrocardiography." © 1957 by McGraw-Hill Inc. Used with permission of McGraw-Hill Book Company.)

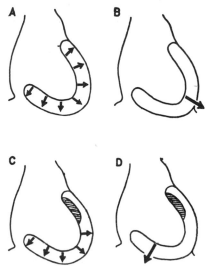

The criteria for Q wave abnormality are outlined in Table 13-1.

QS complexes in leads aVF, III, and II are almost always abnormal. This pattern is generally indicative of inferior infarction with or without left anterior fascicular block, but it is sometimes seen in pulmonary emphysema (Fig. 18-5), left bundle branch block, ventricular preexcitation, and other conditions in the absence of myocardial infarction. Usually the presence of other electrocardiographic abnormalities helps in the differential diagnosis. A QS complex in leads aVF and III associated with a QR or qrS or a small notched initial R wave in lead II suggests the diagnosis of inferior infarction in the presence of left anterior fascicular block (B of Fig. 20-1) if chronic obstructive pulmonary disease can be excluded (Fig. 18-5). The pattern of QS complexes in leads aVF and III without Q waves in lead II is also suggestive of inferior infarction or emphysema, but it may be a normal variant.

It has been widely held by many that respiratory or postural maneuvers may be helpful in deciding whether Q waves or QS complexes are normal or abnormal. As indicated in Chap. 5, the reliability of these maneuvers for this purpose is open to question.

S-T Segment and T Wave Changes

Very early in the course of some cases of anterior myocardial infarction, abnormally tall T waves may occur transiently. Much more often, S-T segment elevation in epicardial leads is the first indication of infarction. The S-T segment is typically convex upward, with slight terminal inversion of the T wave. It may, however, be obliquely elevated. As the S-T segments return to the isoelectric level, deep symmetrically inverted T waves make their appearance. The terms *cove-plane T* and *coronary or Pardee T* are often applied to these T wave changes. The former refers to an inverted T wave which follows an elevated, upwardly convex S-T segment; the latter, to an inverted T wave following an isoelectric but upwardly convex S-T segment. Endocardial leads and epicardial leads located opposite the area of infarction show reciprocal S-T-T changes with the S-T segments depressed and the T waves upright.

TABLE 13-1   CRITERIA FOR Q WAVE ABNORMALITY

Leads	Width	Depth	Q/R Ratio
I, II, aVF	≥0.04 s	≥2 mm	>25%
V_1, V_2, V_3	With few exceptions, Q waves are normally absent in these leads		
V_4, V_5, V_6	≥0.04 s	≥ 2 mm	15%
aVL	≥0.04 s	≥ 2 mm	>50%
III*	≥0.04 s	≥ 2 mm†	>25%

* Abnormal Q_3 not considered pathologic unless associated with abnormal QaVF and preferably also abnormal Q_2.
† Q_3 may sometimes be as much as 6 mm deep normally.

A study by Mills et al. has indicated that the natural history of S-T segment elevation after myocardial infarction is resolution within 2 weeks in 95 percent of inferior infarctions and 40 percent of anterior infarctions. S-T segment elevations persisting more than 2 weeks after infarction did not ordinarily return to baseline levels. Persistent S-T segment elevation was associated with clinically more severe infarctions. It was also found to be a specific but relatively insensitive index of left ventricular asynergy.

Persistent displacement of the S-T segment is found in approximately 60 percent of patients with ventricular aneurysm.

Comments

The electrocardiographic diagnosis of myocardial infarction cannot be established with certainty in the absence of diagnostic alterations of the QRS complex. The diagnosis, however, can be strongly suspected when typical S-T segment or T wave changes, or both, are found in a patient in whom the history and clinical findings are corroborative of myocardial infarction and in whom pericarditis can be ruled out.

It is important to bear in mind that when an infarct is small, intramural, or subendocardial, the electrocardiogram or even serial electrocardiograms may show no specific abnormalities. Under such circumstances, the diagnosis of myocardial infarction, as always, rests on clinical grounds. The absence of pathognomonic electrocardiographic abnormalities, therefore, does not rule out the clinical diagnosis of myocardial infarction.

VECTORELECTROCARDIOGRAPHIC CRITERIA

1 The mean vector for the first 0.04 s of the QRS interval, the *initial 0.04-s vector*, points *away* from the site of the infarct.
2 The *mean T vector* points *away* from the site of the infarct and is more or less parallel to the initial 0.04-s vector.
3 The *S-T vector* due to the current of injury points *toward* the site of the infarct.
4 In many cases, the mean vector for the last 0.04 s of the QRS interval, the *terminal 0.04-s vector*, has an abnormal direction and points *toward* the site of the infarct, indicating the presence of a complicating fascicular block.

EVOLUTION

The various stages in the evolution of a myocardial infarct can usually be demonstrated in serial electrocardiograms taken over a period of time.

In the typical case of myocardial infarction, T wave alterations sometimes appear shortly after the onset. These last from minutes to a few hours and are replaced by S-T segment alterations. Within a period of hours to several days, but sometimes simultaneously, abnormal Q waves or QS deflections appear. Then the S-T segment displacements return gradually to the baseline, and the T waves become inverted. In a matter of weeks, months, or even years, the T waves may gradually revert to normal, which will leave abnormal Q waves or QS deflections as the sole evidence that myocardial infarction has occurred. In some instances, even these may disappear entirely and leave the electrocardiogram devoid of any residual evidence of infarction.

CLASSIFICATION

Infarction may be classified according to its duration as acute, recent, or old. *Acute infarction* is said to be present when the electrocardiogram shows typical S-T segment displacements. *Recent infarction* is diagnosed when typical abnormalities of the QRS complex are combined with typical T wave changes. *Old infarction* is present when only the characteristic abnormalities of the QRS complex are found in the electrocardiogram. A corroborative history of past myocardial infarction is desirable to establish with certainty the electrocardiographic diagnosis of old myocardial infarction.

Since it is often difficult to be certain from a single tracing whether the electrocardiographic signs of infarction are due to a recent process or are the residuals of an old one, sole reliance should not be placed on the above classification to determine the age of an infarct.

The age of an infarct can be estimated best from S-T segment and T wave changes in serial electrocardiograms and by clinical and laboratory data.

LOCALIZATION (FIG. 13-3)

The anatomic localization of infarcts is based on the location of the leads in which diagnostic signs of myocardial infarction occur. It is only the leads in which QRS abnormalities are found that are used for localization. Leads in which only S-T segment and T wave changes occur are ordinarily not employed for this purpose.

DIAGNOSTIC FEATURES OF MYOCARDIAL INFARCTION IN VARIOUS LOCATIONS (TABLE 13-2)

Strictly Anterior or Anteroseptal Infarction (Figs. 13-4, 13-36, 13-37)

The characteristic features are (1) the presence of a normal initial R wave in lead V_1, (2) replacement of the R wave by QS or QR complexes (Q wave

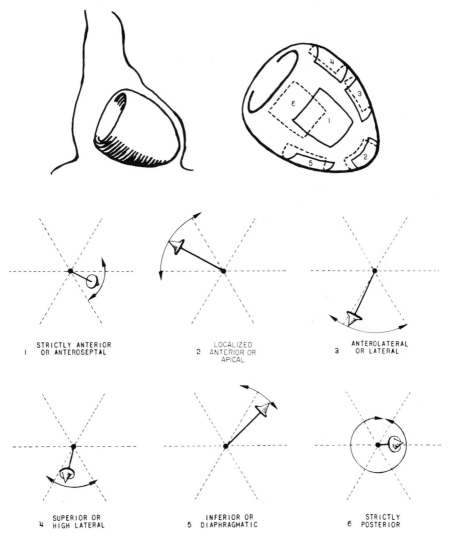

Fig. 13-3 Topography of myocardial infarction.   The lie of the left ventricle in the chest is shown.   The left ventricle is divided into six regions where an infarct may occur.   The initial 0.04-s vector for each of these infarcts is plotted on the triaxial figure.   In 1, abnormal Q waves are present in leads V_1 to V_3, but there are no Q waves in the standard limb leads.   In 2, abnormal Q waves are present in the midprecordial leads.   In 3, abnormal Q waves are seen in leads I, aVL, V_5, and V_6.   In 4, abnormal Q waves are produced in leads aVL and I. In 5, abnormal Q waves occur in leads II, III, and aVF.   In 6, there is typically an abnormally tall and/or broad R wave in lead V_1.   *(Modified from R. P. Grant, "Clinical Electrocardiography."* © 1957 *by McGraw-Hill Inc.   Used with permission of McGraw-Hill Book Company.)*

TABLE 13-2 DIAGNOSTIC FEATURES OF MYOCARDIAL INFARCTION IN VARIOUS LOCATIONS

Criteria for the Diagnosis of Infarction	Leads Showing Diagnostic Abnormalities	S-T-T Changes		
		Acute Infarction	Recent Infarction	Old Infarction
Anteroseptal				
1. RV_1 with Q or QS in V_2 to V_4	V_1–V_4	S-T↑	S-T↕, T↓	S-T↕, T↓ or↑
2. Variant Patterns				
A. Progressive decrease in R, V_1 to V_3 or V_4				
B. Poor R progression in V_1 to V_3 or V_4				
C. qRS in V_1, V_2				
D. QS in V_1 and V_2 or in V_1 to V_3 or V_4				
Localized Anterior				
Q or QS	V_3–V_4	S-T↑	S-T↕, T↓	S-T↕, T↓ or↑
Anterolateral				
Q	V_5–V_6 (I, aVL)	S-T↑	S-T↕, T↓	S-T↕, T↓ or↑
Extensive Anterior				
QS or Q	V_1–V_5 (V_6)	S-T↑	S-T↕, T↓	S-T↕, T↓ or↑
Superior or High Lateral				
Q	I, aVL	S-T↑	S-T↕, T↓	S-T↕, T↓ or↑
Inferior				
Q or QS	II, III, aVF	S-T↑	S-T↕, T↓	S-T↕, T↓ or↑
Strictly Posterior				
RV_1 ≥0.04 s with R/S >1.0 in V_1, V_2	V_1–V_2	S-T↓	S-T↕, T↑	S-T↕, T↑

Key: Q = Abnormal Q wave; QS = QS Deflection; S-T↑ = S-T Elevated; S-T↓ = S-T Depressed; S-T↕ = S-T Isoelectric; T↓ = T Inverted; T↑ = T Upright

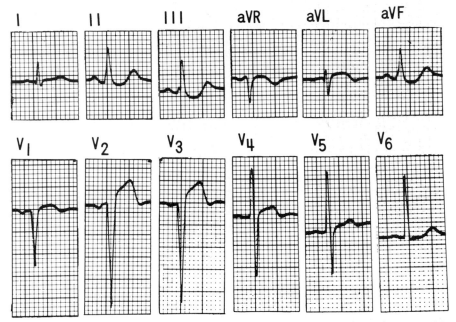

Fig. 13-4 Strictly anterior or anteroseptal myocardial infarction, acute. There are QS complexes in leads V_1 through V_3, with absence of Q waves in V_4 to V_6. The S-T segments are elevated in V_1 through V_5 and in leads I and aVL, which indicates anterior subepicardial injury. Reciprocal S-T segment depression is present in leads II, III, and aVF.

0.04 s wide or amplitude greater than 25 percent of the R wave) in one or more of the next three leads (V_2, V_3, and V_4), and (3) absence of normal septal Q waves in leads V_6, I, and aVL, unless there is anterolateral infarction as well.

Variant patterns include (1) progressive decrease in the amplitude of the R waves in leads V_1 to V_3 or V_4, (2) poor progression of the R waves in these leads, (3) a definite small Q wave preceding an RS complex in lead V_1 or in leads V_1 and V_2, and (4) the presence of a QS complex in leads V_1 and V_2 or in leads V_1 through V_3.

The initial QRS vector points posteriorly.

Apical, Midanterior, or Localized Anterior Infarction (Fig. 13-5)

Abnormal Q waves or QS complexes are present in the midprecordial leads, with preservation of the R waves in the right precordial leads and of normal septal Q waves in leads I, aVL, and V_6. Large apical infarcts are essentially inferolateral infarcts with abnormal Q waves present in the left precordial leads as well as in the standard limb leads.

The very early initial QRS forces (0.01 s) are directed normally in midanterior infarcts, but the remainder of the initial forces are directed

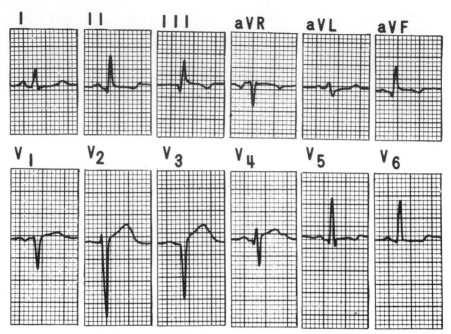

Fig. 13-5   Localized anterior or apical myocardial infarction, acute.   A QS complex is present in lead V_3, and a qrS deflection is seen in lead V_4.   The R waves are preserved in leads V_1 and V_2.   Normal septal Q waves are present in leads V_5 and V_6.   The S-T segment elevation in leads V_1 to V_4 indicates that the infarct is acute.   Residuals of an old inferior myocardial infarction are seen in the inferior extremity leads.

posteriorly in the TP.   When the infarct is large, the initial vector is directed rightward and superiorly in the FP.

Anterolateral or Lateral Infarction (Figs. 13-6, 13-35)

Abnormal Q waves are present in leads V_3 or V_4 to V_6 and usually in leads I and aVL.

The initial QRS vector points inferiorly and rightward.

Superior or High Lateral Infarction (Fig. 13-7)

Abnormal Q waves are present in leads I and aVL.   When the Q waves in these leads exhibit equivocal abnormality, a broad R wave in leads II, III, and aVF has diagnostic significance.

The initial QRS vector points inferiorly and rightward.

Inferior (Posterior in Older Terminology) or Diaphragmatic Infarction (Figs. 13-8, 13-43, 20-3)

Abnormal Q waves or QS deflections are present in leads II, III, and aVF. These abnormalities are often associated with an initial R wave of increased

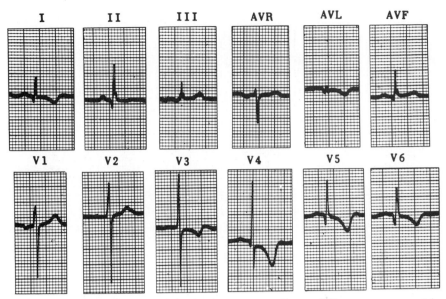

Fig. 13-6 Anterolateral myocardial infarction, recent.   Abnormal Q waves are present in leads I, aVL, V$_5$, and V$_6$.   The S-T segments are more or less isoelectric.   The T waves are symmetrically inverted in leads I, aVL, and V$_3$ to V$_6$.   Both the initial 0.04-s QRS and the T vectors are directed rightward and inferiorly, away from the location of the infarct.

amplitude (greater than 1.0 mm) in lead aVR, a finding which is rather specifically diagnostic of inferior or inferior plus anterior infarction.

The initial QRS vector points superiorly.

Comment   Usually the diagnosis of *acute* inferior infarction presents no problems, because the electrocardiogram reveals not only the QRS abnormalities but also the evolutionary changes in the S-T segments and T waves in leads aVF, III, and II.   However, in the case of *old* inferior infarction, it is another matter.   Studies have revealed that in about 30 to 35 percent of old inferior infarctions, abnormal Q waves are not present in the inferior leads.   A moderate number of such cases actually show small initial R waves in these leads, so that the diagnosis of inferior infarction cannot be made.   Residual Q wave abnormalities occur with the following approximate frequency and distribution in old inferior infarction: all three leads, 15 percent; in lead III only, 25 percent; in aVF alone, 5 to 10 percent; and in leads III and aVF, 25 to 30 percent.   Although the foregoing percentages seem to imply that lead III is the lead of diagnostic preference, this is not true, because lead III is more liable than either lead aVF or lead II to a false-positive interpretation of infarction.   On an overall basis, lead aVF is the preferred diagnostic lead.   It should also be noted that lead III and, to a lesser extent, lead aVF may show abnormal Q waves in chronic obstructive pulmonary disease with or without cor pulmonale, in acute cor pulmonale, in right bundle branch block, and occasionally in left ventricular hypertrophy.

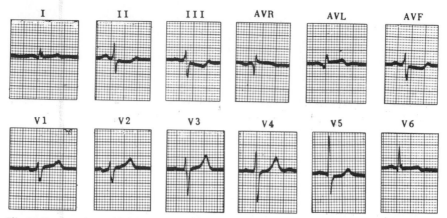

Fig. 13-7 Superior or high lateral myocardial infarction, acute. There are wide Q waves in leads I and aVL and broad R waves in leads III and aVF. The S-T segments are elevated in leads I and aVL, with reciprocal depression in leads II, III, and aVF. The initial QRS vector points inferiorly and rightward; the S-T vector, superiorly.

Precordial S-T segment depression occurs in about half of patients with an initial acute inferior myocardial infarction. Concomitant stenosis of the left anterior descending artery can be detected angiographically in about 50 percent of all patients with inferior infarction whether precordial S-T segment depression is present or not. Patients with inferior infarction with precordial S-T segment depression have been reported to have more extensive left ventricular dysfunction, lower ejection fractions, and a more morbid clinical course. The cause of this phenomenon is not clear. It may represent *mirror imaging* of S-T elevation over the posterior left ventricular wall, additional anterior ischemia, or posterolateral infarction.

Fig. 13-8 Inferior myocardial infarction, old, and digitalis effect. Abnormal Q waves are present in leads II, III, and aVF. The initial QRS vector points superiorly. The contour of the S-T segments is characteristic of digitalis effect.

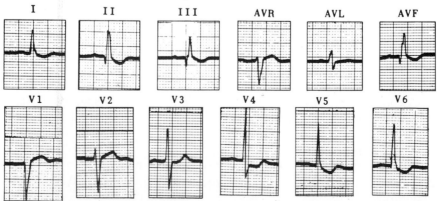

The vectorcardiogram is often superior to the electrocardiogram in the diagnosis of old inferior infarction.

Strictly Posterior, Posterobasal, or Dorsal Infarction (Figs. 13-9, 13-10)

Abnormally tall or broad initial R waves, or both, are present in lead V_1 and in the adjacent right anterior chest leads (V_{3R} and V_2).   The R/S ratio is 1.0

Fig. 13-9   Record A shows strictly posterior myocardial infarction.   There are broad R waves in leads V_{3R}, V_1, and V_2 which were not present in record B, taken 3 years earlier.   Record B is within normal limits.   The patient had a typical clinical picture of myocardial infarction at the time record A was taken.

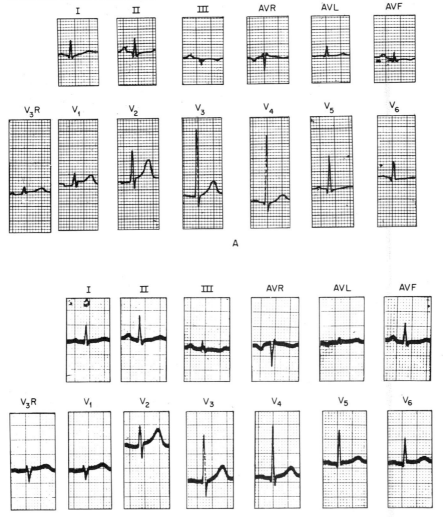

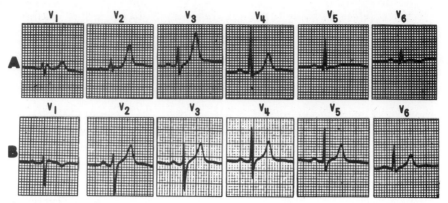

Fig. 13-10   Record *A* shows acute posterobasal myocardial infarction.   There is a broad rSr′ complex in lead V₁ and an Rsr′ deflection in V₂.   The T waves are upright and tall in leads V₂ and V₃.   These changes were not present in record *B*, a routine electrocardiogram taken 1 year previously.

or greater in leads V₁ and V₂.   There is often slurring of the descending limb of the R wave in lead V₁.   Sometimes rR′ or RSR′ deflections are seen in the right precordial leads.

Abnormal Q waves may be found posteriorly between the spine and the left scapula (leads V₈ and V₉).

Abnormal Q waves are absent in the conventional 12-lead electrocardiogram, unless either inferior or lateral myocardial infarction coexists.

During the acute phase of infarction, the S-T segment may be depressed with the T wave upright and tall in the right precordial leads.   This is a reciprocal effect of S-T segment elevation and T wave inversion in posterior leads.

The initial QRS vector points anteriorly.

Other Locations and Combinations of Infarcts (Figs. 13-11, 13-12, 13-26A and B, 19-2)

Infarcts may include or lie between two or more of the six regions listed above.   Thus an infarct situated between locations 1 and 5 in Fig. 13-3 would be called an anteroinferior infarct; one involving regions 1 and 3 would be regarded as an extensive anterior infarct; and one including areas 5 and 3 would be classified as an inferolateral infarct.   Other combinations also occur.

Right Ventricular Infarction (Fig. 13-13)

Pathologic studies have revealed that infarction of the free wall of the right ventricle is present in 14 to 34 percent of patients with transmural left ventricular inferior infarction.   The clinical incidence is reported to be

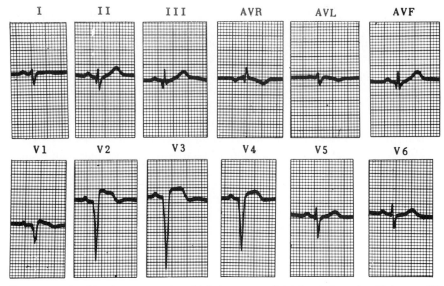

Fig. 13-11 Combined anteroseptal and inferior myocardial infarction, acute. There are QS complexes in leads V₁ to V₄, with elevated S-T segments in these leads. Prominent Q waves are present in leads II, III, and aVF. A routine electrocardiogram taken 3 days previously showed none of these abnormalities and was entirely within normal limits.

Fig. 13-12 Posteroinferolateral myocardial infarction. There are abnormal Q waves in leads I, II, III, aVF, V₅, and V₆. There are broad and tall initial R waves in leads V₃ᵣ, V₁, and aVR. The initial QRS vector is directed anteriorly, superiorly, and rightward, so that from an electrical standpoint, the infarct must involve portions of the posterior, inferior, and lateral walls of the left ventricle.

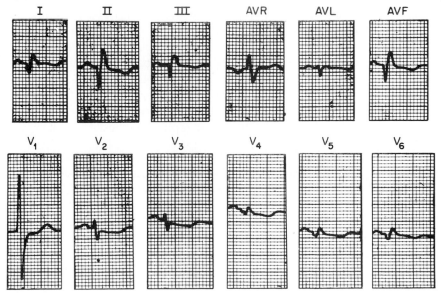

between 25 and 48 percent of such cases. The diagnosis may be suspected clinically when right ventricular failure and arterial hypotension occur in a patient with acute inferior infarction. Chou and his associates have found that acute right ventricular infarction is most commonly manifested electrocardiographically in patients with acute inferior myocardial infarction by the occurrence of transient S-T segment elevation in one or more of the right precordial leads. Braat and his group as well as Croft and his co-workers have confirmed these findings and have concluded that S-T segment elevation of 1.0 mm or more in the right precordial leads (especially V_{4R} to V_{6R}) is a reliable indicator of right ventricular infarction both with respect to sensitivity and specificity.

Correlation of Coronary Arteriographic Findings with the Anatomic Location of Myocardial Infarction

There is good but not absolute correlation between occlusion or marked stenosis of coronary arteries or their branches and the anatomic location of myocardial infarcts. Table 13-3 lists the relationships between infarction in various locations and the coronary vessel(s) most likely to be involved by disease.

SUBENDOCARDIAL INFARCTION

The diagnosis of subendocardial infarction is difficult to establish with certainty. It may be suspected when in association with the typical clinical and laboratory features of myocardial infarction, the electrocardiogram shows evidence of subendocardial ischemia and injury. Thus, depressed S-T segments with terminally upright T waves may make their appearance in some or all of the precordial leads and/or in leads I and aVL and/or in leads II, III, and aVF. Unfortunately, from a diagnostic standpoint, these findings are nonspecific. Not only do they occur in both spontaneous and induced attacks of angina pectoris and in coronary insufficiency, but they are also seen as the initial electrocardiographic manifestations of classic transmural myocardial infarction on occasion.

Sometimes deeply inverted T waves in the precordial leads may be the clue to the presence of left ventricular subendocardial infarction (Fig. 13-14). Such T wave changes have been attributed to a transmural region of myocardial ischemia overlying the subendocardial zone of myocardial infarction. Again, it should be pointed out that the findings are nonspecific, because similar T wave inversions may be seen in angina pectoris, coronary insufficiency, intramural or subepicardial infarction, pericarditis, right ventricular strain, left ventricular strain, acute or chronic cor pulmonale, and other conditions.

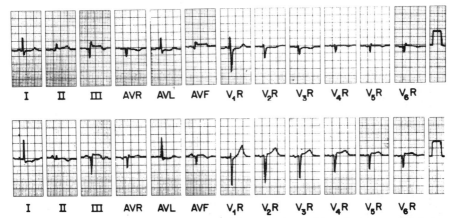

| I | II | III | AVR | AVL | AVF | V₁R | V₂R | V₃R | V₄R | V₅R | V₆R |

Fig. 13-13 Representative tracings from two different patients with acute transmural inferior infarction. In the *upper strip*, the S-T segments are not elevated in the right precordial leads, whereas in the *lower strip* they are elevated in these leads. The precordial S-T segment elevation in the bottom strip is diagnostic of right ventricular infarction. (*From C. H. Croft et al., Detection of Acute Right Ventricular Infarction by Right Precordial Electrocardiography, Am. J. Cardiol.,* 50: 422, 1982. *Used by permission.*)

Fig. 13-14 Myocardial infarction with T wave changes only. The patient had a classic clinical picture of myocardial infarction supported by laboratory evidence. At no time did the electrocardiogram show abnormalities of the initial QRS vector. The T waves are rather deeply and symmetrically inverted in leads I, II, aVL, and V_2 to V_6, which indicates myocardial ischemia.

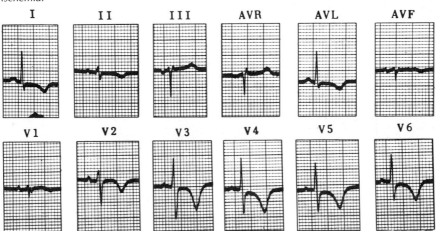

**TABLE 13-3   CORRELATION BETWEEN CORONARY ARTERIOGRAPHIC
FINDINGS AND INFARCT LOCATION***

Infarct Location	Coronary Vessel(s) Usually Involved
Anteroseptal or strictly anterior	Left anterior descending (LAD) branch of left coronary artery (LCA)
Localized anterior	Diagonal branch of LAD or obtuse marginal branch (OM) of left circumflex artery (cfx)
Extensive anterior	LAD and diagonal branch of LCA
Superior or high lateral	Diagonal branch of LAD or high OM branch of left cfx
Inferior	Right coronary artery (RCA) or posterior descending branch of RCA or left cfx
Strictly posterior	Posterior marginal branch of left cfx or distal RCA
Posteroinferior	Posterior marginal branch of left cfx or distal RCA
Posterolateral	Distal circumflex branch of LCA
Posteroinferolateral	Circumflex branch of LCA
Anteroinferior	LAD and sometimes posterior descending branch of RCA

* Courtesy of David Shander, M.D.

ARRHYTHMIAS IN MYOCARDIAL INFARCTION

Arrhythmias are estimated to occur in 90 to 95 percent of patients with myocardial infarctions. Almost any type of arrhythmia may occur. A discussion of the incidence and characteristics of the various arrhythmias in myocardial infarction can be found in almost any textbook of cardiology and hence is not included in this text.

DIAGNOSIS OF MYOCARDIAL INFARCTION IN PACEMAKER PATIENTS

The electrocardiographic diagnosis of myocardial infarction in pacemaker patients is extremely difficult. It can sometimes be detected in nonpaced complexes. Acute myocardial infarction may be suspected when there is marked S-T segment elevation in leads V_1 to V_3 especially if associated with marked increase in latency between the pacemaker stimulus and the onset of the QRS complex. The finding of a notched S wave in leads V_3 to V_5 in patients treated by right ventricular apical pacing may be present in extensive anterior infarction.

VENTRICULAR ANEURYSM (FIG. 13-15)

The diagnosis of ventricular aneurysm may be suspected when, following infarction, the electrocardiogram shows persistent displacement of the S-T segments in association with abnormal Q waves or QS deflections for a period of several weeks or longer.

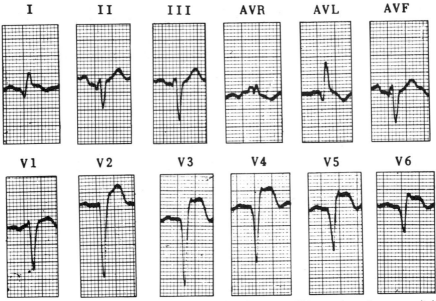

Fig. 13-15   Ventricular aneurysm in a patient with a documented history of anterior myocardial infarction 7 years previously.   The findings of significance are QR complexes in leads I and aVL, QS or Qr complexes from leads V_2 to V_6, elevated S-T segments in the precordial leads, and abnormal left axis deviation.   This would be interpreted as an acute, extensive anterior infarct were it not known that the S-T segment changes had persisted over a period of years. The diagnosis of ventricular aneurysm was confirmed by x-ray.   Left anterior fascicular block is the cause of the abnormal left axis deviation.

DIAGNOSTIC PROBLEMS IN MYOCARDIAL INFARCTION

It is common knowledge that in acute myocardial infarction the initial electrocardiograms may be normal, and it may be a matter of several days before the diagnostic pattern of acute infarction becomes evident.   In some 20 percent or more of cases, the electrocardiogram may remain entirely normal or show nonspecific abnormalities throughout the course of acute infarction.   Moreover, over a period of time, some of the electrocardiographic abnormalities of myocardial infarction may diminish or disappear completely.   It has been estimated that within 1 year after myocardial infarctions as many as 10 percent of patients may have normal electrocardiograms and a further 20 percent may have electrocardiograms no longer diagnostic of infarction.   Thus the diagnosis of old infarction becomes more difficult with the passage of time and may become impossible unless previous tracings are available.   Many silent infarctions are probably not detected at all.

DIFFERENTIAL DIAGNOSIS OF MYOCARDIAL INFARCTION

Electrocardiographic abnormalities that are usually considered diagnostic of myocardial infarction may occur in other disease states and thus lead to erroneous diagnoses.

The differentiation between normal and abnormal Q waves, the problems of inappropriate R wave progression in the right precordial leads, and the significance of QS complexes have been discussed previously.

Left Ventricular Hypertrophy (Figs. 13-16, 13-17)

Left ventricular hypertrophy may present electrocardiographic features that may be mistaken for myocardial infarction. The patterns of poor R wave progression and reversal of the normal R wave trend in the right precordial leads, with or without the presence of QS or QR complexes in these leads, occurs not infrequently in uncomplicated left ventricular hypertrophy,

Fig. 13-16 Left ventricular hypertrophy simulating myocardial infarction. R_{V_1} is slightly taller than R_{V_2}. A QS complex is present in lead V_3. The S wave in lead V_1 is 31 mm, and the R wave in lead aVF is 20.5 mm. The findings in the right precordial leads are strongly suggestive of anteroseptal infarction. However, the patient gave no corroborative history of myocardial infarction. The vectorcardiogram showed only left ventricular hypertrophy. From a patient with essential hypertension and left ventricular enlargement.

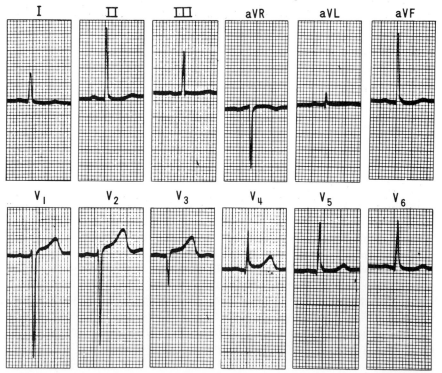

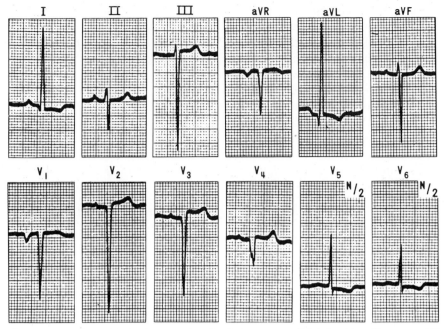

Fig. 13-17 Left ventricular hypertrophy simulating myocardial infarction. There are QS complexes in leads V_1 through V_4 suggestive of anteroseptal myocardial infarction. The high voltage and the strain pattern, as well as the increased P terminal force in lead V_1 (indicative of left atrial abnormality), are diagnostic of left ventricular enlargement. From a 35-year-old woman with rheumatic aortic stenosis, who, at autopsy, showed no evidence of anteroseptal infarction or fibrosis.

particularly when it is caused by diastolic overloading of the left ventricle or aortic valve disease. The differential diagnosis of these changes has been discussed previously. Exaggeration of the Q wave in the left precordial and limb leads may also occur in left ventricular enlargement with septal hypertrophy. In most such cases, the fact that the Q wave is deep rather than wide and is proportionate in size to the R wave (Q/R ratio less than 0.15) helps to identify hypertrophy rather than infarction as the cause of the abnormality. In doubtful cases the vectorcardiogram may be decisive in distinguishing between infarction and hypertrophy or in diagnosing the combination of the two.

Right Ventricular Hypertrophy (Figs. 9-1, 9-3)

In uncomplicated right ventricular hypertrophy or dilatation, or both, the precordial leads often show abnormalities which resemble those associated with anterior infarction. These abnormalities are qR or QR patterns in V_1, localized reduction in the amplitude of the R waves or their replacement by QS deflections in leads at the transition zone, QS patterns in the first three or more precordial leads, persistence of the normal Q wave in the left precordial leads accompanied by reduction in the R wave or exaggeration of the S wave, and S-T segment and T wave changes.   A qR or QR pattern in lead V_1 may suggest right bundle branch block due to septal infarction if the QRS complex is wide.   Myocardial infarction with bundle branch block can usually be recognized by Q waves in association with a late broad R wave in lead V_1 and the presence of wide S waves in leads I and V_5 and V_6.   With respect to the other abnormalities, identification of right ventricular enlargement as the cause is facilitated by the presence of right axis deviation in the limb leads and rS complexes in the left precordial leads.   In problem cases, vectorcardiography may provide the solution.

Diffuse Myocardial Disease (Figs. 13-18 to 13-22)

Diffuse myocardial diseases, including the various types of cardiomyopathy, myocarditis, connective tissue disorders, amyloidosis, sarcoidosis, and others, may produce false patterns of myocardial infarction in the electrocardiogram.

Pseudoinfarction patterns have been observed in various *cardiomyopathies*.   The types of electrocardiographic abnormalities found in these diseases are described in Chaps. 21 and 23.   It is worth noting at this point that pseudoinfarction patterns are a common occurrence in idiopathic hypertrophic subaortic stenosis.

Acute myocarditis shows no specific electrocardiographic pattern. Common findings include arrhythmias and AV conduction defects, bundle branch block, low voltage, and nonspecific ST-T abnormalities.   Abnormal Q waves and ST-T changes simulating acute myocardial infarction sometimes occur.   Such pseudoinfarction patterns are indistinguishable from

Fig. 13-18   Idiopathic hypertrophic subaortic stenosis (proved) simulating myocardial infarction.   The voltage changes suggest left ventricular hypertrophy.   However, the notched QS complexes in leads V_2 and V_3 and the prominent Q waves in leads V_4 to V_6 suggest anterior myocardial infarction.

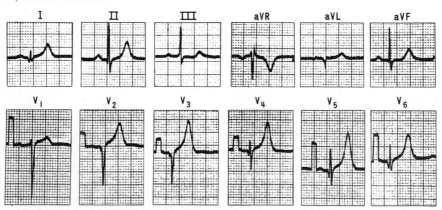

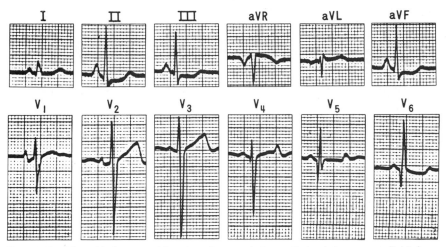

Fig. 13-19 Idiopathic hypertrophic subaortic stenosis (proved) simulating myocardial infarction by the presence of prominent Q waves in leads V_5 and V_6. The diagnosis of left ventricular hypertrophy is suggested by voltage changes and by the criterion $R_{V_5} > R_{V_6}$. Tall and broad P waves are seen in leads II, III, and aVF, and the P terminal force in lead V_1 is increased. These findings indicate either biatrial enlargement or a pseudo P pulmonale pattern caused by left atrial enlargement.

Fig. 13-20 Idiopathic hypertrophic subaortic stenosis simulating inferior myocardial infarction by the presence of deep Q waves in leads II, III, and aVF. The Q waves are also prominent in leads V_5 and V_6. The QRS voltages and the strain pattern are diagnostic of left ventricular hypertrophy.

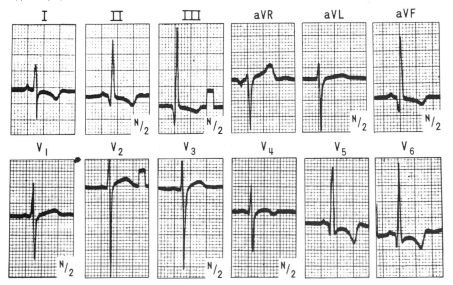

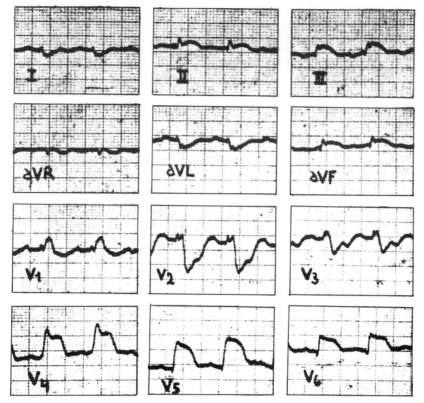

Fig. 13-21   Myocarditis (Chagasic) simulating myocardial infarction or pericarditis.   Right bundle branch block is present.   S-T segment elevations can be seen in leads II, III, aVF, and V₄ to V₆.   Reciprocal depression is noted in leads I, aVL, and V₁ to V₃.   Q wave abnormalities are absent.   (*From M. B. Rosenbaum, Chagasic Myocardiopathy, Progr. Cardiovasc. Dis., 7:* 199, 1964. *Used by permission.*)

those seen in true myocardial infarction.   *Chagasic myocarditis* is usually associated with right bundle branch with or without left anterior fascicular block.   Sometimes there are S-T changes which may simulate myocardial infarction or pericarditis.   Arrhythmias are a common occurrence.   (Fig. 13-21)

   Cardiac amyloidosis may produce pseudoinfarction patterns.   Deep Q waves in leads V₁ to V₃ are found in almost one-half of the cases. Abnormal Q waves are sometimes seen in the inferior limb leads.   Other abnormalities include low voltage, AV and ventricular conduction defects, nonspecific ST-T abnormalities and left axis deviation.

   The electrocardiogram in *Duchenne muscular dystrophy* may simulate the electrocardiographic findings in myocardial infarction.   Typically, there are tall, slender R waves in the right precordial leads with an R/S ratio greater than 1.0.   This abnormality may suggest posterior infarction or right

ventricular hypertrophy.   RSR' complexes are sometimes seen in lead V_1.
Deep, narrow Q waves in the left precordial leads and in one or more of
the limb leads may also suggest myocardial infarction.   Differentiation from
bona fide myocardial infarction is based on the clinical picture and the
fact that R and Q waves, when present, are typically narrow.   Moreover,
in this type of muscular dystrophy, in contrast to the depressed S-T segments
and upright T waves in lead V_1 in acute posterior infarction, the T waves
are upright or inverted in this lead.   Patterns simulating myocardial infarction
are sometimes seen in *Erb's limb girdle dystrophy, myotonia atrophica*, and
Friedreich's ataxia.

   Alcoholic cardiomyopathy is rarely a cause of abnormal Q waves.
Spinous or peaked T waves with a narrow base are common in alcoholics
and tend to persist.   Their relation to alcoholic cardiomyopathy has not
been studied adequately.

   Pseudoinfarctional Q waves are relatively uncommon in *scleroderma*.
The most common abnormalities seen in this disease are low voltage,
nonspecific ST-T changes, AV and ventricular conduction defects, left and
right ventricular enlargement, and arrhythmias.

   Abnormal Q waves occur only rarely in *sarcoidosis*.   Complete heart
block or other AV conduction disturbances, bundle branch block, nonspe-

Fig. 13-22   The electrocardiogram of a 20-year-old man with progressive muscular dystrophy.
Note the tall R waves in lead V_1, and the large Q waves in leads I, aVL, and the left precordial
leads.   Autopsy revealed patchy fibrosis throughout the myocardium.   (*From T-C Chou,
Cardiovasc. Clin., 5(3): 199, 1973.   Used by permission.*)

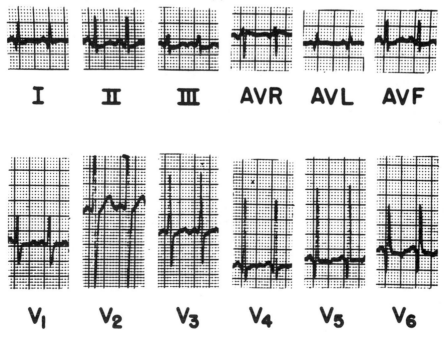

cific ST-T abnormalities, and various arrhythmias are the more common electrocardiographic findings in this disease.

Localized Myocardial Disease

Localized replacement of the myocardium by tumor and other tissues or focal lesions may produce electrocardiographic patterns that mimic myocardial infarction.

The most common abnormalities associated with primary or metastatic cardiac tumors are arrhythmias, AV conduction defects, bundle branch block, and low voltage. Pseudoinfarctional Q waves have been reported in rare instances. Differentiation from myocardial infarction is based primarily on clinical grounds.

Acute Cor Pulmonale (Pulmonary Embolism) (Fig. 18-2)

In acute cor pulmonale, significant Q waves and inverted T waves in leads III and aVF, sometimes associated with similar abnormalities in the right precordial leads, may simulate myocardial infarction. The presence of right axis deviation, an $S_1Q_3T_3$ pattern, transient right bundle branch, clockwise rotation of the heart with a shift of the transition zone to the left, right atrial abnormality, and the right ventricular strain pattern are additional signs found frequently in pulmonary embolism and support this diagnosis rather than that of myocardial infarction.

Pulmonary Emphysema (Fig. 18-3)

When pulmonary emphysema presents electrocardiographically with poor R wave progression or QS deflections in the right precordial leads or both, anterior infarction may be simulated. The diagnosis of emphysema is favored if low-voltage rS complexes in the remaining precordial leads, right or left axis deviation, and/or a rightward P vector with or without right atrial abnormality are also found in the electrocardiogram. The large Q waves in the inferior leads sometimes found in emphysema may imitate, and even be impossible to differentiate from, those found in inferior infarction.

Left Bundle Branch Block (Fig. 11-15)

In left bundle branch block, poor progression of the R waves or the presence of QS complexes or both in the right precordial leads may mimic anteroseptal infarction. Similarly, QS deflections in the inferior limb leads may simulate inferior infarction. The presence of diagnostic signs of left bundle branch block in either the electrocardiogram or vectorcardiogram establishes the correct diagnosis.

Wolf-Parkinson-White Syndrome (Fig. 12-2)

The abnormal Q waves or QS deflections sometimes found in the limb leads or in the right precordial leads in the W-P-W syndrome may be mistaken for myocardial infarction. The presence of short P-R intervals, wide QRS complexes, and delta waves establishes preexcitation as the cause of these changes.

Left Anterior Fascicular Block (Figs. 13-23, 13-24)

Rosenbaum and his associates have reported that the electrocardiographic pattern of a qrS complex in lead V_2 may be found in patients with left

Fig. 13-23 Left anterior fascicular block simulating myocardial infarction. (*A*) The routine electrocardiogram shows abnormal left axis deviation due to left anterior fascicular block, with a QS deflection in lead V_1 and qrS complexes in leads V_2 and V_3. (*B*) The Q waves are absent in the right precordial leads recorded in the fifth interspace. (*C*) The Q waves are more prominent in a recording taken in the third interspace. (*From P. L. McHenry et al., Right Precordial qrS Pattern Due to Left Anterior Hemiblock, Am. Heart J., 81: 498, 1971. Used by permission.*)

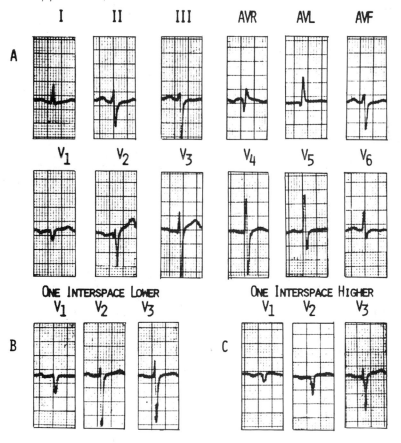

anterior fascicular block in the absence of myocardial infarction. It has been pointed out that anteroseptal infarction and left anterior fascicular block as the cause of this abnormality can be differentiated by recording leads V_1 to V_3 at a lower level. In such low V leads, the noninfarctional Q waves disappear whereas those due to infarction persist.

Hyperpotassemia (Figs. 13-25A and B, 13-26A and B)

In rare instances of hyperpotassemia, the presence of Q waves and S-T-T changes suggestive of subepicardial injury may mimic myocardial infarction. In such cases, the finding of an elevated serum potassium level is diagnostic.

Other Causes

Early repolarization (Fig. 5-15), a normal variant, may be mistaken for subepicardial injury. In early repolarization, the S-T segment, although

Fig. 13-24 Pseudoinfarction pattern produced by left anterior fascicular block, with QS deflections in leads V_1 and V_2 and a qrS complex in lead V_3. In recordings one and two interspaces below the standard precordial leads, the Q waves disappear and are replaced by R waves.

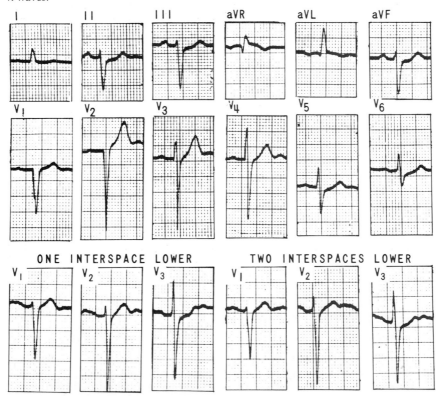

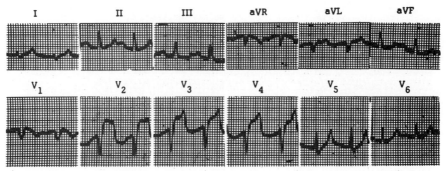

Fig. 13-25A Hyperpotassemia simulating myocardial infarction. The tracing shows a ventricular conduction defect and small R waves, with marked S-T segment elevations in leads V_1 through V_4 suggestive of acute anteroseptal infarction. The serum potassium was 9.6 meq/l. (*From T-C Chou, Pseudo-infarction (Noninfarction Q Waves), Cardiovasc. Clin.*, 5(3): 199, 1973. *Used by permission.*)

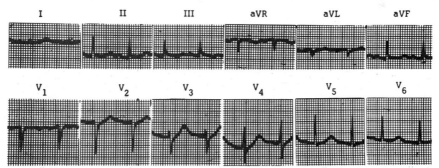

Fig. 13-25B The electrocardiogram recorded from the same patient as in Fig. 13-25A after the serum potassium has returned to normal. The ventricular conduction defect and the S-T segment elevations are no longer present. (*From T-C Chou, Pseudoinfarction (Noninfarction Q Waves), Cardiovasc. Clin.*, 5(3): 199, 1973. *Used by permission.*)

elevated, is typically concave upright and ends in a broad-based, tall, upright T wave. In subepicardial injury, on the other hand, the S-T segment is usually convex upward and terminates in an inverted T wave. The fixed nature of the S-T segment changes in serial tracings, the absence of abnormal Q waves, and the clinical picture are helpful in establishing the diagnosis of early repolarization in problem cases and in ruling out myocardial infarction or pericarditis. (See also pp. 324–325.)

Athletes not uncommonly show electrocardiographic abnormalities simulating myocardial infarction (Figs. 13-27, 13-28, 13-29). These include S-T segment and J point elevations usually distributed over the lateral precordial leads as well as leads II, III, and aVF. Diagnostic problems may be especially difficult when the S-T segment is bowed upward and accompanied by an inverted T wave. Occasionally, abnormal Q or QS waves are seen which mimic myocardial infarction. Other electrocardi-

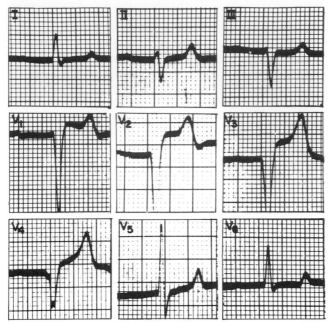

Fig. 13-26A Hyperpotassemia simulating acute anteroseptal myocardial infarction. There is loss of the R waves and S-T segment elevation in leads V₂ to V₄. The serum potassium was 6.6 meq/l. (*From C. R. VanderArk, F. Ballantyne, III, and E. W. Reynolds, Jr., Electrolytes and the Electrocardiogram, Cardiovasc. Clin., 5(3): 269, 1973. Used by permission.*)

Fig. 13-26B The electrocardiogram recorded from the same patient as in Fig. 13-26A after treatment for hyperpotassemia. The serum potassium was 5.2 meg/l. The changes suggestive of infarction have resolved. (*From C. R. VanderArk, F. Ballantyne, III, and E. W. Reynolds, Jr., Electrolytes and the Electrocardiogram, Cardiovasc. Clin., 5(3): 269, 1973. Used by permission.*)

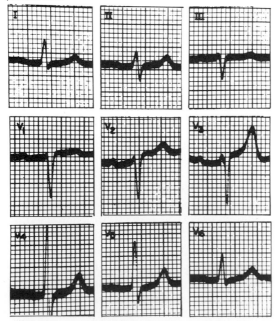

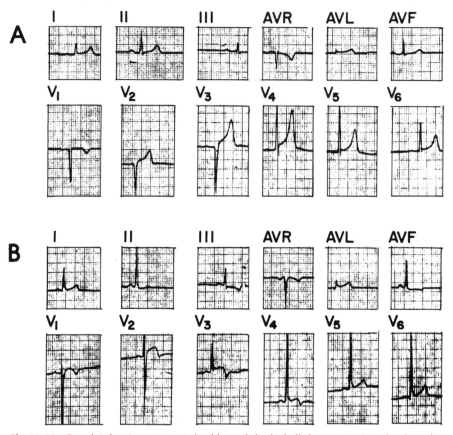

Fig. 13-27   Pseudoinfarction patterns in healthy male basketball players.   (A) Sinus bradycardia and QS complexes in leads V_1 and V_3 accompanied by tall, peaked T waves in the mid and lateral precordial leads.   (B) Increased QRS voltage and S-T segment elevation in the precordial leads.   There is also terminal T wave inversion in leads V_1 to V_4.   (*Reprinted by permission from J. Lichtman et al., Electrocardiogram of the Athlete, Arch. Intern. Med., 32: 763, November 1973. Copyright 1973, American Medical Association.*)

ographic abnormalities that have been observed in athletes include sinus bradycardia, sinus arrhythmia, AV junctional rhythm, first- and second-degree block, T wave abnormalities, and signs consistent with atrial or ventricular enlargement.

Pneumothorax, both spontaneous and artificial, especially if left-sided, may produce electrocardiographic changes simulating infarction (Figs. 13-30A and B.)   Right axis deviation, a reduction in QRS voltage, and T wave inversions in the precordial leads may occur.   Sometimes there is a decrease or loss of the R waves in the precordial leads which may mimic anterior infarction.   These findings have been reported to be normalized when the electrocardiogram is recorded with the patient in the upright position.

Central nervous system lesions, notably subarachnoid hemorrhage, may produce electrocardiographic abnormalities simulating myocardial infarction (Fig. 21-7). The changes usually consist of S-T segment elevations or depressions, large upright or inverted T waves, prolonged Q-T intervals, prominent U waves, and sometimes abnormal Q waves.

Myocardial contusion, caused by nonpenetrating injury of the chest, may produce nonspecific ST-T abnormalities, AV block, and ventricular conduction defects. Sometimes when hemorrhage and necrosis are extensive, Q wave changes indistinguishable from those due to infarction may be observed in the electrocardiogram (Fig. 13-31).

Miscellaneous conditions: Several cases have been reported in which abnormal electrocardiograms diagnostic of infarction were recorded in

Fig. 13-28 Pseudosubepicardial injury patterns in healthy male athletes. (*A*) Tall R waves with elevated S-T segments in the precordial leads. (*B*) T wave inversion is seen in leads V₁ to V₃. First-degree AV block, high QRS voltage, and a right ventricular conduction defect are also present. (*Reprinted by permission from J. Lichtman et al., Electrocardiogram of the Athlete, Arch. Int. Med., 132: 763, November 1973. Copyright 1973, American Medical Association.*)

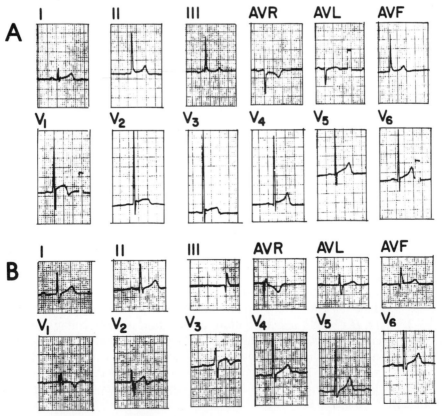

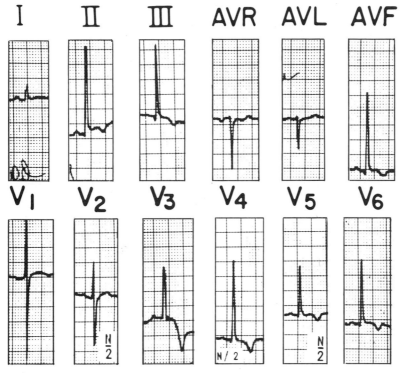

Fig. 13-29 Electrocardiogram from a 19-year-old male athlete without heart disease. The voltage changes are consistent with biventricular enlargement. The S-T changes are suggestive of subepicardial injury.

Fig. 13-30A Spontaneous pneumothorax. Abnormal QS complexes with slight S-T elevation are present in leads V_1 through V_4. The T waves are inverted in leads III and aVF. The changes in the precordial leads resemble those of acute anteroseptal myocardial infarction. From a 26-year-old man with massive left-sided pneumothorax. (*From T-C Chou, Pseudoinfarction (Noninfarction Q Waves), Cardiovasc. Clin.,* 5(3): 199, 1973. *Used by permission.*)

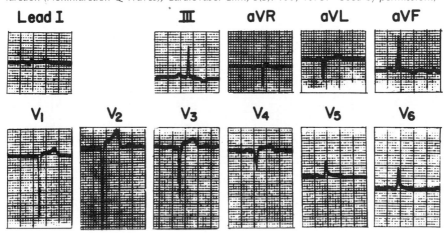

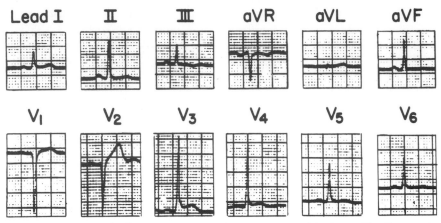

Fig. 13-30B Same patient as in Fig. 13-30A after reexpansion of the lung. The Q waves in leads V$_2$ through V$_4$ have disappeared. (*From T-C Chou, Pseudo-infarction (Noninfarction Q Waves), Cardiovasc. Clin., 5(3): 199, 1973. Used by permission.*)

healthy young men with normal coronary arteriograms. No cause for these changes was found, nor was heart disease present.

Transitory Q wave abnormalities have also been recorded during bouts of tachycardia, in Prinzmetal's angina, and in coronary insufficiency.

Reversal of the right and left limb leads is a common technical error which may cause the appearance of spuriously abnormal Q waves in lead I and bring the unwary to an erroneous diagnosis of infarction (Fig. 13-32). Prominent Q waves may appear in lead I in dextrocardia.

Fig. 13-31 Electrocardiographic changes suggestive of anterior and inferior myocardial infarction in a patient who sustained nonpenetrating trauma to the chest. (*From T-C Chou, Pseudoinfarction (Noninfarction Q Waves), Cardiovasc. Clin., 5(3): 199, 1973. Used by permission.*)

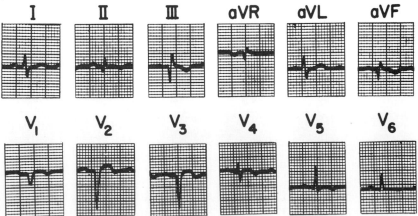

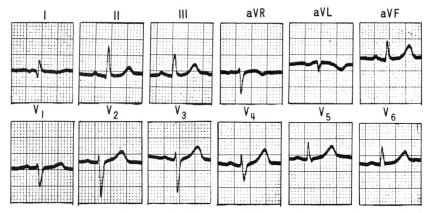

Fig. 13-32 Reversal of the right and left arms resulting in a pattern suggestive of superior myocardial infarction. The clue to the technical error is the presence of a negative P wave in lead "I" and a positive P wave in lead "aVR."

Electrocardiograms typical of myocardial infarction have been recorded in patients critically ill with acute pancreatitis, pneumonia, and similar disorders associated with shock and severe metabolic stress.

Pes excavatum and the straight back syndrome are sometimes associated with pseudoinfarction patterns, as is the mitral valve prolapse syndrome.

DIFFERENTIAL DIAGNOSIS OF STRICTLY POSTERIOR MYOCARDIAL INFARCTION

The differential diagnosis of strictly posterior myocardial infarction is discussed separately from other types of infarction because it presents special problems.

Abnormally tall and/or broad R waves in lead V_1 are not pathognomonic of strictly posterior infarction, since they may also occur in right ventricular hypertrophy, right bundle branch block, ventricular preexcitation, and occasionally in normal individuals. The W-P-W syndrome usually presents no diagnostic difficulties, because its features are distinctive (short P-R, wide QRS, and delta wave). Since right bundle branch block itself is often associated with broad R and R' waves in lead V_1, the differential diagnosis between the two is exceedingly difficult. However, absence of a wide S wave in lead I rules out right bundle branch block as a cause of a prominent R' wave in lead V_1. The tall, broad R wave of right ventricular hypertrophy is often associated with right ventricular strain and right axis deviation. On the other hand, the dominant R wave of posterobasal infarction is usually associated with S-T segment depression and upright T waves in the right precordial leads and with an axis to the left of $+45°$, a finding unusual in right ventricular hypertrophy. The broad R wave found in normal subjects tends to occur in association with an electrical axis to the right of +45°. The more vertical the electrical axis, the more likely is the normal occurrence of an 0.04-s R wave in lead V_1. The presence in the electrocardiogram of signs of inferior or lateral infarction increases the likelihood that a dominant R wave in lead V_1 is due to dorsal infarction rather than to other causes.

Other conditions which may be associated with tall R waves in the right precordial leads include asymmetric septal hypertrophy, congenital dextroversion, Duchenne muscular dystrophy, right bundle branch block, and, rarely, chronic constrictive pericarditis.

Comments

S-T segment and T wave changes in any of the aforementioned conditions may mimic those found in myocardial infarction. Sole reliance should not be placed on S-T-T changes for the diagnosis of infarction.

Sometimes, if premature systoles are present in the electrocardiogram, the diagnosis of myocardial infarction may be established from the configuration of the ectopic beats. To be diagnostic of infarction, premature systoles, whether ventricular or supraventricular, must have a QR and not a QS morphology and must be recorded in ventricular epicardial leads, not in leads overlying the atria.

MYOCARDIAL INFARCTION WITH PERICARDITIS

See Chap. 15 on pericarditis.

MYOCARDIAL INFARCTION WITH FASCICULAR BLOCK
(FIGS. 13-33, 13-34)

Many cases of myocardial infarction show alterations in the direction of the terminal 0.04-s QRS vector in addition to the characteristic deformity of the initial 0.04-s vector. Whereas the latter points away from the location of the infarct, the former points toward it.

Two explanations have been offered for the mechanism of the terminal vector deformity. One view holds that the normal radial spread of excitation is blocked by the infarct, so that any viable muscle overlying the infarct can be stimulated only by circuitous pathways. This region of the heart is thus the last to be depolarized. The other view holds that the terminal vector deformity is the result of a specific block in either the anterior or posterior division of the left bundle branch. An infarct located in the region of the anterior division blocks these fibers so that excitation takes place via the posterior division, which results in terminal forces that are

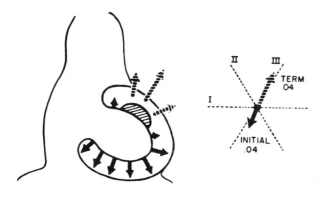

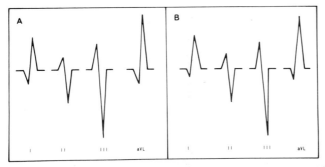

Fig. 13-33 Schematic representation of the mechanism of the initial and terminal QRS vector deformity of lateral infarction with left anterior fascicular block. (A) The standard limb leads show abnormal Q waves in leads aVL and I.   The terminal forces are directed leftward and superiorly.   The initial 0.04-s and terminal 0.04-s QRS vectors are widely separated.   The QRS loop, if plotted, is inscribed in a CCW manner. (B) Variant pattern of lateral infarction in which the Q wave is not abnormally wide in leads I and aVL.   However, the R waves are broad in leads II and III, which has the same diagnostic significance.   The terminal forces are directed leftward and superiorly.   The initial 0.04-s and terminal 0.04-s QRS vectors are widely separated.   The QRS loop is rotated CCW. (*Modified from R. P. Grant, Left Axis Deviation: An Electrocardiographic-Pathologic Correlation Study, Circulation, 14: 233, 1956. Used by permission of the American Heart Association, Inc.*)

directed leftward and superiorly.   On the other hand, an infarct located in the region of the posterior division blocks these fibers so that stimulation takes place via the anterior division, which results in terminal forces that point inferiorly and rightward.   Thus fascicular block may complicate anterior or inferior myocardial infarction.

Left anterior fascicular block is seen most commonly with anteroseptal or localized anterior infarction, but it also occurs with anterolateral or superior infarction.

The basic vectorcardiographic features of myocardial infarction with

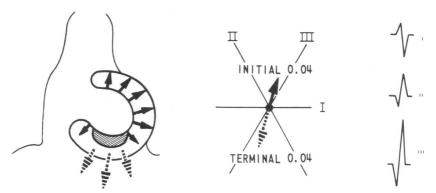

Fig. 13-34 Schematic representation of the mechanism of the initial and terminal QRS vector deformity of inferior infarction with left posterior fascicular block. The standard leads show QR patterns in leads II and III, and an RS pattern in lead I. The initial 0.04-s QRS vector is directed leftward and superiorly; the terminal 0.04-s QRS vector, rightward and inferiorly; and the angle between the two is abnormally wide.

fascicular block, according to Grant, are (1) an abnormality of the initial QRS forces characteristic of myocardial infarction, so that they point away from the site of infarction, (2) an abnormality of the terminal QRS forces, so that they point opposite to the initial forces, and (3) little or no prolongation of the QRS interval.

The term *peri-infarction block* has been used (notably by Grant) to describe what is now considered a fascicular block complicating myocardial infarction. However, other writers have used the same term to describe other conduction disturbances observed in myocardial infarction. It is the opinion of most authorities that the term peri-infarction or postinfarction block should be discarded in favor of a specific designation of the underlying conduction disturbance (e.g., left anterior fascicular block). If this is not possible, a diagnosis of a nonspecific intraventricular or intramural (intramyocardial) block should be made.

Diagnosis of Anterior Infarction with Left Anterior Fascicular Block (Figs. 13-33, 13-35, 13-36, 13-37)

1   The initial 0.04-s QRS vector in the frontal plane is directed rightward and inferiorly, which results in abnormal Q waves in leads aVL and I and an initial broad R wave in leads II, III, and aVF. Abnormal Q waves may also appear in the left precordial leads. In anteroseptal and localized anterior infarction, abnormal Q waves are found in the precordial leads but not in the limb leads. The initial 0.04-s QRS vector in the frontal plane will then be normal. Occasionally, in anterolateral or superior infarction, the Q waves will not be abnormally wide in leads aVL, I, or the left precordial leads. In such instances, the presence of

broad (0.04 s), slurred R waves in the inferior limb leads, even in the absence of diagnostic Q waves in the left precordial leads or lead aVL, or both, is diagnostic of lateral infarction.

2   The terminal QRS vector in the frontal plane (usually the mean QRS vector as well) is directed leftward and superiorly to $-45°$ or more.

3   The angle between the initial and terminal 0.04-s QRS vectors is 110° or more in the frontal plane.

4   Leads I and aVL thus show a qR or QR pattern; leads II, III, and aVF usually show an rS pattern; and lead aVR, a positive terminal deflection.

5   If the terminal QRS vector is also anteriorly directed, there may be an R' wave in lead V_1, V_2, or V_3.

6   The QRS interval is usually normal or slightly prolonged.

Diagnosis of Inferior Infarction with Left Anterior Fascicular Block (Figs. 13-39, 13-40, 13-41, 13-42)

Since left anterior fascicular block produces initial R waves in leads II, III, and aVF, previous inferior infarction may be concealed when the block develops because Q waves are partially or completely obliterated (Figs.

Fig. 13-35   Anterolateral myocardial infarction with left anterior fascicular block. Abnormal Q waves are present in leads I, aVL, V_5, and V_6. In addition, there is abnormal left axis deviation. Thus the initial and terminal 0.04-s QRS vectors point in almost opposite directions, a finding diagnostic of anterolateral infarction with left anterior fascicular block. The S waves are unusually deep in leads V_2 and V_3, suggesting the diagnosis of left ventricular enlargement as well. The tall R wave in V_1 may represent a reciprocal effect on the deep Q wave in the left precordial leads or may indicate coexisting posterobasal infarction.

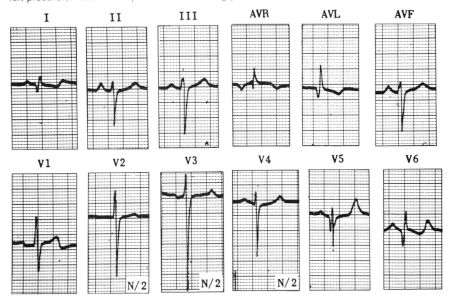

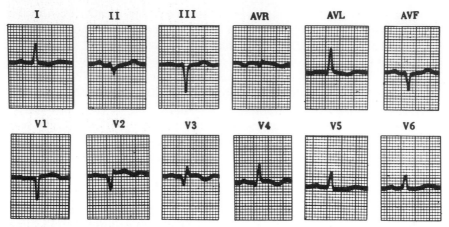

Fig. 13-36 Anteroseptal myocardial infarction with left anterior fascicular block. The former is manifested by the presence of a QS complex in lead V_1 and QR patterns in leads V_2 to V_4; the latter, by the abnormal left axis deviation.

13-37, 13-38).   Conversely, inferior infarction may actually mask preexisting left anterior fascicular block by causing the initial R waves in the inferior leads to disappear (Fig. 13-40).   It has been reported that if patients with right bundle branch block are excluded, abnormal left axis deviation accompanied by a positive terminal deflection in leads aVL and aVR, and a negative terminal deflection in lead II is diagnostic of left anterior fascicular block in the presence or absence of coexistent inferior myocardial infarction.

Although it is usually possible to diagnose the coexistence of inferior infarction and left anterior fascicular block, the diagnostic changes may be quite subtle.   Therefore, the inferior leads should always be scrutinized carefully for clues to the diagnosis of inferior infarction whenever left anterior fascicular block is present.   Clues to this diagnosis are a qrS complex or a tiny, bifid or notched, initial R wave in lead II (Fig. 13-39). Small Q waves preceding the rS complexes in leads III and aVF may also be significant (Fig. 13-37).

The presence of QS complexes in leads II, III, and aVF makes the differential diagnosis between isolated inferior myocardial infarction and inferior infarction with left anterior fascicular block very difficult.   The presence of even a tiny late R wave in these leads is strong evidence against the diagnosis of left anterior fascicular block, because a late R wave in these leads indicates that the terminal forces are directed inferiorly and not superiorly as they should be in left anterior fascicular block.   On the other hand, as indicated above, the presence of a small bifid or notched initial R wave or a qrS complex in lead II strongly suggests the diagnosis of inferior myocardial infarction with left anterior fascicular block (Fig. 20-1B).   In most cases of old inferior myocardial infarction presenting with QS complexes in leads II, III, and aVF, the additional diagnosis of left anterior fascicular block appears to be justified if there is a positive terminal deflection in leads aVL and aVR. Inferior infarction with left anterior fascicular block may be mimicked by chronic obstructive pulmonary disease (Fig. 18-5).

Warner and his associates have proposed the following criteria for the diagnosis of combined inferior myocardial infarction and left anterior fascicular block: (1) leads aVR and aVL both end in R waves, with the peak of the terminal R wave in lead aVR occurring later than the peak of the terminal R wave in lead aVL; (2) a Q wave of any magnitude is present in lead II. They believe that the performance of these criteria is superior to that of previously proposed criteria.

Diagnosis of Inferior Infarction with Left Posterior Fascicular Block (Figs. 13-34, 13-38, 11-22, 11-23, 20-1B)

1 The initial 0.04-s QRS vector in the frontal plane is directed leftward and superiorly, which results in abnormal Q waves in the inferior extremity leads.
2 The terminal 0.04-s QRS vector in the frontal plane is directed inferiorly and sometimes rightward.
3 The angle between the initial and terminal 0.04-s QRS vector is 110° or more in the frontal plane.

Fig. 13-37 Superoanteroseptal myocardial infarction with left anterior fascicular block, left ventricular enlargement, and first-degree AV block. The superior component of the infarct is shown by the presence of abnormal Q waves in leads I and aVL and broad R waves in leads III and aVF. The QS complexes in leads V_1 and V_2 and the QR pattern in lead V_3 are indicative of the anteroseptal component of the infarct. The initial and terminal QRS vectors are widely separated. The diagnosis of left ventricular enlargement is suggested by high voltage of the R wave in lead aVL and increased voltage of the sum of the R_1 and S_3 waves. The P-R interval is prolonged at 0.22 s.

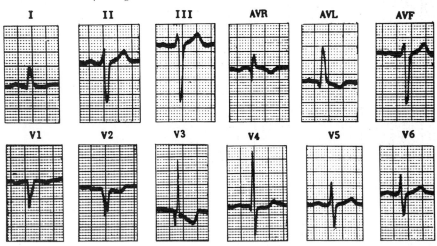

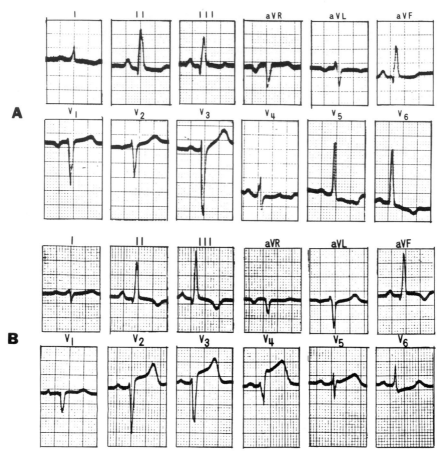

Fig. 13-38 (*A*) Old inferior myocardial infarction with left ventricular enlargement and a nonspecific ST-T abnormality. (*B*) Same patient as in *A* during a later episode of acute anteroseptal myocardial infarction. There is poor R wave progression from V₁ to V₄, with elevated S-T segments in these leads. However, there is now right axis deviation in the frontal plane (about +105°) with a qR pattern in leads II, III, and aVF, which indicates concomitant left posterior fascicular block. The T wave inversions in leads II, III, and aVF are consistent with inferior wall ischema.

4   There is thus a wide Q wave with a QR pattern in leads II, III, and aVF. Leads I and aVL usually show an rS or RS pattern.
5   Leads V₁ and V₂ usually show deep S waves, but a terminal R′ wave does not occur.
6   The QRS interval is usually normal or slightly prolonged.

Comments

Monofascicular and bifascicular blocks may occur in myocardial infarction. The incidence of these abnormalities in the series of 250 cases reported by

Marriott and Hogan is as follows: isolated left anterior fascicular block, 11.2 percent; left anterior fascicular block with right bundle branch block, 4 percent; left posterior fascicular block with right bundle branch block, 0.8 percent; isolated right bundle branch block, 12.4 percent; and left bundle branch block alone, 11.6 percent. In some cases it was not possible to determine whether the fascicular block preceded or followed the onset of myocardial infarction.

Anterior (especially anteroseptal) myocardial infarction may cause transient or permanent left anterior fascicular block, right bundle branch

Fig. 13-39 Inferior myocardial infarction masked by probable incomplete left anterior fascicular block. (A) Old inferior infarction manifested by prominent Q waves in leads III and aVF. There are S-T segment elevations in leads V₁ to V₄, with T wave inversion in leads V_2 to V_5. The findings are consistent with acute anterior subepicardial injury and compatible with the clinical diagnosis of acute myocardial infarction. In B a tracing taken 2 days after A. The axis had shifted leftward, and aside from tiny Q waves in leads III and aVF, the evidence of previous inferior myocardial infarction has disappeared. The probable cause is incomplete left anterior fascicular block. In subsequent tracings (not shown), the left axis deviation disappeared and the Q waves in leads III and aVF reappeared.

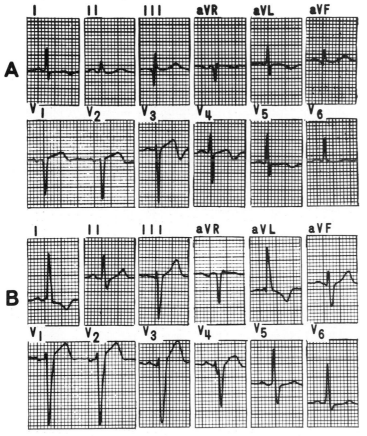

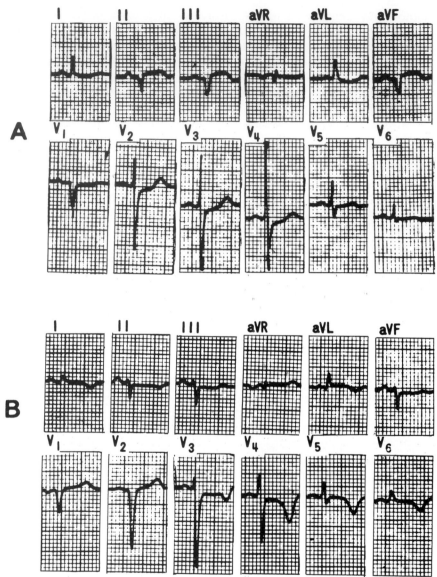

Fig. 13-40 Inferior myocardial infarction masked by left anterior fascicular block. In A, recent inferior myocardial infarction is evidenced by QS complexes and elevated S-T segments in leads II, III, and aVF. In B, recorded one year later during an episode of acute anterior myocardial infarction, the QS complexes in leads II, III, and aVF have been replaced by rS deflections, obliterating evidence of the previous inferior myocardial infarction.

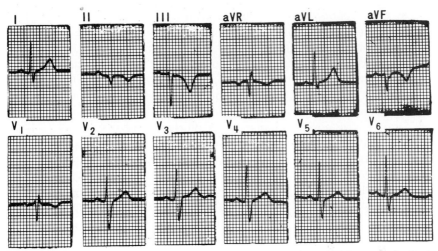

Fig. 13-41   Recent inferior myocardial infarction superimposed on old left anterior fascicular block.   The only evidence of the recent inferior myocardial infarct is the tiny notched R wave in lead II and the T wave inversions in the inferior extremity leads.

block, or both.   These conduction abnormalities may or may not precede the onset of infarction.

Many cases of inferior infarction present not only with the initial QRS vector deformity of infarction but also with an inferior and rightward terminal QRS vector deformity, which produces late R waves in leads II, III, and aVF and a prominent S wave in lead I.   Most authorities believe that this terminal vector deformity represents left posterior fascicular block. Others believe that it results from a localized block due to infarction unless the R_2 and R_3 are quite tall.

Rosenbaum and his associates have indicated that while right bundle branch block and left anterior fascicular block, or both, are relatively common in anterior infarction, left posterior fascicular block is much less common in inferior infarction.   The combination of anterior and inferior myocardial infarction is more likely to cause left posterior fascicular block than inferior infarction alone (Fig. 13-38).

Although fascicular block may simulate or conceal myocardial infarction, it does not ordinarily interfere with the diagnosis of infarction.

When left anterior fascicular block exhibits small Q waves in leads V_1 to V_3, anteroseptal infarction is simulated (Figs. 13-23, 13-24).   However, noninfarctional Q waves tend to disappear in chest leads recorded at a lower level, while those caused by myocardial infarction persist in the lower V leads.

Left anterior fascicular block may mimic superior infarction when the Q wave in aVL shows borderline abnormality, and anterolateral infarction when the left chest leads show small R waves and deep S waves.

In left posterior fascicular block with right bundle branch block, a deep Q wave in lead V_1 is not uncommon in the absence of infarction.

In left anterior fascicular block, an anteroseptal myocardial infarct may be concealed (by changing QS to rS complexes) if the chest leads are taken slightly below the conventional level; in left posterior fascicular block, if recorded above this level. The recording of high and low V leads will usually obviate these diagnostic dilemmas.

Since left anterior fascicular block produces initial R-waves in leads II, III, and aVF, previous inferior infarction may be concealed when the block develops, because Q waves are partially or completely obliterated (Figs. 13-39, 13-40). When inferior infarction is superimposed on left anterior fascicular block abnormal Q waves may sometimes fail to appear (Fig. 13-41). Conversely, inferior infarction may actually mask preexisting

Fig. 13-42 Recent inferior infarction masking preexisting left anterior fascicular block. *A*, recorded during acute anteroseptal infarction, reveals left anterior fascicular block. At a later time, *B*, acute inferior infarction has developed. The rS complexes in leads II, III, and aVF have been replaced by QS deflections. A lateral component to the inferior infarct may be present (QR complexes in leads V_5 and V_6)

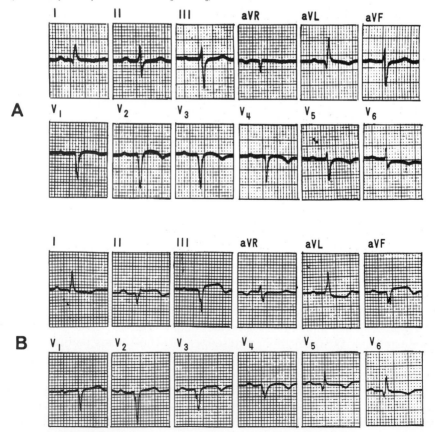

left anterior fascicular block by causing the initial R waves in the inferior leads to disappear (Fig. 13-42).   Although it is usually possible to diagnose the coexistence of inferior infarction and left anterior fascicular block, the diagnostic changes may be quite subtle.   Therefore the inferior leads should always be scrutinized carefully for clues to the diagnosis of inferior infarction whenever left anterior fascicular block is present.   Clues to the diagnosis of inferior infarction are QR or qrS complexes or a tiny bifid or notched initial R wave in lead II (Fig. 13-41).   Small Q waves preceding the rS complexes in leads III and aVF may also be significant (Fig. 13-39).

The presence of QS complexes in leads II, III, and aVF makes the differential diagnosis between isolated inferior myocardial infarction and inferior infarction with left anterior fascicular block very difficult.   The presence of even a tiny late R wave in these leads is strong evidence against the diagnosis of left anterior fascicular block, because a late R wave in these leads indicates that the terminal forces are directed inferiorly and not superiorly as they should be in left anterior fascicular block.   On the other hand, the presence of a small bifid or notched initial R wave, a QR deflection, or a qrS complex in lead II strongly suggests the diagnosis of inferior myocardial infarction with left anterior fascicular block (Figs. 13-41, B of 20-1).   In most cases of old inferior myocardial infarction presenting with QS complexes in leads II, III, and aVF, the additional diagnosis of left anterior fascicular block may be mimicked by chronic obstructive pulmonary disease (Fig. 18-5).

Anterolateral infarction with left anterior fascicular block is usually manifested by abnormal Q waves in the left precordial leads and usually in leads aVL and I, in addition to abnormal left axis deviation.   This initial vector deformity produces broad (0.04-s) R waves in leads II, III, and aVF. Sometimes increased duration of these R waves may occur in anterolateral or superior infarction without the appearance of abnormal Q waves in lead aVL or the left precordial leads.   Such wide R waves should be considered diagnostic of infarction even if abnormal Q waves are not present in other leads (Fig. 13-33).

MYOCARDIAL INFARCTION WITH BUNDLE BRANCH BLOCK

In right bundle branch block, the QRS vectors during the first 0.04 to 0.06 s of the QRS interval are not affected by the block.   Therefore, when anteroseptal, anterolateral, or inferior infarction coexists with right bundle branch block, the direction of the initial QRS vectors is changed by the infarct, as one would expect.   But since infarcts in these locations have no effect on the ventricular forces produced late in the QRS interval, the characteristic terminal QRS vector deformity of right bundle branch block is unaltered.   Therefore it is usually possible to diagnose coexisting myocardial infarction and right bundle branch block: the former on the basis of the initial 0.04-s QRS vector deformity, the latter on the basis of the terminal 0.04-s QRS vector deformity. The diagnosis of coexisting posterobasal infarction and right bundle branch block, on the other hand, is the one exception to the rule. The problem with this combination is that both strictly posterior infarction and right bundle branch block displace the QRS vectors in the same general anterior direction. Since it is virtually impossible to separate the effects of one from the other in the QRS complex, the electrocardiographic diagnosis of dorsal infarction in the presence of right bundle branch block is exceedingly difficult, if not impossible.

Wilson et al. long ago pointed out that in the presence of left bundle branch block it is seldom possible to make the diagnosis of myocardial infarction from the electrocardiogram alone. The reason for this is that in left bundle branch block, because the ventricular septum is depolarized from right to left, the initial 0.04-s QRS vector is always directed leftward. This is true whether infarction of the free ventricular wall is present or not. The diagnostic sign of infarction—an abnormal initial 0.04-s QRS vector— is thus lost. Stated otherwise, abnormal Q waves do not appear in the left precordial or extremity leads in left bundle branch block even in the presence of infarction. However, the effect of an anterolateral infarct may become manifest during the latter half of the QRS interval, when activation of the free left ventricular wall takes place. The failure of the infarcted region to generate electrical potentials during this period permits other forces, directed away from the infarct, to become preponderant. The orientation of these forces is such that a terminal S wave is often inscribed in lead V_6, and sometimes also in lead I. On the other hand with extensive infarction of the interventricular septum, the initial QRS vector abnormality of infarction may become evident in the electrocardiogram. This happens when the initial right-to-left septal depolarization of left bundle branch block is eliminated by the infarct so that right ventricular forces become dominant early in the QRS interval. Their rightward direction results in progressive diminution in the height of the R wave in leads V_1 to V_4 and in the inscription of Q waves in leads V_6, I, and aVL. However, once activation of the left ventricular wall begins, the remaining QRS vectors are directed leftward and posteriorly, which causes terminal R waves to be projected on leads I, aVL, and V_6 and final S waves to be recorded in the right precordial leads.

Anterior Myocardial Infarction with Right Bundle Branch Block
(Fig. 13-43)

Conventional Criteria

1   The duration of the QRS complex is 0.12 s or more.
2   Lead I and the left precordial leads show wide final S waves.
3   In anteroseptal infarction with right bundle branch block, the right-sided precordial leads from V_1 to V_3 or V_4 show diagnostic signs of infarction.

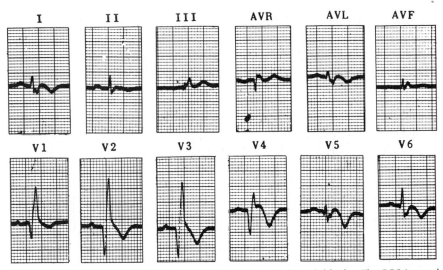

Fig. 13-43 Anterior myocardial infarction and right bundle branch block. The QRS interval is prolonged. There are wide S waves in leads I, V_5, and V_6. QR complexes with late R waves are seen in leads V_1 to V_4.

There is loss of the initial R waves in these leads. However, the QRS patterns are modified by the presence of right bundle branch block, so that in addition to the abnormal Q waves, tall late R waves appear in these leads. When the infarct is more extensive, abnormal Q waves may also appear in leads I and aVL and the left precordial leads.

Vectorelectrocardiographic Criteria

1   The initial 0.04-s QRS vector points away from the site of infarction and so produces abnormal Q waves in the precordial and limb leads.
2   The terminal QRS vector points rightward and anteriorly, which produces a wide S wave in lead I and a terminal R' wave in lead V_1.

Inferior Myocardial Infarction with Right Bundle Branch Block
(Fig. 13-44)

Conventional Criteria

1   The duration of the QRS complex is 0.12 s or more.
2   The precordial electrocardiogram shows the pattern of right bundle branch block.
3   Diagnostic signs of inferior infarction are found in leads II, III, and aVF.

Vectorelectrocardiographic Criteria

1   The initial 0.04-s QRS vector points superiorly, which produces abnormal Q waves in leads II, III, and aVF.

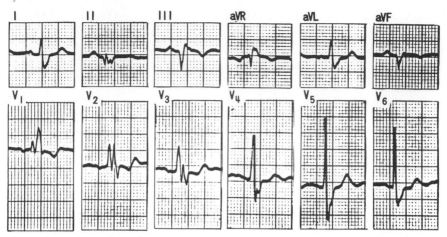

Fig. 13-44   Recent inferior myocardial infarction with right bundle branch block.   There are deep, wide Q waves in leads II, III, and aVF, with inverted T waves in leads III and aVF.   The QRS duration is 0.16 s, with a wide S wave in leads I, V_5, and V_6 and an RsR' pattern in lead V_1.   The R wave in lead V_5 exceeds 20 mm, which suggest. concomitant left ventricular enlargement.

2   The terminal 0.04-s QRS vector points rightward and anteriorly, which produces a wide S wave in lead I and a terminal R' wave in lead V_1.

Myocardial Infarction with Left Bundle Branch Block

Acute Myocardial Infarction (Figs. 13-45, 13-46, 13-47)   Myocardial infarction in the presence of left bundle branch block may be suspected when S-T and T vector abnormalities characteristic of infarction are found in a tracing showing left bundle branch block.   This does not occur too often, because in left bundle branch block the secondary S-T and T vector abnormalities have such magnitude that they are rarely altered even by myocardial injury and ischemia.

The appearance of S-T segment elevation either in the left precordial leads or in leads II, III, and aVF is suggestive, respectively, of anterolateral or inferior myocardial infarction.   Positive S-T displacement in the right precordial leads is much more difficult to evaluate, since S-T segment elevation in these leads may occur in uncomplicated left bundle branch block alone.   Elevation of the S-T segment of more than 2 mm concordant to the main deflection of the QRS complex or more than 7 mm discordant to the main deflection is considered significant.   The presence of T wave inversion in the right precordial leads in left bundle branch block is suggestive of anterior myocardial ischemia.   Similarly, inferior myocardial ischemia is suggested by the presence of T wave inversion in leads II, III, and aVF.

Positive T waves in leads with positive main deflections may also be significant.

Infarction of the Free Wall of the Left Ventricle   In some cases of lateral wall infarction, an RS pattern may appear in leads I, aVL, V_5, and V_6. Caution should be exercised in considering this pattern diagnostic of myocardial infarction, because it may also occur in uncomplicated left bundle branch block when the transition zone is displaced leftward.   The configuration of the T wave may be helpful.   When the RS pattern is transitional, the T wave in this lead is usually upright.   On the other hand, when the RS pattern is due to infarction, the T wave is usually inverted.

Anterior Infarction (Fig. 13-47)   The diagnosis of anterior infarction in the presence of left bundle branch block may be suspected if in addition to the features of left bundle branch block, the electrocardiogram shows one or more of the following findings:

1   The presence of Q waves that are 0.04 s or more in width in leads I, V_5, or V_6, particularly in association with an R wave in lead V_1.   Wide Q waves in lead aVL and Q waves of lesser duration in lead I may sometimes occur in left bundle branch block in the absence of infarction. However, abnormal Q waves are rarely seen in lead V_5 or V_6 in left bundle branch block without associated infarction.
2   Notching of 0.05 s in duration in the ascending limb of the S wave in lead V_3 or V_4 and notching of the ascending limb of the R wave in lead I, aVL, or V_6 are sometimes seen with anterior infarction.
3   Progressive diminution in the height of the R wave from leads V_1 to V_4.

Inferior Myocardial Infarction (Figs. 13-48, 13-49)   According to some authorities, the combination of inferior myocardial infarction and left bundle branch block may be suspected if in addition to the features of left bundle branch block, the electrocardiogram shows (1) Q waves or QS complexes

Fig. 13-45   Left bundle branch block with acute anterior subepicardial injury.   There is S-T segment elevation in leads I, aVL, V_5, and V_6, with reciprocal S-T segment depression in leads II, III, and aVF.   From a patient with preexisting left bundle branch block.   The recording was taken early in the course of acute myocardial infarction.

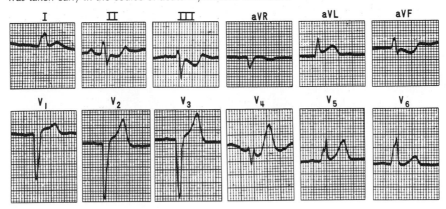

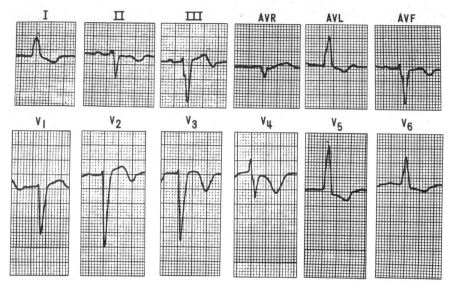

Fig. 13-46   Left bundle branch block with anterior and inferior myocardial ischemia. Recorded from a patient with preexisting left bundle branch block during the course of acute myocardial infarction.

Fig. 13-47   Anterior myocardial infarction and left bundle branch block.   The QRS interval is markedly prolonged.   The R waves in leads V_3 and V_4 are smaller than those in lead V_2. There is a broad notch on the ascending limb of the S wave in lead V_4.   Abnormal Q waves are present in leads I, aVL, V_5, and V_6.   There are slurred, late R waves in leads V_5 to V_7. An alternative diagnosis for this electrocardiogram is anterolateral myocardial infarction with left anterior fascicular and intramural block.

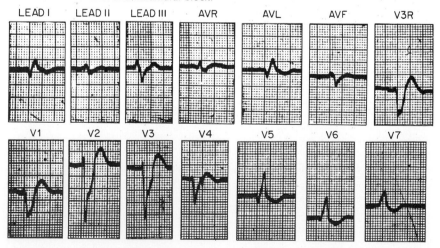

in leads II, III, and aVF or (2) notched R or R' waves in leads III and aVF. These criteria are tenuous, because similar abnormalities may occur in left bundle branch block in the absence of inferior infarction.

THE VECTORCARDIOGRAM IN MYOCARDIAL INFARCTION

Anteroseptal Myocardial Infarction (Fig. 13-50)

1   The 0.02QRS vector is displaced posteriorly and leftward in the TP.
2   There is CCW inscription of the QRS loop in the TP.   The initial component, however, may rotate CW.

Fig. 13-48   (A) Old inferior infarction manifested by deep Q waves in leads II, III, and aVF. (B) Same patient as in A after the development of left bundle branch block.   There are now QS complexes in leads II, III, and aVF.   The findings are otherwise typical of left bundle branch block.   Small Q waves are present in leads I, aVL, V₅, and V₆.   This may occur in uncomplicated left bundle branch block.

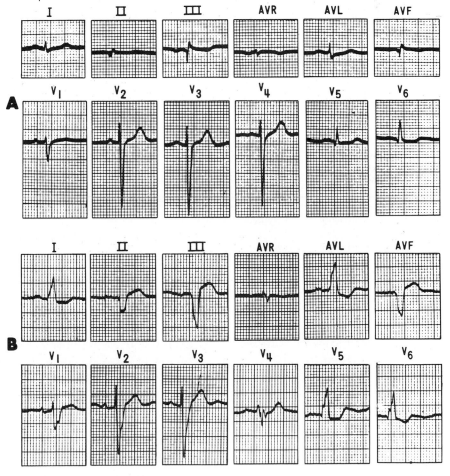

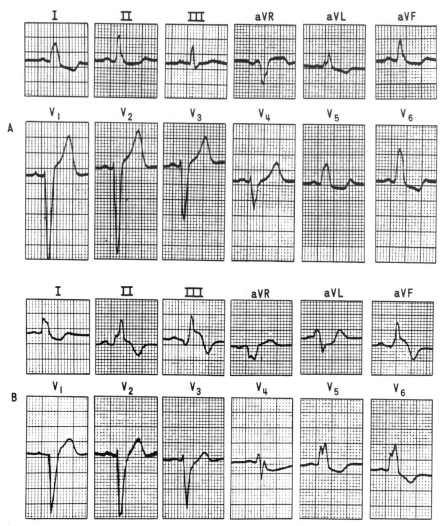

Fig. 13-49 (A) Left bundle branch block. (B) Same patient as in A, recorded 3 months later during an acute episode of myocardial infarction. There are wide Q waves in leads III and an aVF and S-T segment elevation with T wave inversion in leads II, III, and aVF. The left bundle branch block pattern persists.

3 The 0.02QRS vector is displaced posteriorly and usually inferiorly in the LSP. There is usually CCW inscription of the QRS loop in this plane. A CW inscription of the QRS loop in the LSP suggests coexisting inferior infarction.

4 The QRS loop is normal in the FP.

Localized Anterior Infarction (Fig. 13-51)

1 The 0.01QRS vector is normal and is directed rightward and anteriorly in the TP. The 0.02QRS vector is oriented posteriorly and to the left.

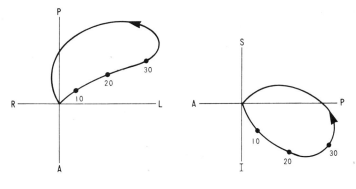

TRANSVERSE PLANE   LEFT SAGITTAL PLANE

Fig. 13-50 The vectorcardiogram in anteroseptal myocardial infarction. The numbers indicate the time in milliseconds after the beginning of the QRS loop. Described in text.

2 In the LSP, the 0.01QRS vector is directed anteriorly and superiorly, but the 0.02QRS vector is displaced posteriorly and inferiorly. Inscription of the main body of the loop is usually CCW.

3 The QRS loop is normal in the FP.

Anterolateral or Lateral Myocardial Infarction (Fig. 13-52)

1 In the TP, the 0.01QRS vector is usually inscribed normally, but the 0.02QRS vector is displaced rightward and posteriorly. There is CW rotation of the QRS loop in the TP.

2 In the LSP, inscription of the QRS loop is CCW or CW. The CW rotation of the loop in this plane suggests coexisting inferior infarction.

3 In the FP, there is rightward displacement of the 0.022QRS vector. There is always CCW rotation of the QRS loop in this plane, even if it

Fig. 13-51 Vectorcardiogram in localized anterior myocardial infarction. The 10-ms vector is directed anteriorly, which indicates that the initial septal forces are present. However, the 20-ms vector is displaced posteriorly because of infarction of the apical region of the left ventricle.

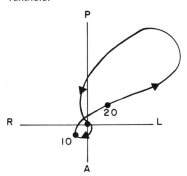

TRANSVERSE PLANE

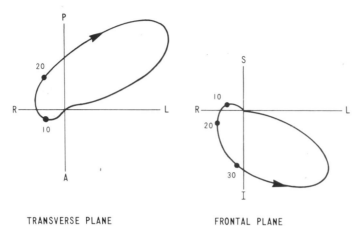

TRANSVERSE PLANE   FRONTAL PLANE

Fig. 13-52 The vectorcardiogram in anterolateral or lateral myocardial infarction. The numbers indicate the time in milliseconds after the beginning of the QRS loop. Described in text.

is directed vertically. (In normals, whenever the maximum FP QRS vector is to the right of +40°, inscription of the loop is CW.)

Superior or High Lateral Myocardial Infarction (Fig. 13-53)

1 In the Tp, the 0.01QRS and 0.02QRS vectors are directed rightward and anteriorly. Inscription of the QRS loop in this plane is more frequently CCW than CW, but figure-of-eight patterns are commonly observed with both types of rotation.
2 In the FP, the 0.01QRS and 0.02QRS vectors show rightward displacement. There is usually CCW rotation of the QRS loop in this plane.

Extensive Anterior Infarction (Fig. 13-54)

The vectorcardiogram combines the features of anteroseptal and anterolateral myocardial infarction. In the TP, there is absence of the initial vectors anteriorly. The QRS loop is rotated CW.

Inferior or Diaphragmatic Myocardial Infarction (Fig. 13-55)

1 In the FP, generally CW early superior QRS forces must be present; i.e., forces which are initially superior (rightward or leftward) or inferior and completely rightward for not more than 0.010 s prior to becoming superior. The superior forces must cross the X axis to the left of the 0 point, or, less commonly, the entire efferent limb is found superior to the X axis.

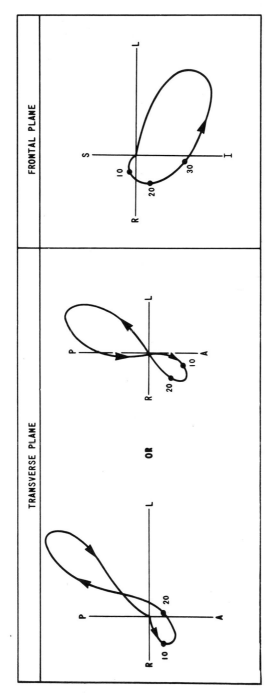

Fig. 13-53 The vectorcardiogram in superior or high lateral myocardial infarction. The numbers indicate the time in milliseconds after the beginning of the QRS loop. Described in text.

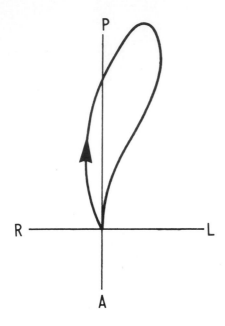

TRANSVERSE PLANE

Fig. 13-54   The vectorcardiogram in extensive anterior myocardial infarction.   The QRS loop presents a combination of the features of anteroseptal and anterolateral infarction.

2   In addition, one of the following conditions must be fulfilled:

a   The time from the 0 point to the leftward X intersect is at least 0.025 s and the distance from the 0 point to the leftward X intercept is at least 0.3 mV.

b   Orientation of the maxQRS vector in the FP is less than 15°.

c   The ratio of the maximum superior force to the maximum inferior force is at least 1:5.

3   The 0.025QRS vector is displaced superiorly in the LSP.   Rotation of the QRS loop may be CW or CCW.   The CW rotation is usually associated with coexisting anterior infarction or left ventricular hypertrophy.

4   Anterior forces of 0.5 mV or more which are equal to or exceed the posterior forces and which have a duration of 45 ms or more suggest coexisting posterior infarction.

5   When definite initial QRS vector criteria for inferior infarction are not met, there may be characteristic mid to late changes in the FP QRS loop which suggest the diagnosis.   These alterations consist of large "bites" of unexpected directional deviations of the terminal QRS forces (Young et al.).

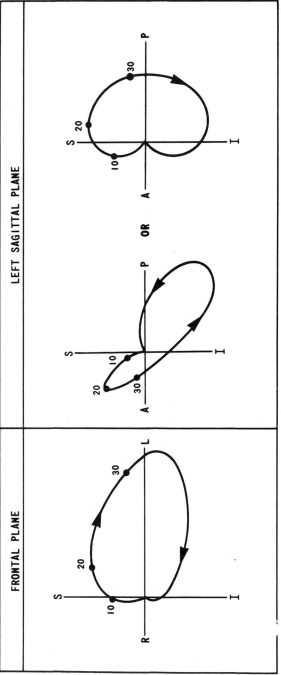

Fig. 13-55 The vectorcardiogram in inferior or diaphragmatic myocardial infarction. Two types of QRS loop pattern may be found in the LSP. A CW rotation of the loop in the LSP is usually associated with coexisting anterior infarction or left ventricular hypertrophy. The numbers indicate the time in milliseconds after the beginning of the QRS loop.

Strictly Posterior, Posterobasal, or Dorsal Myocardial Infarction
(Fig. 13-56)

1   The QRS loop is displaced anteriorly in the TP so that at least one-half to two-thirds of the loop area is located anterior to the 0 to 180° axis.
2   The early QRS vectors are little affected, but the 0.04QRS, the maxQRS, and the 0.06QRS vectors are oriented more anteriorly than in the normal.
3   Rotation of the QRS loop in the TP is usually CCW; less often, it is figure of eight or CW.
4   Hoffman et al. have recommended that the diagnosis of posterobasal infarction in the TP be based on the presence of all the following signs:
a   Maximum anterior voltage of 0.5 mV or more.
b   Location of the half-area vector at 10° or more anterior to the 0 to 180° axis.
c   An anterior accession time (the time required for the peak anterior voltage to be recorded) of 30 ms or more.
d   Total duration of the anterior QRS forces of 42 ms or more.
5   No appreciable changes are noted in the FP, which helps to differentiate true posterior infarction from right ventricular hypertrophy.

Inferolateral Myocardial Infarction (Fig. 13-57)

1   The initial rightward QRS forces exceed 0.022 s, and their magnitude is increased (>0.16 mV) in the TP.   The inscription of the QRS loop is CCW.
2   The initial QRS forces exceed 0.025 s and are directed rightward and superiorly in the FP.   Rotation of this vector and of the afferent limb is usually CW.
3   The duration and amplitude of the initial superior QRS forces is increased in the LSP, as in inferior infarction.

Myocardial Infarction with Fascicular Block (Fig. 13-58)

The presence of left anterior fascicular block does not ordinarily alter the vectorcardiographic criteria for either anterior or inferior myocardial infarction.

When left anterior fascicular block and true posterior infarction coexist, the 0.04-s QRS vector in the TP is oriented anteriorly and leftward and rotation of the loop is usually CCW in this plane.

The association of inferior infarction and left posterior fascicular block is characterized by initial QRS vector deformities typical of inferior infarction and rightward displacement of the afferent limb and terminal deflections as seen in left posterior fascicular block.

The features most useful for the diagnosis of inferior infarction with left anterior fascicular block in the frontal plane are superior displacement

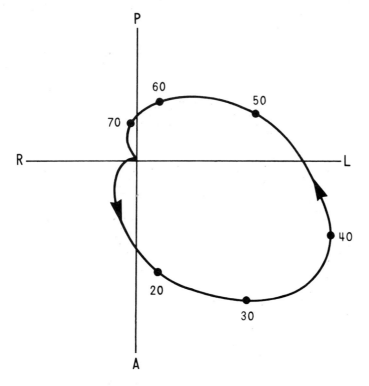

TRANSVERSE PLANE

Fig. 13-56 The vectorcardiogram in strictly posterior, posterobasal, or dorsal myocardial infarction. The numbers indicate the time in milliseconds after the beginning of the QRS loop. Described in text.

Fig. 13-57 Vectorcardiogram in inferolateral myocardial infarction. In the FP, the initial superior QRS forces exceed 25 ms. The QRS loop is rotated CW. In the TP, the initial rightward forces (which are greater than 0.16 mV) exceed 22 ms. The QRS loop is inscribed in CCW manner.

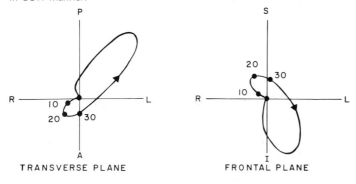

TRANSVERSE PLANE   FRONTAL PLANE

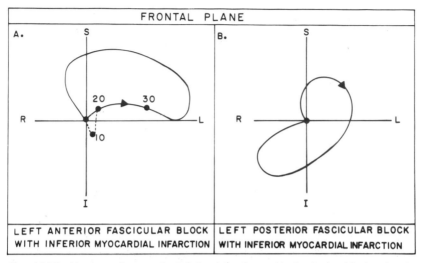

Fig. 13-58 Vectorcardiogram in inferior infarction with fascicular block. In *A*, with concomitant left anterior fascicular block, the initial 20- to 30-ms forces are displayed superiorly and rotated CW. The remainder of the loop is also displaced superiorly but is rotated CCW. Occasionally the very early QRS vectors (10 ms) may be directed inferiorly (dotted line), producing tiny R waves in the inferior leads, but the remainder of the loop is displaced superiorly. *B* shows the initial QRS vector deformities typical of inferior infarction and the rightward displacement of the afferent limb and terminal deflections which are characteristic of left posterior fascicular block.

with CW rotation of the initial QRS forces (20 to 30 ms) and CCW rotation of the remainder of the loop, which is also displaced superiorly. Occasionally the very early QRS vectors (10 ms) may be directed inferiorly but the remainder of the loop superiorly. When this occurs, rS deflections may be seen in the inferior limb leads.

Slowing of the terminal QRS deflection lasting 30 ms or more is common in myocardial infarction.

Myocardial Infarction with Right Bundle Branch Block

1 There are abnormalities of the initial QRS vectors indicative of myocardial infarction.
2 There are abnormalities of the terminal QRS vectors indicative of right bundle branch block.

Myocardial Infarction with Left Bundle Branch Block

Myocardial infarction coexisting with left bundle branch block may be suspected if in addition to the findings of left bundle branch block, certain atypical features, as outlined below, are noted.

Infarction of the Interventricular Septum   Complete loss of the initial anterior forces or rightward and anterior displacement of these forces in the TP suggests coexisting septal infarction.

Infarction of the Free Wall of the Left Ventricle   Rightward displacement of the afferent limb, usually with CCW inscription of the QRS loop in the TP, suggest concomitant infarction of the left ventricular free wall, as does uniform slow inscription of the entire loop or the presence of large bites in the loop.

Inferior Infarction   Superior displacement and irregular inscription of the frontal QRS loop suggest coexisting inferior infarction.

Vectorcardiographic Differential Diagnosis of Myocardial Infarction

Anteroseptal Myocardial Infarction versus Left Ventricular Hypertrophy

1   In the TP, the 0.02QRS vector is always anteriorly directed in left ventricular hypertrophy and posteriorly directed in anteroseptal infarction. The direction of the 20-ms vector thus permits differentiation between the two.
2   When the 20-ms vector is displaced posteriorly because of anterior infarction, coexisting left ventricular hypertrophy may be diagnosed if the 30-ms and maxQRS vectors also show abnormal posterior displacement and the magnitude of the maxQRS vector is increased.

Strictly Posterior Myocardial Infarction versus Right Ventricular Hypertrophy

1   Diagnostic problems arise because both conditions are characterized by anterior displacement of the QRS loop in the TP.   A CCW rotation of such an anteriorly directed loop favors the diagnosis of infarction, and CW rotation favors right ventricular hypertrophy.
2   In right ventricular hypertrophy, the maxQRS vector in the TP is usually directed to the right of the 50° axis (H° − 50°); in dorsal infarction, it is generally located to the left of this axis.
3   The T vector in the TP is usually directed anteriorly in posterior infarction and posteriorly and leftward in right ventricular hypertrophy.
4   The magnitude of the terminal rightward deflection exceeds 1.0 mV in right ventricular hypertrophy and is usually less in posterobasal infarction.
5   In the FP, right axis deviation is the usual finding in right ventricular hypertrophy.   In uncomplicated posterobasal infarction, the axis is either normal or deviated to the left.

Anterior Infarction with Left Anterior Fascicular Block versus Left Bundle Branch Block

1   In the TP, the initial QRS vectors are directed rightward and then posteriorly in anterior infarction with left anterior fascicular block; in left bundle branch block, they are directed anteriorly and leftward.
2   In anterior infarction with left anterior fascicular block, the terminal forces are always opposite to the initial forces. They are directed leftward, superiorly, and posteriorly. The terminal slowing lasts 30 ms or more. In left bundle branch block, the characteristic slowing occurs in the mid and terminal portions of the loop. The terminal vector is directed leftward and posteriorly.

REFERENCES

Benchimol, A.: "Vectorcardiography," Williams & Wilkins, Baltimore, 1973.
——— and K. B. Desser: Advances in Clinical Vectorcardiography, *Am. J. Cardiol.*, 36: 76, 1975.
——— and ———: The Electrovectorcardiographic Diagnosis of Posterior Wall Myocardial Infarction, *Cardiovasc. Clin.*, 5(3): 183, 1973.
———, J. E. Lasry, and F. R. Carvalho: The Ventricular Premature Contraction: Its Place in the Diagnosis of Ischemic Heart Disease, *Am. Heart J.*, 65: 334, 1963.
Bisteni, A., G. A. Medrano, and D. Sodi-Pallares: Ventricular Premature Beats in the Diagnosis of Myocardial Infarction, *Brit. Heart J.*, 23: 521, 1961.
Braat, S., P. Brugada, J. Conegracht, F. Bär, and H. Wellens: The Value of Right Precordial Leads in Detection of Right Ventricular Infarction, *Circulation*, (Supp. II) 64: 309, 1981.
Burns-Cox, C. J.: The Occurrence of a Normal Electrocardiogram after Myocardial Infarction, *Am. Heart J.*, 75: 572, 1968.
Castle, C. H., and W. M. Keane: Electrocardiographic "Peri-infarction Block": A Clinical and Pathologic Correlation, *Circulation*, 21: 403, 1965.
Chapman, M. G., and M. L. Pearce: Electrocardiographic Diagnosis of Myocardial Infarction in the Presence of Left Bundle Branch Block, *Circulation*, 16: 558, 1957.
Chou, T-C: Pseudo-infarction (Non-infarction Q Waves), *Cardiovasc. Clin.*, 5(3): 199, 1973.
———, R. A. Helm, and S. Kaplan: "Clinical Vectorcardiography," Grune & Stratton, New York, 1974.
———, J. Van Der Bel-Kahn, J. Allen, L. Brockmeier, and N. O. Fowler: Electrocardiographic Diagnosis of Right Ventricular Infarction, *Am. J. Med.*, 70: 1175, 1981.
Cook, R. W., J. E. Edwards, and R. D. Pruitt: Electrocardiographic Changes in Acute Subendocardial Infarction, *Circulation*, 98: 603, 613, 1958.
Croft, C. H., P. Nicod, J. R. Corbett, S. E. Lewis, R. Huxley, J. Mukharji, J. T. Wilkerson, and R. E. Rude: Detection of Acute Right Ventricular Infarction by Right Precordial Electrocardiography, *Am. J. Cardiol.*, 50: 421, 1982.
———, W. Woodward, P. Nicod, J. R. Corbett, S. E. Lewis, J. T. Wilkerson, and

R. E. Rude: Clinical Implications of Anterior S-T Segment Depression in Patients with Acute Inferior Myocardial Infarction, *Am. J. Cardiol.*, 50: 428, 1982.

Doucet, P., J. Walsh, and E. Massie: A Vectorcardiographic Study of Right Bundle Branch Block with the Frank System: Clinical Correlation with Myocardial Infarction, *Am J. Cardiol.*, 16: 342, 1965.

——, ——, and ——: A Vectorcardiographic and Electrocardiographic Study of Left Bundle Branch Block with Myocardial Infarction, *Am. J. Cardiol.*, 17: 171, 1966.

Durrer, D., A. A. W. Van Lier, and J. Büller: Epicardial and Intramural Excitation in Chronic Myocardial Infarction, *Am. Heart J.*, 68: 765, 1964.

Goldberger, A. L.: "Myocardial Infarction—Electrocardiographic Differential Diagnosis," C. V. Mosby Company, St. Louis, 1979.

Grant, R. P.: "Clinical Electrocardiography," McGraw-Hill, New York, 1957.

——: Peri-infarction Block, *Prog. Cardiovasc. Dis.*, 2: 237, 1959.

—— and R. H. Murray: QRS Complex Deformity of Myocardial Infarction in the Human Subject, *Am. J. Med.*, 17: 587, 1954.

Gunnar, R. M., R. J. Pietras, J. Blackaller, S. E. Dadmun, P. B. Szanto, and J. R. Tobin, Jr.: Correlation of Vectorcardiographic Criteria for Myocardial Infarction with Autopsy Findings, *Circulation*, 35: 158, 1967.

Hattori, V., D. S. Berman, J. Maddahi, and M. Pichler: Acute Inferior Myocardial Infarction: Precordial ST-Segment Depression, *Primary Cardiology*, 9: 173, 1983.

Hoffman, I., R. C. Taymor, and A. Gootnick: Vectorcardiographic Residua of Inferior Infarction, *Circulation*, 29: 562, 1964.

——, ——, M. H. Morris, and I. Kittell: Quantitative Criteria for the Diagnosis of Dorsal Infarction Using the Frank Vectorcardiogram, *Am. Heart J.*, 70: 295, 1965.

Hugenholtz, P. G., C. E. Forkner, Jr., and H. D. Levine: A Clinical Appraisal of the Vectorcardiogram in Myocardial Infarction: II. The Frank System, *Circulation*, 24: 825, 1961.

Libanoff, A. J. G. M. Boiteau, and B. J. Allenstein: Diaphragmatic Myocardial Infarction with Peri-infarction Block, *Am. J. Cardiol.*, 12: 772, 1963.

Likoff, W., B. Segal, and L. Dreifus: Myocardial Infarction Patterns in Young Subjects with Normal Coronary Arteriograms, *Circulation*, 26: 373, 1962.

McConahay, D. R., B. D. McCallister, F. J. Hallermann et al.: Comparative Quantitative Analysis of the Electrocardiogram and the Vectorcardiogram, *Circulation*, 42: 245, 1970.

Marriott, H. J. L.: "Workshop in Electrocardiography," Tampa Tracings, Oldsmar, Fla., 1972.

—— and P. Hogan: Hemiblock in Myocardial Infarction, *Chest*, 58: 342, 1970.

—— and R. Slonim: False Patterns of Myocardial Infarction, *Heart Bull.*, 16: 71, 1967.

Martinez, A.: Aberrant Ventricular Conduction in the Diagnosis of Myocardial Infarction, *Am. J. Cardiol.*, 14: 352, 1964.

Massie, E., and T. J. Walsh: "Clinical Vectorcardiography and Electrocardiography," Year Book, Chicago, 1960.

Mathur, V. S., and H. D. Levine: Vectorcardiographic Differentiation between Right Ventricular Hypertrophy and Posterobasal Myocardial Infarction, *Am. J. Cardiol.*, 17: 131, 1966.

Mills, R. M., E. Young, R. Gorlin, and M. Lesch: Natural History of S-T Segment Elevation After Acute Myocardial Infarction, *Am. J. Cardiol.*, 35: 609, 1975.

Myers, G. B.: QRS-T Patterns in Multiple Precordial Leads That May Be Mistaken for Myocardial Infarction, *Circulation*, 1: 844, 860, 1950.

———, H. A. Klein, and T. Hiratzka: Correlation of Electrocardiographic and Pathologic Findings in Large Anterolateral Infarcts, *Am. Heart J.*, 37: 205, 1949.

———, ———, and ———: Correlation of Electrocardiographic and Pathologic Findings in Posterolateral Infarction, *Am. Heart J.*, 38: 837, 1949.

———, ———, and B. E. Stofer: Correlation of Electrocardiographic and Pathologic Findings in Anteroseptal Infarction, *Am. Heart J.*, 36: 535, 1948.

Perloff, J. K.: The Recognition of Strictly Posterior Myocardial Infarction by Conventional Scalar Electrocardiography, *Circulation*, 30: 706, 1964.

Pruitt, R. D., D. W. Curd, Jr., and R. Leachman: Simulation of Electrocardiograms of Apicolateral Myocardial Infarction by Myocardial Destructive Lesions of Obscure Etiology (Myocardiopathy), *Circulation*, 25: 506, 1962.

Pryor, R: Recognition of Myocardial Infarction in the Presence of Bundle Branch Block, *Cardiovasc. Clin.*, 6(1): 255, 1974.

Rosenbaum, M. B., M. V. Elizari, and J. O. Lassari: "The Hemiblocks," Tampa Tracings, Oldsmar, Fla., 1970.

Rubin, I. L., H. Gross, and E. M. Vigliano: Transitory Abnormal Q Waves during Coronary Insufficiency, *Am. Heart J.*, 71: 254, 1966.

Scott, R. C.: Left Bundle Branch Block: A Clinical Assessment, *Am. Heart J.* 70: 535, 691, and 813, 1965.

Shah, P. K., and D. S. Berman: Implications of Precordial S-T Segment Depression in Acute Inferior Infarction, *Am. J. Cardiol.*, 48: 1167, 1981.

Shettigar, V. R., H. N. Hultgren, J. F. Pfeifer, and M. J. Lipton: Diagnostic Value of Q-Waves in Inferior Myocardial Infarction, *Am. Heart J.*, 88: 170, 1974.

Starr, J. W., G. S. Wagner, V. S. Behar, A. Watson II, and J. C. Greenfield: Vectorcardiographic Criteria for the Diagnosis of Inferior Infarction, *Circulation*, 49: 829, 1974.

Surawicz, B., R. G. Van Horne, J. R. Urbach, and S. Bellet: QS- and QR-Pattern in Leads V_3 and V_4 in Absence of Myocardial Infarction: Electrocardiographic and Vectorcardiographic Study, *Circulation*, 12: 391, 1955.

Tavel, M. E., and C. Fish: Abnormal Q Waves Simulating Myocardial Infarction in Diffuse Myocardial Diseases, *Am. Heart J.*, 68: 534, 1964.

Verhave, J. H.: Electrocardiograms Simulating Myocardial Infarction, *Rocky Mt. Med.*, 61: 40, 1964.

Warner, R. A., N. E. Hill, S. Mookherjee, and H. Smulyan: Improved Electrocardiographic Criteria for the Diagnosis of Left Anterior Hemiblock, *Am. J. Cardiol.*, 51: 723, 1983.

Wasserburger, R. H., D. H. White, and E. R. Lindsay: Noninfarctional $QS_{II, III, AVF}$ Complexes as Seen in the Wolff-Parkinson-White Syndrome and Left Bundle Branch Block, *Am. Heart J.*, 64: 617, 1962.

Wilson, F. N., F. F. Rosenbaum, F. D. Johnston, and P. S. Barker: The Electrocardiographic Diagnosis of Myocardial Infarction Complicated by Left Bundle Branch Block, *Arch. Inst. Cardiol.*, Mex., 14: 201, 1945.

Young, E., H. D. Levine, P. S. Vokonas et al.: The Frontal Plane Vectorcardiogram in Old Inferior Myocardial Infarction, *Circulation*, 42: 1143, 1970.

CHAPTER 14

TRANSIENT MYOCARDIAL ISCHEMIA AND INJURY; EXERCISE ELECTROCARDIOGRAPHY

ANGINA PECTORIS (FIGS. 14-1, 14-2)

The electrocardiographic patterns of spontaneous or induced attacks of angina pectoris are produced by transient subendocardial ischemia and injury or by subepicardial or transmural ischemia. One or more of the following findings may be noted during these attacks:

1 Depressed S-T segments that are characteristically horizontal or downward sagging, followed by terminally upright T waves, in some or all of the precordial leads and/or in leads I and aVL and/or in leads II, III, and aVF.
2 Inverted T waves in some or all of the precordial leads and/or in leads I and aVL and/or in leads II, III, and aVF.
3 Arrhythmias, including conduction defects and ventricular premature systoles.
4 In rare instances, the electrocardiographic patterns are produced by transient subepicardial injury. This is called the *variant pattern of angina pectoris* (Prinzmetal's angina). It is manifested by S-T segment elevations with terminally inverted T waves in one or more leads overlying the injured region.

The duration of the electrocardiographic changes is brief, usually lasting only a matter of minutes.

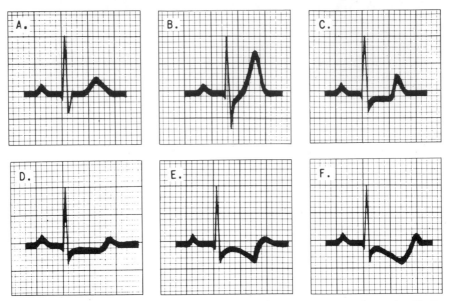

Fig. 14-1   Schematic representation of the types of ischemic S-T segment depression (C, D, E, F) encountered in angina pectoris, coronary insufficiency, subendocardial infarction, and positive Master tests.   Record A is a normal control electrocardiogram.   Record B illustrates the type of junctional S-T segment depression often found in normal persons after a Master test.

The resting electrocardiogram in patients with angina pectoris is frequently normal, but may show specific or nonspecific abnormalities or present evidence of previous myocardial infarction.

ACUTE AND SUBACUTE CORONARY INSUFFICIENCY— INTERMEDIATE CORONARY SYNDROME, PREINFARCTION ANGINA, UNSTABLE ANGINA, ETC. (FIGS. 14-3, 14-4)

This is a clinical syndrome intermediate between angina pectoris and myocardial infarction, characterized electrocardiographically by evidence

Fig. 14-2   Variant pattern of angina pectoris.   Monitor lead.   (A) Recorded during an attack of angina.   There is S-T segment elevation.   (B) Recorded after anginal pain had subsided.

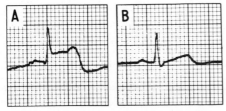

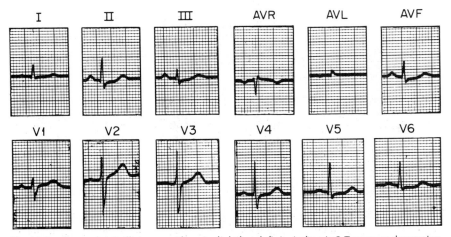

Fig. 14-3 Coronary insufficiency. There is slight but definite ischemic S-T segment depression in leads II, III, aVF, V₅, and V₆. The S-T segment changes in this patient disappeared after a few days and were not accompanied by either clinical or laboratory evidence of myocardial infarction. Similar S-T segment abnormalities may occur in angina pectoris and subendocardial infarction. The S-T segment depression in all these conditions may be more pronounced than those illustrated.

of subendocardial ischemia and injury or by subepicardial or transmural ischemia. The findings are thus similar to those encountered in subendocardial infarction and angina pectoris, but in contradistinction to the latter condition in which the electrocardiographic abnormalities last only minutes, in coronary insufficiency they are apt to persist for longer intervals, often for hours, days, or even weeks.

EXERCISE ELECTROCARDIOGRAPHY

Exercise testing with continuous electrocardiographic monitoring both during and after exercise is a useful procedure in the diagnosis of both overt and latent coronary artery disease and in the evaluation of cardiovascular performance. Exercise testing may be performed by walking a treadmill, pumping a stationary bicycle, or climbing stairs. A physician should always be present and supervise the performance of an exercise test.

The procedure favored by many experts is a multistage treadmill test that encompasses submaximal and maximal exercise. The national experience in a survey of 170,000 exercise tests (Rochmis and Blackburn) reveals morbidity and mortality rates of 2.4 and 1.0 per 10,000 tests, respectively. Treadmill and bicycle ergometer studies are not readily available in many communities and are not inexpensive. The Master two-step test is a possible substitute under these conditions. It is easily performed

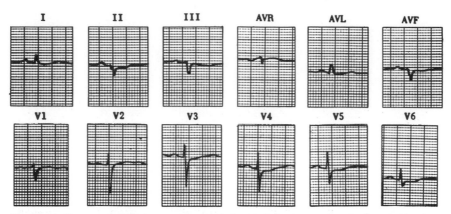

Fig. 14-4 Coronary insufficiency. There is ischemic S-T segment depression in leads II, III, aVF, and V_3 to V_7. The electrocardiographic changes appeared after an episode of retrosternal pain of about 30-min duration and disappeared after 5 days. There was no clinical or laboratory evidence of myocardial infarction. The patient had sustained an inferior myocardial infarct several months previously and was asymptomatic until the pain recurred.

in the physician's office and is fairly reliable provided that a rapid heart rate can be obtained (110 to 120 or more beats per minute).

Indications and contraindications for exercise tests are considered later in this chapter.

THE MASTER TWO-STEP TEST (FIGS. 14-1, 14-5, 14-6)

Procedure

The test is generally performed according to the method and technique described by Master. The two-step apparatus consists of two steps 9 in. high, about 10 in. deep, and 20 to 24 in. wide. With the patient under essentially basal conditions, a control electrocardiogram is taken. The patient then makes a number of trips over the steps. During exercise the extremity electrodes are left in place, with the lead wires attached. The number of trips to be performed is shown in Table 13 in the Appendix, according to the patient's age, sex, and weight. The single test (one-half the charted trips) is performed in $1\frac{1}{2}$ min; the double test, in 3 min. One ascent and one descent are counted as one trip. The patient should always turn toward the examiner at the end of each trip to avoid dizziness. The test should be discontinued promptly if the patient complains of chest pain or other discomfort during the procedure.

When the exercise is completed, the patient lies down and electrocardiograms are taken immediately and at 2-min intervals thereafter for 6 min and until the electrocardiogram has returned to the resting condition. Leads II, aVF, V_4, V_5, and V_6 are most useful in evaluating the response to exercise.   The single most informative lead is V_5.   The most important postexercise tracing is the one recorded *immediately* after exercise.

Standards for Interpretation

There are no criteria for an abnormal response to exercise that are accepted by all authorities.   The consensus is that ischemic S-T segment depression following exercise is the single most reliable criterion.   In evaluating S-T segment depression, ischemic depression must be differentiated from depression limited to the junction between the QRS complex and the S-T segment, because junctional, or J, depression is a frequent finding in normal individuals both during and after exercise.   The adjunctive use of the Q-X/Q-T ratio, as described below, has been suggested by Lepeschkin as being of diagnostic aid in the evaluation of S-T depression and has been adopted also by Master.

The P-R segment is the reference level for determining junctional or S-T segment depression.

The Q-T ratio is obtained by dividing the actually measured Q-T interval by the corrected Q-T interval (Q-Tc).   Q-Tc is determined by the formula Q-Tc $= 0.4\sqrt{R\text{-}R}$, in which R-R is the R-R interval measured in seconds. The Q-T ratio can be determined more easily by using the Q-T calculator devised by William Welsh and manufactured by Bowen and Company, Bethesda, Md.   A Q-T ratio of 1.08 or greater after exercise is considered abnormal; a Q-T ratio of 1.07 or less is within normal limits.

Fig. 14-5   Methods of measuring S-T segment depression.   Point O is the point of intersection of a tangent to the terminal portion of the P-R segment with a vertical line passing through the S-T segment junction J.   True depression of the junction corresponds to the distance O-J.   Point X is the point of intersection of the S-T segment with a line connecting the points of origin, Q, of two consecutive QRS complexes.   The horizontal distance Q-X is expressed as a percentage of the Q-T interval.   (*From E. Lepeschkin, Exercise Tests in the Diagnosis of Coronary Heart Disease, Circulation,* 22: 986, 1960. *Used by permission of the American Heart Association, Inc.*)

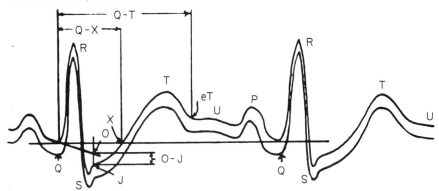

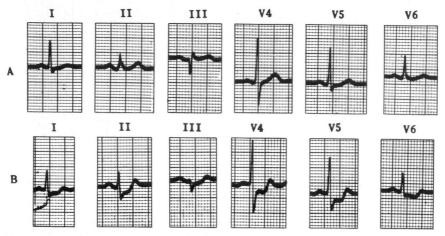

Fig. 14-6 Positive Master test. Record *A* shows a normal control electrocardiogram. Record *B*, taken immediately after exercise while the patient was experiencing anginal pain, shows ischemic S-T segment depression in all the leads.

The Q-X/Q-T ratio, expressed as a percentage, is determined by measuring the interval from the beginning of the QRS to the point where the end of the S-T segment returns to the isoelectric level, Q-X, dividing this by the measured Q-T interval, and multiplying by 100. Normally this ratio is less than 50 percent.

The reliability of the Q-X/Q-T ratio is open to question.

Criteria for a Positive Test

The single most reliable criterion is horizontal or downward-sagging S-T segment depression 1.0 mm or more in depth, with a duration of at least 0.08 s. This is called *ischemic depression*. The greater the degree of depression, the more significant is the finding. Q-X/Q-T ratios exceeding 50 percent and Q-T ratios that are 1.08 or more are further evidence of the abnormality of this type of S-T segment depression.

According to some authorities, junctional (J) S-T depression that is 2 mm or more (in relation to the P-R segment) is also abnormal, as is junctional depression less than 2 mm, provided the Q-X/Q-T ratio exceeds 50 percent and the Q-T ratio is equal to or greater than 1.08. Stuart and Ellestad have presented evidence that S-T depression which slopes upward but is at least 1.0 mm below the reference level at a point 0.08 s after J is indicative of a positive response. Upsloping S-T depression should not be confused with isolated J-point depression, which is commonly regarded as a non-ischemic or innocent electrocardiographic manifestation. Kattus believes that J-point depression may be a manifestation of myocardial ischemia, but it cannot be interpreted with reliability unless confirmatory evidence is obtained: the presence of typical anginal pain, regression of the J depression by sublingual nitroglycerin while exercise is continued, the eventual emergence of a typical ischemic pattern either during or after exercise, or the demonstration of significant arterial obstruction.

Sometimes the ischemic response emerges only in the recovery period after exercise. Hence recordings should be continued for at least 6 min after exercise is completed. This should also be done to ensure that no serious arrhythmia has occurred.

An ischemic response is sometimes manifested by elevation of the S-T segment rather than by its depression. Reversal of the T wave polarity, changes in the QRS-T angle, and inversion of the T wave may be evidence of a positive test but cannot be regarded as reliable indicators of myocardial ischemia.

A wide variety of supraventricular arrhythmias may be noted in the process of stress testing. These include wandering atrial pacemaker, sinus arrhythmia, short runs of paroxysmal atrial or junctional tachycardia, and rarely, atrial fibrillation and flutter, SA block, and sinus arrest.

Conduction defects such as AV or bundle branch block may occur during the course of exercise testing and are generally regarded as evidence of a positive test.

Ventricular arrhythmias are a frequent occurrence, especially in the postexercise period. Debate continues on the significance of exercise-induced ventricular extrasystoles as indicators of the presence of organic heart disease. Although ventricular arrhythmias may be provoked by exercise in normal subjects, it is apparent from most studies that they occur more frequently in the presence of organic heart disease. Ventricular ectopic beats which occur with minor increases in heart rate or which demonstrate high frequency, a multifocal pattern, or repetitive firing are particularly suggestive of cardiac disease.

The ischemic electrocardiographic response may be obscured by bundle branch block and healed myocardial infarction. Digitalis administration is associated with a high incidence of false-positive tests. Its use should probably be discontinued for at least 2 to 3 weeks before an exercise test is performed. False-positive ischemic responses may be found also in patients taking potassium-depleting drugs and in patients with hyperadrenergic states, pes excavatum, or short P-R intervals. Exercise testing may also be misleading in women under the age of 40 years. In this group the incidence of coronary artery disease is remarkably low, but false-positive S-T segment depression is not uncommon.

Comments

Positive exercise tests are considered indicative of coronary artery disease, although it is recognized that false-positive tests occur in normal subjects and in patients with rheumatic or other types of heart disease, including the congenital varieties. A negative test does not exclude the diagnosis of coronary artery disease.

Many authorities have questioned the validity of the testing procedure devised by Master. They feel that standardization of exercise should be based upon a challenge to the coronary circulation and not upon a challenge to the skeletal muscle, as in the Master two-step test. In the Master two-step test, the levels of exercise are prescribed on the basis of age, sex, and weight of the individual. Since the heart rate during exercise is a more valid index of cardiac stress, these authorities favor a graded exercise test which produces a heart rate of approximately 85 percent of the mean predicted maximal heart rate for the subject's age. The test may be stair climbing, treadmill walking, or cycling.

A study by Schweitzer et al. comparing the two-step and maximal exercise test in coronary artery disease has revealed the following: (1) In the majority of cases of chest pain, the sensitivity and specificity of the two-step and maximal exercise tests for coronary artery disease are similar. (2) Patients with an inadequate increase in the heart rate after the two-step test should continue the test until higher heart rates are achieved (110 to 120 beats per minute) or perform a maximal exercise test. (3) The electrocardiogram should be recorded with the patient in the supine position after exercise if a maximal exercise test is used, since an ischemic response may not appear until the recovery period. It was found that some patients with a positive maximal exercise test had a negative two-step test. The combination of a positive two-step test and a negative maximal exercise test occurred less frequently but could be obviated by lead selection and supine recordings in the postexercise period. From the analysis of the results, it was noted that neither the two-step test nor the maximal exercise test is of great help in the diagnosis of coronary artery disease in patients with single-vessel disease. Both tests, however, are more sensitive in multivessel disease.

It is worth noting that interpretation of exercise tests in the presence of an abnormal control electrocardiogram is much more difficult than when it is normal.

Recording both the exercise and the postexercise electrocardiograms yields a higher percentage of positive responses than either procedure alone.

Exercise tests are valuable for epidemiologic studies and as screening procedures. Asymptomatic "healthy" individuals with positive tests have a statistically higher mortality rate than those with negative tests.

Graded exercise tests have proved to be of great value not only in diagnosis but in assessing functional capacity following recovery from myocardial infarction and as a guide to work classification.

GRADED EXERCISE TESTS

Most authorities believe that graded exercise tests (e.g., multistage treadmill tests) give a higher percentage of true-positive diagnoses than the Master test.

The methodology, protocols, and procedures for the performance of graded exercise tests are beyond the scope of this text. This information is readily available from other sources.

Indications

The exercise electrocardiographic test is primarily indicated for the confirmation of coronary artery disease and in the differential diagnosis of chest pain of uncertain origin. It may be useful in detecting latent ischemic heart disease, in determining the effect of exercise on cardiac arrhythmias, and in discovering a possible cause for symptoms which may be related to exercise (e.g., syncope, palpitation, etc.). It is useful in the evaluation of functional capacity in patients with coronary artery disease and in the evaluation of the efficacy of medical and surgical treatment of this disease. It may be valuable in the assessment of rehabilitation programs for the evaluation of cardiac drugs, and as a screening procedure.

Contraindications

Absolute contraindications to exercise electrocardiography include acute myocardial infarction, preinfarction or unstable angina, acute myocarditis or pericarditis, serious cardiac arrhythmias (e.g., atrial fibrillation), second- or third-degree AV block, congestive heart failure, severe pulmonary hypertension, and significant anemia. Acute illnesses such as infectious serious noncardiac diseases, drug intoxication, and electrolyte abnormalities are also contraindications.

Relative contraindications include aortic stenosis, left main coronary artery disease, severe hypertension, asymmetric septal hypertrophy, S-T segment depression in the resting electrocardiogram, and limiting neurological or musculoskeletal impairments.

Limitations

The exercise test is of little or no diagnostic value in patients receiving digitalis or some other drugs, and with hypopotassemia. The test also has limited or no diagnostic significance in patients with previous myocardial infarction, mitral valve prolapse, the W-P-W syndrome, congenital heart disease, cardiomyopathy, and left bundle branch block. Its diagnostic significance in severe left ventricular hypertrophy is uncertain.

Electrocardiographic Criteria for a Positive Test

1   The single most reliable criterion is horizontal or downward sloping S-T segment depression of 1.0 mm or more with a duration of 0.08 s or more. The P-R segment is the reference level for determining S-T segment displacement.

2   Upsloping S-T segment depression of 2.0 mm or more that is greater than 0.08 s in duration from the J point is similarly considered a positive response.

3   Horizontal or upsloping S-T segment elevations equal to or greater than 1.0 mm are also abnormal.

4   Other findings that are strongly suggestive of a positive test include:

a   Inverted U waves

b   Multifocal ventricular premature systoles, frequent or groups of ventricular extrasystoles, and ventricular tachycardia

c   Increased R wave amplitude (of disputed significance)

d   An abnormal Q-X/Q-T ratio, as indicated earlier in this chapter

Other Abnormal Responses to Exercise Tests of Clinical Significance

1   Hemodynamic changes, such as:

a   Slowing of the heart rate or failure to achieve the targeted heart rate not attributable to drugs

b   The occurrence of progressive hypotension during exercise

c   The development of excessive hypertension during exercise

2   Clinical findings, such as:

a   The occurrence of typical angina, dyspnea, pallor, cyanosis, and claudication

b   The appearance of S_3 or S_4 heart sounds, the development of heart murmurs, and the occurrence of pulsus alternans

Findings of Little or no Diagnostic Significance

1   Minor cardiac arrhythmias, occasional premature beats, supraventricular arrhythmias, first- or second-degree AV block, type I.

2   The development of bundle branch block.

3   Alternations in the morphology of the P and T waves.

4   Junctional S-T segment depression less than 2.0 mm with a duration less than 0.08 s.

Indications for Termination of the Test

1   Progressive fall in blood pressure or heart rate during continued exercise.

2   The development of extreme elevations in systolic and diastolic blood pressure during the performance of the test.

3   Progressively severe anginal pain.

4   Increased frequency of ventricular premature systoles or their occurrence in pairs or groups during continued exercise.

5   The occurrence of ventricular tachycardia, atrial tachycardia, atrial fibrillation, or flutter.

6 The development of severe S-T segment depression.
7 Increasing dyspnea, fatigue, faintness, and pallor.
8 The test should always be terminated at the request of the patient regardless of the circumstances surrounding the request.

Causes of False-Positive Exercise Tests

1 Drugs such as digitalis, diuretics, and antidepressants.
2 Certain types of heart disease: the W-P-W syndrome, mitral valve prolapse, nonischemic cardiac disease.
3 Electrolyte abnormality, notably hypopotassemia.
4 Preexisting left bundle branch block, nonspecific ST-T abnormalities, and ventricular hypertrophy.
5 Miscellaneous conditions: hyperventilation, vasomotor lability, anemia, and hypoxemia.
6 A false-positive test is not uncommonly seen in some healthy women.

Causes of False-Negative Exercise Tests

1 Drugs such as nitroglycerin, some antianginal agents, propranolol, procainamide, quinidine, and tricyclic antidepressants.
2 Preexisting coronary artery disease.
3 Inadequate testing.

Clinical Significance

Maximal exercise testing has a sensitivity of about 70 percent and a specificity approaching 90 percent in the detection of latent or overt coronary artery disease.

An abnormal response to exercise when screening asymptomatic individuals, notably men, identifies those at high risk for developing coronary artery disease. Potential candidates for routine screening include pilots, firemen, policemen, truckdrivers, railroad engineers, etc. Persons undertaking vigorous exercise programs should probably be screened, particularly if middle-aged or older. Those with hypertension, a strong familial history of coronary artery disease, and hyperlipidemia are also potential candidates for exercise testing.

Stress scintigraphy with thallium-201 appears to be more sensitive and more specific for the diagnosis of ischemic heart disease than stress electrocardiography alone.

REFERENCES

Bellet, S., O. F. Muller, D. LaVan, G. J. Nichols, and A. B. Herring: Radioelectrocardiography during Exercise in Patients with the Anginal Syndrome: Use of Multiple Leads, *Circulation*, 29: 366, 1964.

Blackburn, H., and R. Katigbak: The Exercise ECG Test: At What Intervals to Record after Exercise, *Am. Heart J.*, 67: 186, 1964.

———— and ————: What Electrocardiographic Leads to Take after Exercise, *Am. Heart J.*, 67: 184, 1964.

Chung, E. K. (ed.): "Exercise Electrocardiography: Practical Approach," Williams & Wilkins Company, Baltimore, 1979.

————, B. M. Cooke, Jr., and P. S. Greenberg: Stress Testing: Clinical Application and Predictive Capacity, *Progr. Cardiovasc. Dis.*, 21: 431, 1979.

De Maria, A. N., et al.: Disturbances of Cardiac Rhythm and Conduction Induced by Exercise: Diagnostic, Prognostic and Therapeutic Implications, *Am. J. Cardiol.*, 33: 732, 1974.

Ellestad, M. H.: "Stress Testing: Principles and Practice," 2d ed., F. A. Davis Company, Philadelphia, 1980.

Fentz, V., and J. Gormsen: Electrocardiographic Patterns in Cerebrovascular Accidents, *Circulation*, 25: 22, 1962.

Friedberg, C. K., H. L. Jaffe, L. Pordy, and K. Chester: The Two-step Exercise Electrocardiogram: A Double-blind Evaluation of Its Use in the Diagnosis of Angina Pectoris, *Circulation*, 26: 1254, 1962.

Gazes, P. C., M. R. Culler, and J. K. Stokes: The Diagnosis of Angina Pectoris, *Am. Heart J.* 67: 830, 1964.

Hellerstein, H. K., G. B. Prozaw, I. M. Liebow, A. E. Doan, and J. A. Henderson: Two-step Exercise Test as a Test of Cardiac Function in Chronic Rheumatic Heart Disease and in Arteriosclerotic Heart Disease with Old Myocardial Infarction, *Am. J. Cardiol.*, 7: 234, 1961.

Kattus, A. A.: Exercise Electrocardiography: Recognition of the Ischemic Response, False Positive and Negative Patterns, *Am. J. Cardiol.*, 33: 721, 1974.

Kawai, C., and H. N. Hultgren: The Effect of Digitalis upon the Exercise Electrocardiogram, *Am. Heart J.*, 68: 409, 1964.

Lepeschkin, E.: Exercise Tests in the Diagnosis of Coronary Heart Disease, *Circulation*, 22: 986, 1960.

———— and B. Surawicz: Characteristics of True-positive and False-positive Results of ECG Master Two-step Exercise Tests, *New Engl. J. Med.*, 258: 511, 1958.

Master, A. M.: The Master Two-step Test, *Am. Heart J.*, 75: 809, 1968.

Mattingly, T. W.: The Postexercise Electrocardiogram: Its Value in the Diagnosis and Prognosis of Coronary Arterial Disease, *Am. J. Cardiol.*, 9: 395, 1962.

Prinzmetal, M., R. Kennamer, R. Merliss, T. Wada, and N. Bor: Angina Pectoris: I. A. Variant Form of Angina Pectoris, *Am. J. Med.*, 27: 375, 1959.

Robb, G. P., and H. H. Marks: Postexercise Electrocardiogram in Arteriosclerotic Heart Disease, *J.A.M.A.*, 200: 110, 1967.

Rochmis, P., and H. Blackburn: Exercise Tests: A Survey of Procedures, Safety, and Litigation Experience in Approximately 170,000 Tests, *J.A.M.A.*, 217: 1061, 1971.

Roman, L., and S. Bellet: Significance of the QX/QT Ratio and QT Ratio (QTr) in the Exercise Electrocardiogram, *Circulation*, 32: 435, 1965.

Scherf, D.: The Electrocardiographic Exercise Test, *J. Electrocardiol.*, 1: 141, 1968.

Schweitzer, P., V. M. Jelinek, M. V. Herman, and R. Gorlin: Comparison of the Two-step Test and Maximal Exercise Tests in Patients with Coronary Artery Disease, *Am. J. Cardiol.*, 33: 797, 1974.

Sheffield, L. T., J. H. Holt, and I. J. Reeves: Exercise Graded by Heart Rates in Electrocardiographic Testing for Angina Pectoris, *Circulation*, 32: 622, 1965.

Simonson,E.: Use of the Electrocardiogram in Exercise Tests, *Am. Heart J.*, 66: 552, 1963.

Stuart, R. J., Jr., and M. H. Ellestad: Upsloping S-T Segments in Exercise Stress Testing, *Am. J. Cardiol.*, 37: 19, 1976.

Vakil, R. J.: Intermediate Coronary Syndrome, *Circulation*, 24: 557, 1961.

CHAPTER 15

PERICARDITIS

ACUTE PERICARDITIS (FIG. 15-1)

Typical electrocardiographic changes are found in about 80 percent of patients with acute pericarditis. In the remainder, the electrocardiogram is normal or shows only nonspecific abnormalities.

The electrocardiographic diagnosis of acute pericarditis is based primarily on sequential changes in the S-T segments and T waves. In acute pericarditis, the S-T vector is typically increased in a direction more or less parallel to the mean QRS vector. Thus the S-T segment is elevated in leads with upright QRS complexes and depressed, if at all, in leads with negative QRS complexes such as aVR, V_1, and sometimes V_1, V_2, and aVL. The reciprocal S-T segment changes seen in myocardial infarction do not occur. The T vector tends to parallel the S-T vector, but when the S-T segment becomes isoelectric, the T vector shifts to an opposite direction. (See Fig. 8-3.) Surawicz and Lasseter have attributed the S-T segment deviations to a current of injury resulting from pressure by fluid or fibrin on the myocardium, and the T wave changes to a superficial myocarditis.

S-T Segment and T Wave Abnormalities

The characteristic changes can be divided into four stages.

First Stage This phase usually begins within 10 days of the onset of acute pericarditis and lasts from 2 days to 2 weeks. The earliest change is elevation of the S-T junction and of the S-T segment in leads facing the epicardial surfaces of the heart.   These include leads I, II, III, aVF, and V_3 to V_6.   In cavity leads such as aVR (and sometimes V_1, V_2, and/or aVL), there is S-T segment depression.   There is a lack of the reciprocal changes which generally occur in myocardial infarction.   The T wave may decrease in amplitude, but its direction remains concordant with that of the S-T segment.   The S-T segments are characteristically concave upward but may be either straight or obliquely elevated.   The Q-Tc is generally normal.

Second Stage   During this phase, which lasts from a few days to several weeks, the S-T segments and T waves begin to return to the baseline. According to some authorities, the Q-Tc increases during this stage.   Others, however, maintain that the Q-Tc remains normal.   Sometimes a small notch is seen in the T wave summit in one or more leads.   Some electrocardiographers consider this finding almost characteristic of pericarditis.   By the time the S-T segments become isoelectric, the T waves may begin to flatten, show terminal negativity, or remain isoelectric with the S-T segment so that there is a continuous, flat S-T-T interval.

Third Stage   During this phase, which usually begins at the end of the second or third week and lasts from a week or two to several months, the T waves become clearly inverted in epicardial leads, with corresponding elevation in cavity leads.

Fourth Stage   During this phase there is gradual resolution of the T wave changes.   This stage may last as long as 3 months.   The T waves become less inverted, approach the isoelectric line, and eventually become normal.

QRS Complexes

The QRS complex may show no alteration.   When pericarditis is accompanied by effusion, there is characteristically decreased voltage of the QRS complexes due to the short-circuiting effect of the effusion.   Occasionally, the QRS complexes may decrease in amplitude in the absence of effusion. There may be persistence of the S waves when the S-T segment is elevated. This is in contrast to their disappearance when the S-T segments are elevated because of myocardial infarction.

P Waves

The P waves are generally unaltered but may decrease in amplitude with effusion.   If the atrial myocardium is injured by the inflammatory process, signs of atrial injury may occur. (See page 134.)

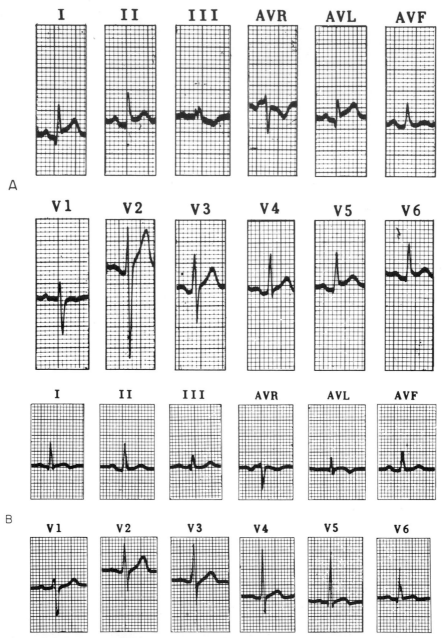

Fig. 15-1 Acute pericarditis. (*A*) One day after the onset. The S-T segments are elevated in leads I, II, aVL, and aVF and in the precordial leads but are depressed in leads aVR and III. (*B*) Twelve days after the onset. The S-T segments are now almost isoelectric, but the contours are still abnormal in many of the leads. There is T wave inversion in leads I, aVL, V$_5$, and V$_6$. In both (*A*) and (*B*), the P-R segments are elevated in lead aVR and depressed in leads II, aVF, and V$_2$ to V$_6$.

P-R Segment Changes

Shifts of the P-R segment are almost as characteristic of acute pericarditis as the classic S-T segment changes.   The P-R segment deviations probably represent subepicardial atrial injury.   They occur in the first and second stages of acute pericarditis, or both.   The P-R segment vector, which is opposite to the mean P vector, is directed rightward, superiorly, and posteriorly.   This results in elevated P-R segments in lead aVR, and negative

Fig. 15-1 (*Continued*)   (*C*) Seven weeks after the onset.   The T waves are now more inverted in leads I, aVL, and V₄ to V₆.   (*D*) Twelve weeks after the onset.   There is still slight T wave inversion in leads I and aVL, and the contour of the S-T segments in lead I and the left precordial leads is not quite normal.   In (*C*) and (*D*), P-R segment changes are no longer present.   Resolution of all the S-T segment and T wave abnormalities in acute pericarditis may take several months even though all clinical evidence of the disease has disappeared.

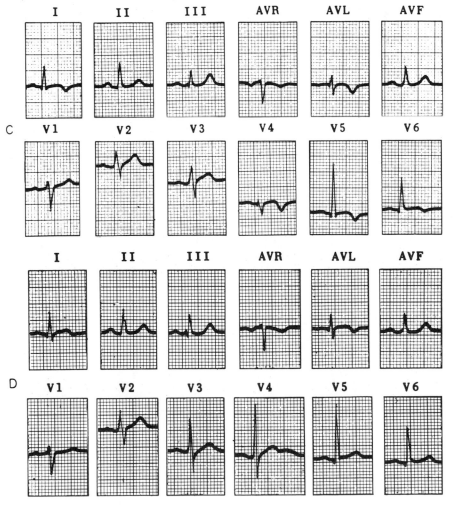

P-R segments in leads aVF, II, and in the precordial leads. On occasion, the P-R segments are elevated in lead V_1 but not in leads V_2 to V_6.

Other Findings

1 Some cases of pericarditis show normal electrocardiograms; others may show atypical findings.
2 The cardiac rhythm is usually a sinus tachycardia. Occasional cases may develop rhythm or conduction abnormalities.
3 Electrical alternans may be present when pericardial effusions are large. Two forms of this phenomenon are seen in pericarditis:
a Electrical alternans limited to the ventricles
b Total electrical alternation of the heart

PERICARDIAL EFFUSION

Low voltage of the QRST complex is the most consistent abnormality in pericardial effusion. The S-T-T changes of pericarditis may be noted. Total electrical alternation of the heart involving P waves as well as the QRST complexes is virtually pathognomonic of large pericardial effusions.

CHRONIC CONSTRICTIVE PERICARDITIS

The electrocardiographic changes are not diagnostic. The following abnormalities may be noted:

1 Low voltage of the QRS complexes.
2 Flattened or inverted T waves in the precordial and limb leads.
3 Fixed electrical position of the heart which does not change with position or respiration. This is not a reliable sign, since it occurs in some normal individuals.
4 The P wave is notched or wide, especially in leads I and II, resembling the P mitrale pattern.
5 Atrial fibrillation. This arrhythmia occurs in about one-third of the cases.

Differential Diagnosis

1 The differential diagnosis between acute pericarditis and myocardial infarction is outlined in Table 15-1.
2 Electrocardiographic mimicry between early repolarization and acute pericarditis requires differentiation between the two conditions. The diagnosis of early repolarization is favored by P-R segment and S-T

**TABLE 15-1   DIFFERENTIAL DIAGNOSIS OF PERICARDITIS AND
MYOCARDIAL INFARCTION**

Characteristic	Pericarditis	Infarction
Evolution of electrocardio-graphic changes	Rapid	Slow
Distribution of electrocardiographic changes	Widespread—many leads	Localized—fewer leads
Reciprocal changes in standard limb leads	Absent	Present
Q wave abnormalities	Absent	Present
Characteristics of the S-T segments and T waves	S-T less elevated, T waves usually not inverted until S-T is isoelectric, T less deeply inverted	S-T more elevated, T wave begins to invert before S-T is isoelectric, T more deeply inverted
Q-Tc	Normal	Often prolonged
Residual ECG changes	Unusual	Present in majority

segment deviations confined to either the precordial or limb leads, a vertical S-T vector located to the right of the T vector, an elevated S-T segment in lead V_1 and the right precordial leads, but an isoelectric S-T segment in lead V_6. The diagnosis of acute pericarditis is supported by the presence of P-R segment and S-T segment deviations in both the limb and precordial leads with a horizontal S-T vector located to the left of the T vector, S-T segment depression in lead V_1 and an elevated S-T segment in lead V_6. Serial electrocardiograms show evolutionary ST-T changes in pericarditis, but the ST-T changes in early repolarization remain unchanged over long periods of time.

Ginzton and Laks have shown that the ST/T ratio in lead V_6 is a most reliable discriminator between acute pericarditis and early repolarization. They found that an ST/T ratio ≥ 0.25 in this lead is virtually diagnostic of pericarditis. If lead V_6 is unavailable, a similar ratio in lead V_5, V_4, or I is also highly suggestive of acute pericarditis rather than the normal variant.

3 Other conditions with S-T segment deviations, such as ventricular aneurysm, left ventricular strain, and left bundle branch block, must also be differentiated from pericarditis. In ventricular aneurysm, the S-T segment elevations are accompanied by Q wave abnormalities and remain unchanged in serial electrocardiograms over a long period of time. Reciprocal elevation of the S-T segments in the right precordial leads is often found in left ventricular enlargement (with "strain") and left bundle branch block. The depression of the S-T segment in the left precordial leads and the overall stability of the S-T displacements help to distinguish these conditions from acute pericarditis.

PERICARDITIS COMPLICATING MYOCARDIAL INFARCTION

Anterior or Anterolateral Infarction plus Pericarditis

When anterior or anterolateral infarction occurs, any or all of leads I and aVL, and the precordial leads, commonly show abnormal Q waves, elevation of the S-T segment, and T wave changes.   Leads aVF and III show a normal QRS pattern and reciprocal depression of the S-T segment.   When anterior or anterolateral infarction is complicated by pericarditis, the S-T segment in leads aVF, III, and II, instead of being depressed, becomes elevated, with concomitant depression of the S-T segment in lead aVR.

Inferior Infarction plus Pericarditis

When inferior infarction occurs, leads aVF, III, and II show abnormal Q waves, elevation of the S-T segment, and T wave changes.   Leads aVL and I show a normal QRS pattern and reciprocal depression of the S-T segment. The precordial leads show normal or depressed S-T segments.   When inferior infarction is complicated by pericarditis, the S-T segment in leads aVL and I, instead of being depressed, becomes elevated.   The precordial leads (V_3 to V_6) also show upward displacement of the S-T segments.   Lead aVR shows S-T segment depression.

ACUTE HEMOPERICARDIUM

In acute hemopericardium secondary to rupture of the heart or aorta, the electrocardiogram may show the following findings: sinus bradycardia, AV junctional rhythm, electromechanical dissociation, electrical alternans, S-T segment elevation or depression, and reversal of the polarity of the T waves.

REFERENCES

Bellet, S., and T. M. McMillan: Electrocardiographic Patterns in Acute Pericarditis, *Arch. Intern. Med.*, 61: 381, 1938.

Fowler, N. O.: The Electrocardiogram in Pericarditis, *Cardiovasc. Clin.*, 5(3): 255, 1973.

Friedman, H. S., L. A. Kuhn, and A. M. Katz: Clinical and Electrocardiographic Features of Cardiac Rupture Following Acute Myocardial Infarction *Am. J. Med.*, 50: 709, 1971.

Ginzton, L. E. and M. M. Laks: The Differential Diagnosis of Acute Pericarditis from the Normal Variant: New Electrocardiographic Criteria, *Circulation*, 65: 1004, 1982.

Hull, E.: The Electrocardiogram in Pericarditis, *Am. J. Cardiol.*, 7: 21, 1961.

London, R. E., and S. B. London: The Electrocardiographic Sign of Acute Hemo-pericardium, *Circulation*, 25: 780, 1962.

Nizet, P. M., and H. J. L. Marriott: The Electrocardiogram and Pericardial Effusion, *J.A.M.A.*, 198: 189, 1966.

Spodick, D. H.: "Acute Pericarditis," Grune & Stratton, New York, 1959.

———: "Chronic and Constrictive Pericarditis," Grune & Stratton, New York, 1964.

———: Electrocardiogram in Acute Pericarditis, *Am. J. Cardiol.*, 33: 470, 1974.

———: Differential Characteristics of the Electrocardiogram in Early Repolarization and Acute Pericarditis, *New Eng. J. Med.*, 295: 523, 1976.

Surawicz, B., and K. C. Lasseter: Electrocardiogram in Pericarditis, *Am. J. Cardiol.*, 26: 471, 1970.

CHAPTER 16

EFFECT OF CERTAIN DRUGS ON THE ELECTROCARDIOGRAM

DIGITALIS (FIGS. 9-1, 10-15, 13-8, 16-1, 24-19, 24-33, 24-34, 24-46, 24-54, 24-59, 24-64, 24-88, 24-90)

Digitalis produces significant changes in the electrocardiogram. However, it is important to bear in mind that not infrequently there is relatively poor correlation between the electrocardiographic findings and the dosage of digitalis. It is also important to know that the effect of digitalis on the electrocardiogram is much less pronounced when the control electrocardiogram is normal than when it is abnormal.

Theoretical Considerations

Digitalis hastens the recovery process in the ventricular myocardium, particularly in the subendocardial region where it is normally the longest. At first, the early repolarization forces increase in magnitude and so cause the S-T vector to rotate gradually away from the mean QRS vector. This causes the depression of the S-T segment in epicardial leads with upright QRS complexes. At the same time, the T vector decreases in magnitude but is not altered in direction. This results in the flattening of the T waves in epicardial leads. Later, when digitalis completely reverses the direction of repolarization, the S-T and T vectors both point in the opposite direction to that of the mean QRS vector. The S-T segment becomes depressed, with the T wave inverted and merged with the S-T segment in epicardial

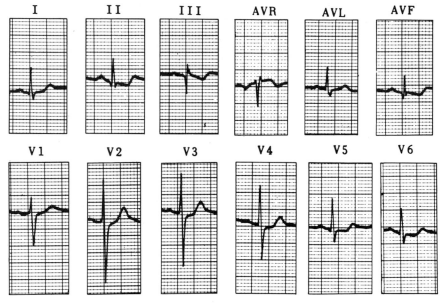

Fig. 16-1   Digitalis effect.   The S-T segments are depressed and concave upward.   The T waves are of decreased amplitude.   The Q-T interval is shortened.

leads with upright QRS complexes.   The Q-T interval is shortened as a result of the acceleration or the repolarization process in the ventricles.

Digitalis inhibits both the SA and AV junctional pacemakers and depresses both SA and AV conductivity.   It prolongs the refractory period of the AV node.   By its direct action it depresses atrial conductivity, but by its vagal activity it shortens the refractory period of atrial muscle and thus enhances its conductivity.   Digitalis depresses atrial excitability but increases ventricular excitability.   Digitalis in excessive or toxic doses may enhance the rhythmicity of secondary pacemakers and produce ectopic rhythms.

Effect on the Normal Electrocardiogram

Digitalis produces the following changes in the normal electrocardiogram:

1   In leads in which the QRS complex is predominantly upright, the earliest effect is downward displacement of the S-T junction and a decrease in the amplitude and duration of the T wave.   The S-T segment is concave upward.
2   In the next stage there is further depression of the S-T segment, so that the obliquity of its downward portion is increased.   The T wave becomes diphasic, with its proximal part inverted and its disal part upright.   The

angle between the terminal portion of the S-T segment and the T wave approaches 90°.

3   Finally the S-T segment becomes markedly depressed and slopes downward in a straight line. The T wave is merged with the S-T segment and is completely inverted.

4   The Q-Tc interval is shortened. This is a consistent and early finding.

5   There is a slight increase in the U wave amplitude.

6   The changes produced by digitalis are usually more pronounced in leads II, III, aVF, and the left precordial leads than in lead I and the right precordial leads. The presence of S-T segment depression or diphasic T waves in the right precordial leads helps to differentiate digitalis effect from the pattern of left ventricular hypertrophy and strain. In the latter, the depressed S-T segments and inverted T waves in the left precordial leads are associated with reciprocal elevations in the right-sided leads. However, digitalis may sometimes produce S-T segment elevation without appreciable lowering of the T wave in these leads.

7   Digitalis may occasionally produce two atypical T wave patterns: a pointed, inverted T wave similar to that seen in ischemia or pericarditis; and peaking of the terminal portion of the T wave, sometimes, but not always, related to hyperpotassemia or other abnormalities.

Effect on the Abnormal Electrocardiogram

Digitalis produces changes in the abnormal electrocardiogram which are similar to those noted in the normal one. To some extent, the changes produced by it depend on the initial direction of the T wave. When the T wave is upright or flat, it may become inverted. When the T wave is slightly inverted, it may become less inverted or even upright.

Digitalis does not change the direction of the S-T segments or T waves in ventricular hypertrophy, bundle branch block, or myocardial infarction. However, it may accentuate the changes already present and change the shape of the S-T segment or T wave to the typical digitalis contour.

Therapeutic Effects

1   S-T segment changes.

2   T wave alterations.

3   Shortening of the Q-T interval.

4   Prolongation of the P-R interval.

5   In atrial fibrillation, digitalis may slow the ventricular rate or even terminate the arrhythmia.

6   In rapid atrial rhythms, digitalis may stop the arrhythmia, continue it, or accelerate it. Thus atrial tachycardia may go on to flutter, to fibrillation, and eventually to sinus rhythm.

Toxic Effects

1   Paroxysmal atrial tachycardia with irregular ventricular response (PAT with block).
2   Nonparoxysmal AV junctional tachycardia with AV dissociation.
3   SA block.
4   Second- and third-degree AV block.
5   Ventricular premature systoles, often with bigeminy.
6   Multifocal ventricular premature systoles.
7   Runs of ventricular premature systoles.
8   Ventricular paroxysmal tachycardia.
9   Bidirectional tachycardia.
10 Ventricular fibrillation.
11 Digitalis may cause almost any other type of arrhythmia or conduction defect with the exception of intraventricular conduction defects, type II second-degree AV block, parasystole, and multifocal atrial tachycardia.
12 In atrial fibrillation, digitalis overdosage may result in the sequential development of a slowed ventricular response, AV junctional escapes, nonparoxysmal AV junctional tachycardia, exit block in the preceding arrhythmia, and bidirectional tachycardia.

QUINIDINE (FIG. 16-2)

Quinidine is a cardiac depressant.   Its principal electrophysiologic effects are as follows: (1) little or no change in the sinus rate; (2) depression of atrial automaticity, excitability, and conductivity and prolongation of its refractory period; (3) little or no effect on conduction through the AV junction; (4) depression of automaticity, slowing of conduction velocity, and prolongation of the refractory period in the His-Purkinje system; and (5) depression of ventricular conductivity and excitability.   There is some evidence that quinidine may have a vagolytic effect, but this is uncertain. It also has antifibrillatory action.

Therapeutic Effects

1   Notching, flattening or inversion of the T waves, usually associated with both increased duration of the T waves and increased amplitude of the U waves
2   Prolongation of the Q-Tc interval
3   Absence of S-T segment elevation or depression
4   Slight widening and notching of the P waves
5   Slight prolongation of the P-R interval

Digitalis and quinidine in combination produce depressed S-T seg-

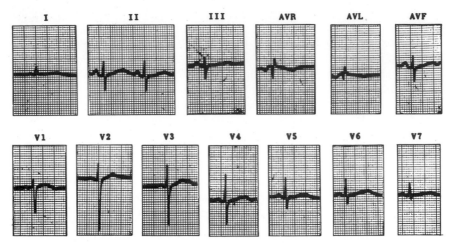

Fig. 16-2 Quinidine effect.   The Q-T interval is prolonged, the T waves are flattened, and the U waves are prominent.

ments, low T waves, and prominent U waves.   This pattern is indistinguishable from that produced by hypopotassemia.

Toxic Effects

The toxic effects of quinidine may or may not be dose-dependent.   Sinus bradycardia and widening of the QRS complexes are dose-related, but ventricular dysrhythmias are not strictly related to dosage.   The ventricular arrhythmias caused by quinidine are probably caused by reentry rather than increased automaticity.

1   Varying degrees of AV block.
2   Atrial slowing, intraatrial block, and atrial standstill.
3   Marked prolongation of the Q-T interval.
4   Widening of the QRS complex without any change in its contour or in the direction of the mean QRS vectors, or production of conventional bundle branch block.   When the intraventricular conduction time is normal, a 50 percent increase in the width of the QRS interval is dangerous and may herald the appearance of ventricular tachycardia or fibrillation.   In patients with bundle branch block, a 25 percent increase in the QRS duration has similar significance.
5   Ventricular arrhythmias, such as premature systoles, tachycardia, and fibrillation.

PROCAINAMIDE

The effects of procainamide are similar to those produced by quinidine.   It has no significant effect on heart rate.   It reduces cardiac excitability and increases the effective refractory period of the atria, ventricles, and His-Purkinje system. The automaticity of the His-Purkinje system is depressed. By virtue of direct effects, conductivity is reduced, leading to prolongation of the P-R and QRS intervals. Procainamide also tends to reduce vagal tone. In toxic doses, procainamide may produce ventricular extrasystoles, tachyarrhythmias, high degree of AV block, and asystole.

LIDOCAINE

Lidocaine has little or no effect on sinus rhythm, AV, or intraventricular conduction. Lidocaine acts more powerfully on the ventricles than on the atria. It depresses automaticity in the His-Purkinje fibers, raises the excitability threshold of both the atria and ventricles, and decreases the capacity of ventricular fibers to respond to repetitive stimulation.

Therapeutic doses of lidocaine have no significant effect on the P wave, P-R interval, QRS complex, Q-Tc interval, or the morphology of the T wave. In some instances it may detrimentally slow the heart rate in sinus bradycardia, SA block, and AV block.

PHENYTOIN (DIPHENYLHYDANTOIN)

Phenytoin depresses ventricular automaticity and may enhance AV conduction but has little or no effect on intraventricular conduction or the sinus rate. Phenytoin is useful in the treatment of digitalis toxicity because it abolishes both the ventricular arrhythmias and the AV conduction abnormalities produced by the glycoside. These effects contrast with those of procainamide and similar agents, which, although suppressing ventricular ectopy, exacerbate the AV conduction defect. However, phenytoin is contraindicated in complete heart block because of its depressant effect on ventricular automaticity.

Conflicting reports on the effects of phenytoin on the electrocardiogram have been reported by different investigators. Some investigators have observed very slight prolongation of the P-R interval and decreased amplitude of the T waves. Others have stated that the drug either does not change or shortens the QRS duration and that the P-R and Q-Tc intervals are reduced.

The intravenous administration of 150 to 250 mg of phenytoin has been reported to produce bradycardia, AV block, asystole, and ventricular fibrillation in some patients with severe heart disease and congestive heart failure.

PROPRANOLOL

Propranolol, a beta-adrenergic blocking agent, by reversing catecholamine effects, slows the rate of discharge of the SA node, decreases conduction velocity and increases the refractory period in the AV node, and reduces ventricular excitability.   It also has a negative inotropic effect.

In the electrocardiogram, the most striking effect with moderate to large doses of the drug is the production of sinus bradycardia, often with slight prolongation of the P-R interval.   The Q-Tc interval is usually shortened, and the height of the T wave is frequently increased.   Propranolol slows the ventricular response in atrial fibrillation and flutter by prolonging the effective refractory period of the AV node.

High degrees of AV and SA block have been reported following the intravenous or oral administration of propranolol in some patients, particularly those with preexisting disease of the conduction system or those who are on digitalis therapy.

SYMPATHOMIMETIC DRUGS

There are individual differences among the sympathomimetic drugs in their ability to stimulate alpha and beta receptors.   In general, these drugs tend to produce the following effects: (1) enhancement of pacemaker activity; (2) a tendency to restore excitability to normal levels if it is depressed; and (3) generally an increase in conduction velocity in the atria, ventricles, and His-Purkinje system.   There are no specific electrocardiographic effects.   The intravenous infusion of norepinephrine or isoproterenol in customary therapeutic dosage is often associated with increased P wave amplitude, depression of the P-R segment, slight shortening of the P-R and QRS intervals, and variable T wave changes.

ATROPINE

Atropine is a parasympathetic blocking agent.   In very small doses (less than 0.3 to 0.6 mg), it may slow the heart rate.   In larger doses, it produces bradycardia followed by tachycardia.   After intravenous administration, in doses of 0.8 to 1.2 mg, atropine may produce the following arrhythmias: AV dissociation, atrial arrhythmias, wandering pacemaker, and sometimes second-degree AV block.

PSYCHOTROPIC AGENTS (PHENOTHIAZINES AND ANTIDEPRESSANT DRUGS)

The phenothiazines and the antidepressant group of drugs (e.g., the dibenzazepine deviates such as amitriptyline and imipramine) tend to impair intracardiac conduction.   With excessive dosage, the S-T segments may become depressed and the T waves flat or inverted.   Prolongation of the

TABLE 16-1 EFFECTS OF NEWER ANTIARRHYTHMIC DRUGS ON ECG INTERVALS AND ON EFFECTIVE REFRACTORY PERIOD*

Agent (Class)	Atria	Atrioventricular Node	P-R or A-H Interval	His-Purkinje System	QRS Interval†	Ventricular Muscle	Q-Tc Interval	Accessory Pathway in Preexcitation
Aprindine hydrochloride (1)	Lengthen	Lengthen	Lengthen	Lengthen	Lengthen	Lengthen	0	Lengthen
Mexiletine hydrochloride (1)	0	±	0	Lengthen	Lengthen	Lengthen	0	Lengthen
Tocainide hydrochloride (1)	0	±	0	Lengthen	Lengthen	Lengthen	0	Lengthen
Ethmozin hydrochloride (1)	0	0	0	Lengthen	Lengthen	Lengthen	0	Lengthen
Lorcainide hydrochloride (1)	±	±	±	Lengthen	Lengthen	Lengthen	0	Lengthen
Encainide hydrochloride (1)	Lengthen	Lengthen	Lengthen	Lengthen	Lengthen	Lengthen	0	Lengthen
Flecainide acetate (1)	0	0	0	Lengthen	Lengthen	Lengthen	0	Lengthen
Acecainide hydrochloride (1)	?	±	0	Lengthen	Lengthen	Lengthen	Lengthen	Lengthen
New β-blockers (2)	±	Lengthen	Lengthen	0	0	0	0	0
Amiodarone hydrochloride (3)	Lengthen	Lengthen	Lengthen	Lengthen	0	Lengthen	Lengthen	Lengthen
Verapamil hydrochloride (4)	0	Lengthen	Lengthen	0	0	0	0	±
Diltiazem hydrochloride (4)	0	Lengthen	Lengthen	0	0	0	0	±
Nifedipine (4)	0	0	0	0	0	0	0	0

* The data shown for some of the agents are preliminary and may require revision in light of further investigations. Plus or minus indicates variable effect but not significant; 0, no effect.
† The effect on the QRS duration may not be apparent except when recorded at fast paper speeds and at high drug concentrations.
SOURCE: K. Nademanee and B. N. Singh: Advances in Antiarrhythmic Therapy, J.A.M.A., 247: 217, 1982. Used by permission.

Q-Tc interval, prominence of the U waves, AV and intraventricular conduction defects, and cardiac arrhythmias may also occur.

EFFECT OF VARIOUS DRUGS ON CARDIAC CONDUCTION

His bundle recordings in conjunction with atrial pacing have revealed the following effects of various drugs on the conduction system:

Digitalis increases the A-H interval but does not affect the H-V interval. Propranolol has similar actions. Atropine decreases the A-H interval but interval. Diphenylhydantoin either shortens or has no effect on the A-H interval and has either no effect on or decreases the H-V interval. Lidocaine has no appreciable effect on either the A-H or H-V intervals. Procainamide may increase or have no effect on the A-H interval but increases the H-V interval. Diphenylhydantoin either shortens or has no effect on the A-H interval and leaves the H-V interval unaltered.

The effects of some of the newer drugs on ECG intervals and on the effective refractory period are listed in Table 16-1.

The effect of drugs on normal and anomalous conduction in the preexcitation syndrome is discussed in Chap. 12.

REFERENCES

Bellet, S.: "Clinical Disorders of the Heart Beat," 3d ed., Lea & Febiger, Philadelphia, 1971.

Broome, R. A., E. H. Estes, Jr., and E. S. Orgain: The Effects of Digitoxin upon the Twelve Lead Electrocardiogram, *Am. J. Med.*, 21: 237, 1956.

Denes, P., and K. M. Rosen: His Bundle Electrograms: Clinical Applications, *Cardiovasc. Clin.*, 6(1), 69, 1974.

Gianelly, R., and D. C. Harrison: Drugs Used in the Treatment of Cardiac Arrhythmias, *Disease-A-Month*, January 1969.

Helfant, R. H., S. H. Lau, S. I. Cohen, and A. N. Damato: Effects of Diphenylhydantoin on Atrioventricular Conduction in Man, *Circulation*, 36: 686, 1967.

———, B. J. Scherlag, and A. N. Damato: The Electrophysiologic Properties of Diphenylhydantoin Sodium as Compared to Procaine Amide in the Normal and Digitalis-intoxicated Heart, *Circulation*, 36: 108, 1967.

Irons, G. V., Jr., and E. S. Orgain: Digitalis-induced Arrhythmias and Their Management, *Progr. Cardiovasc. Dis.*, 8: 539, 1966.

Kastor, J. A., and P. M. Yurchak: Recognition of Digitalis Intoxication in the Presence of Atrial Fibrillation, *Ann. Intern. Med.*, 67: 1045, 1967.

Kayden, H. J.: The Current Status of Procaine Amide in the Management of Cardiac Arrhythmias, *Progr. Cardiovasc. Dis.*, 3: 331, 1960-1961.

Lieberman, N. A., R. S. Harris, R. I. Katz, H. M. Lipschultz, M. Dolgin, and V. J. Fisher: The Effects of Lidocaine on the Electrical and Mechanical Activity of the Heart, *Am. J. Cardiol.*, 22: 375, 1968.

Marriott, H. J. L.: Rational Approach to Quinidine Therapy, *Mod. Concepts Cardiovasc. Dis.*, 31: 745, 1962.

Pick, A.: Digitalis and the Electrocardiogram, *Circulation*, 15: 603, 1957.

Scherlag, B. J., R. H. Helfant, and A. N. Damato: The Contrasting Effects of Diphenylhydantoin and Procaine Amide on AV Conduction in the Digitalis-intoxicated and the Normal Heart, *Am. Heart J.*, 75: 200, 1968.

Sokolow, M.: Therapy of Cardiac Arrhythmias with Quinidine, *Am. Heart J.*, 42: 771, 1951.

Stern, S., and S. Eisenberg: The Effect of Propranolol (Inderal) on the Electrocardiogram of Normal Subjects, *Am. Heart J.*, 77: 192, 1969.

Surawicz, B., and K. C. Lasseter: Effect of Drugs on the Electrocardiogram, *Progr. Cardiovasc. Dis.*, 13: 26, 1970.

CHAPTER 17

EFFECT OF ELECTROLYTE ABNORMALITIES ON THE ELECTROCARDIOGRAM

Electrolyte disturbances may produce significant alterations in the electro-cardiogram. The effects produced by electrolyte abnormalities depend on the relative concentrations of the individual ions to one another at the cellular level as well as the absolute levels of each in the serum. The correlation between the electrocardiogram and the clinical state of the patient is sometimes better than that between the electrocardiogram and the serum levels. In general, the precordial leads are more useful than the limb leads in the detection of electrolyte imbalance, and serial electrocardiographic changes are much more significant than the findings in a single electrocardiogram.

HYPERPOTASSEMIA (FIGS. 17-1 TO 17-4)

The following more or less sequential electrocardiographic changes are seen in hyperpotassemia:

1 Progressive increase in the amplitude of the T waves, which become tall, thin, and peaked. This is the earliest change associated with potassium intoxication. At this stage, the Q-T interval may be normal, shortened, or prolonged.
2 With advancing intoxication, there may occur decreased amplitude of the R wave with concomitant increased depth of the S wave, S-T segment depression, and prolongation of the QRS and P-R intervals.

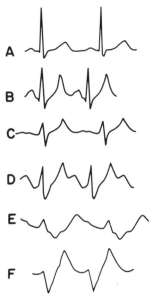

Fig. 17-1 Electrocardiographic changes of hyperpotassemia.   *A* is a normal tracing.   *B* through *F* are arranged to illustrate serial changes of elevated potassium levels.   (*From C. R. VanderArk, F. Ballantyne, III, and E. W. Reynolds, Jr., Electrolytes and the Electrocardiogram, Cardiovasc. Clin.*, 5(3): 269, 1973.   *Used by permission.*)

Fig. 17-2 Typical narrow, symmetrical, tall, and peaked T waves of hyperpotassemia.   The serum K^+ was 6.2 meq/l.

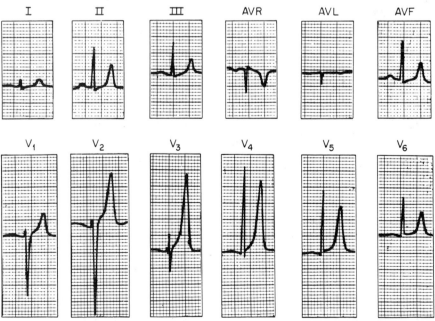

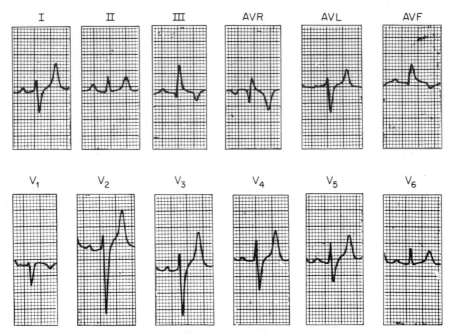

Fig. 17-3 Hyperpotassemia in a 15-year-old boy with a serium K^+ of 8.0 meq/l. The P-R interval is 0.20 s, the QRS duration 0.11 s. Both are slightly prolonged for a child of this age. Although the T waves are not particularly tall, they are narrow, symmetrical, and peaked.

3 As hyperpotassemia increases still further, the P wave increases in duration while decreasing in amplitude, the QRS and P-R intervals lengthen even more, and the Q-T interval becomes prolonged.

4 Eventually the P wave disappears. Sinoventricular rhythm may supervene. However, a slow, irregular idioventricular rhythm may occur at this stage.

5 In succeeding stages there occurs a progressive widening of the QRS complex and T wave with obliteration of the S-T segment, so that the T wave originates from the S wave. Eventually the QRST complex is replaced by a smooth diphasic or sine curve.

6 The final stage is ventricular tachycardia, ventricular flutter, ventricular fibrillation, or ventricular standstill.

7 At any time during the sequence, ventricular premature systoles or ventricular escape beats may develop.

The electrocardiographic effects are enhanced by concomitantly depressed serum sodium and/or calcium levels and are antagonized by concomitantly normal serum levels for sodium or calcium or both.

Comments

The sequential changes of hyperpotassemia are usually characteristic but variant patterns may occur.

The effects of hyperpotassemia on cardiac rhythm are complex. Almost any arrhythmia may occur. A mild to moderate rise in serum K$^+$ may shorten the P-R interval, but progressive increases in the serum concentration of this ion generally slow AV conduction and produce complete heart block. Sinus bradycardia, sinus arrest, and a slow idioventricular rhythm may be found in some cases of hyperpotassemia, but in others progressive sinus tachycardia, frequent premature beats, ventricular tachycardia, and fibrillation may be observed.

The intraventricular conduction defect in hyperpotassemia is usually diffuse and uniform, but complete right or left bundle branch block may occur. Hyperpotassemia has been reported to cause both right and left axis deviation.

Fig. 17-4 Hyperpotassemia. There is atrial standstill. The QRS complexes are widened markedly. There is almost complete obliteration of the S-T segment. The Q-T interval is prolonged. The electrical axis is deviated leftward. The serium K$^+$ was 9.9 meq/l. The patient expired shortly after the electrocardiogram was taken.

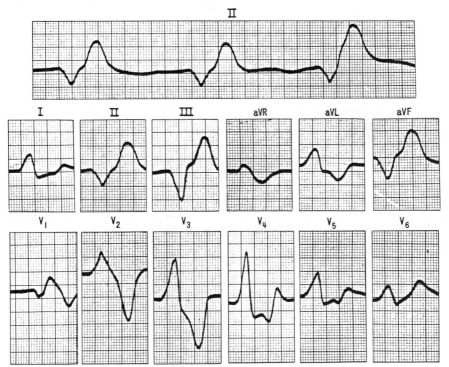

The typical T wave changes of hyperpotassemia may be masked by the prior administration of digitalis. In patients receiving digitalis, the proximal T wave inversion and the low amplitude terminal T wave of digitalis effect may be "normalized" when hyperpotassemia develops. It is only during the more advanced stages of potassium intoxication that the typical T wave changes may become apparent. Hyperpotassemia has also been reported to reverse the polarity of the T waves in the left ventricular strain pattern.

Although the S-T segment is usually depressed in hyperpotassemia, there are some cases in which S-T segment elevation may occur and thereby simulate the pattern of subepicardial injury. In rare instances, the presence of abnormal Q waves together with the ST-T changes of subepicardial injury may mimic myocardial infarction (Figs. 13-25A and B, 13-26A and B).

The tall precordial T waves of hyperpotassemia must be distinguished from those sometimes seen in cerebrovascular accidents, posterior subepicardial ischemia, anterior subendocardial ischemia, and some normal persons.

HYPOPOTASSEMIA (Figs. 17-5, 17-6)

In hypopotassemia, the electrocardiographic changes listed below are not necessarily sequential.

1   Lowering, flattening, or inversion of the T wave as well as widening and occasional notching of the T wave.
2   A Q-T interval which is generally at the upper limits of normal or is slightly prolonged.
3   Depression of the S-T segment, which often develops a troughlike appearance. The S-T segment change may also resemble the change produced by digitalis. Attention to the Q-T interval may help differentiate between the two. If the Q-T interval is short, digitalis is the more likely cause; if it is lengthened, hypopotassemia is the more likely cause.
4   If not previously present, a U wave may appear; if previously present, the U wave becomes broader and taller. This gives the T-U segment a double contour. Occasionally the T wave becomes notched. When it does, and if a U wave is present also, the T-U segment shows a triple contour.

The question whether the second of a pair of summits is the second notch of a T wave or is a U wave may be resolved by measuring the time between the two summits. If this period measures less than 40 percent of the time from the beginning of the QRS complex to the second summit, it is the second notch of a T wave; if more than 40 percent, it is a U wave.

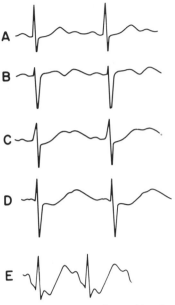

Fig. 17-5 Electrocardiographic changes of hypopotassemia. *A* is a normal tracing with a typical U wave. *B* through *E* are arranged to illustrate serial changes of hypopotassemia. *(From C. R. VanderArk, F. Ballantyne, III, and E. W. Reynolds, Jr., Electrolytes and the Electrocardiogram, Cardiovasc. Clin., 5(3): 269, 1973. Used by permission.)*

Fig. 17-6 Hypopotassemia. The U waves are large and the T waves flattened. The T/U ratio is less than 1.0 in leads II and V_3. U_{V_3} exceeds 2 mm. The S-T segments have a shallow, troughlike appearance in the limb leads. The serum K^+ was 2.2 meq/l.

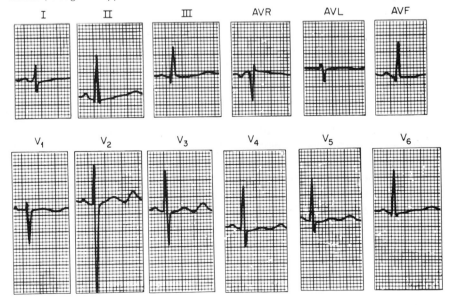

5   Various arrhythmias and conduction disturbances, including prolongation of the P-R interval, AV junctional rhythm, and supraventricular
tachycardia, may occur whether or not the patient has been digitalized.
On the other hand, arrhythmias or conduction defects resulting from
digitalis intoxication may be induced in patients previously successfully
carried on maintenance doses of digitalis without toxicity when these
patients become hypopotassemic.   These arrhythmias include premature
systoles, AV junctional tachycardia, AV dissociation, and paroxysmal
atrial tachycardia with block.

Criteria for the Diagnosis of Hypopotassemia (Weaver and Burchell)

These criteria are based on various combinations of the following signs:

1   A T/U value of 1.0 or less in lead II or V_3
2   A U wave amplitude of more than 0.5 mm in lead II or more than 1.0
mm in lead V_3
3   S-T segment depression of 0.5 mm or more in lead II or in leads V_1, V_2
and V_3

These abnormalities are assigned values according to the following
table:

Electrocardiographic Signs	Value
T/U 1.0 or less in lead II	1
T/U, 1.0 or less in lead V_3	1
U_2, 0.6–1.4 mm	1
U_2, 1.5 mm or more	2
U_{V_3}, 1.1–1.9 mm	1
U_{V_3}, 2.0 mm or more	2
S-T depression of 0.5 mm or more in lead II or leads V_1 to V_3	1

These values are then added.   The electrocardiographic diagnosis is
based on the following scores:

0–1   Nondiagnostic
2   Suggestive
3–7   Characteristic

The above criteria pertain only to normotensive subjects.   A negative
score or even a normal electrocardiogram does not exclude hypopotassemia,
nor does an electrocardiogram which fulfills the established criteria necessarily indicate hypopotassemia.

Comment

The major problem in the electrocardiographic diagnosis of hypopotassemia is the frequent production of similar changes by drugs or disease states in which the serum potassium is normal.   Several examples can be cited: sinus bradycardia with large U waves; hypertension, left ventricular hypertropy, or both, with prominent U waves (suggesting hypopotassemia secondary to primary aldosteronism, diuretic therapy, or other causes); drug effects, notably quinidine, quinidine in combination with digitalis; procainamide, and phenothiazine derivatives; cerebrovascular accidents; and the prolonged Q-T interval syndrome.

HYPERCALCEMIA (FIGS. 17-7, 17-8)

1   There is shortening to the Q-oTc interval (the interval from the beginning of the Q wave to the onset of the T wave corrected for the heart rate). The degree of shortening is inversely proportional to the serum calcium level up to values of 20 mg/100 ml.
2   There is shortening of the Q-Tc interval (the corrected Q-T interval) inversely proportional to the serum calcium level up to values of 16 mg/100 ml.   At levels greater than this, prolongation of the Q-Tc interval may occur because of prolongation of the T wave.
3   As already indicated, in some instances of hypercalcemia, widening and rounding of the T wave may occur at very high levels of serum calcium.

Fig. 17-7   Hypercalcemia.   There is shortening of the Q-Tc interval.   The Q-oT segment is virtually absent, and the U wave is prominent in lead V_2.   The serium calcium was 17.2 mg/100 ml.   (*Redrawn from D. Bronsky, A. Dubin, S. S. Waldstein, and D. S. Kushner, Calcium and the Electrocardiogram: II.   The Electrocardiographic Manifestations of Hyperparathyroidism and of Marked Hypercalcemia from Various Other Etiologies, Am. J. Cardiol., 7: 833, 1961. Used by permission.*)

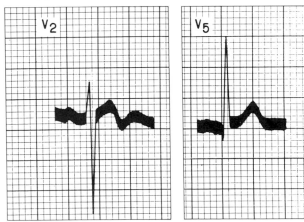

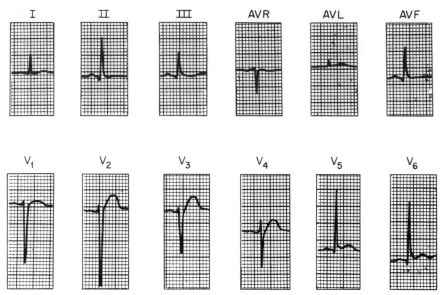

Fig. 17-8 Hypercalcemia.   There is shortening of the Q-Tc interval and virtual absence of the Q-oT segment.   The serum Ca^{++} was 18.7 mg/100 ml.

Comment

According to Wortsman and Frank, shortening of the Q-T interval, long regarded as the classical diagnostic sign of hypercalcemia, is unreliable for the diagnosing of chronic hypercalcemia.   After correction for all factors that may alter the Q-T interval, they concluded that the absolute Q-T interval remains normal in most patients with severe hypercalcemia.

HYPOCALCEMIA (FIGS. 17-9, 17-10)

1   There is prolongation of the Q-oTc interval (the interval from the beginning of the Q wave to the onset of the T wave, corrected for the heart rate), causing prolongation of the Q-Tc interval (the corrected Q-T interval).   The degree of prolongation is inversely proportional to the serum calcium level.

2   In approximately half the cases, the T waves appear normal.   Symmetrical late T wave inversion is the abnormality seen most commonly, but tall, peaked T waves also are observed.

MAGNESIUM

According to Surawicz, it is unlikely that an abnormal plasma level of magnesium can be detected electrocardiographically.

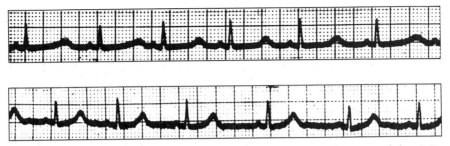

Fig. 17-9 Hypocalcemia. *Upper tracing:* Hypocalcemia with prolongation of the Q-Tc interval due to prolongation of the Q-oTC interval. The serium calcium was 4.2 mg/100 ml. *Lower tracing:* The same patient after correction of the hypocalcemia. The electrocardiogram is now normal.

Hypermagnesemia

In experimental studies, large doses of magnesium have been reported to slow conduction velocity. This is manifested electrocardiographically by an increase in the P-R interval and the QRS duration and, occasionally, by SA and AV block, but without any change in the Q-T interval. Clinically, hypermagnesemia is usually found in patients with renal failure. Its effect,

Fig. 17-10 Hypocalcemia. The T waves are deeply inverted in leads V_1 through V_3. Slight T wave inversion is also present in leads II, III, and aVF. The serum Ca^{++} was 3.8 mg/100 ml.

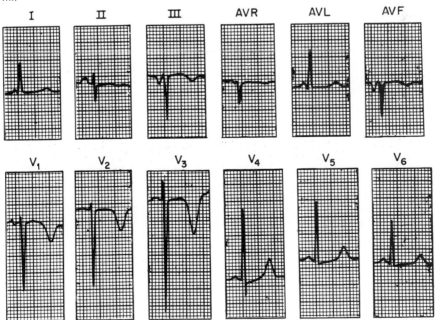

however, is usually masked by other electrolyte abnormalities, although it may augment the changes of hyperpotassemia.

Hypomagnesemia

Moderate magnesium deficiency in animals and humans has been reported to produce slight narrowing of the QRS complexes and tall T waves of normal width. The Q-T interval remains normal. Since marked magnesium deficiency is associated with potassium depletion, the electrocardiogram of severe hypomagnesemia is indistinguishable from that of hypopotassemia.

ACIDOSIS AND ALKALOSIS (FIG. 17-11)

Acidosis per se may cause the T waves to be tall and peaked, resembling the T waves of hyperpotassemia even in the presence of hypopotassemia. Actually, hyperpotassemia is commonly associated with acidosis.

Alkalosis per se may lower the T waves and prolong the Q-T interval even when the calcium levels are normal. Hypopotassemia is commonly associated with alkalosis.

Fig. 17-11 Metabolic alkalosis. The Q-T interval is prolonged. The T and U waves are merged. The pH was 7.64. The serum K^+ and Ca^{++} were normal.

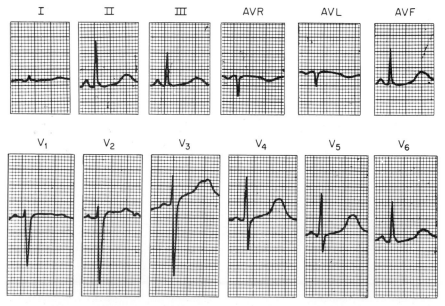

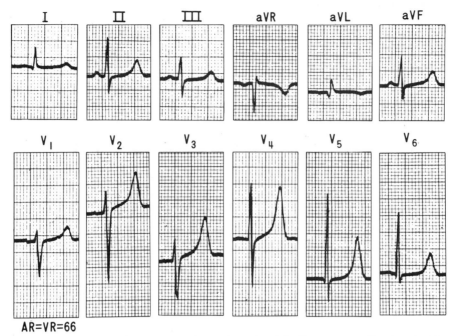

AR=VR=66

Fig. 17-12 Uremia. The Q-T interval is prolonged and the T waves are tall and peaked in the precordial leads, which denote hypocalcemia and hyperpotassemia, respectively.

UREMIA (FIG. 17-12)

The most characteristic electrocardiographic feature of uremia is the combination of a prolonged Q-T interval (due to hypocalcemia) with tall T waves (due to hyperpotassemia or acidosis or both).

REFERENCES

Bellet, S.: The Electrocardiogram in Electrolyte Imbalance, *Arch. Intern. Med.*, 96: 618, 1955.

Bronsky, D., A. Dubin, S. S. Waldstein, and D. S. Kushner: Calcium and the Electrocardiogram, *Am. J. Cardiol.*, 7: 823, 833, and 840, 1961.

Dreifus, L. S., and A. Pick: A Clinical Correlative Study of the Electrocardiogram in Electrolyte Imbalance, *Circulation*, 14: 815, 1956.

Langendorf, R., and C. L. Pirani: The Heart in Uremia: An Electrocardiographic and Pathologic Study, *Am. Heart J.*, 33: 282, 1947.

Surawicz, B.: Electrolytes and the Electrocardiogram, *Am. J. Cardiol.*, 12: 656, 1963.

———: Relationship between Electrocardiogram and Electrolytes, *Am. Heart J.*, 73: 814, 1967.

————, H. A. Braun, W. B. Crum, R. L. Kemp, S. Wagner, and S. Bellet: Quantitative Analysis of the Electrocardiographic Pattern of Hypopotassemia, *Circulation,* 16: 750, 1957.

———— and E. Lepeschkin: The Electrocardiogram in Hyperpotassemia, *Heart Bull.,* 10: 66, 1961.

———— and ————: The Electrocardiographic Pattern of Hypopotassemia with or without Hypocalcemia, *Circulation,* 8: 801, 1953.

VanderArk, C. R., F. Ballentyne, III, and E. W. Reynolds: Electrolytes and the Electrocardiogram, *Cardiovasc. Clin.,* 5 (3): 269, 1973.

Weaver, W. F., and H. B. Burchell: Serum Potassium and the Electrocardiogram in Hypokalemia, *Circulation,* 21: 505, 1960.

Wortsman, J., and S. Frank: The QT Interval in Clinical Hypercalcemia, *Clin. Cardiol.,* 4: 87, 1981.

CHAPTER 18

PULMONARY DISEASE

PULMONARY EMBOLISM AND ACUTE COR PULMONALE

Acute cor pulmonale may be produced by any condition which causes sudden pulmonary hypertension. While the most common cause by far is pulmonary embolism, other conditions such as acute respiratory failure, asthma, and acute pulmonary edema may produce it.

Pulmonary embolism is commonly, but not invariably, associated with electrocardiographic abnormalities which tend to appear early and are transient. None of the electrocardiographic changes are pathognomonic, but when interpreted in relation to the clinical findings, they furnish strong corroborative evidence for the diagnosis.

Electrocardiographic Findings (Figs. 18-1, 18-2)

1   The electrocardiogram may be normal or may be abnormal because of preexisting disease.
2   Sinus tachycardia is the usual rhythm. Other rhythm disturbances are uncommon.
3   As a result of right ventricular dilatation, the mean electrical axis may become more vertical or shift rightward (right axis deviation), with the extremity leads showing an S_1Q_3 pattern consisting of
a   A deep S wave in lead I
b   A prominent Q wave and an inverted T wave in lead III

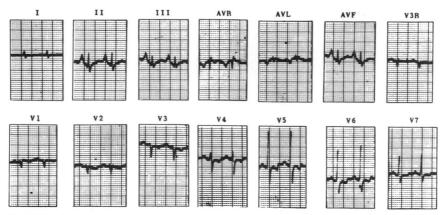

Fig. 18-1   Acute cor pulmonale.   There is sinus tachycardia, an S_1Q_3 pattern in the standard leads, P pulmonale, an rSr' pattern in leads V_{3R} to V_2, and S-T segment and T changes in the precordial leads.

   c Depression of the S-T segment in lead II and often in lead I, with a staircase ascent of the S-T segment in lead II

      This pattern occurs not only in acute cor pulmonale, but also in normal persons.   It resembles the pattern seen in inferior myocardial infarction, in which, however, abnormal Q waves are usually found not only in lead II, but also in leads III and aVF.   In acute cor pulmonale, on the other hand, abnormal Q waves do not generally occur in lead II, and even the Q wave in leads III and aVF may not be abnormally wide.

4 Also as a result of right ventricular dilatation, the precordial leads may exhibit one or more of the following patterns:

a T wave inversions in the right precordial leads

b Complete or incomplete right bundle branch block

c A QR or QS pattern in leads V_{3R}, V_1, and V_2, with negative T waves in these leads simulating anteroseptal infarction

d Clockwise rotation of the heart with a shift of the transition zone to the left, with the appearance of rS or RS patterns in most or all of the precordial leads

5 A recent study has shown that a leftward shift of the QRS axis occurs twice as frequently as a rightward shift, and abnormal left axis deviation is twice as common as right axis deviation.

6 Low voltage of the frontal plane QRS complexes may occur.

7 Right atrial abnormality (P pulmonale) is observed in some instances.

8 An $S_1S_2S_3$ pattern is seen on occasion.

9 The most common electrocardiographic manifestations of acute pulmonary embolism are nonspecific T wave changes (chiefly inversion) and nonspecific S-T segment abnormalities (depression or, less frequently, elevation).

Diagnosis

The following patterns are strongly suggestive, if not diagnostic, of acute cor pulmonale:

1 $S_1Q_3T_3$ pattern with T wave inversion in the right precordial leads
2 S_1T_3 pattern or T wave inversion in lead III and the right precordial leads
3 $S_1Q_3T_3$ pattern with right bundle branch block

The diagnosis is less secure in the absence of these abnormalities, which, unfortunately, are found in only 25 to 35 percent of cases.

Differential Diagnosis

Chronic Cor Pulmonale   Common to both acute and chronic cor pulmonale are T wave inversions in the right precordial leads, an S_1T_3 pattern, clockwise rotation of the heart, and a vertical electrical axis.   In chronic cor pulmonale, signs of right atrial and right ventricular enlargement may also occur.   These are usually not present in acute cor pulmonale.   The electrocardiographic abnormalities are usually quite transient in acute cor pulmonale and stable in chronic cor pulmonale.

Acute Myocardial Infarction   Either anteroseptal or inferior myocardial infarction may be misdiagnosed when pulmonary embolism is present. The presence of abnormal, persistent Q wave changes and evidence of subepicardial injury favor the diagnosis of myocardial infarction.

Fig. 18-2   Acute cor pulmonale manifested by right ventricular dilatation with a QR pattern in leads V_{4R} through V_3 and subendocardial anoxemia with S-T segment depression in the left precordial leads.   There is an S_1Q_3 pattern in the limb leads, with the electrical axis at $+100°$. Q waves are present in leads III and aVF but not in lead II (in contrast to myocardial infarction, in which abnormal Q waves are usually found in all three leads).

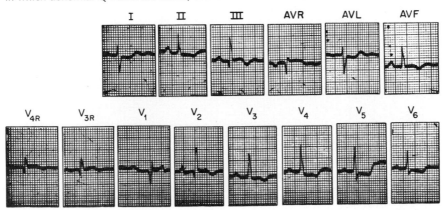

CHRONIC OBSTRUCTIVE PULMONARY DISEASE
AND CHRONIC COR PULMONALE

Various electrocardiographic patterns can occur in chronic obstructive pulmonary disease (and other diffuse lung diseases) with or without cor pulmonale. The electrocardiographic differentiation between chronic obstructive pulmonary disease (e.g., emphysema) with cor pulmonale and without it may be difficult or impossible. Criteria for the diagnosis of cor pulmonale in the presence of emphysema are listed later in this chapter.

Electrocardiographic Findings
(Figs. 9-1, 10-11, 11-7, 18-3, 18-4, 18-5, 18-6, 20-2, 21-1)

1 A rightward shift in the P vector to +70 to +90°, resulting in tall, peaked P waves in leads II, III, and aVF (P ≥ 2.5 mm). This may be found in emphysema without cor pulmonale.
2 Right axis deviation to +90° or more.
3 A shift in the transition zone to the left in the precordial leads, with the appearance of QS, rS, or RS patterns in most or all of the precordial leads.
4 An S_1Q_3 pattern in the extremity and precordial leads.
5 Low voltage of the extremity and precordial leads.
6 An $S_1S_2S_3$ syndrome.
7 Signs of right ventricular enlargement.
8 Right bundle branch block.
9 Right bundle branch block plus right ventricular enlargement.

Fig. 18-3 Emphysema with cor pulmonale. An unusual example with QS complexes in leads V_1 through V_5. There is low voltage in both the extremity and precordial leads.

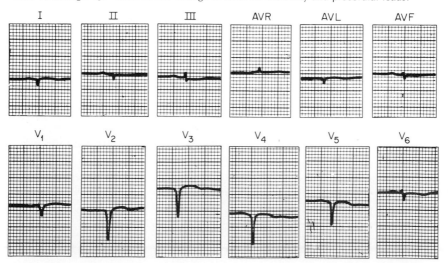

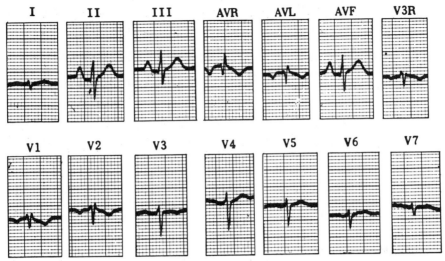

Fig. 18-4 Emphysema with cor pulmonale and right atrial enlargement. The P waves are tall and show a vertical axis. An $S_1S_2S_3$ pattern is present. The mean electrical axis of the QRS complex is indeterminate. rSr' complexes are seen in leads V_{3R} through V_5. The other precordial leads show rS patterns.

10 T wave inversion in the right precordial leads.
11 Abnormal left axis deviation (pseudo left axis deviation)

It should be noted that emphysema (with or without cor pulmonale) and acute cor pulmonale show electrocardiographic similarities. The differentiation depends on the transient nature of the electrocardiographic abnormalities in acute cor pulmonale. The electrocardiographic diagnosis of emphysema is not too reliable in the presence of myocardial infarction and vice versa.

Criteria for the Diagnosis of Chronic Obstructive Pulmonary Disease

1 A mean QRS axis in the limb leads of $+70$ to $+110°$, an $S_1S_2S_3$ pattern, or (pseudo) left axis deviation superior to $-30°$
2 Evidence of right atrial abnormality: P wave axis in the limb leads greater than $+70$ or $+75°$, P amplitude in leads II, III, aVF ≥ 2.5 mm, or $V_1 \geq 1.5$ mm, or both
3 Posterior displacement of the mean QRS axis in the horizontal plane:
a QS complexes in the right-sided precordial leads succeeded by rS deflections in leads farther to the left, or
b rS complexes across most or all of the precordial leads, or
c An R/S ratio of less than 1.0 in lead V_4 or in leads farther to the left
4 Low voltage of the QRS complexes (0.7 mV) in the limb leads and lead V_6

The greater the number of such abnormalities in a tracing, the greater the likelihood that chronic obstructive pulmonary disease is present.

Chronic Obstructive Pulmonary Disease with Right Ventricular Hypertrophy (Cor Pulmonale)

1 Electrocardiographic evidence of chronic obstructive pulmonary disease is present.
2 Additionally, one or more of the following abnormalities is noted:
a The mean QRS axis $\geqq +110°$.
b Lead V_1 shows a qR, R, or Rs complex or an rsR′ pattern with an R′/S ratio greater than 1.0 However, an rSr′ pattern or a slurred S wave in lead V_1, although suggestive, is not diagnostic of early right ventricular hypertrophy.

Fig. 18-5 Tracing in a patient with chronic obstructive pulmonary disease with cor pulmonale. There is right atrial enlargement. QS complexes are present in leads II, III, and aVF, simulating those seen in inferior myocardial infarction with left anterior fascicular block. A QR pattern is present in lead V_1, with prominent S waves in the remaining precordial leads—findings diagnostic of right ventricular enlargement. The patient had no clinical evidence of coronary artery disease. QS complexes in the inferior leads may occur in chronic lung disease in the absence of inferior myocardial infarction, left anterior fascicular block, or both. The large P terminal force in lead V_1 is a common finding in chronic obstructive pulmonary disease in the absence of left atrial enlargement.

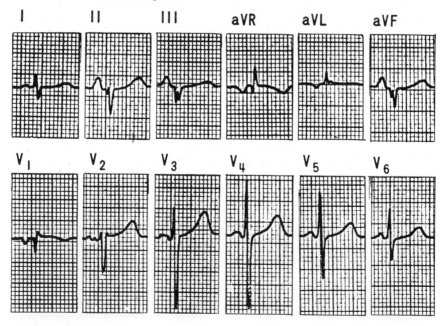

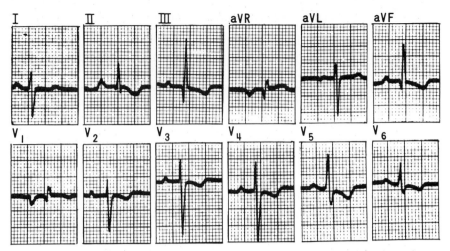

Fig. 18-6 Abnormal right axis deviation (about +125°) in a patient with cor pulmonale. In the limb leads, the deep S wave in lead I and the qR patterns in leads II, III, and aVF simulate left posterior fascicular block and inferior myocardial infarction. The qR pattern in lead V₁ is diagnostic of right ventricular enlargement. The large P terminal force in lead V₁ is a common finding in chronic pulmonary disease in the absence of left atrial abnormality.

Fig. 18-7 The vectorcardiogram in emphysema. There is posterior displacement of a CCW QRS loop in the transverse plane.

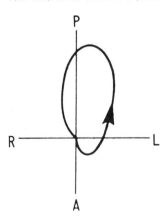

TRANSVERSE PLANE

Vectorcardiogram in Pulmonary Emphysema (Fig. 18-7)

Typically, there is posterior displacement of the QRS loop in the TP, which is inscribed in CCW fashion. In the LSP, inscription of the loop is CCW. Inscription in the FP is CW or CCW. Usually the loop is vertically placed in this plane. The P loops often show the characteristics of right atrial enlargement.

REFERENCES

Burch, G. E., and N. P. DePasquale: The Electrocardiographic Diagnosis of Pulmonary Heart Disease, *Am. J. Cardiol.,* 11: 622, 1963.

Fowler, N. O., C. Daniels, R. C. Scott, B. S. Faustino, and M. Gueron: The Electrocardiogram in Cor Pulmonale with and without Emphysema, *Am. J. Cardiol.,* 16: 500, 1965.

Lynch, R. E., P. D. Stein, and T. A. Bruce: Leftward Shift of Frontal Plane QRS Axis as a Frequent Manifestation of Acute Pulmonary Embolism, *Chest,* 61: 443, 1972.

Oram, S., and P. Davies: The Electrocardiogram in Cor Pulmonale, *Progr. Cariovasc. Dis.,* 9: 341, 1967.

Scott, R. C.: The Electrocardiogram in Pulmonary Emphysema and Cor Pulmonale, *Am. Heart J.,* 61: 843, 1961.

Selvester, R., and H. B. Rubin: New Criteria for the Electrocardiographic Diagnosis of Emphysema and Cor Pulmonale, *Am. Heart J.,* 69: 437, 1965.

Spodick, D. H.: Electrocardiographic Studies in Pulmonary Disease, *Circulation,* 20: 1067, 1073, 1959.

Stein, P. D., et al.: The Electrocardiogram in Acute Pulmonary Embolism, *Progr. Cardiovasc. Dis.,* 17: 247, 1975.

Walsh, T. J.: The Vectorcardiogram in Cor Pulmonale, *Progr. Cardiovasc. Dis.,* 9: 363, 1967.

Wasserburger, R. H., J. R. Kelly, H. K. Rasmussen, and J. J. Juhl: The Electrocardiographic Pentaology of Pulmonary Emphysema, *Circulation,* 20: 831, 1959.

Zuckerman, R., E. Cabera, B. L. Fishleder, and D. Sodi-Pallares: Electrocardiogram in Chronic Cor Pulmonale, *Am. Heart J.,* 35: 421, 1948.

CHAPTER 19

RIGHT AXIS DEVIATION

Right axis deviation is present when the mean electrical axis lies between +91 and −90°.

Abnormal right axis deviation is present in adults when the mean electrical axis lies between +110 and −90°. Right axis deviation with the mean electrical axis between +90 and +110° may be abnormal but is frequently a normal variant, particularly in young adults or in asthenic persons.

Abnormal right axis deviation is present in children when the mean electrical axis lies to the right of +120° in children from 3 months to 16 years of age. In infants below 1 month of age, marked right axis deviation may occur normally, and it is difficult to define standards of abnormality. In infants between 1 and 3 months of age, abnormal right axis deviation is probably present if the mean electrical axis lies to the right of +140°.

CAUSES OF RIGHT AXIS DEVIATION

1 Right axis deviation is a *normal variant* in children, young adults, and asthenic individuals (Fig. 19-1).
2 It is seen in *pulmonary emphysema with or without cor pulmonale* (see Figs. 10-11, 18-6).
3 It occurs occasionally in *superior or anterolateral myocardial infarction* when the initial and mean QRS vectors are rotated rightward. Leads

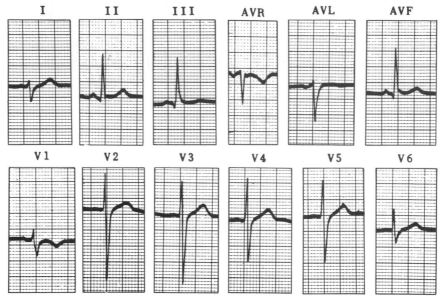

Fig. 19-1   Right axis deviation (about +105°) in a young adult without heart disease.   The electrocardiogram is normal.

Fig. 19-2   Extensive anterior myocardial infarction with abnormal right axis deviation (+130°) resulting from the presence of an unusually deep Q wave in lead I.

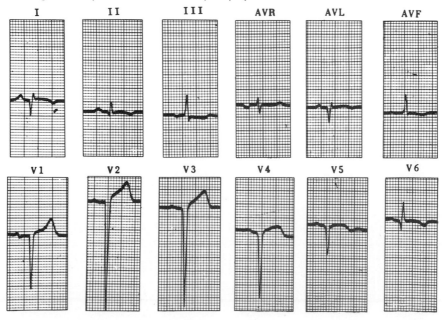

I and aVL then show unusually deep and broad Q waves (Figs. 19-2, 19-3).

4   Its most frequent cause is *right ventricular enlargement* (see Figs. 10-8, 10-9, 10-11, 23-4), which is usually associated with one or more of the following: abnormal right axis deviation of the mean QRS vector, a rightward and anteriorly directed initial QRS vector, a rightward and anteriorly directed terminal QRS vector.   From a pattern standpoint, there is no Q_2 and no Q_3 or a Q_3 that is less than 0.04 s wide.   The reader is referred to the section on right ventricular enlargement in Chap. 10 for further details.

5   Another cause of right axis deviation is *acute cor pulmonale* (see Fig. 18-2), which may be associated with a variety of electrocardiographic findings, as described in the section on acute cor pulmonale in Chap. 18.   In this condition, the electrocardiographic changes are transitory. From a vector standpoint, the initial QRS vector is directed somewhat superiorly and the mean QRS vector is vertical or rightward.   Occasionally, the terminal vector may point rightward and anteriorly.   The S-T vector points away from the right ventricle, and the T vector is normal unless ischemia is present.   From a pattern standpoint, there is frequently a prominent S_1 and often an abnormal Q_3 but no Q_2; also, the S-T segments in the right precordial leads are depressed, but the T waves are upright or inverted.

6   *Left posterior fascicular block* is another cause of right axis deviation (Figs. 11-22, 11-23).   It is characterized by an initial 0.02-s QRS vector that is directed leftward and superiorly, producing 0.02-s R waves in leads aVL and I and 0.02-s Q waves in leads, II, III, and

Fig. 19-3 Extensive anterior and superior myocardial infarction with abnormal right axis deviation (about +120°) due to a qrS deflection in lead I.   This finding, together with the presence of a QS deflection in lead aVL, is indicative of destruction of the lateral free wall of the left ventricle.

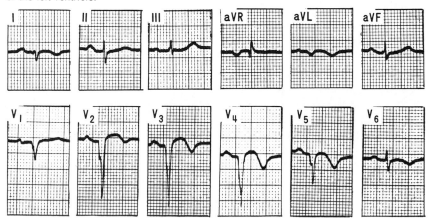

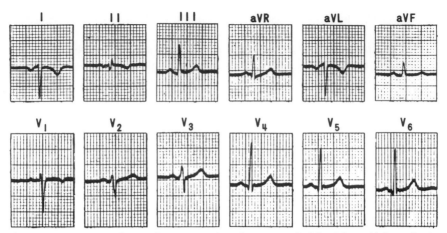

Fig. 19-4 Factitious right axis deviation resulting from reversal of the right and left arm leads. Lead I is the mirror image of the correct lead I; leads II and III are reversed; lead aVR is really lead aVL; and lead aVL is really lead aVR. The precordial leads are unaffected. The negative P and T waves in lead I are also the result of the technical error.

aVF. The main and terminal QRS forces are oriented inferiorly and to the right (beyond +90 and usually close to +120°), producing an S wave in leads aVL and I and rather tall R waves in leads II, III, and aVF. The QRS loop rotates CW in the frontal plane. The diagnosis of left posterior fascicular block is clinical as well as electrocardiographic. It is necessary to exclude a vertical heart, emphysema, right ventricular enlargement, and lateral infarction as causes of the right axis deviation.

7 *Inferior myocardial infarction with left posterior fascicular block* (Figs. 13-32, 13-36) is also a cause of right axis deviation. From a vector standpoint, it is characterized by an initial vector that is directed leftward and markedly superiorly and a terminal vector that points inferiorly and rightward, which produce right axis deviation. The angle between the initial and terminal vectors is 110° or more. The S-T vector points toward the infarct, the T vector away from it. From a pattern standpoint, there are abnormal Q waves in leads II, III, and aVF and rS patterns in leads I and aVL. An R′ wave does not occur in lead V₁. The right axis deviation that may complicate inferior myocardial infarction is probably due to a conduction defect involving the posterior division of the left bundle branch. Excitation spreads inferiorly and rightward from the fibers of the anterior division, which results in right axis deviation of the terminal QRS vector.

8 Right axis deviation is a common finding in *dextrocardia*.

9 *Reversal of the right and left arm leads* may produce factitious right axis deviation (Fig. 19-4).

10 Right axis deviation has been reported in *hyperpotassemia*.

11 Right axis deviation may be found in *right bundle branch block* and rarely in *left bundle branch block*. Its diagnostic significance in the presence of these entities is discussed in Chap. 11.

CHAPTER 20

LEFT AXIS DEVIATION

Left axis deviation is present when the mean electrical axis lies between +29 and −89°.

Abnormal left axis deviation is present in adults when the mean electrical axis lies between −30 and −89°. Left axis deviation with the mean electrical axis between +29 and −29° is a normal variant in adults and merely indicates a horizontal axis.

Abnormal left axis deviation is present in children when the mean electrical axis lies to the left of +60° in the first week of life, to the left of +20° from 1 week to 3 months of age, and to the left of 0° from 3 months to 16 years of age.

In this chapter, the term *left axis deviation* is used to designate abnormal left axis deviation even when the qualifying adjective is omitted.

CAUSES OF ABNORMAL LEFT AXIS DEVIATION

1 *Left anterior fascicular block* (see Figs. 11-20, 11-21, 20-1A) is the most common cause of abnormal left axis deviation. It is characterized by an initial 0.02-s QRS vector in the frontal plane that is directed inferiorly and rightward, producing 0.02-s Q waves in leads aVL and I and 0.02-s R waves in leads II, III, and aVF. A terminal positive deflection is seen in leads aVL and aVR. The mean and terminal QRS forces in the frontal plane are directed leftward and superiorly to −45° or more, resulting in deeps waves in leads II, III, and aVF. The QRS

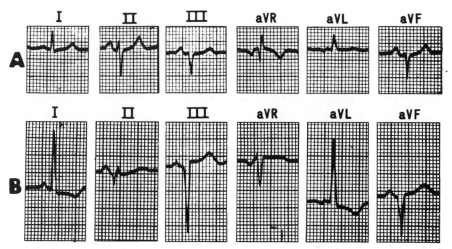

Fig. 20-1   Abnormal left axis deviation due to left anterior fascicular block (*A*) compared with abnormal left axis deviation due to inferior myocardial infarction with left anterior fascicular block (*B*).   Note that in lead II there is an rS complex in *A* and a QR deflection in *B*.

loop rotates CCW in the frontal plane.   To make the diagnosis of left anterior fascicular block with certainty, anomalous atrioventricular excitation, emphysema, right ventricular apical pacing, hyperpotassemia, and inferior myocardial infarction should be excluded as causes of the abnormal left axis deviation.   The $S_1S_2S_3$ syndrome may mimic left anterior fascicular block or vice versa.   In the $S_1S_2S_3$ syndrome, S_2 is usually greater than S_3, whereas in left anterior fascicular block S_3 is usually deeper than S_2.

2   *Anterior myocardial infarction with left anterior fascicular block* is a common and important cause of left axis deviation (see Figs. 13-33, 13-35, 13-36, 13-37).   From the vector standpoint, it is characterized by a terminal QRS vector that is directed leftward and superiorly.   The initial QRS vector points away from the location of the infarct.   The angle between the initial and terminal QRS vectors is 110° or more.   From a pattern standpoint, with the exception of anteroseptal infarcts, which produce no Q wave abnormalities in the limb leads, there are abnormal Q waves in leads I and aVL and/or an initial R wave, 0.04 s or more wide, in leads II, III, and aVF.   These leads thus show rS patterns.   The findings in the precordial leads depend on the location of the infarct.   An R' wave is present in lead V_1 or V_2 if the terminal vector is also directed anteriorly.

3   *Left ventricular hypertrophy* is often complicated by abnormal left axis deviation (see Figs. 10-4, 11-21).   The mechanism is probably left anterior fascicular block due to myocardial fibrosis.   The electrocar-

diogram shows diagnostic signs of left ventricular enlargement. The angle between the initial and terminal vectors is narrow.

4 *Chronic coronary artery disease* may cause left axis deviation even in the absence of myocardial infarction (see Figs. 11-20, 20-1A). The mechanism is probably block of the anterior division of the left bundle branch. The angle between the initial and terminal QRS vectors is narrow, and voltage abnormalities of left ventricular enlargement are lacking, although S-T and T vector abnormalities resembling the left ventricular strain pattern may occur.

5 Some cases of *pulmonary emphysema* are associated with left axis deviation (see Fig. 20-2). The mechanism in this condition is not completely understood but is probably extracardiac, hence the designation pseudo left axis deviation for this abnormality in emphysema (see also page 203).

From a vector standpoint, the angle between the initial and terminal QRS vectors is narrow, but occasionally it may be wide. Associated electrocardiographic findings may be helpful in establishing emphysema as the cause of left axis deviation: low voltage in the limb and precordial leads, predominantly negative QRS complexes in the precordial leads, a rightward P vector, and the P pulmonale pattern.

6 *Diffuse myocardial diseases* (cardiomyopathy, amyloidosis, myocarditis, etc.) are infrequent causes of abnormal left axis deviation because of their relative rarity, but left axis deviation occurs commonly in these entities.

7 *Inferior infarction* may be associated with left axis deviation due to left

Fig. 20-2 Pseudo left axis deviation (about −90°) due to emphysema. There is low voltage in the extremity leads and in lead V_6. The P vector points inferiorly. The combination of a vertical axis of the P wave and left axis deviation of the QRS complex, especially when associated with low voltage in leads I and V_6 and right atrial abnormality, should suggest the diagnosis of emphysema.

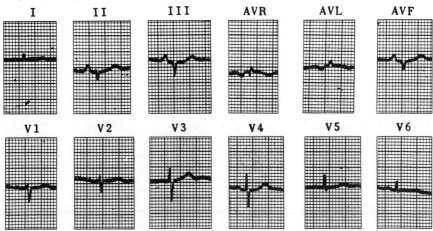

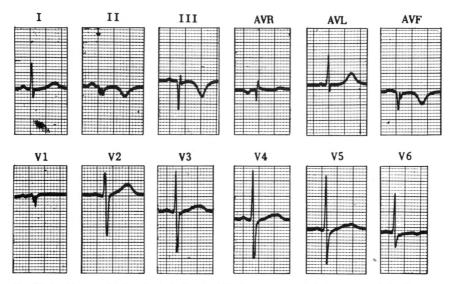

Fig. 20-3   Abnormal left axis deviation ($-40°$) due to recent inferior myocardial infarction. There are abnormal Q waves and inverted T waves in leads II, III, and aVF.

anterior fascicular block when the initial QRS vector is directed markedly superiorly and leftward and the terminal QRS vector likewise points leftward (see Figs. 13-40A, 13-41, 20-1B). This is sometimes the result of multiple infarctions but may also occur in large diaphragmatic infarcts. From a pattern standpoint, there are deep and wide QS deflections in leads III and aVF, with a QR or qrS pattern in lead II. Inferior infarction may cause left axis deviation in the absence of left anterior hemiblock if there are unusually deep Q waves in the inferior leads (Fig. 20-3).

8 Left axis deviation may also occur in *congenital heart disease* in such malformations as ostium primum defects (see Fig. 23-6), atrioventricularis communis, tricuspid atresia, single ventricle, left ventricular endocardial fibroelastosis, ventricular septal defects, coarctation of the aorta, anomalous origin of the left coronary artery from the pulmonary trunk, large pulmonary AV fistula, and aortic stenosis A conduction defect in the left ventricle or a congenital anomaly of the conduction system may be responsible for the left axis deviation in some of these conditions.

9 Other causes of left axis deviation include *hyperpotassemia, the W-P-W syndrome, acute pulmonary embolism,* Lev's disease, some neuromuscular diseases, right ventricular ectopic rhythms.

10 Left axis deviation may be found in either *right or left bundle branch block* (see Figs. 11-15, 11-24 to 11-26). Its diagnostic significance in the presence of these entities is discussed in Chap. 11.

11   Epidemiologic studies have shown that abnormal left axis deviation is fairly common among apparently *healthy people*. While this finding may be an indicator of latent coronary artery disease, it is also possible that it may be a benign comcomitant of aging. Actuarial data suggest that persons with left axis deviation alone have no significant excess mortality in general or a higher proportion of cardiac deaths in particular when compared with persons at standard risk.

REFERENCES

Banta, H. D., J. C. Greenfield, Jr., and E. H. Estes, Jr.: Left Axis Deviation, *Am. J. Cardiol.*, 14: 330, 1964.

Corne, R. A., T. W. Parkin, R. O. Brandenburg, and A. L. Brown, Jr.: Significance of Marked Left Axis Deviation: Electrocardiographic-Pathologic Correlative Study, *Am. J. Cardiol.*, 15: 605, 1965.

Curd, G. W., Jr., W. M. Hicks, Jr., and F. Gyorkey: Marked Left Axis Deviation: Indication of Cardiac Abnormality, *Am. Heart J.*, 62: 462, 1961.

Eliot, R. S., W. A. Millhon, and J. Millhon: The Clinical Significance of Uncomplicated Marked Left Axis Deviation in Men without Known Diseases, *Am. J. Cardiol.*, 12:767 1963.

Entman, M. L., E. H. Estes, Jr., and D. B. Hackel: The Pathologic Basis of the Electrocardiographic Pattern on Parietal Block, *Am. Heart J.*, 74:202, 1967.

Grant R. P.: "Clinical Electrocardiography," McGraw-Hill, New York, 1957.

———: Left Axis Deviation, *Mod. Concepts Cardiovasc. Dis.*, 27: 437, 1958.

Libanoff, A. J.: Marked Left Axis Deviation, *Am. J. Cardiol.*, 14: 339, 1964.

Ostrander, L. D.: Left Axis Deviation: Prevalence Associated Conditions, and Prognosis, *Ann. Intern. Med.*, 75: 23, 1971.

Pryor, R., and S. G. Blount, Jr.: The Clinical Significance of True Left Axis Deviation: Left Intraventricular Blocks, *Am. Heart J.* 72: 391, 1966

Saka, S. K., and C. Fisch: The Electrocardiogram and Vectorcardiogram with Abnormal Left Axis Deviation, *J. Electrocardiol.*, 1: 199, 1968.

Yano, K., G. M. Peskoe, et al.: Left Axis Deviation and Left Anterior Hemiblock among 8,000 Japanese-American Men, *Am. J. Cardiol.*, 35: 809, 1975.

CHAPTER 21

MISCELLANEOUS DISORDERS

$S_1S_2S_3$ SYNDROME (FIGS. 18-4, 21-1 TO 21-5)

The $S_1S_2S_3$ syndrome is characterized by the following electrocardiographic findings: (1) predominantly negative deflections of the S wave type in the three standard limb leads, with the S wave greater or equal to the R wave in each lead, (2) a normal QRS interval, and (3) usually an R' wave in lead V_1.

From a vector standpoint it simply means that the terminal QRS vector is directed rightward and superiorly and usually anteriorly.

The $S_1S_2S_3$ pattern may occur as a normal variant, particularly in young people. The electrocardiogram then is otherwise normal, and the electrical axis is usually indeterminate. More frequently the $S_1S_2S_3$ syndrome is indicative of abnormality. It is seen in right ventricular enlargement due to congenital heart disease, especially in complete transposition of the great vessels, tetralogy of Fallot, and ventricular septal defect. It is observed in emphysema with or without cor pulmonale and sometimes in other types of acquired heart disease with right ventricular enlargement. Lastly, it may occur in myocardial infarction in the absence of a complicating acute cor pulmonale.

The $S_1S_2S_3$ syndrome sometimes may have to be differentiated from left anterior fascicular block. When this problem arises, an S_2 that is greater than S_3 supports the diagnosis of the $S_1S_2S_3$ syndrome. Conversely, when S_3 is deeper than S_2, the diagnosis of left anterior fascicular block is more likely.

HYPOTHERMIA (FIG. 21-6)

During hypothermia, characteristic changes occur in the electrocardiogram. As the temperature decreases, there is progressive slowing of the sinus rate, T wave inversion, and prolongation of the P-R, QRS, and Q-T intervals. Atrial flutter and fibrillation are seen frequently. Ventricular premature systoles and ventricular fibrillation may also occur. However, the most distinctive electrocardiographic feature of hypothemia is the presence of a slow, usually positive wave, called the *J deflection*, or *Osborn wave*, which is inscribed during the terminal portion of the QRS complex. It is found consistently when body temperatures are below 25°C. The origin of this deflection is unknown.

CARDIOMYOPATHY

Almost any type of electrocardiographic abnormality may be seen in cardiomyopathies. The electrocardiogram is abnormal in almost every case.

Fig. 21-1 $S_1S_2S_3$ syndrome due to emphysema and cor pulmonale with right atrial enlargement. There are deep S waves in all three standard limb leads. The P pulmonale pattern is present. There are rS complexes in the precordial leads.

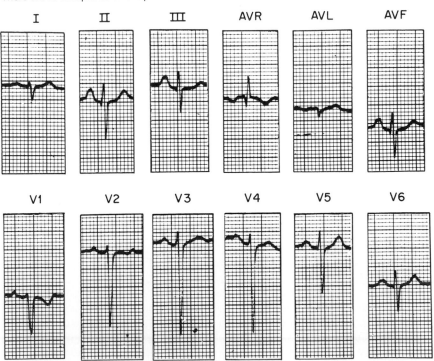

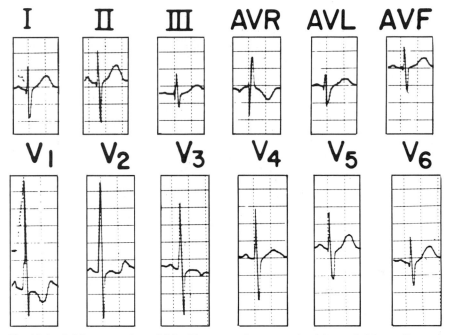

Fig. 21-2 $S_1S_2S_3$ pattern in a child with a secundum type of atrial septal defect. Signs of right ventricular enlargement (tall R wave in lead V_1 and deep S waves in leads V_5 and V_6) are also present.

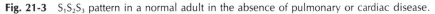

Fig. 21-3 $S_1S_2S_3$ pattern in a normal adult in the absence of pulmonary or cardiac disease.

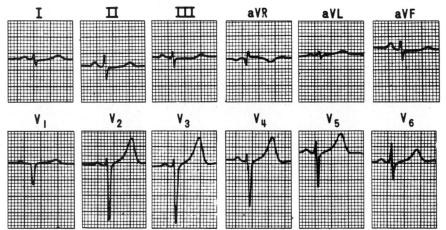

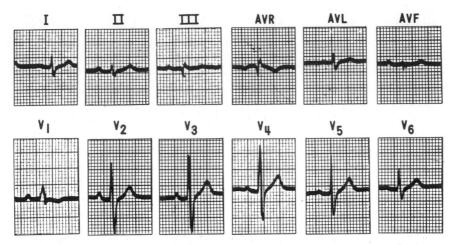

Fig. 21-4 $S_1S_2S_3$ pattern in 50-year-old man with mitral stenosis and right ventricular hypertrophy. There is a broad R wave in lead V_1 with an R/S ratio greater than 1.0.

1   Abnormalities of the P wave occur in 30 to 84 percent of cases. The most common abnormality is a broad, notched P wave with an increased P terminal force in lead V_1 that suggests left atrial abnormality or enlargement, or an intraatrial conduction defect. Patterns of right or combined atrial enlargement are seen less commonly.

2   Incomplete AV block is fairly frequent, but complete AV block is uncommon except in Chagas' disease. A short P-R interval may be seen in glycogen storage disease.

3   The preexcitation syndrome has been reported in familial forms of cardiomyopathy.

4   Left ventricular enlargement is quite common, but right ventricular

Fig. 21-5 $S_1S_2S_3$ pattern in a patient with extensive anterior myocardial infarction. There was no evidence of complicating pulmonary disease, acute cor pulmonale, or right ventricular hypertrophy.

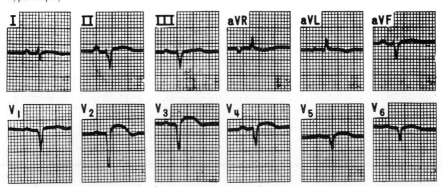

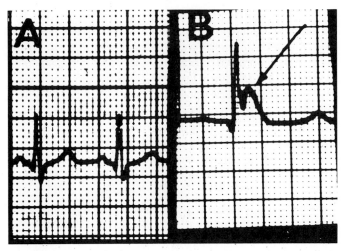

Fig. 21-6 Hypothermia. (A) Control tracing. The body temperature is 101.5°F. (B) Recording from the same patient as in A at a time when the body temperature was 78°F. Note the broad QRS complexes and the prolongation of the P-R interval. The arrow points to the J deflection, or Osborn wave.

enlargement is infrequent except in restrictive cardiomyopathies and endomyocardial fibrosis.

5 Pseudoinfarction patterns are seen frequently in idiopathic hypertrophic subaortic stenosis (Figs. 13-18 to 13-20,) amyloidosis, and to a lesser extent in Duchenne's muscular dystrophy, alcoholic cardiomyopathy, and other myocardoses.

6 Low voltage is often seen in idiopathic cardiomyopathy, amyloidosis, and endomyocardial fibrosis.

7 All types of ventricular conduction defects, especially left bundle branch block, left anterior fascicular block, and bifascicular block, are often noted.

8 Nonspecific S-T-T abnormalities are present in virtually all cases.

9 Almost any type of arrhythmia may occur, but ventricular premature systoles and atrial fibrillation are the most common dysrhythmias.

10 Distinctive electrocardiographic features are found in certain types of cardiomyopathy. *Idiopathic hypertrophic subaortic stenosis* is discussed in Chap. 23. In *cardiac amyloidosis*, generally a disease of the elderly, low voltage of the QRS complexes (especially in the limb leads), left axis deviation, QS or rS complexes in the right precordial leads, atrial arrhythmias, and varying degrees of AV block are characteristic findings. The diagnostic features of *Duchenne's muscular dystrophy* are tall R waves in the right precordial leads, abnormal Q waves in the limb and left precordial leads, and both supraventricular and ventricular arrhythmias. *Glycogen storage disease* is typified by high voltage of the QRS complexes and a short P-R interval. In *African*

endomyocardial fibrosis, low voltage of the QRS complexes in the limb leads and signs of right ventricular enlargement are a frequent occurrence. In *Chagas'* disease, which is a panmyocarditis, the usual findings are right bundle branch block with left anterior fascicular block; less commonly, left posterior fascicular block; and least commonly, left bundle branch block or nonspecific ventricular conduction defects. Complete AV block may occur. Ventricular extrasystoles and atrial arrhythmias are common. Abnormal Q waves and symmetrically inverted T waves are sometimes observed. In severe, acute Chagas' disease, right bundle branch block and a monophasic pattern of subepicardial injury may be recorded (Fig. 13-21). *Friedreich's ataxia* is characterized by T wave changes, especially in leads II, III, and aVF, nonspecific S-T-T abnormalities, signs of isolated or biventricular hypertrophy, bundle branch block, AV conduction disturbances, and arrhythmias such as inappropriate sinus tachycardia, premature beats, atrial fibrillation, and atrial paroxysmal tachycardia.

ELECTROCARDIOGRAPHIC CHANGES AFTER CEREBROVASCULAR ACCIDENTS AND NEUROSURGICAL PROCEDURES (FIGS. 21-7, 21-8)

Electrocardiographic abnormalities may occur after cerebrovascular accidents and various neurosurgical procedures. However, they have been reported predominantly in patients with subarachnoid hemorrhage. The mechanism of these changes is unknown. They may be seen in the absence of both associated heart disease and electrolyte imbalance. The electrocardiographic abnormalities are described in this section because they are often mistaken for those produced by ischemic heart disease.

1   The abnormalities are usually most clearly demonstrable in leads I, aVL, and V_4 to V_6.
2   Usually the T waves are predominantly affected. They may be flattened but more often are abnormally broad and deeply inverted, with contours that are strongly suggestive of ischemia. Large positive T waves may also be noted.
3   Ischemic S-T segment changes, marked prolongation of the Q-T interval, large U waves, and abnormal Q waves may also be seen.
4   The abnormalities appear to be reversible and usually subside spontaneously over a period of time.

THE MITRAL VALVE PROLAPSE SYNDROME

The mitral valve prolapse syndrome is a relatively common disorder found in about 6 percent of healthy young women. It is characterized by the

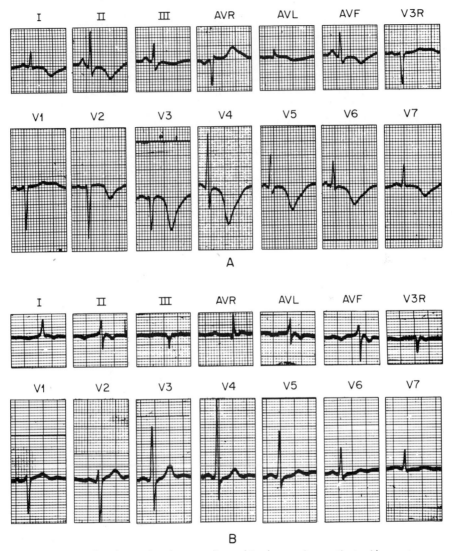

Fig. 21-7 Record *A* shows the electrocardiographic changes in a patient with spontaneous subarachnoid hemorrhage but without clinical evidence of heart disease. The Q-T interval is markedly prolonged. There are wide, deeply inverted T waves in the precordial and extremity leads. The patient recovered. Record *B*, taken a few months later, is entirely within normal limits.

occurrence of midsystolic clicks and/or late systolic or holosystolic murmurs. The prolapse involves usually either the posterior leaflet or both leaflets. Involvement of the anterior leaflet alone is less common. Myxomatous degeneration of the leaflets is the most characteristic histologic finding. The syndrome is sometimes associated with other cardiac diseases.

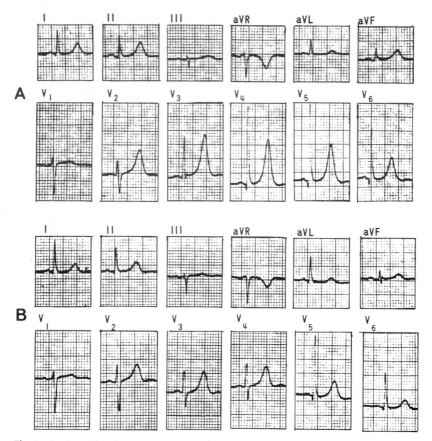

Fig. 21-8   Record *A* shows tall precordial T waves in a patient with spontaneous subarachnoid hemorrhage.   Record *B*, taken five days later, shows complete resolution of the T wave changes.

Electrocardiographic Findings

1   The most typical changes are flattened or inverted T waves in leads II, III, and aVF with or without nonspecific S-T segment depression. Sometimes, the T wave changes are confined to the precordial leads; less commonly, they are diffuse.

2   Prominent U waves and slightly prolonged Q-T intervals may occur.

3   In rare instances, abnormal Q waves and S-T segment elevations suggestive of myocardial infarction have been described.

4   Ventricular preexcitation seems to occur more frequently than would be expected in a comparable population.

5   Cardiac arrhythmias occur in routine resting electrocardiograms in about 50 percent of cases.   Premature ventricular systoles are the most common arrhythmia.   They may be unifocal or multifocal, exhibit group beating, or occur in pairs.   Paroxysmal ventricular tachycardia and

ventricular fibrillation sometimes occur and may produce syncope and even sudden death.   Atrial premature beats, supraventricular tachycardia, atrial fibrillation, sinus node dysfunction, and AV block are also seen.

6   False-positive exercise tests.

PECTUS EXCAVATUM

Although cardiac dysfunction is rare in this disorder, the electrocardiogram may mimic organic heart disease.   The following findings have been observed:

1   An entirely negative P wave in lead V_1.
2   An rSr′ pattern in lead V_1; less commonly, a Qr pattern in this lead.
3   Abnormal Q waves simulating anterior or inferior myocardial infarction, especially the former.   T wave inversions may also be present.
4   Paroxysmal supraventricular tachycardias have been reported in some cases.
5   False-positive exercise tests have also been noted.

STRAIGHT BACK SYNDROME

Most of the electrocardiographic findings are probably related to cardiac displacement. An rSr′ pattern in V_1, nonspecific T wave changes, abnormal left axis deviation, and pseudoinfarction patterns have been described.

ELECTROCARDIOGRAPHIC POOR OR REVERSED R WAVE PROGRESSION IN THE RIGHT PRECORDIAL LEADS (FIGS. 10-4, 10-11, 13-15, 18-4, 21-9, 21-10, 21-11)

Electrocardiograms showing poor or reversed R wave progression occur in approximately 8 percent and 2 percent, respectively, of routine tracings recorded in hospitalized patients.

Poor R wave progression (PRWP) is considered to be present if the absolute magnitude of the R wave is 3.0 mm or less in V_3 and the R wave in lead V_2 is equal to or smaller than the R wave in lead V_3.   In the series reported by Zema and Kligfield, the causes of PRWP were as follows: normal variant, 38 percent; anterior myocardial infarction, 35 percent; left ventricular hypertrophy, 14 percent; and right ventricular hypertrophy, 13 percent.

PRWP may also be observed in diffuse pulmonary disease (in the presence or absence of cor pulmonale), left bundle branch block, left

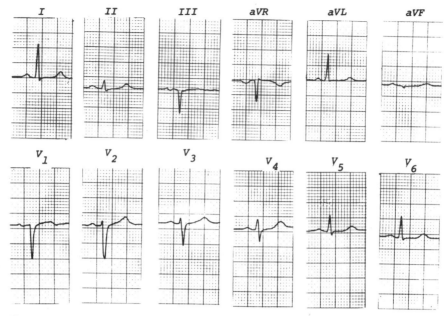

Fig. 21-9 Poor R wave progression in a healthy young woman.

anterior fascicular block, diffuse or localized myocardial disease (e.g., cardiomyopathy, myocarditis, scleroderma, neuromuscular disorders), mitral valve prolapse, and idiopathic hypertrophic subaortic stenosis.

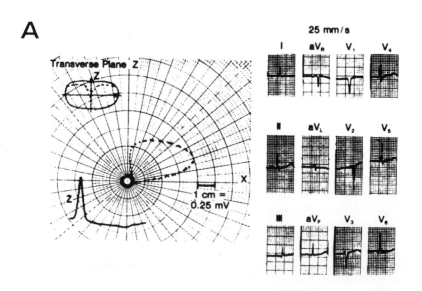

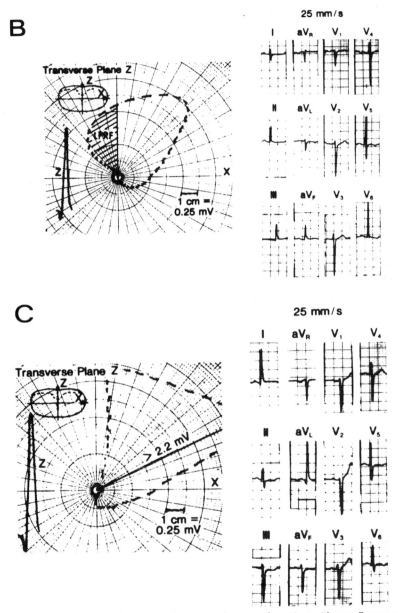

Fig. 21-10 Electrocardiogram and vectorcardiogram of a patient with poor R wave progression due to anterior myocardial infarction (*A*), right ventricular hypertrophy (*B*), and left ventricular hypertrophy (*C*). (*From M. J. Zema and P. Kligfield, Arch. Intern. Med., 142: 1145, 1982. Copyright 1982 by the American Medical Association. Used by permission.*)

Diagnostic Approach

Rule out precordial lead misplacement as a possible cause of the electrocardiographic abnormality.

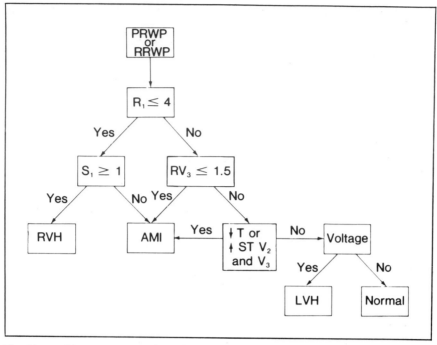

Fig. 21-11   Diagnostic approach to the patient with poor R wave progression. PRWP = poor R wave progression. RRWP = reversed R wave progression. RVH = right ventricular hypertrophy. LVH = left ventricular hypertrophy. AMI = anterior myocardial infarction. (*From M. J. Zema and P. Kligfield, Arch. Intern. Med., 142: 1145, 1982. Copyright 1982 by the American Medical Association. Used by permission.*)

Exclude left bundle branch block, localized or diffuse myocardial disease, cardiomyopathy, and the other conditions listed above as diagnostic possibilities. (See Differential Diagnosis of Myocardial Infarction, Chap. 13.)

The criteria which follow have been suggested by Zema and his coworkers as helpful in establishing the probable cause of poor or reversed R wave progression. The presence of Q waves or QS complexes and low voltage in leads V_2 and V_3 must be excluded.

1   If the R wave in lead V_3 is 1.5 mm or less or if the R wave in lead I is no greater than 4.0 mm, the most likely diagnosis is anterior myocardial infarction. This diagnosis is further supported by the presence of S-T segment elevation (greater than 2 mm) or T wave inversion, or both, in leads V_2 and V_3. When the R wave in lead V_3 exceeds 2 mm, poor R wave progression caused by anterior myocardial infarction is unlikely. Reversed R wave progression, as previously indicated, is more common in anterior myocardial infarction.

2   If the R wave in lead I is 4.0 mm or less and the S wave in this lead is

at least 1.0 mm deep, right ventricular enlargement (most often cor pulmonale) is the most likely cause.

3   If the criteria in 1 or 2 are not met, left ventricular enlargement is the most appropriate diagnosis provided voltage criteria for his condition are fulfilled. If, in addition to left ventricular enlargement, the R wave in lead V_3 is 1.5 mm or less, concomitant anterior myocardial infarction is likely to be present.

Reversed R wave progression (RRWP) is described as the presence of decreasing R wave amplitudes in consecutive right precordial leads so that the R wave in lead V_2 is less than the R wave in lead V_2, and/ or the R wave in lead V_4 is less than the R wave in lead V_3. The R wave voltage in lead V_3 or V_4 is 3.0 mm of less. Reversal of the normal R wave trend is more common in anterior myocardial infarction, but is not pathognomonic of this disorder since it may occur in left ventricular enlargement (see Fig. 13-16) and some of the other conditions listed in the preceding paragraph.

4   In the absence of the criteria described in 1, 2, and 3, the most probable cause for PRWP is a normal variant.

Comments

In the author's experience, chronic obstructive pulmonary disease with or without cor pulmonale is more commonly a cause of PRWP than right ventricular enlargement. The presence of rS complexes in all of the standard precordial leads is typical of chronic pulmonary disease. It should be emphasized that incorrect precordial electrode placement is commonly responsible for the pattern of PRWP in routine tracings.

The criteria of Zema and Kligfield have an acceptable degree of sensitivity and specificity, but often no definite etiologic diagnosis can be made with certainty.

REFERENCES

Bahl, O. P., and E. Massie: Electrocardiographic and Vectorcardiographic Patterns in Cardiomyopathy, *Cardiovasc. Clin.*, 4 (1): 95, 1972.

Bekheit, S., and A. Ali: QT Interval in Idiopathic Prolapsed Mitral Valve, *Am. J. Cardiol.*, 41: 374, 1978.

Burch, G. E., R. Myers, and J. A. Abildskov: A New Electrocardiographic Pattern Observed in Cerebrovascular Accidents, *Circulation*, 9: 719, 1954.

———— and J. H. Phillips: The Large Upright T Wave as an Electrocardiographic Manifestation of Intracranial Disease, *Southern Med. J.*, 61: 331, 1968.

DeLeon, A. C., J. K. Perloff, H. Twigg, and M. Majd: The Straight Back Syndrome, Clinical Cardiovascular Manifestations, *Circulation*, 32: 193, 1965.

DeMaria, A. N., E. A. Amsterdam, L. A. Vismara, A. Neumann, and D. T. Mason: Arrhythmias in the Mitral Valve Prolapse Syndrome, *Ann. Intern. Med.*, 84: 656, 1976.

deOliveira, J. M., M. P. Sambhi, and H. A. Zimmerman: The Electrocardiogram in Pectus Excavatum, *Br. Heart J.*, 20: 495, 1958.

Elisberg, E. I.: Electrocardiographic Changes Associated with Pectus Excavatum, *Ann. Intern. Med.*, 49: 30, 1958.

Engel, P. J., B. L. Alpert, J. H. Triebwasser, and M. C. Lancaster: Exercise Testing in Mitral Valve Prolapse, *Am. J. Cardiol.*, 41: 430, 1978.

Moeler, J. H., R. D. White, R. C. Anderson, and P. Adams Jr.: Significance of the $S_1S_2S_3$ Electrocardiographic Pattern in Children, *Am. J. Cardiol.*, 16: 524, 1965.

Trevino, A., B. Razi, and B. M. Beller: The Characteristic Electrocardiogram of Accidental Hypothermia, *Arch. Intern. Med.*, 127: 470, 1971.

Zema, M. J. and P. Kligfield: ECG Poor R Wave Progression—Review and Synthesis, *Arch. Intern. Med.*, 142: 1145, 1982.

CHAPTER 22

THE NORMAL ELECTROCARDIOGRAM IN INFANTS AND CHILDREN

The evolution of the electrocardiogram in infancy and childhood is a dynamic process, dramatic during the first week of life and more gradual thereafter. At birth, there is a relative or even an absolute right ventricular preponderance. As the child grows older the relative sizes of the right and left ventricles eventually reach adult proportions. The evolutionary changes in the QRS complex and T wave which take place during childhood mirror the gradual regression of right ventricular preponderance and the eventual emergence of left ventricular dominance.

Figures 22-1 and 22-2 are examples of a normal electrocardiogram in a newborn infant and a child, respectively.

P WAVE

The mean P vector in the frontal plane ranges widely in normal infants and children (Table 22-1).

The P wave is upright in leads I, II, and aVF, inverted in lead aVR, and variable in leads III and aVL. The P wave is usually upright in the precordial leads during infancy and diphasic in the older child. The maximum P amplitude is 2.5 mm. The duration of the P wave is usually less than 0.07 s up to 1 year of age and less than 0.09 s up to the age of 14 years.

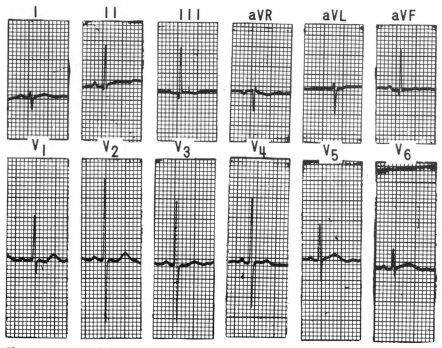

Fig. 22-1 A normal electrocardiogram in a one-day-old infant. There is right axis deviation (+105°). There is right ventricular preponderance, with dominant R waves in the precordial leads. The positive T wave in lead V_1 is a normal finding at this age.

P-R INTERVAL

The P-R interval increases primarily with age rather than with changes in heart rate.

QRS COMPLEX

During the first week of life the full-term infant's electrocardiogram shows right ventricular dominance. In the precordial leads, a monophasic R wave is commonly present in leads V_{4R} and V_1, the R/S ratio is greater than 1.0 in lead V_1, and an rS complex is seen in lead V_6. The R wave tends to decrease and the S waves to increase in size as the electrode is moved to the left. The mean QRS axis in the frontal plane at this time is generally rightward, averaging between +128° and +137°. Low voltage is commonly present during the first day of life, but persistence of this finding is unusual.

The premature infant's electrocardiogram is frequently indistinguishable from that of the full-term infant. Occasionally the premature infant may show low voltage in all leads, a wide range of the QRS axis in the frontal

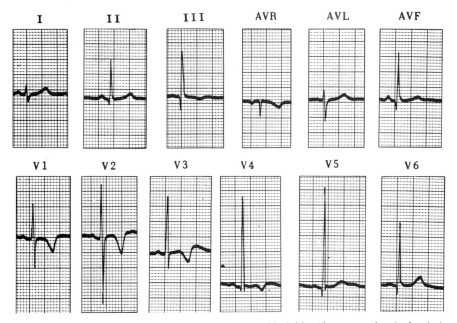

Fig. 22-2 A normal electrocardiogram in a 6-year-old child. The mean electrical axis is vertical. There is a normal juvenile T wave pattern. The voltages are within normal limits for a child of this age.

plane, and left ventricular dominance in the precordial leads, with an R/S ratio equal to or less than 1.0 in lead V_1 and a qR pattern in V_6. The R wave progression in the precordial leads may resemble the adult pattern.

By 3 months of age, the R and S waves in the normal child become equiphasic in the right-sided precordial leads. The R wave then increases, and the S wave decreases as the electrode is moved to the left. The left-sided precordial leads may show deep, narrow Q waves.

TABLE 22–1   THE MEANS OF P AND QRS VECTORS IN NORMAL INFANTS AND CHILDREN

Age	P axis			QRS axis		
	Average	Minimum	Maximum	Average	Minimum	Maximum
0–24 hours	60	−30	90	137	75	190
1 day–1 month	58	0	120	115	−5	190
1–6 months	56	30	90	72	35	135
6 months–1 year	55	−30	75	64	30	135
1–12 years	50	−30	75	66	−15	120
12–16 years	54	0	90	66	−15	110

SOURCE: Modified from R. F. Ziegler, "Electrocardiographic Studies in Normal Infants and Children," Charles C Thomas, Publisher, Springfield, Ill., 1951.

The amplitude of the R wave in lead V_1 exceeds that of lead V_6 from birth to 6 months of age. From 6 months to 1 year, the R waves are approximately equal in amplitude. After 1 year of age, the amplitude of the R wave in lead V_6 exceeds that of lead V_1.

As noted above, the mean QRS vector at birth is markedly rightward, more or less parallel to the lead I axis. By the age of 3 months it is more vertical and perpendicular to the lead I axis and this points inferiorly. By adolescence the mean QRS vector is rotated slightly leftward, often parallel to the lead II axis. From the late teens until the third decade of life the mean QRS vector becomes more vertical again. Normal values for the mean QRS axis at various ages are listed in Table 22-1.

By the age of 5 years, the precordial electrocardiogram basically resembles that of the adult (Fig. 22-2).

The crista pattern, consisting of an R' wave in lead V_1 or V_3, or both, with a normal QRS interval is a frequent normal variant in children.

The maximum normal duration of the QRS complex is 0.08 s under 3 years of age, 0.09 s between 3 and 12 years, and 0.10 s above the age of 12.

S-T SEGMENT

Upward displacement of the S-T segment, not exceeding 2 mm, may be seen in the limb leads. After 1 year of age, the S-T segment may be elevated as much as 3 mm in the right precordial leads normally.

T WAVE

During the first week of life the T waves undergo striking changes. At birth, the T wave is upright in the limb leads (leads I and aVL) and in the precordial leads. During the phase between 1 and 6 hours after birth, the T wave becomes inverted in leads I, aVL, and V_6 and shows increased positivity in the right precordial leads. From 3 to 7 days after birth, the T wave becomes upright in leads I, II, aVF, and V_6 and inverted in leads aVR, V_{4R}, and V_1 but is variable in leads III and aVL. Persistence of an upright T wave in lead V_1 beyond 3 to 4 days, and certainly after 7 to 10 days, is abnormal.

After the first few days of life the T wave is usually inverted from leads V_1 to V_4 or even farther to the left. This pattern may persist until the child is 3 to 5 years of age. By the age of 10 the T wave usually assumes the adult form, but the juvenile T wave pattern may sometimes persist into early adult life normally. The juvenile T wave is usually less than 3 mm deep. As the electrode position is moved from right to left, a negative or diphasic T wave does not become more negative in any lead immediately to the left except in lead V_2. In infancy and early childhood the T vector tends to point leftward and posteriorly until the age of 10 years, when it becomes more anteriorly directed.   The maximum amplitude of the T wave in the precordial leads is 8 mm whether it is positive or negative.

HEART RATE

The heart rate is quite variable, especially in newborn infants.   Rates less than 100 per minute are not uncommon in normal newborn infants.   After the first day of life, sinus tachycardia with heart rates of 180 or more beats per minute is not unusual.

QRS-T ANGLE

The QRS-T angle in children is often quite wide normally.   It may be 90° or more in either the FP or TP.

Normal values for the various deflections and intervals in children have been described in the sections dealing with the P wave, QRS complex, S-T segment, T wave, and electrical axis in Chap. 5.   The reader is referred to these sections and to the tables in the Appendix for further details.

Criteria for the diagnosis of atrial and ventricular enlargement are found in the sections dealing with these entities.

REFERENCES

Borkow, A. M., et al.: The Superior QRS Axis in Ostium Primum ASD: A Proposed Mechanism, *Am. Heart J.,* 90: 215, 1975.

Gasul, B. M., R. A. Arcilla, and M. Lev: "Heart Diseases in Children," Lippincott, Philadelphia, 1966.

Hait, G., and B. M. Gasul: The Evolution and Significance of T Wave Changes in the Newborn during the First Seven Days of Life, *Am. J. Cardiol.,* 12: 494, 1963.

James, F. W., and S. Kaplan: The Normal Electrocardiogram in the Infant and Child, *Cardiovasc. Clin.,* 5 (3): 295, 1973.

Keith, J. D., R. D. Rowe, and P. Vlad: "Heart Disease in Infancy and Childhood," 3d ed., Macmillan, New York, 1978.

Liebman, J., and R. Plonsey: Electrocardiography, in F. H. Adams (ed.): "Moss' Heart Disease in Infants, Children, and Adolescents," 3d ed., Williams & Wilkins, Baltimore, 1983.

Nadas, A. S., and D. C. Fyler: "Pediatric Cardiology," 3d ed., Saunders, Philadelphia, 1972.

Walsh, S. Z.: Evolution of the Electrocardiogram of Healthy Premature Infants during the First Year of Life, *Acta Paediat.* (Scand.), suppl. 145: 1963: 1.

Wenger, N. K., W. L. Watkins, and J. W. Hurst: A Preliminary Study of the Electrocardiogram of the Normal Premature Infant, *Am. Heart J.,* 62: 304, 1961.

Ziegler, R. F.: "Electrocardiographic Studies in Normal Infants and Children," Charles C Thomas, Springfield, Ill., 1951.

CHAPTER 23

THE ELECTROCARDIOGRAM IN CONGENITAL HEART DISEASE

A detailed discussion of the electrocardiographic findings in congenital heart disease is beyond the scope of this text. Only the salient features of the more common anomalies are presented.

UNCOMPLICATED DEXTROCARDIA WITH SITUS INVERSUS (FIG. 23-1)

1 Lead I shows inverted P waves and usually inverted QRS complexes and T waves. This pattern is the mirror image of the usual one found in lead I. The complexes in leads aVR and aVL are interchanged, as are those in leads II and III.
2 The precordial patterns are reversed. Precordial leads taken over the right chest (V_{3R} to V_{6R}) show complexes of the type usually recorded from the left side of the chest and vice versa. There is usually a progressive increase in the amplitude of the R waves from lead V_1 to lead V_{5R} or V_{6R}.

DEXTROVERSION (FIG. 23-2)

Dextroversion of the heart is almost invariably associated either singly or in combination with other cardiac anomalies, such as corrected transposition of the great vessels, pulmonic stenosis, atresia or hypoplasia of the pulmonary artery, and ventricular or atrial septal defects.

1   Lead I shows an upright P wave together with small Q and R waves.
2   The right precordial leads show R or RS deflections, while the left precordial leads show small Q and R waves.

CONGENITALLY CORRECTED TRANSPOSITION OF THE GREAT VESSELS

1   Varying degrees of AV block, including first-, second-, and third-degree block, occur in over 75 percent of cases.   Paroxysmal tachycardia, ventricular preexcitation, and atrial fibrillation may occur.

Fig. 23-1   Uncomplicated dextrocardia.

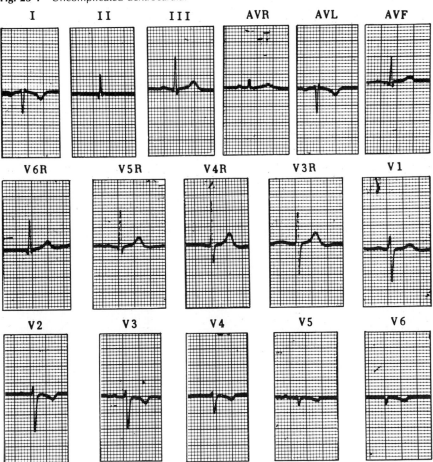

2   Left atrial or right atrial enlargement may occur, depending on the existence and severity of associated defects.
3   When the arterial ventricle is dominant, left axis deviation occurs; when the venous ventricle is dominant, the axis is vertical or deviated to the right.
4   Because septal depolarization proceeds from right to left and superiorly, Q waves are usually but not invariably present in the right precordial leads and absent in the left chest leads.   Prominent Q waves are generally found in lead III but are almost always absent in lead I.
5   The T waves are generally upright in the precordial leads, with T_{V1} taller than T_{V6}.

EBSTEIN'S ANOMALY (FIG. 23-3)

1   With few exceptions there is right axis deviation.
2   Signs of right atrial enlargement with unusually tall and peaked P waves are seen.   The P waves are frequently broad.
3   Prolongation of the P-R interval is the rule during sinus rhythm.
4   A characteristic finding is the presence of atypical complete or incomplete right bundle branch block with wide, multiphasic QRS complexes of low voltage in most, if not all, of the precordial leads.   Many cases

Fig. 23-2   Dextroversion with probable biventricular enlargement.

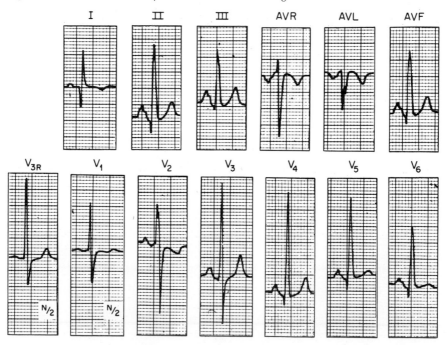

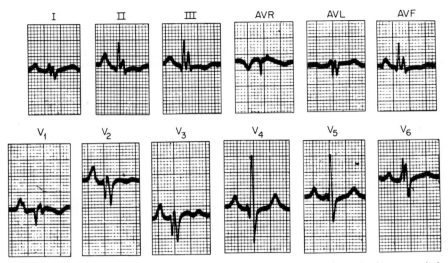

Fig. 23-3 Ebstein's anomaly. There are wide, bizarre QRS complexes in the precordial leads. The P waves are abnormally broad and tall, which indicates biatrial enlargement.

show qR patterns and T wave inversions in lead V_1 and in other right-sided chest leads.

5　Ventricular preexcitation, almost always of the Type B variety, is seen in 5 to 10 percent of cases.

6　Arrhythmias, including paroxysmal atrial fibrillation, flutter, and tachycardia, as well as premature systoles are observed frequently.

CONGENITAL AORTIC STENOSIS (SUPRAVALVULAR, VALVULAR, AND DISCRETE SUBVALVULAR)

1　The electrocardiogram is of no assistance in distinguishing between supravalvular, valvular, and subvalvular (discrete) aortic stenosis.

2　The electrocardiogram may be normal.

3　The P waves are usually normal, but left atrial enlargement may be found in about 25 percent of cases.

4　Left ventricular enlargement and strain are eventually present in most cases and are typically manifested by tall R waves and ST-T changes in leads II, III, aVF, as well as in the left precordial leads.

5　The mean frontal QRS axis is normal in the vast majority of cases.

IDIOPATHIC HYPERTROPHIC SUBAORTIC STENOSIS (FIGS. 13-18 TO 13-20)

1　The electrocardiogram is usually abnormal.

2　Left atrial and combined atrial enlargement are observed commonly.

3 Abnormal Q waves or QS complexes simulating myocardial infarction are found in almost half the cases with the familial form of the disease and in about 15 percent of the remainder.

4 The vast majority of cases show evidence of left ventricular hypertrophy.

5 Almost all cases have S-T segment depression and widening of the QRS-T angle in the frontal and transverse planes.

6 Abnormal left axis deviation occurs in 15 to 20 percent of cases.

7 Ventricular preexcitation is reported to occur in about one-fourth of cases, but this has been questioned by some authorities.

AORTIC ATRESIA

1 Right axis deviation is present.

2 Right ventricular enlargement is present.

COARCTATION OF THE AORTA

1 The electrocardiogram may be normal when coarctation is mild.

2 The P waves are usually normal, but left atrial enlargement may occur in long-standing coarctation.

3 Signs of left ventricular enlargement eventually appear in most cases. Prominent ST-T abnormalities, however, are infrequent in uncomplicated coarctation. Signs of right ventricular enlargement may sometimes be seen in infants with heart failure or preductal coarctation.

4 The mean QRS axis is usually normal, although left axis deviation occurs occasionally in older patients and right axis deviation is sometimes seen in children below 6 months of age with heart failure or preductal coarctation.

PRIMARY ENDOCARDIAL FIBROELASTOSIS

1 Sinus rhythm is the rule, although premature beats, paroxysmal supraventricular and ventricular tachycardias, and complete heart block may occur.

2 The P-R interval is usually normal but may be slightly prolonged.

3 Ventricular preexcitation sometimes occurs.

4 The P waves may be normal or may show left atrial, right atrial, or biatrial enlargement.

5 Left ventricular enlargement is a characteristic feature of the dilated type of primary endocardial fibroelastosis; right ventricular enlargement, of the contracted form of the disease.

CONGENITAL PULMONIC STENOSIS WITH AN INTACT VENTRICULAR SEPTUM (FIG. 10-9)

1 The electrocardiogram may be normal when the stenosis is mild.
2 Right atrial enlargement is usually present. Tall, peaked P waves are common as the severity increases. Giant P waves are found occasionally.
3 The P-R interval is usually normal but may be prolonged occasionally.
4 Right axis deviation is present unless the stenosis is mild. The degree of right axis deviation tends to vary with the severity of the stenosis.
5 Signs of right ventricular enlargement are present. A variety of QRS configurations may be seen in lead V_1, including rSr', rsR', a monophasic R, and qR patterns.
6 T wave inversions are frequently observed in the right precordial leads and in leads II, III, and aVF. These T wave changes in association with right axis deviation and tall 0.04-s R waves in lead V_1 are indicative of severe pulmonic stenosis (i.e., the right ventricular pressure exceeds systemic pressure). In children with mild pulmonic stenosis, upright T waves in the right chest leads may be the only abnormality present.

TETRALOGY OF FALLOT (FIGS. 10-8, 23-4)

1 The P waves are normal in about one-half of the cases. The remainder show either peaked P waves of normal amplitude or, less commonly, P waves of increased amplitude.
2 The P-R interval is usually normal.
3 Right axis deviation is present.
4 The right precordial leads show evidence of right ventricular enlargement. The usual finding is a tall R wave or variant R pattern (rR, Rs, or RS) in lead V_1. Complexes of the rS type with deep S waves are often seen in leads V_2 and V_3. In a small percentage of cases, the right precordial leads show an rsR' pattern with a normal QRS duration or a qR complex.
5 The T wave in lead V_1 is normally upright in the newborn infant, but it is invariably inverted by the third or fourth day of life and remains inverted until the age of 12 years. A positive T wave in lead V_1 in children with a tetralogy of Fallot is indicative of right ventricular enlargement. A negative T wave in lead V_1 in children with this anomaly is indicative of fairly marked right ventricular enlargement.

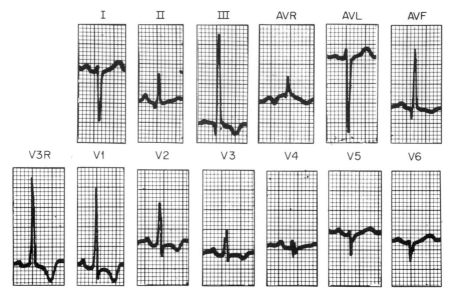

Fig. 23-4   Tetralogy of Fallot in a 13-year-old child.   There is abnormal right axis deviation (+125°).   Tall R waves and inverted T waves are seen in the right precordial leads.   The R/S ratio in leads V₅ and V₆ is less than 1.0.   The degree of right ventricular hypertrophy is marked.   Compare with Fig. 10.8.

ATRIAL SEPTAL DEFECT (FIGS. 10-10, 21-2, 23-5, 23-6)

1   The P wave is usually normal in uncomplicated atrial septal defects but is sometimes peaked in lead II in the presence of right atrial abnormality.

2   The mean P vector in ostium secundum defects is directed inferiorly and leftward.   In sinus venosus defects, the P vector tends to shift leftward, resulting in inverted P waves in lead III and isoelectric, diphasic, or inverted P waves in lead aVF.

3   The P-R interval is often prolonged.

4   The right precordial leads show evidence of right ventricular enlargement.   The usual finding is an rSr' or an rsR' complex with a normal QRS interval, attributed to hypertrophy of the outflow tract of the right ventricle.   With the advent of pulmonary hypertension, the rSr' complexes in lead V₁ are replaced by tall R' waves and shallower S waves. An rR, qR, or monophasic R wave may appear as the severity of the right ventricular hypertrophy increases.   These complexes may be accompanied by T wave inversions in the right precordial leads.

5   In uncomplicated ostium secundum atrial septal defect, the left precordial leads generally show small or absent Q waves, R waves of relatively low voltage, and somewhat prominent S waves.

6   In ostium secundum defects, the mean QRS vector shows right axis

deviation, with the QRS vector loop below the isoelectric line and inscribed in a CW direction.

ENDOCARDIAL CUSHION DEFECTS

1 The common patterns of endocardial cushion defects consist of the complete defect or a combination of an ostium primum atrial septal defect with a cleft mitral valve.
2 Sinus rhythm is usually present, but the incidence of prolongation of the P-R interval is comparatively high. Atrial arrhythmias are common, and complete AV block is noted occasionally.
3 Signs of right atrial, left atrial, or biatrial enlargement may be observed.
4 The right precordial leads show QRS patterns like those found in ostium secundum defects. However, the left precordial leads may show signs of left ventricular enlargement when marked mitral regurgitation or a large ventricular septal defect, or both, are present.
5 In endocardial cushion defects the mean QRS vector typically shows left axis deviation, with the QRS vector loop above the isoelectric line and inscribed in a CCW direction. The mechanism of the left axis deviation is not established. It has been attributed to left anterior fascicular block by some writers and to early activation of the poster-

Fig. 23-5 The FP vector loop in atrial septal defects.   (*A*) Ostium secundum defect.   The loop is oriented inferiorly (right axis deviation) and is inscribed in a CW manner. (*B*) Ostium primum defect and atrioventricularis communis.   The loop is superiorly oriented (left axis deviation) and is inscribed in a CCW fashion.

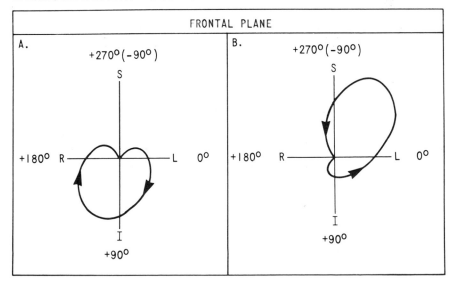

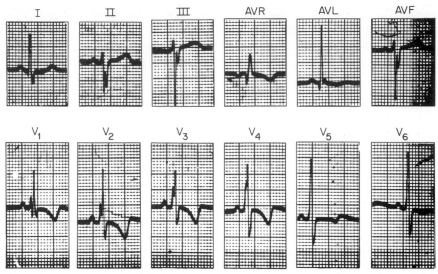

Fig. 23-6 Ostium primum defect and atrioventricularis communis. There is abnormal left axis deviation. The QRS loop is located superiorly and is inscribed in a CCW direction. There is basically an RSR' complex in lead V₁ with a tall secondary R wave, indicating right ventricular enlargement.

obasal region of the left ventricle through an abnormally short posterior fascicle by others.

ANOMALOUS PULMONARY VENOUS CONNECTION

Partial

When less than half of the pulmonary venous blood enters the right atrium and there are no major cardiac anomalies, the electrocardiogram is usually normal.

Total

1   When total anomalous pulmonary venous connection is associated with increased pulmonary blood flow and relatively normal pulmonary arterial pressure, the electrocardiogram is similar to that found in uncomplicated atrial septal defects with large left-to-right shunts.
2   In the presence of pulmonary hypertension, signs of right atrial enlargement are commonly seen. Signs of right ventricular enlargement are almost always present in the right precordial leads, which show rsR', qR, or monophasic R patterns. The left precordial leads display rS complexes.
3   Right axis deviation is usually present.

4   When right ventricular hypertrophy is severe, T wave inversions appear in the right precordial leads and in leads II, III, and aVF. Early in life, positive T waves may be present in the right precordial leads.

VENTRICULAR SEPTAL DEFECT

1   The electrocardiogram may be normal if the defect is small and the hemodynamic disturbance is minimal. The electrocardiographic findings depend primarily on the site of the defect and the pulmonary vascular resistance.
2   Sinus rhythm is usually present.
3   The P-R interval is generally normal. Prolongation of this interval occurs but is uncommon.
4   In the presence of large left-to-right shunts, left atrial enlargement is usually found. Signs of right atrial or biatrial enlargement may appear when pulmonary hypertension coexists with large shunts.
5   The QRS axis is frequently normal but may be deviated rightward as the pulmonary vascular resistance increases, so that right axis deviation or an $S_1S_2S_3$ pattern appears. Left axis deviation occurs in about one-fifth of the cases, usually in isolated ventricular septal defects of the "endocardial cushion" variety.
6   With large left-to-right shunts, left ventricular enlargement is the rule when pulmonary vascular resistance is high, and signs of right ventricular enlargement may appear. Combined ventricular enlargement is not an uncommon pattern in large shunts with elevated pulmonary arterial pressures. In infants and young children, combined ventricular hypertrophy may be manifested by large equiphasic RS complexes in two or more limb leads and in the midprecordial leads (Katz-Wachtel phenomenon).

PATENT DUCTUS ARTERIOSUS

1   The electrocardiogram may be normal when the ductus is small.
2   In patent ductus arteriosus with left-to-right shunt, the following may be noted:
a   Left atrial enlargement or, when pulmonary hypertension is present, biatrial enlargement.
b   Prolongation of the P-R interval (10 to 20 percent of cases).
c   Left ventricular enlargement, usually with the patterns of diastolic overloading of the left ventricle.
d   Normal electrical axis of the QRS complex.
e   Sinus rhythm; but atrial fibrillation may be found in older patients with large shunts.

3 When patent ductus arteriosus with a left-to-right shunt is associated with pulmonary hypertension, electrocardiographic evidence of biventricular enlargement is generally present. The Katz-Wachtel phenomenon, consisting of large equiphasic RS complexes in the limb and midprecordial leads, may be seen.

4 In patent ductus arteriosus with right-to-left shunt, right atrial and right ventricular enlargement as well as right axis deviation are present. The persistence of a qR pattern in the left precordial leads in such cases is a residual of the previous left ventricular enlargement.

ANOMALOUS LEFT CORONARY ARTERY ARISING FROM THE PULMONARY ARTERY (FIG. 23-7)

1 Sinus rhythm is usually present.

2 Left ventricular enlargement is almost always found.

3 Also, in the majority of cases, signs of anterolateral myocardial infarction are observed, with deep Q waves in leads I, aVL, V_5, and V_6, usually associated with S-T segment or T wave changes, or both, in these leads.

4 Left axis deviation may occur in older patients and is also sometimes seen in infants.

Fig. 23-7 Anomalous origin of the left coronary artery from the pulmonary artery. The electrocardiogram shows evidence of anterolateral myocardial infarction, with deep Q waves in leads I, aVL, V_5, and V_6. (*From D. C. Sabiston, Jr., C. A. Neill, and H. B. Taussig, The Direction of Blood Flow in Anomalous Left Coronary Artery Arising from the Pulmonary Artery, Circulation, 22: 591, 1960. Used by permission of the American Heart Association, Inc.*)

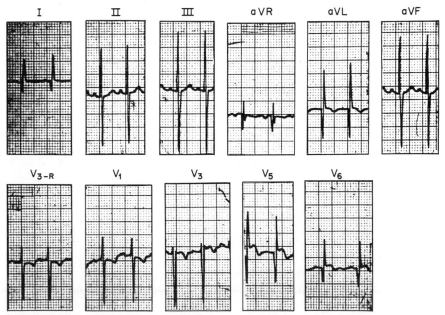

PULMONARY ATRESIA WITH AN INTACT VENTRICULAR SEPTUM

1 The electrocardiographic findings depend on the size of the right ventricle and the age of the patient.
2 Although the P wave may be normal initially, evidence of right atrial enlargement develops in days to weeks.
3 The P-R interval is usually normal.
4 The mean QRS axis is normal or deviated to the right. The QRS loop is inscribed in a CW manner.
5 When the right ventricle is small, the electrocardiogram is dominated by signs of left ventricular enlargement.
6 When the right ventricle is large, right axis deviation appears and signs of right ventricular enlargement are not only evident but may dominate the electrocardiogram.

TRICUSPID ATRESIA (FIG. 23-8)

1 Signs of right atrial enlargement are almost always present, and signs of left atrial enlargement may be present also. The P waves are usually tall and notched in leads I and II, with the first peak taller than the second (P tricuspidale).
2 Signs of isolated right atrial enlargement at an early stage may be the result of a foramen ovale that is too small. Later, the additional appearance of signs of left atrial enlargement is considered good evidence of adequate patency of the foramen ovale.
3 The P-R interval is usually normal, but it may be prolonged or even shortened.
4 Abnormal left axis deviation is found in 75 to 85 percent of patients, with the QRS loop rotated CCW in the frontal plane. A normal axis or right axis deviation is more likely to occur when tricuspid atresia is associated with transposition of the great vessels.
5 The QRS pattern in the precordial leads resembles that of an adult rather than a child. Signs of left (but not right) ventricular enlargement are usually evident in both the precordial and the limb leads.

SINGLE VENTRICLE

1 Sinus rhythm is the rule.
2 The P waves generally show right atrial enlargement.
3 The P-R interval is usually normal but is sometimes prolonged.
4 With transposition of the great vessels, right ventricular enlargement, associated with a qR or rsR' pattern in the right precordial leads and large diphasic complexes in the left precordial leads, is the usual finding. Left axis deviation is not uncommon.

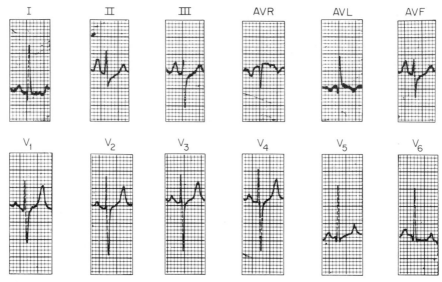

Fig. 23-8   Tricuspid atresia in a 6-month-old infant.   The electrical axis is about − 10°.   This is abnormal for a child of this age.   There is also right atrial enlargement.

5   Without transposition of the great vessels, there are usually rS complexes and upright T waves in all the precordial leads.

COMPLETE TRANSPOSITION OF THE GREAT VESSELS

1   Transposition with a large ventricular septal defect and a low pulmonary vascular resistance shows the following findings:

a   Right atrial enlargement and often left atrial enlargement as well.

b   A normal or slightly prolonged P-R interval.

c   Right axis deviation in most cases. When left axis deviation is present, tricuspid atresia or an overriding tricuspid valve is usually associated. A normal axis is uncommon.

d   Combined ventricular enlargement as a rule.

e   Generally, absence of deeply inverted T waves in the right precordial leads and the presence of upright T waves in leads V_5 and V_6. However, unusual T wave patterns sometimes occur, consisting of a negtive T wave in lead V_6 and a positive T wave in lead V_1 or positive T waves in both these leads with T_{V1} greater than T_{V6}.

2   Transposition with a large ventricular septal defect and increased pulmonary vascular resistance may cause the pattern of right ventricular enlargement to emerge and become dominant.

3   Transposition with severe pulmonic stenosis and a large ventricular septal defect produces signs of right atrial and right ventricular enlargement as well as marked right axis deviation.

4 Transposition with an isolated large atrial septal defect is characterized by right axis deviation, right atrial enlargement, and right ventricular enlargement.   Tall R waves and upright T waves are usually seen in the right precordial leads in association with rS complexes and positive T waves in the left-sided leads.

TRUNCUS ARTERIOSUS

1 Truncus arteriosus with large pulmonary arteries generally shows the following findings:
a Sinus rhythm.
b A normal or slighly prolonged P-R interval.
c Right atrial and sometimes also left atrial enlargement.
d Slight right axis deviation.
e All gradations of biventricular enlargement and only rarely evidence of isolated chamber hypertrophy.   Usually, however, right ventricular enlargement is dominant because the right ventricular pressure is at systemic levels.   When the pulmonary blood flow is large, signs of diastolic overloading of the left ventricle become more prominent.
2 Truncus arteriosus with absent or hypoplastic pulmonary arteries shows right atrial enlargement, right axis deviation, and predominant right ventricular enlargement.

REFERENCES

Benchimol, A., and E. G. Lucena: Vectorcardiography in Congenital Heart Disease with the Use of the Frank System, *Brit. Heart J.*, 27: 236, 1965.
Beregovich, J., S. Bleifer, E. Donoso, and A. Grishman: The Vectorcardiogram and Electrocardiogram in Persistent Common Atrioventricular Canal, *Circulation*, 21: 63, 1960.
———, ———, ———, and ———: The Vectorcardiogram and Electrocardiogram in Ventricular Septal Defect, *Brit. Heart J.*, 22: 205, 1960.
Braunwald, E., C. T. Lambrew, A. G. Morrow, G. E. Pierce, S. D. Rockoff, and J. Ross, Jr.: Idiopathic Hypertropic Subaortic Stenosis, *Circulation*, 30, Suppl. 4. November, 1964.
Burch, G. E., and N. P. DePasquale: "Electrocardiography in the Diagnosis of Congential Heart Disease," Lea & Febiger, Philadelphia, 1967.
Gasul, B. M., R. A. Arcilla, and M. Lev: "Heart Disease in Children," Lippincott, Philadelphia, 1967.
Keith, J. D., R. D. Rowe, and P. Vlad: "Heart Disease in Infancy and Childhood," 3d ed., Macmillan, New York, 1978.
Nadas, A. S., and D. C. Fyler: "Pediatric Cardiology," 3d ed., Saunders, Philadelphia, 1972.
Perloff, J. K.: "The Clinical Recognition of Congenital Heart Disease," 2d ed., Saunders, Philadelphia, 1978.

Pryor, R., G. M. Woodwork, and S. G. Blount, Jr.: Electrocardiographic Changes in Atrial Septal Defects: Ostium Secundum Defect versus Ostium Primum (Endocardial Cushion) Defect, *Am. Heart J.*, 58: 689, 1959.

Sodi-Pallares, D. (ed.): Symposium on Electrocardiography in Congenital Heart Disease, *Am. J. Cardiol.*, 21: 617, 773, 1968.

———, B. Portillo, F. Cisneros, M. V. de la Cruz, and A. G. Acosta: Electrocardiography in Infants and Children, *Pediat. Clin. N. Am.*, 5: 87, 1958.

CHAPTER 24

THE ARRHYTHMIAS

PHYSIOLOGIC BASIS OF CARDIAC ARRHYTHMIAS

Introduction

The presentation of cellular electrical activity in Chap. 1 was based on physical mechanisms originally proposed many years ago. As a working hypothesis, this membrane theory is useful in explaining the derivation of the various components of the electrocardiogram. However, as a working concept of cellular electrophysiology, it is inadequate for explaining the genesis of cardiac arrhythmias.

The biochemical and bioelectrical phenomena involved in the activity of cardiac muscle fibers are rather complex, but they provide an insight into the mechanisms of impulse information and conduction within the heart. Knowledge of these phenomena thus provides a physiologic basis for understanding the mechanisms of cardiac arrhythmias.

The Transmembrane Potentials of Cardiac Cells (Fig. 24-1)

Figure 24-1 is a schematic representation of the intracellular or transmembrane potentials of a cardiac cell in the resting state and during depolarization and repolarization.

When a microelectrode pierces the membrane of a resting cardiac muscle fiber, a steady potential difference of -90 mV is recorded because the interior of the cell is negative with respect to the exterior. This is the transmembrane resting potential RP.   When the cell is activated by a propagated impulse, the intracellular potential increases rapidly to a value of approximately +30 mV, which produces an upstroke.   Repolarization then sets in.   Three phases can be recognized: an initial phase of rapid repolarization carrying the intracellular potential down to almost the zero level; a second phase of slow repolarization, the so-called "plateau"; and a final phase of rapid repolarization, the downstroke.   The time between the onset of activation and the return to the resting state is the duration of the transmembrane action potential AP.   The various slopes of the action potential have been designated as phases 0, 1, 2, 3, and 4.   Phase 0 represents depolarization; phases 1, 2, and 3, repolarization; and phase 4, electrical diastole.   The upstroke is related to the initial deflection of the QRS complex; the plateau, to the S-T segment; and the downstroke, to the T wave.

The cell membrane is a semipermeable barrier to ionic exchange. Outside of the cell the concentration of sodium ions Na^+ is great and that of potassium ions K^+ is low.   Within the cell the predominant cation is K^+, the amount of Na^+ being very small.   When a stimulus is applied to

Fig. 24-1   Diagrammatic representation of the transmembrane action potential and unipolar electrogram recorded from an isolated preparation of cardiac muscle.   Depolarization and the various phases of repolarization are designated by the symbols 0, 1, 2, 3, and 4.   Shown on the right are the changes in transmembrane potential produced by subthreshold and threshold stimuli.   Stimulus c is sufficient to produce a local response which reaches threshold TP and merges with the upstroke of the action potential.   (*From B. F. Hoffman, P. F. Cranefield, and A. G. Wallace, Physiologic Basis of Cardiac Arrhythmias, Mod. Concepts Cardiovasc. Dis., 35: 103, 1966.   Used by permission of the American Heart Association, Inc.*)

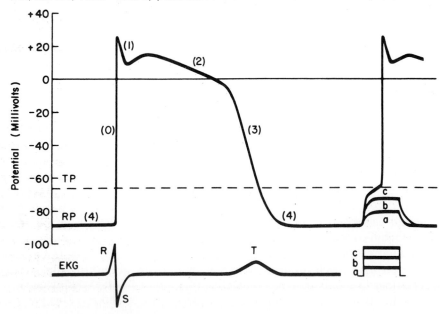

a resting cell, the permeability of the cell membrane to the passage of ions is increased.   As a result, sodium diffuses into the cell along its electro-chemical gradient.   The influx of Na^+ ions into the cell causes an abrupt change in the intracellular potential to a positive value (phase 0).   Membrane permeability for K^+ ions increases shortly after the Na^+ ions begin to enter the cell.   Then K^+ ions leave the cell because the intracellular concentration of this cation is greater than its extracellular concentration.   When the outward diffusion of K^+ ions exceeds the inflow of Na^+ ions, repolarization begins.   The efflux of K^+ ions from the cell is associated with the fall in potential during phases 1 and 2.   During the plateau, there is a relatively steady membrane potential, presumably associated with reduced membrane permeability for both Na^+ and K^+.   The termination of the plateau and the downstroke have been attributed to increased conductance of the membrane for K^+, with a consequent greater outflow of K^+ ions.   During phase 4, Na^+ ions are restored to the surface of the cell and K^+ ions to its interior by means of the sodium pump.

In the past decade, the concept has emerged that the currents underlying the action potential include calcium as well as sodium and potassium ions. It has been demonstrated that a fast sodium inward current is responsible for the rapid upstroke of the cardiac action potential and that a second, slower inward current (carried by calcium and sodium ions) is responsible for the plateau phase of repolarization.   Both currents are found in the specialized conducting tissues as well as in ordinary atrial and ventricular muscle cells.   The fast current is regulated primarily by the extracellular concentration of sodium ions; and the slow current, by the extracellular concentration of calcium ions.

Experimental data suggest that primary pacemaker cells, like those found in the SA node, depend for their action potentials on a slow inward flow of calcium ions.   Normal sinus rhythm and normal AV conduction are maintained primarily, if not exclusively, by slow channel mechanisms. Calcium currents may also be involved in the genesis of some of the arrhythmias seen in myocardial infarction, digitalis toxicity, and other conditions.

The Basis for Normal Cardiac Automaticity (Fig. 24-2)

On the basis of their physiologic properties and histologic characteristics, cardiac cells may be classified as either specialized or nonspecialized. Ordinary atrial and ventricular muscle fibers are considered nonspecialized. Although capable of conducting impulses, they are incapable of initiating them.   The capacity for impulse formation is an exclusive property of automatic cells found in the specialized tissues of the heart.   Groups of such automatic cells are distributed in the SA node, in areas about the great veins, in the vicinity of the coronary sinus, in the specialized tracts of the atria, in Bachmann's bundle, in the interatrial septum, at the junction

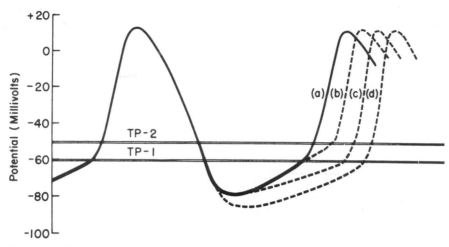

Fig. 24-2 Diagrammatic representation of transmembrane potentials from a single fiber in the sinoatrial node. On the right, the progression from (a) to (b), (c), and (d) illustrates the mechanisms by which the rate of firing of a normally automatic fiber is altered. In (b), a shift in the threshold potential from TP-1 to TP-2 delays firing and widens the cycle length. In (c), a decrease in the slope of spontaneous diastolic depolarization without a change in threshold delays firing and widens the cycle length. In (d), a shift in the maximal level of resting potential (e.g., hyperpolarization), without a change in threshold or slope of spontaneous diastolic depolarization, delays firing and widens the cycle length. *(From B. F. Hoffman, P. F. Cranefield, and A. G. Wallace, Physiologic Basis of Cardiac Arrhythmias, Mod. Concepts Cardiovasc. Dis., 35: 103, 1966. Used by permission of the American Heart Association, Inc.)*

of the pulmonary veins with the left atrium, in the left AV ring, in the bundle of His, in the bundle branches, and in the peripheral Purkinje system. There are pacemaker cells in the bundle of His, in the NH region of the AV node, and possibly some in the AN region, but none in the main body of the AV node (N region). Under appropriate conditions any one of these automatic cells may demonstrate automatic activity and act as a pacemaker of the heart. The term *pacemaker* thus applies to the anatomic site at which an impulse arises. Automatic cells may function either as true pacemakers or as latent pacemakers.

Recordings of transmembrane potentials from automatic cells differ from those of ordinary muscle fibers in one respect (Fig. 24-2). During phase 4, there is no constant resting potential. Instead, as soon as phase 3 is ended, slow spontaneous depolarization carries the transmembrane potential to a critical level called the *threshold potential*. When this value is reached, an action potential is initiated. Thus the mechanism for the automaticity of these specialized cells is spontaneous diastolic (phase 4) depolarization.

Most specialized cardiac fibers are automatic and therefore self-excitatory. Under normal conditions, the nonspecialized fibers of the myocardium are not automatic. Nonautomatic cells are activated by a propagated impulse or some other stimulus.   An impulse arriving at such a cell causes a current to flow across the cell membrane.   When the resting potential, which is ordinarily constant, is thereby raised to the threshold level (about -65 mV), an action potential is initiated.   Each action potential, in turn, generates a new action potential in adjacent fibers which have as yet not been activated.   Excitation is thus self-propagating and continues until the entire heart has been activated.

Disturbances in Impulse Formation

From an electrophysiologic standpoint, cardiac arrhythmias may be classified as either disturbances of impulse formation or disturbances of impulse conduction, or combinations of the two.

Normally, impulse formation is initiated by the SA node.   After the heart has been completely activated, slow diastolic depolarization probably proceeds simultaneously in several groups of automatic cells.   But because the slope of diastolic depolarization is steepest in the fibers of the SA node, threshold potentials are attained earlier in this region than at other pacemaker sites.   Once threshold potentials have been reached, the SA node fires the impulse.   The impulse is then propagated to the remainder of the heart. Other potential pacemakers are discharged by the propagated impulse before intracellular potentials can rise to threshold, so that the SA node is normally the dominant pacemaker of the heart.

The rate of discharge of any pacemaker depends on three variables: the slope of spontaneous diastolic depolarization, the maximum diastolic potential at the end of repolarization (hyperpolarization), and the magnitude of the threshold potential.   A decrease in the slope of diastolic depolarization, an increase in the maximal diastolic potential, or a rise in the threshold potential, operating independently or concurrently, will increase the cycle length and thus slow the pacemaker.   Opposite changes in these variables will shorten the cycle length and accelerate the pacemaker.

Any factor which decreases the automaticity of one fiber or increases the automaticity of another may cause the site of impulse formation to shift from the former to the latter.   If the two fibers are in close proximity, this change may be manifested only as a change in rate.   If the fibers are more widely separated, changes in both the rate and site of the pacemaker can be recognized.

The most frequent cause of changes in either the rate or the site of a pacemaker is the action of autonomic agents.   Automatic cells in different parts of the heart differ in their responsiveness to the neurotransmitters, acetylcholine and norepinephrine.   Vagal activity, by liberating acetylcholine, decreases the slope of diastolic depolarization and increases the maximal diastolic potential in the automatic cells of the SA node and in other atrial foci.   Because the effect is most marked in the SA node, pacemaker activity may shift to an ectopic focus in the atria.   Further vagal stimulation may completely arrest automatic activity in all the sinus and atrial fibers. However, because the automaticity of the fibers in the His-Purkinje system is not affected by acetylcholine, pacemaking activity will shift to this locus with the production of *escape* rhythms. The likelihood of escape rhythms from this site is enhanced by circulating catecholamines and by the reflex liberation of norepinephrine, both of which increase the slope of phase 4 depolarization in these fibers.

Other environmental factors may influence the rhythmicity of automatic cells. Hypothermia reduces the slope of diastolic depolarization of all automatic fibers and thus slows the heart rate. A rise in temperature has an opposite effect. Hypoxemia, hypercapnia, and stretch act to increase the rate of diastolic depolarization in automatic cells. These factors may be responsible for the frequent occurrence of arrhythmias in patients suffering from hypoxemia, hypercapnia, and congestive heart failure.

Other factors may influence automaticity by altering the threshold potential. An increase in extracellular calcium concentration elevates the threshold potential and reduces the firing rate of a pacemaker. A decrease in extracellular calcium concentration has an opposite effect. The passage of weak depolarizing currents across the membrane of Purkinje fibers increases the slope of diastolic depolarization. It is thus possible that electrotonic currents from ischemic lesions of the myocardium (as in myocardial infarction) may similarly enhance the automaticity of adjacent Purkinje fibers and initiate ectopic rhythms.

Most ectopic rhythms result from enhanced automatic activity in latent pacemaker foci with or without depression of the automaticity of the normal pacemaker. These arrhythmias include those produced by digitalis toxicity, sympathomimetic agents, hypoxemia, ischemia, hypercapnia, and reduction in the extracellular concentrations of calcium or potassium. In some instances more than one factor may be operative. Thus the increased automaticity of the Purkinje fibers resulting from digitalis excess may be further enhanced by decreased extracellular concentrations of potassium.

Afterpotentials may possibly be a cause of ectopic impulse formation. Afterpotentials appear as oscillations of the membrane potential after repolarization. If the oscillations are of sufficient magnitude to reach the threshold level, isolated beats or sustained arrhythmias may occur. In addition, delayed repolarization and persistent depolarization have been invoked as possible causes of arrhythmias, on the assumption that the flow of current from such cells may reexcite fibers that have already repolarized.

In addition to automaticity, abnormal impulse generation in cardiac cells may be dependent on afterdepolarizations. The nondriven rhythmic impulses dependent on afterdepolarizations are called *triggered impulses* or *triggered activity*. The relation between triggered activity and clinical arrhythmias is largely speculative.

Disturbances in Impulse Conduction

The two major determinants of impulse conduction are the rate of depolarization and the amplitude of the action potential. A decrease in the slope of the upstroke or in the height of the action potential reduces conduction velocity. Most often, these changes are produced by a decrease in the resting potential at the time of excitation. Many factors may reduce the resting potential. An elevated extracellular potassium concentration, for example, lowers transmembrane potential, which reduces the rate of rise and the height of the action potential so that conduction is slowed. When extracellular potassium levels are markedly elevated, the excitability of some cardiac muscle fibers may even be arrested completely. Normally, during the repolarization of a muscle fiber, the transmembrane potential is lower than during the resting phase. Slowing of conduction or block thus may occur whenever an impulse arrives at fibers which are incompletely repolarized following a preceding beat. The ventricular conduction defects (aberrant ventricular conduction) found in some supraventricular arrhythmias are probably caused by this mechanism.

Decremental Conduction (Fig. 24-3)

Decremental conduction is a physiologic property of some cardiac fibers in the SA and AV nodes and in the His-Purkinje system. In these fibers, the amplitude of the action potential and the rate of depolarization decrease progressively from cell to cell so that the resultant stimulus becomes weaker as it is propagated. Excitation of more distal fibers then depends on the number of participating proximal fibers. The impulse may fade out completely when the strength of the stimulus proximally becomes insufficient to elicit a response in the distal fibers even if they are still excitable. This type of conduction is called *decremental conduction*. It is not the result of refractoriness or loss of excitability in the fibers distal to the excitation wave. Decremental conduction is the mechanism responsible for the normal delay in conduction through the AV node and for the prolonged AV conduction time of early atrial premature beats. It may also be responsible for other abnormalities. These will now be considered.

It is well known that AV junctional escape beats often show aberrant ventricular conduction. Since these beats occur after long pauses, the aberration cannot be explained by incomplete recovery of excitability in the His-Purkinje fibers. A different mechanism must be operative. If during the long pause, slow diastolic depolarization of the Purkinje fibers develops, the transmembrane potential will be reduced at the time of arrival of the escaping AV junctional beats. Because the transmembrane potential is thus decreased at the time of excitation, the action potential in the Purkinje fibers will show a decreased rate of depolarization, conduction velocity will be slowed, and the pattern of ventricular activation will be altered. Aberration of escape beats has also been attributed to conduction by a pathway different from the normal (namely, the paraspecific fibers of Mahaim).

An accentuation of the normal decremental conduction through the AV node is the probable explanation of first-degree AV block.

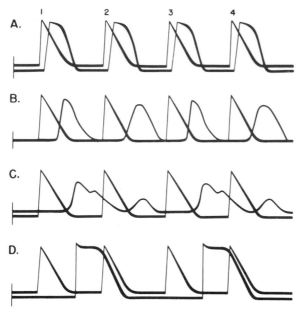

Fig. 24-3 Tracings of transmembrane action potentials recorded from a single fiber of the atrium and from fibers of the AV node and His bundle, showing decremental conduction during a sustained supraventricular tachycardia. (A) Atrium and atrial margin of the node. (B) Atrium and middle node. (C) Atrium and lower node. (D) Atrium and His bundle. The same atrial fiber was employed in all records. Note that during the second and fourth beats, the abortive responses in the lower node fail to produce a His bundle response. This is 2:1 AV heart block resulting from complete decrement of beats 2 and 4 within the node. Beats 2 and 4 also are concealed responses. Note the relative loss of resting membrane potential from the fibers in the middle and lower nodal areas, panels B and C. The resting potential of fibers in the His bundle, panel D, is normal. (From B. F. Hoffman, P. F. Cranefield, and A. G. Wallace, Mod. Concepts Cardiovasc. Dis., 35: 107, 1966. Used by permission of the American Heart Association, Inc.)

Type I AV block (Wenckebach phenomenon) has been attributed to decremental conduction in the AV node, particularly in the N region. In Type II AV block the conduction disturbance is situated in the more peripheral ramifications of the AV conduction system. The mechanism is probably a transient but complete decrement of conduction in both bundle branches, or in one bundle branch if the other is already blocked.

Inhomogeneous Conduction

Normally, conduction in the AV junction is homogeneous; that is, there is synchronous activation of the fibers in the AN and N regions of the node, so that the wave front arriving at the NH region is smooth. Successful AV conduction may then be anticipated. On the other hand, when the rate of depolarization is reduced and conduction is slowed, excitation spreads through the fibers inhomogeneously.   The resultant wave front is irregular, and it may then be incapable of eliciting a response in the NH region. Thus AV transmission may fail.

Inhomogeneous conduction may occur in the AV junction because of the existence of two different functional pathways for impulse transmission in this structure, one of which conducts more rapidly than the other.   If conduction velocity is reduced in both pathways or in the slower pathway alone, the progressive deterioration of the wave front which follows may eventually lead to failure of conduction.

Supernormality

Supernormality is a fundamental property of specialized atrial fibers and the His-Purkinje system but does not appear to be a property of the AV node under normal or pathologic circumstances (Childers).

The supernormal phase of excitability is a brief interval near the end of the T wave during which subthreshold stimuli may evoke a response. In microelectrode recordings of specialized atrial and Purkinje fibers it corresponds to a small dip in the trailing foot of the action potential.

The supernormal phase of conductivity is a short period of paradoxically improved conduction which may occur during the absolute and relatively refractory periods following excitation.   Conduction occurs only during a short period, and both earlier and later impulses are blocked or are conducted with greater delay.   Supernormal conduction appears to occur only in hearts in which AV conduction is impaired or blocked.   The supernormal phase of conductivity ordinarily coincides with the U wave or the distal limb of the T wave.

Although supernormal conduction and excitability have been demonstrated in vitro, the existence of true supernormal conduction in the intact human heart has not yet been proved.   According to Josephson and Seides, apparent supernormal conduction can be explained by physiologic mechanisms including: (1) the gap phenomenon, a zone in the cardiac cycle during which premature atrial impulses fail to evoke ventricular responses while atrial beats of greater and lesser prematurity are conducted to the ventricles; (2) peeling back of the refractory period by premature stimulation; (3) shortening of refractoriness by changes in the preceding cycle length; (4) the Wenckebach phenomenon in the bundle branches; (5) bradycardia-dependent blocks; (6) summation; and (7) dual AV nodal pathways.   Supernormal conduction is also discussed later in this chapter.

Concealed Conduction

Concealed conduction is the term applied to the partial penetration of the AV conduction pathways by antegrade or retrograde impulses.   Impulses which enter the AV junction but do not emerge from it are not recorded by the electrocardiogram. Their conduction is thus concealed. Concealed conduction may result from any one or a combination of the factors causing block: refractory tissue, decremental conduction, or inhomogeneous conduction. It has been suggested that the concealment of conduction in cardiac tissue may prove to be similar to, if not identical with, Wedensky inhibition. This phenomenon may be defined as an increase in the threshold of excitation distal to an area of block as a result of an impulse proximal to the region of the block.

Unidirectional Block and Macroreentry in the AV Junction (Figs. 24-68, 24-125)

Block is a common phenomenon in many regions of the heart. When it occurs in the AV node or the His-Purkinje system, clinical AV block is usually recognizable. However, it is possible for block to be so localized that adjacent tissues can conduct normally. When this happens, *unidirectional* block may ensue and set the stage for reentry.

Reciprocal rhythm is an example of an arrhythmia produced by unidirectional block and reentry within the AV junction. To explain reciprocal rhythm it is necessary to postulate the existence of dual (or multiple) pathways for impulse transmission in the AV junction. Recently it has been demonstrated experimentally that when the right side of the AV node is blocked unidirectionally, inhomogeneity of conduction permits the passage of an impulse through the left side of the node to the ventricles and its reentry and retrograde transmission through the right side of the node. It would thus appear that reciprocal rhythms probably result from functional longitudinal dissociation of the AV junctional tissues due to inhomogeneous conduction, unidirectional block, and reentry.

Reentry has been established as the mechanism for the overwhelming majority of paroxysmal supraventricular tachycardias. Reentry may occur in the SA and AV nodes, the atria, the ventricles, and by an accessory pathway in addition to the normal AV nodal pathway.

Unidirectional Block without Reentry

The mechanism of unidirectional block without reentry, as evidenced by the retrograde conduction of idioventricular beats to the atria in the presence of advanced AV block, is not understood. It may be a form of unidirectional block in the AV node, resulting from different degrees of decrement in the antegrade and retrograde conduction pathways.

Local Unidirectional Block and Microreentry

Unidirectional block at the Purkinje-ventricular junction and microreentry may play a role in the genesis of ventricular premature beats and certain

self-sustaining ventricular tachyarrhythmias.   These mechanisms are explained in Fig. 24-4.

As illustrated in the diagram, premature beats may occur as a result of
reexcitation by the normal impulse or as a result of reentry and reexcitation.
Some self-sustaining arrhythmias may also be the result of persistent reentry
and reexcitation.

Combined Disturbances of Impulse Formation and Conduction

Cardiac arrhythmias may result from combined disturbances of impulse
formation and conduction.   Parasystole and ectopic rhythms with exit
block are examples of such dysrhythmias.

Automatic fibers possessing high degrees of automaticity generally
show lowered maximal diastolic potentials, a smaller action potential
amplitude, and a slower rate of depolarization than other fibers.   Under
conditions which lower the threshold potential sufficiently, phase 4 depolarization in specialized fibers exhibiting increased automaticity may not
only initiate an ectopic beat but at the same time cause the spread of the
impulse to be decremental.   The ectopic focus is thus surrounded by a
region in which conduction is impaired.   This mechanism may cause both
entrance and exit block.

In ectopic tachycardias with exit block, the cause of the block is also
believed to be decremental conduction.   The occurrence of decremental
conduction is favored by the lowered amplitude of the action potential and
the slow rate of depolarization in the fibers of the ectopic focus.

Relationship between the Electrocardiogram and the
Action Potentials of Cardiac Cells

Electrophysiologic studies (Surawicz and his associates), based on simultaneous recordings of the electrocardiogram with the ventricular transmembrane action potential in isolated rabbit hearts and with monophasic action
potentials in humans, suggest the following relationships:

1   Decreased upstroke velocity of the action potential is associated with
    decreased conduction velocity and uniform widening of the QRS
    interval.
2   The end of the ventricular action potential roughly coincides with the
    end of the T wave.
3   Shortening of the action potential is accompanied by a corresponding
    shortening of the Q-T interval; its lengthening, by prolongation of the
    Q-T interval.
4   The duration of the plateau is related to the duration of the S-T segment:
    a prolonged plateau is associated with a long S-T segment; a shorter
    one, with a shortened S-T segment.

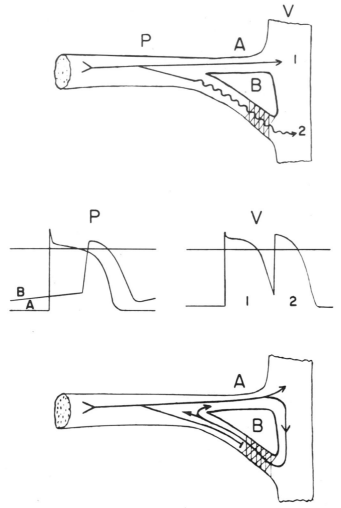

Fig. 24-4 Diagrammatic representation of arrhythmias due to delayed conduction and unidirectional block. The upper drawing represents a peripheral part of the Purkinje system P and attached ventricular muscle V. In branch A, conduction proceeds at normal velocity, and the action potential is shown by trace A. In branch B, conduction velocity is reduced and unidirectional block is present in the hatched area. The locally recorded action potential is shown by trace B. The action potential in branch A elicits the ventricular action potential 1; the slowly propagating action potential in B initiates the second ventricular action potential 2.

The lower drawing shows, by the direction of the arrows, a possible mechanism for production of a self-sustaining arrhythmia. Here the direction of unidirectional block is opposite to that in the upper drawing. (*From B. F. Hoffman, The Electrophysiology of Heart Muscle and the Genesis of Arrhythmias, in L. S. Dreifus, and W. Likoff, eds., "The Mechanisms and Therapy of Cardiac Arrhythmias," Grune & Stratton, Inc., New York, 1966. Used by permission.*)

5 Abolition of the plateau by increased velocity of the initial phase of repolarization is associated with disappearance of the isoelectric interval of the S-T segment and S-T segment deviation.

6 Abrupt transition from phase 2 to phase 3 and increased slope of phase 3 is accompanied by increased amplitude and decreased duration of the T wave. A more uniform, flattened repolarization slope is associated with decreased T wave amplitude.

7 Prolongation of the terminal phase of repolarization is accompanied by increased amplitude of the U wave.

These relationships may be expected when ventricular activation is unaltered and when the action potentials affect all ventricular fibers in the same manner.

The Refractory Period (Figs. 24-5, 24-6)

After stimulation, heart muscle is completely unresponsive to further stimulation for a brief period of time. This is the absolute refractory period. It normally coincides with the time between the beginning of the QRS complex and a portion of the upstroke of the T wave. The absolute refractory period is followed by a relative refractory period, during which the heart gradually recovers its excitability and conductivity. Stimulation during this period must be greater than normal to elicit a response, and the response is usually below normal. The relative refractory period coincides with the interval beginning at a point on the descending limb of the T wave and terminating with the end of the T wave. Following the relative refractory period, there is a supernormal phase of excitability, coinciding with the afterpotentials and the inscription of the U wave, when the threshold for stimulation is lowered. Between the absolute and relative refractory periods there is a critical phase, the so-called "vulnerable" period, which represents an interval of 20 to 40 ms coinciding with the uppermost portion of the T wave, during which an impulse may or may not be initiated or conducted. It is also the period in the cardiac cycle in which ventricular tachycardia or fibrillation may be most easily produced by a strong electrical stimulus. The stimulus may be from an intrinsic source such as a ventricular premature systole or from an extrinsic source such as a pacemaker. During the vulnerable period, maximal electrical nonuniformity in the ventricular muscle is present. In other words, the ventricular muscle cells are at varying stages of recovery: some fibers are completely repolarized, others only partially repolarized, and still others completely refractory. Stimulation during this stage results in nonuniform conduction, with some areas of slowed conduction or actual block, setting the stage for repetitive reentrant excitation. Myocardial ischemia enhances electrical nonuniformity during the vulnerable period, which explains the grave importance of ventricular extrasystoles in acute myocardial infarction.

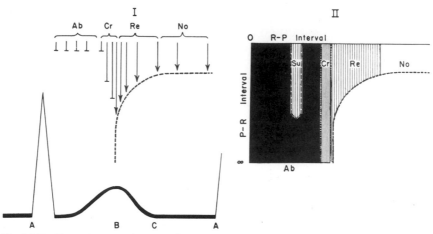

Fig. 24-5 Two schematic diagrams illustrating the method of constructing the recovery curve of conductivity of the AV junction by relating R-P and P-R intervals. Diagram I schematically relates the recovery curve to the ventricular electrocardiogram. The absolute refractory period of the AV junction is defined on the electrocardiogram by A-B; the relative refractory period, by B-C; and the nonrefractory period, by C-A. In the upper portion of the diagram, the arrowheads to the right of B are connected by the curvilinear dashed line, which shows the progressive shortening of the P-R interval during the course of the relative refractory period Re. When the P-R interval becomes stabilized, as indicated by the constant length of the arrows, the nonrefractory phase No begins and continues to the end of the cycle. To the left of B, beginning at A, is the absolute refractory phase Ab, during which impulses are not transmitted to the AV junction. This is indicated by the absence of an arrowhead and by an inverted T symbol ⊥. The transition between Ab and Re is not sharp, but gradual. This short transitional period is the critical phase Cr, during which the impulse may or may not penetrate the AV junction to varying degrees—indicated by elongation of the vertical limb of the inverted T symbol—and may even reach the ventricles after a long delay (longest arrow). The supernormal phase is not considered in this diagram.

Diagram II shows the same events by relating the P-R to the R-P interval. The symbols Ab, Cr, Re, and No are the same as in Diagram 1. The lines bounding the critical phase Cr are dotted to indicate the ill-defined limits of this transitional phase. In addition, the rarely encountered phase of supernormality Su, which appears only when the AV junction is abnormally depressed, is shown here within the absolute refractory period Ab. It may also be located within the relative refractory phase Re. (*From L. N. Katz and A. Pick, "Clinical Electrocardiography: Part I. The Arrhythmias," Lea and Febiger, Philadelphia, 1956. Used by permission.*)

Slow heart rates also seem to create a greater disparity in the normal recovery process and thus may predispose to ectopic impulse formation. For this reason, simply increasing the heart rate may eliminate the ventricular premature beats and tachyarrhythmias which occur in the setting of sinus bradycardia.

Patients with congenitally prolonged Q-T intervals are at greater risk than normal persons of developing ventricular tachyarrhythmias. In these individuals, the normal AV conduction delay may be insufficient to prevent an ectopic impulse from reaching the ventricles during the vulnerable period of the antecedent T wave and initiating ventricular tachycardia or fibrillation.

Certain drugs such as quinidine, procainamide, and the phenothiazines may increase the risk of ventricular fibrillation during the vulnerable period by slowing conduction, altering the duration of the refractory period, and increasing the difference between the durations of refractory periods in the Purkinje and the ventricular fibers.

Fig. 24-6 An identical diagrammatic representation of the duration of the refractory phases of the AV junction in the various types of AV block, as compared with the normal.   The entire length of each bar represents the duration of the cycle.   The heavily shaded part of each bar represents the absolute refractory phase, the lightly shaded part represents the relative refractory phase, and the unshaded part represents the portion of the cycle where AV conduction is unimpeded.

The bars I, II, III, IV, and V represent, respectively, the normal state and the states in first-degree, in Type I second-degree, in Type II second-degree, and in complete AV block.

Normally (bar I), at rates between 60 and 100, the absolute A-B and relative B-C refractory periods are of about the same duration and together occupy less than half the cycle.

In first-degree AV block (bar II), the absolute refractory phase A-B is unchanged but the relative refractory phase may occupy the entire cycle B-C' or extend into any portion thereof, between C and C'.

In Type I second-degree AV block (bar III), both the absolute and the relative refractory phases are prolonged to equal or unequal degrees.   Thus in the diagram the absolute refractory phase is prolonged from A-B to A-B' and the relative refractory phase from B'-C, which equals B-C in I, to B'-C'.   Obviously, B' and C' may be projected toward the right to any degree, provided both phases are prolonged.

In Type II second-degree AV block (bar IV), only the absolute refractory phase is prolonged, the relative refractory phase remaining unchanged.   Thus in the diagram the absolute refractory phase is prolonged from A-B to A-B', and B'-C equals B-C in bar I.   Obviously, B' may be projected toward the right almost up to, but not to, the end of the cycle.

In complete AV block (bar V), the absolute refractory phase occupies the entire cycle A-B' instead of its usual duration A-B.   Consequently there is no relative refractory phase.

In the electrocardiogram, a normal P-R is the index of unimpeded AV conduction, a prolonged P-R is the index of the relative refractory period, and a dropped ventricular beat (a P wave not accompanied by its expected QRST) is the index of the absolute refractory phase of the AV junction.

(From L. N. Katz and A. Pick, "Clinical Electrocardiography: Part I. The Arrhythmias," Lea & Febiger, Philadelphia, 1956. Used by permission.)

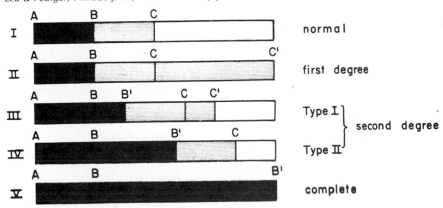

The vulnerable period of the atria occurs at the time of the atrial T wave. Stimulation of the atria at this time by intrinsic (atrial premature beats) or extrinsic electrical stimuli may produce atrial fibrillation.

The length of the refractory period depends to a large extent on the preceding cycle length. The shorter the cycle length, the faster the heart rate and the shorter the refractory period; the longer the cycle length, the slower the heart rate and the longer the refractory period. This rule holds within limits. The refractory period is normally longest in the AV node, shortest in atrial muscle, and intermediate in duration in ventricular muscle.

Refractoriness of cardiac muscle is defined by the response of that tissue to the introduction of premature stimuli. Cardiac electrophysiologists recognize three measurements: the relative, effective, and functional refractory periods. Further details can be found in textbooks of cardiac electrophysiology.

CLINICAL CLASSIFICATION OF THE ARRHYTHMIAS

Although from an electrophysiologic standpoint the cardiac arrhythmias may be classified as disturbance in impulse formation or in conduction, or combinations of the two, clinically it is more convenient to base the classification of arrhythmias on their origin (atrial, ventricular, etc.) and their mode of appearance (tachycardia, premature beats, fibrillation, etc.).

Recently much emphasis has been placed on the presumed mechanisms of the cardiac arrhythmias. This type of information may ultimately have important clinical significance (e.g., in dictating the choice of an appropriate agent for prophylaxis or treatment).

The known causes of arrhythmias include automaticity, fibrillation, block, and reentry. Examples of automatic rhythms include sinus and escape rhythms, wandering pacemaker, ectopic atrial tachycardia, accelerated idioventricular and His bundle rhythms, and parasystole. Atrial and ventricular fibrillation are obvious examples of fibrillatory mechanisms. They are probably produced by firing of the respective chambers by premature beats or external electrical impulses during the vulnerable period. Arrhythmias due to block include SA block, intraatrial block, AV block (both nodal and infranodal), and intraventricular block. Reentry has been established as the cause of most paroxysmal supraventricular tachycardias, reciprocal beats, tachycardias in the preexcitation syndrome, coupled premature beats, and many cases of ventricular tachycardias. At the time of this writing, the mechanism of atrial flutter, multifocal atrial tachycardia, multifocal ventricular beats, and multifocal ventricular tachycardia is still under investigation. Reentry may occur in the SA and AV nodes, the His-Purkinje system, the ventricles, and by an accessory atrioventricular pathway, in addition to the normal AV conduction pathway.

TERMINOLOGY

Because of wide acceptance and common usage, the terms *arrhythmia* and *dysrhythmia* are used interchangeably with *disorder of the heart beat*, even though semantically the first two terms imply an irregularity in rhythm.

The terms *tachycardia* and *bradycardia* present problems in usage. This author concurs with others who believe that the criteria for rapid or slow rates should relate to the norm for any given pacemaker rather than to some arbitrary rate. For example, the proper designation of an idioventricular rhythm with a rate exceeding 50 beats per minute is idioventricular tachycardia, even though the rate may be less than 100 per minute.

The term *allorhythmia* refers to a regularly recurrent irregularity of rhythm.

LADDER DIAGRAMS (FIGS. 24-7, 24-8)

The AV ladder diagram, originally devised by Sir Thomas Lewis, is a valuable technique for the graphic demonstration of atrial, AV junctional, and ventricular activity. When properly employed, it not only promotes a better understanding of arrhythmias but may be indispensable in elucidating the mechanism of complex arrhythmias.

Fig. 24-7 Construction of AV ladder diagrams. (*A*) The electrocardiogram is mounted. (*B*) The AV diagram is placed beneath it. The P waves and QRS complexes are drawn in the A and V levels, respectively. (*C*) The lines are drawn from the A to the V level to indicate AV conduction. The atrial and ventricular cycle lengths and the P-R interval are expressed in hundredths of a second.

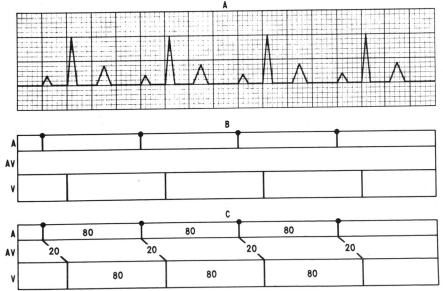

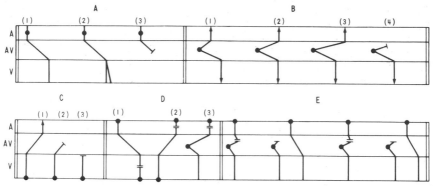

Fig. 24-8   Representative examples of the AV ladder diagram in various conditions.   (*A*) Atrial premature systoles: (1) with normal conduction, (2) with aberrant ventricular conduction, (3) nonconducted.   (*B*) AV junctional premature systoles: (1) upper, (2) middle, (3) lower, (4) AV junctional premature systole with blocked retrograde conduction.   (*C*) Ventricular premature systoles: (1) with retrograde atrial conduction, (2) with partial penetration of the AV junction, (3) blocked at the AV junction.   (*D*) (1) Ventricular fusion between a sinus and an ectopic ventricular impulse, (2) atrial fusion between a sinus and a retrograde atrial impulse of ectopic ventricular origin, (3) atrial fusion between sinus and a retrograde atrial impulse of AV junctional origin.   (*E*) AV dissociation: the third and sixth ventricular impulses are ventricular captures, the sinus rate is slower than the ventricular rate, and the ventricular pacemaker is located in the AV junction.

Procedure

1   The electrocardiogram to be analyzed is mounted.

2   The AV diagram is drawn or placed beneath the electrocardiogram.   In the diagram, A represents atrial activation, V represents ventricular activation, and AV represents impulse conduction or formation in the AV junction.   When dealing with disturbances in SA conduction, the letters S, SA, and A are substituted for A, AV, and V, respectively, S representing impulse formation in the SA node; SA, sinoatrial conduction; and A, atrial activation.

3   The P waves are drawn in the A level, with the beginning of each P wave used as the reference point.   A similar procedure is followed in the V level with respect to the QRS complex.   Appropriate lines are then drawn from the A to the V level when conduction is antegrade and in the reverse direction when conduction is retrograde.   Some authorities slant the lines to indicate the approximate duration of the complexes, but this is not necessary.   Although atrial and ventricular activity are recorded in the electrocardiogram, AV junctional activity is not.   Therefore what takes place in the AV junction can only be surmised or inferred.

4   Certain symbols are employed to designate specific events.   A dot is used to depict the site of impulse formation but may be omitted if this is apparent from the drawing.   Aberrant ventricular conduction, fusion,

partial penetration of an impulse, block, and interference are indicated by the notations shown in the accompanying diagram (Fig. 24-8).

ECTOPIC BEATS AND RHYTHMS

Beats or rhythms initiated in foci outside of the SA node are called *ectopic beats* and *ectopic rhythms,* respectively.

When the SA node is depressed or its impulses are blocked, subsidiary pacemakers take over and produce *passive* ectopic or escape rhythms. At other times, because of enhanced automaticity, these latent pacemakers may spring into action and produce *active* ectopic rhythms.

Escape beats and rhythms may be atrial (rarely), AV junctional, or ventricular in origin. Continuous escape of an AV junctional pacemaker is called *AV junctional rhythm.* Continuous ventricular escape is called *ventricular* or *idioventricular rhythm.*

Active ectopic beats and rhythms include premature systoles and the ectopic tachycardias. These dysrhythmias may be of supraventricular or ventricular origin.

PREMATURE SYSTOLES

The terms *premature systole, premature contraction, premature beat, ectopic beat,* and *extrasystole* are used interchangeably even though they are not exactly synonymous.

Premature systoles are *early* ectopic beats. They occur before the arrival of the next normally conducted impulse. However, all premature beats are not necessarily ectopic (e.g., capture beats), nor are all ectopic beats necessarily premature (e.g., escape beats).

The ectopic focus or foci from which premature systoles arise may be located in the SA node, atria, AV junction, bundle of His, or ventricles.

The term *coupling* or *coupling interval* refers to the period of time between the normal beat and the extrasystolic beat which follows it.

Interpolated premature systoles are extrasystoles which, although interposed between two sinus beats, do not replace a beat or disturb the sinus cycle. Interpolated extrasystoles are most frequently ventricular, less often AV junctional, and rarely atrial in origin. Prolongation of the P-R interval of the postectopic sinus impulse is common because of retrograde concealed conduction (see section on Concealed Conduction).

Except when interpolated, premature systoles are followed by *compensatory* or *noncompensatory pauses.* A pause is considered compensatory if the pause following a premature beat is of sufficient duration to make the P-P interval between the two normal beats which flank the extrasystole twice the basic P-P interval. In other words, the intervals preceding and following the premature beat, plus the time occupied by the premature beat, when added together, equal two sinus cycles. Pauses of lesser duration are noncompensatory pauses. The type of pause following a premature systole depends mainly on whether the sinus pacemaker is discharged by the premature impulse. If the SA node is discharged, for example, by an atrial premature beat (P′), it would seem logical that the postectopic pause (P′-P interval) should be exactly the same as the normal sinus cycle (P-P interval). However, two factors prevent this from occurring: (1) The P′-P interval is lengthened by the time it takes the extrasystole to discharge the atrium, travel to and discharge the SA node, and reemerge to the atrium. (2) Premature discharge of a pacemaker such as the SA node depresses its rhythmicity and thereby delays the appearance of the next impulse. Thus, if the sinus node is discharged by a premature beat, the pause following the premature beat is longer than the normal sinus cycle but is usually not compensatory. On the other hand, if the sinus pacemaker is not disturbed by the premature beat, the pause is usually compensatory unless the premature beat is interpolated. The duration of a pause cannot be measured accurately when the basic rhythm is irregular, as in sinus arrhythmia.

Ventricular premature systoles are characteristically followed by compensatory pauses, because the discharge of the sinus pacemaker is usually not disturbed by the ectopic beats. The mechanism is interference between the sinoatrial and ventricular impulses in the AV junction. Compensatory pauses may also occur if interference takes place elsewhere in the heart (at the sinoatrial, atrial, or ventricular levels). Noncompensatory pauses may follow ventricular premature systoles which are conducted in retrograde fashion to the atria. When this occurs, the SA node is discharged prematurely, resulting in a noncompensatory postectopic pause. However, even with retrograde atrial activation and premature discharge of the sinus pacemaker, the pause is sometimes compensatory. This can happen if the inhibitory effect of the ectopic impulse on the SA node is so prolonged that a compensatory or even longer pause ensues. When the basic cardiac rhythm is AV junctional or ventricular, compensatory pauses rarely follow ventricular extrasystoles, since they almost invariably discharge the dominant pacemaker.

The duration of the postectopic pause is quite variable following AV junctional premature systoles. When the ascending impulse from the AV junction fails to discharge the sinus pacemaker, either because of sinoatrial, atrial, or AV junctional interference or because retrograde conduction is completely blocked, the postectopic pause is fully compensatory. Noncompensatory pauses occur when the sinus node is activated prematurely by retrograde conduction of the impulse through the atria.

The pause following an atrial premature systole is usually noncompensatory, because the atrial impulse discharges the SA node prematurely. The postectopic pause, although longer than the sinus cycle, is noncompensatory. However, compensatory pauses may sometimes follow atrial premature beats which so depress the sinus pacemaker that there is a significant delay in the appearance of the next sinus beat. This may happen with early or late atrial premature beats. If an atrial extrasystole occurs very late in diastole, it may fail to discharge the sinus pacemaker because of sinoatrial interference, but it will also prevent the sinus impulse from activating the atria. If conditions are suitable, the next sinus impulse will arrive on time and depolarize the atria. This is the explanation for interpolated atrial extrasystoles.

From the foregoing, it is apparent that the duration of the postectopic pause is of limited help in identifying the site of origin of premature systoles.

Premature systoles may give rise to group beating, such as bigeminy, trigeminy, and quadrigeminy.

All premature beats may affect subsequent impulse formation and conduction. They may also be responsible for reciprocal beats or rhythms.

Occasionally, the first or the first few P waves of the sinus beats which follow a premature systole may have a different configuration from other sinus P waves in the tracing (Fig. 24-9). This is most apt to occur after atrial premature contractions, less often after AV junctional beats, and least often after ventricular extrasystoles. It may be the result of a shift in the pacemaker to another site in the SA node or atria or may result from aberrant atrial conduction.

Mechanism of Premature Systoles

Various theories have been proposed to explain the genesis of premature systoles. There is no evidence that all extrasystoles are caused by the same

Fig. 24-9 Aberrant atrial conduction. A sinus beat is followed by an atrial premature systole and a pause. The P wave of the postectopic beat is different in configuration from that of the other sinus beats in the record as a result of aberrant atrial conduction or because of a shift in the location of the atrial pacemaker.

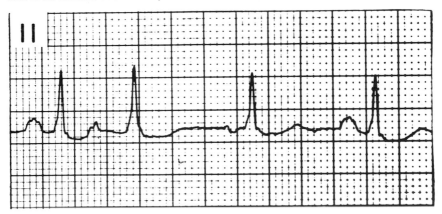

mechanism, and it may well be that different mechanisms are operative under different conditions. The mechanisms that have been proposed include microreentry with unidirectional block, ectopic focal impulse formation, ectopic enhancement (Wedensky facilitation), parasystole, negative afterpotentials, and circus movements.

Etiology

Premature systoles may occur in both health and disease. They are the most frequent of all cardiac arrhythmias.

Clinical Significance

Differentiation between premature systoles occurring in normal and diseased hearts is not always possible. The features listed below may be helpful in this regard:

Ventricular Premature Systoles

1 Ventricular premature beats with a QRS duration of 0.18 s or more suggest myocardial abnormality.
2 Ventricular extrasystoles that have variable coupling and variable interectopic intervals are more apt to be associated with cardiac disease.
3 Multiform or multifocal ventricular premature systoles are invariably indicative of abnormality.
4 Variable coupling and marked multiformity denote the presence of a serious arrhythmic state and a predisposition to grave ventricular arrhythmias.
5 Ventricular extrasystoles with the configuration of left bundle branch block and a vertical or rightward axis occur most frequently in normal persons. In the presence of heart disease, however, extrasystoles with the contour of right bundle branch block are found more often.
6 Ventricular premature beats of bizarre configuration with multiple notching and slurring (bizarre depolarization) or primary S-T-T changes (bizarre repolarization) or both are considered by Soloff to be significant. According to him, they are almost always found in association with heart disease.
7 Any premature beat, whether ventricular or supraventricular with aberrant ventricular conduction, is usually diagnostic of myocardial infarction if the ectopic beat presents a basic QR morphology in ventricular epicardial leads (D of Figs. 24-13 and 24-15).
8 Bidirectional ventricular extrasystoles usually are diagnostic of digitalis intoxication.
9 Ventricular premature beats with bigeminy are often, but not always, a sign of digitalis toxicity.

10 Ventricular extrasystoles occurring during the vulnerable phase (at or near the peak of the T wave) of the preceding beat (Figs. 24-97, 24-104, 24-190) may result in ventricular tachycardia or fibrillation and sudden death. When ventricular premature systoles have a Q-R/Q-T ratio of less than 0.85, the likelihood of this occurrence is greatly increased. In the formula, the Q-R interval is measured from the beginning of the QRS complex to the R wave of the premature beat; the Q-T interval, in the usual manner.

Atrial Premature Systoles Atrial premature systoles may occur in health as well as disease. Occasional atrial extrasystoles usually have little clinical significance and are seen in normal individuals. Frequent and persistent atrial premature systoles, runs of atrial extrasystoles, and multifocal atrial premature beats are generally associated with organic heart disease, chronic lung disease, or both.

AV Junctional Premature Systoles AV junctional premature systoles occur less frequently than those of ventricular or atrial origin, but like them they may occur in health as well as in disease.

Miscellaneous Observations

1 There is rarely coexistence of atrial and ventricular premature beats in the same patient in the absence of heart disease.
2 Exercise and tachycardia tend to abolish ectopic beats in both normal and diseased hearts. Their failure to do so cannot be considered abnormal, nor can an increased frequency of premature beats following exercise necessarily be regarded as significant.
3 Alteration in the direction or voltage of the T wave in the sinus beat following a ventricular extrasystole, the so-called "postextrasystolic" T wave change, may occur in the presence or absence of cardiac disease. The frequency of this change depends on the length of the preceding compensatory pause, shorter pauses favoring its occurrence.

Sinus Premature Systoles (Fig. 24-10)

1 Sinus premature systoles are extremely rare.
2 The premature P wave is identical in contour to the normal sinus P wave.
3 The coupling intervals of the premature beats are usually constant.
4 The pause after the premature systole is always noncompensatory.
5 Sinus premature systoles should be differentiated from the following:
a Atrial premature systoles, in which the P waves are different in contour from the normal sinus P waves.
b Sinus arrhythmia, in which the relationship to the respiratory cycle is apparent from the gradual increase or decrease in the cycle length.

Lead II

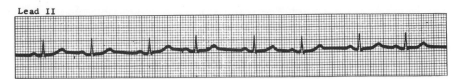

Fig. 24-10   Sinus premature systoles with bigeminy versus 3:2 SA block. Each pair of sinus impulses is followed by a pause. Two interpretations are possible: (1) The coupled beat is a sinus premature systole, or (2) it is the second beat in a three-beat Wenckebach period, the third of which is dropped (3:2 SA block).

c   3:2 SA block, which may present a most difficult or impossible problem. When 3:2 SA block is uncomplicated the distinction is not difficult, because the pause is equal to twice the normal P-P interval. However, when 3:2 SA block is of the Wenckebach type, the pause is less than the sum of two normal cycles. Under these circumstances, the diagnosis cannot be resolved unless sinus rhythm returns. According to Schamroth, with sinus extrasystoles the cycle length during sinus rhythm will equal the longer P-P interval during bigeminal rhythm, whereas in 3:2 SA block the cycle length during sinus rhythm will equal the shorter P-P interval during bigeminal rhythm.

Atrial Premature Systoles
(Figs. 24-8A, 24-9, 24-11, 24-12, 24-13A and C)

1   The ectopic P wave (called P′ wave) is premature.
2   The contour of the P′ wave is abnormal with respect to the sinus P wave. The nearer the origin to the SA node, the closer the resemblance of the ectopic to the sinus P wave. The opposite is also true: the farther the origin from the SA node, the greater the abnormality in its configuration. Ectopic beats arising low in the atrium, near the AV node, are often retrograde in contour (inverted in leads II, III, and aVF). A P′ wave occurring early in ventricular diastole may be superimposed on the preceding T wave and is easily overlooked unless searched for carefully.
3   The P′-R interval is usually as long as or longer than the sinus P-R interval, but it may be shorter.
4   The coupling interval of atrial premature beats may be constant or inconstant.
5   Atrial premature systoles that are multifocal have two or more P′ waves with different configurations.
6   The QRST complexes may be normal, aberrant, or absent (no QRS complex follows the P′ wave). The P′ waves are usually followed by QRST complexes. However, if the atrial premature beats occur early in ventricular diastole, when the AV conduction system is still completely refractory from previous sinus stimulation, ventricular conduc-

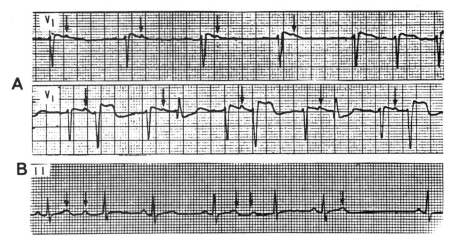

Fig. 24-11 Atrial premature systoles. (*A*) *Upper strip:* Nonconducted atrial premature systoles, indicated by arrows. *Lower strip:* Atrial extrasystolic bigeminy with alternating patterns of left and right bundle branch block aberrancy. The arrows point to the P' waves. (*B*) Multiple atrial premature systoles. When paired, the initial ectopic impulse is nonconducted, but the second is conducted at a prolonged P-R interval because of concealed conduction of the first premature beat. The mechanism in a similar situation is diagramed in Fig. 24-141.

tion will fail (nonconducted or blocked atrial premature systoles). When there is partial recovery in the AV conduction system, an atrial premature beat may be transmitted but at a prolonged AV conduction time, or it may be conducted aberrantly through the ventricles, or both may occur. The degree of ventricular aberration is determined by the length of the preceding cycle and the prematurity of the beat. As a rule, the longer the preceding cycle and the more premature the beat, the more marked is the aberration. Exceptions, however, occur.

Fig. 24-12 Atrial premature systoles. The premature beats are identified by the letter P'. The first premature beat is superimposed on the preceding T wave, and its QRS complex is markedly aberrant. The second premature beat occurs later in the cycle, so there is a lesser degree of aberration of the QRS complex. The pauses following the premature systoles are not compensatory.

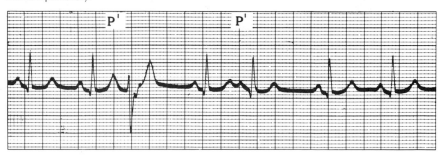

Sometimes, a very early premature beat is not conducted aberrantly. This happens when the beat encounters so much AV nodal delay that the His-Purkinje system is no longer refractory at the time of arrival of the impulse.

7 The pause following the premature beat is usually noncompensatory, but exceptions occur.

8 Atrial premature systoles are only rarely interpolated.

9 Spontaneous (or artificially induced) atrial premature beats may initiate atrial fibrillation. The propensity of an atrial premature systole to initiate fibrillation is related to its relative prematurity, expressed as a coupling index based on the following formula (Killip and Gault):

$$\text{Coupling index} = \frac{\text{coupling interval}}{\text{preceding cycle length}} = \frac{P_2\text{-}P'}{P_1\text{-}P_2}$$

where P′ represents the atrial extrasystole, P_2 the impulse preceding atrial discharge, and P_1, the atrial discharge immediately preceding P_2.

When the coupling index is less than 0.50, the chance of atrial fibrillation is high; when it is greater than 0.60, the chance of atrial fibrillation is small.

10 Atrial premature systoles may affect conduction of subsequent beats. When two or more atrial premature beats occur in succession, an early beat may penetrate the AV junction but fail to reach the ventricles (concealed conduction). In so doing, it leaves the AV junction partially refractory, so that conduction of the following P wave is slowed.

11 An early atrial extrasystole may conduct slowly through the AV junction to the ventricles and then return to the atria by an alternate pathway

Fig. 24-13 Premature systoles. (A) Atrial bigeminy. Each sinus beat is followed by an atrial ectopic beat. The P′ waves of the first and third atrial premature systoles deform the T waves of the preceding sinus beats. Both of these are conducted aberrantly. The ventricular cycle preceding the third atrial premature beat is longer than that preceding the second. Also, the second atrial extrasystole occurs later in the cycle than either the first or the third atrial ectopic beats. Aberrant ventricular conduction of atrial premature systoles is determined by the prematurity of the ectopic beat and the length of the preceding ventricular cycle. The aberrantly conducted beats show a right bundle branch block morphology. (B) An AV junctional premature systole. The P′-R interval is 0.09 s. The pause following the beat is not compensatory. (C) An atrial premature systole with a P′-R interval of 0.12 s followed by a noncompensatory pause. (D) An atrial premature systole (the P′ wave is superimposed on the T wave of the preceding beat) showing aberrant ventricular conduction with a QR morphology. This is considered virtually diagnostic of myocardial infarction. (E) A late diastolic premature systole occurring after inscription of the normal sinus P wave. (F) A ventricular premature systole with retrograde atrial conduction. An inverted P wave follows the ectopic impulse.

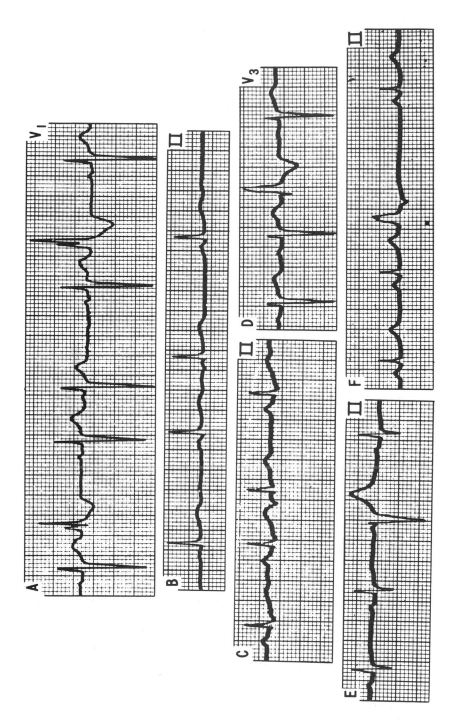

and produce an atrial echo (also called a *reciprocal beat* or *return extrasystole*).

12   Interpolation of atrial extrasystoles occurs but is a rarely observed phenomenon.

Atrioventricular Junctional Premature Systoles
(Figs. 24-8B, 24-13B, 24-14, 24-15A and B)

1   The P' waves occur before, during, or after the QRS complexes.
2   When identifiable, the P' waves are abnormal and retrograde in contour (inverted in leads II, III, and aVF and upright in aVR).
3   The P'-R interval is 0.10 s to negative.
4   The coupling interval is usually constant.
5   The QRST complexes, although of essentially normal outline and duration (0.10 s or less), are often slightly aberrant.
6   The duration of the postectopic pause is variable. The pause is fully compensatory if retrograde conduction of the extrasystole is blocked or interfered with. The pause is noncompensatory when the retrograde impulse discharges the SA node prematurely. There is no pause if the premature beat is interpolated.

Fig. 24-14   AV junctional premature systoles (JPS). (*A*) The configuration of the premature beat is identical with that of the conducted sinus beats. The pause is compensatory. (*B*) A slightly aberrant premature systole is followed by a retrograde P wave. The pause, in spite of retrograde atrial activation, is compensatory.

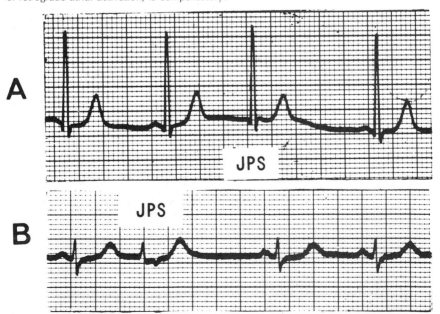

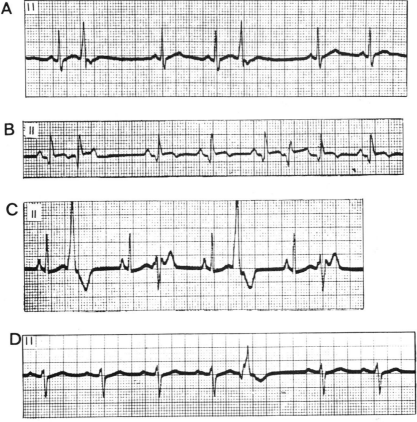

Fig. 24-15 AV junctional and ventricular premature systoles. (*A*) AV junctional premature systoles (the second and fifth ventricular complexes) show only slight aberration and are followed by retrograde P waves. The pauses are noncompensatory. (*B*) AV junctional premature systoles (the second and sixth ventricular complexes) in a patient with acute inferior myocardial infarction. The second ectopic beat is interpolated. (*C*) Extrasystolic bigeminy due to bifocal ventricular premature systoles. (*D*) A ventricular premature beat (fifth ventricular complex) shows a QR morphology considered to be diagnostic of myocardial infarction.

7   AV junctional premature systoles are occasionally interpolated. Like other extrasystoles, they may produce echo beats.

Ventricular Premature Systoles
(Figs. 5-42, 24-8C, 24-13F, 24-15C and D, 24-16 to
24-28, 24-31, 24-60, 24-61, 24-63, 24-64)

1   There are premature, bizarre QRST complexes which are not preceded by premature P waves. The QRST complex of the ectopic beat is usually dissociated from the sinus P wave. However, retrograde conduction to the atria from such beats is not uncommon.

I I

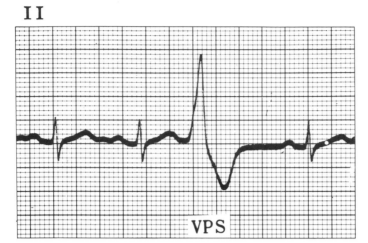

VPS

Fig. 24-16   Ventricular premature systole followed by a fully compensatory pause.   The premature beat is wide and aberrant and is not preceded by a premature P wave.

2   The QRS complexes are abnormally wide (0.12 s or more) and bizarre, with the T wave opposite to the main ventricular deflection.

3   Premature beats with identical contour and coupling are unifocal in origin.   Premature beats with identical contour but variable coupling are often parasystolic.   Premature beats with variable contour but fixed coupling are probably unifocal but are often described as multiform. The different configuration of the beats is explained by variable transmission through the ventricles.   Premature beats with both variable

Fig. 24-17   Ventricular premature systoles of unifocal origin with bigeminy due to digitalis intoxication.   The ectopic beats are preceded by normal P waves appearing as a slur on the upstroke of the deflections.

LEAD II

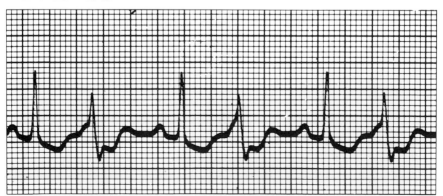

LEAD II

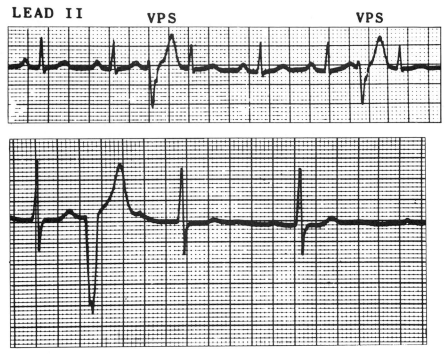

Fig. 24-18 Interpolated premature systoles. *Upper tracing:* Two interpolated ventricular premature systoles. The basic rhythm is not disturbed. *Lower tracing:* An interpolated ventricular premature systole causing prolongation of the P-R interval of the first postectopic sinus beat as a result of the retrograde concealed conduction.

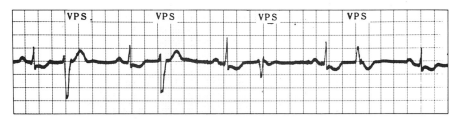

Fig. 24-19 Multiform ventricular premature systoles with bigeminy due to digitalis intoxication.

Fig. 24-20 Ventricular premature systoles with trigeminy.

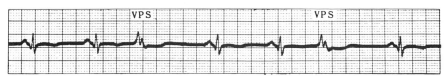

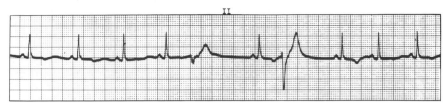

Fig. 24-21 Postextrasystolic T wave change. The fifth and seventh ventricular beats are ventricular premature systoles. The T wave of the sinus beat following each premature systole is more deeply inverted than other beats in the record.

Fig. 24-22 Ventricular premature systoles (the second beat in each lead) arising from the Purkinje network of the left posterior fascicle, displaying a pattern of right bundle branch block with left anterior fascicular block. The sinus beats show left bundle branch block. (*From M. B. Rosenbaum, Classification of Ventricular Extrasystoles According to Form, J. Electrocardiol., 2: 289, 1969. Used by permission.*)

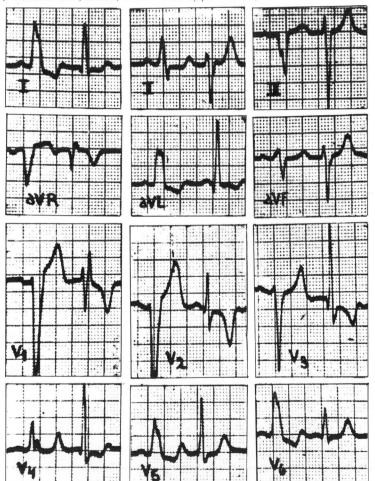

contour and variable coupling are usually multifocal but are commonly described as multiform.

4   Ventricular premature systoles may be interpolated, may cause the echo phenomenon, and may produce ventricular as well as atrial fusion beats.

5   The site of origin of ventricular premature systoles can usually be determined from their appearance.   Right ventricular extrasystoles generally produce a left bundle branch block pattern, and left ventricular

Fig. 24-23   Ventricular premature systoles arising from the Purkinje plexus of the left anterior fascicle, displaying a pattern of right bundle branch block with left posterior fascicular block. (*From M. B. Rosenbaum, Classification of Ventricular Extrasystoles According to Form, J. Electrocardiol., 2: 289, 1969.   Used by permission.*)

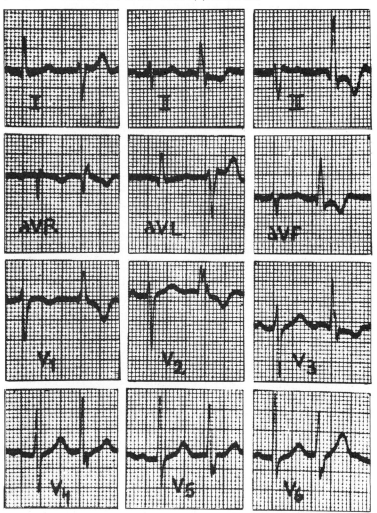

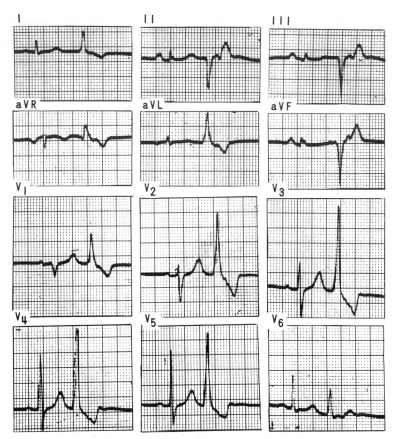

Fig. 24-24 Ventricular extrasystoles arising from the base of the left ventricle, but posteriorly. The premature beats are upright in all the precordial leads. A retrograde P wave follows each extrasystole. The axis of the ectopic beats is directed superiorly and leftward in the limb leads.

extrasystoles a right bundle branch block pattern. Extrasystoles arising from the posterior wall of the left ventricle display the pattern of right bundle branch block with left anterior fascicular block, and those arising from its anterior wall display the pattern of right bundle branch block with left posterior fascicular block. Basal extrasystoles show upright QRS complexes in all or nearly all the precordial leads. In the extremity leads, such beats show the pattern of left anterior fascicular block if they arise posteriorly and that of left posterior fascicular block if they arise anteriorly. Apical extrasystoles produce negative QRS complexes in all or nearly all the precordial leads. In the extremity leads the QRS axis of such beats is directed rightward and superiorly if they arise from the posterior aspect of the apex, rightward and inferiorly if they arise from its anterior aspect.

According to Rosenbaum, right ventricular extrasystoles in normal hearts show a left bundle branch block pattern which differs from that found in abnormal hearts in the following respects: (1) the initial forces are directed anteriorly, resulting in tall and broad R waves in leads V_1 to V_3; (2) the main QRS forces are directed inferiorly; and (3) the QRS loop is inscribed in a CCW manner in the transverse plane.

Ventricular extrasystoles with relatively narrow QRS complexes arise proximally in the conduction system. The subject of narrow ventricular ectopic beats and rhythms is discussed later in this chapter under the heading Fascicular Beats and Rhythms.

Fig. 24-25 Ventricular premature beats arising from the base of the left ventricle, but anteriorly. The extrasystoles are upright in all the precordial leads. Their axis in the limb leads is directed rightward and inferiorly. (*From M. B. Rosenbaum, Classification of Ventricular Extrasystoles According to Form, J. Electrocardiol., 2: 289, 1969. Used by permission.*)

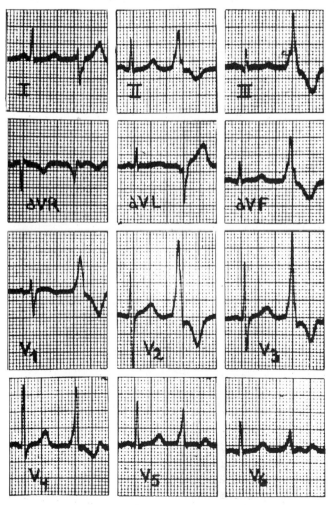

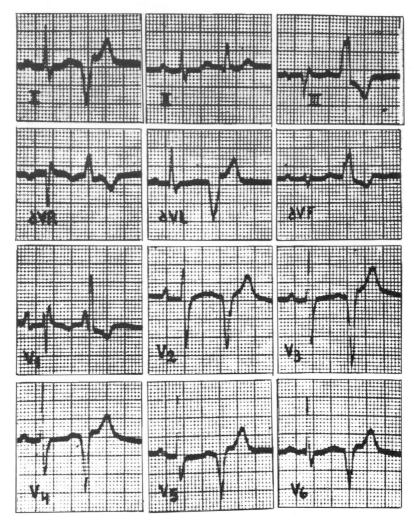

Fig. 24-26   Ventricular premature systoles arising from the anterior aspect of the apex of the left ventricle.   The extrasystoles are downward in all the precordial leads except lead V_1.   In the limb leads, their axis is directed rightward and inferiorly.   (*From M. B. Rosenbaum, Classification of Ventricular Extrasystoles According to Form, J. Electrocardiol., 2: 289, 1969. Used by permission.*)

6   The pause following ventricular premature systoles is usually compensatory unless either the beat is interpolated or the sinus pacemaker is discharged as a result of retrograde atrial activation.   However, compensatory pauses may occur even in the presence of retrograde atrial activation.

Differential Diagnosis of Premature Systoles

1   If the QRST complex of a premature beat is essentially of normal configuration, the beat is supraventricular in origin.

2   If the QRST complex of a premature beat is abnormally wide, the beat
is ventricular or supraventricular with aberrant ventricular conduction.

3   If the QRST complex of a premature beat is preceded by an abnormal
P wave at a normal or prolonged P-R interval, the ectopic beat is of
atrial origin.   If the P' wave is retrograde in contour and the P'-R
interval is 0.10 s or less, the beat is of AV junctional origin.   If the P'
wave is retrograde in contour but the P'-R interval is 0.12 s or more,
the beat is of atrial origin.

4   If the QRST complex of a premature beat is abnormally wide and is not

Fig. 24-27   Ventricular premature systoles arising from the posterior aspect of the apex of the
left ventricle.   The extrasystoles are downward in all the precordial leads except lead V_1.
Their axis is directed superiorly and rightward in the extremity leads.   (*From M. B. Rosenbaum,
Classification of Ventricular Extrasystoles According to Form, J. Electrocardiol., 2: 289, 1969.
Used by permission.*)

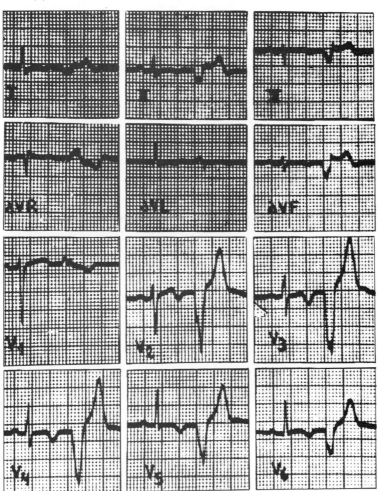

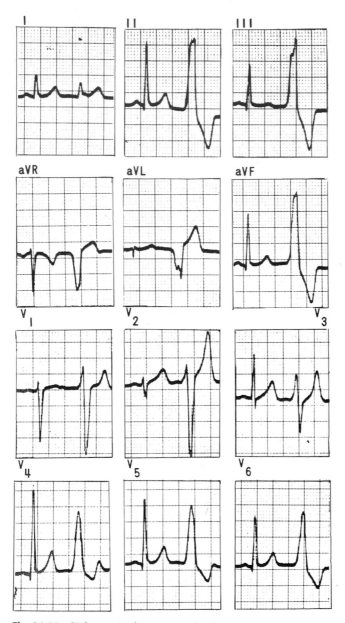

Fig. 24-28   Right ventricular extrasystoles from a normal person.   The premature beats show the patterns of left bundle branch block in the precordial leads, but the R waves in leads V_1 to V_3 are tall and broad.   Their axis in the frontal plane is normal in this instance, but right ventricular extrasystoles in normal hearts often show a mean QRS vector that is directed inferiorly.

preceded by an ectopic P wave, the beat is either ventricular or AV junctional with aberrant ventricular conduction. Usually the two are indistinguishable. Differentiation between them is sometimes possible if there is retrograde conduction to the atria. If the QRS-P′ interval is 0.10 s or less, the beat is AV junctional in origin. If the interval is longer, it is not possible to determine whether the beat is ventricular or whether it is AV junctional with delayed retrograde conduction.

5 If the pause following a premature systole is compensatory, it is most often a ventricular extrasystole; less often it is an AV junctional extrasystole with retrograde block or interference; and only rarely is it atrial in origin. If the pause is noncompensatory, the premature beat is either atrial or AV junctional in origin, although on occasion it may be a ventricular extrasystole with retrograde atrial activation.

6 Ventricular or AV junctional premature systoles occurring late in diastole after the inscription of the normal P wave may be mistaken for atrial premature systoles. However, the QRS complexes of the last are preceded by premature ectopic P waves and those of the first two by correctly timed normal P waves.

ESCAPE BEATS (FIGS. 24-40, 24-56 to 24-59, 24-115, 24-176)

1 Escape beats are *late* ectopic beats that follow a pause *longer* than the normal cycle length (in contrast to premature beats, which are *early* ectopic beats). Escape beats are most often of AV junctional origin. Ventricular escape beats occur less often. Atrial or sinus escape beats are rare.

2 Atrioventricular junctional escape beats have the characteristics of AV junctional premature systoles except that they are delayed. Usually AV junctional escape beats are not accompanied by retrograde P waves. However, the escape beat is sometimes preceded by a nonconducted sinus P wave. Classic AV junctional escape beats without aberration probably arise from the bundle of His; they show a configuration that is similar to or identical with that of conducted beats. Aberration of AV junctional escapes, however, is common and its degree variable. Potential mechanisms of aberration of escape beats include origin in Mahaim fibers, a ventricular fascicular origin, functional dissociation within a bundle branch, Wedensky facilitation, supernormality of intraventricular conduction, spontaneous phase 4 depolarization, and incomplete recovery. In the two latter instances it is assumed that aberration occurs because the cells in which they originate conduct abnormally. Functional aberrancy based on incomplete recovery of the conduction fibers cannot account for aberrancy in slow junctional rhythms. Phase 4 depolarization may explain aberrancy in slow heart rates but cannot account for the fusion complexes seen so frequently in these rhythms.

According to the Sherf and James concept of synchronized sino-ventricular conduction (discussed in Chap. 2), AV junctional beats produce ventricular aberration by a desynchronization of the normal sequence of depolarization in the AV junctional area and its distal branches, except when the ectopic junctional focus is fortuitously located directly on the axis of normal depolarization. At present this is based only on deductive reasoning.

Studies have disclosed that aberrancy in junctional beats usually shows features of incomplete or complete right bundle branch block and a leftward or rightward shift of the QRS axis in the frontal plane. With the use of His bundle electrography, aberrant AV junctional escape beats have been shown, in several cases, to originate in one of the two fascicles of the left bundle branch: in the anterior fascicle for beats displaying right axis deviation and in the posterior fascicle for beats displaying left axis deviation. A fascicular origin also provides a satisfactory explanation for the fusion complexes so frequently seen in these rhythms.

3   The escape interval is usually fairly constant and corresponds to the cycle length of the AV junctional or ventricular pacemaker.

4   Ventricular escape beats have the characteristics of ventricular premature systoles except that they are delayed.

5   Escape beats in atrial fibrillation are recognized as long, essentially equal pauses. Escape beats may occur singly or in groups. Although the intervals are usually longer than other cycle lengths in the record, they need not be exactly equal, because concealment of fibrillatory waves may result in unexpected postponement of escape. The escape beats may resemble the normally conducted beats, or they may be aberrant.

CAPTURE BEATS (FIGS. 24-79, 24-95, 24-96, 24-98, 24-116 to 24-120, 24-122, 24-129, 24-148, 24-149)

In AV dissociation, different pacemakers control the atria and ventricles so that they beat independently. Because the temporal relationship between the two rhythms varies, impulses originating in one of the pacemakers may occur at a time when the AV junction is not refractory and capture the chambers controlled by the other pacemaker. Beats produced by this mechanism are called *capture(d) beats*. Ventricular captures occur much more frequently than atrial captures. The contour of ventricular captures may be helpful in determining the site of the ventricular pacemaker. The reader is referred to the section on AV dissociation in this chapter for further details.

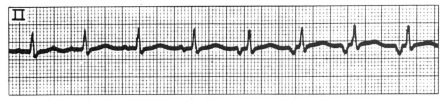

Fig. 24-29 Wandering pacemaker. The third, fourth, and fifth P waves are atrial fusion beats. The contours of these beats are intermediate between those of the first two P waves and those of the sixth, seventh, and eighth P waves.

FUSION, COMBINATION, OR SUMMATION BEATS

Fusion, combination, or summation beats occur when two separate impulses discharge the atria or ventricles simultaneously. The superimposition of P waves on QRST complexes in the electrocardiogram is not fusion.

Atrial Fusion Beats (Figs. 24-29, 24-83, 24-118, 24-134)

Atrial fusion beats occur when two impulses of different origin stimulate the atria simultaneously. The contour of the P wave of the fusion beat is intermediate between the contours of the P waves produced by each impulse. Atrial fusion beats may be seen when the pacemaker wanders between the SA and AV nodes. It may also occur from the fusion of the sinus impulse either with an ectopic atrial impulse or with a retrograde impulse of AV junctional or ventricular origin.

Ventricular Fusion Beats (Figs. 24-8, 24-58, 24-95, 24-96, 24-98, 24-106, 24-107, 24-109, 24-110, 24-111C, 24-114, 24-136 to 24-138, 24-188, 24-193)

Ventricular fusion beats occur when two impulses of different origin stimulate the ventricles simultaneously. The contour of the QRST complex of the fusion beat is intermediate between the contours of the QRST complexes produced by each impulse. Ventricular fusion beats usually result from the simultaneous discharge of the ventricles by impulses of supraventricular and ectopic ventricular origin. Simultaneous activation of the ventricles by two ventricular impulses may also cause fusion beats.

Fusion beats occur in ventricular preexcitation when atrial impulses are conducted simultaneously through both the normal and the accessory pathways.

Diagnosis of Ventricular Fusion Beats (Marriott et al.)

1 The contour and duration of the fusion beat must be intermediate between those of the competing pacemakers. The duration of the QRS complex of the fusion beat is not more than 0.06 s longer than that of the sinus QRS complex.

2   The fusion beat must occur at a time when impulses from both pacemakers may be expected.

3   The P-J interval of the fusion beat must be longer than the P-R interval of the supraventricular beat, because for fusion to occur, the SA impulse must have time to reach the ventricles before they are completely activated by the ectopic center.

4   The P-R interval of the fusion beat may be equal to, or not more than 0.06 s shorter than, the P-R interval of the conducted beat. This is because it takes no longer than 0.06 s for an ectopic ventricular beat to depolarize the ventricles and thus prevent the descent of a supraventricular impulse.

5   The initial vector of the fusion beat may or may not be different from that of the supraventricular beat, depending on whether the supraventricular or ventricular beat depolarizes the ventricles first. When the P-R interval of the fusion beat is shortened, the ectopic beat will activate the ventricles first and the initial vector of the fusion beat will differ from that of the conducted beat.

6   In all fusion beats, the terminal vector differs from that of the supraventricular beats, because it is inscribed by the ectopic impulse alone or by the two impulses simultaneously.

Exceptions to these criteria may occur in the presence of ventricular conduction defects and during Wenckebach periods.

ABERRANT CONDUCTION

Aberrant Ventricular Conduction (Figs. 5-40, 5-42, 24-12, 24-13A and D, 24-15A, 24-30, 24-31, 24-42, 24-51, 24-63 to 24-66, 24-116D, 24-129, 24-131, 24-149)

Aberrant ventricular conduction of supraventricular impulses is defined as the abnormal spread of excitation through the ventricles because of partial refractoriness of the intraventricular conduction pathways. It is manifested by alterations in the contour and duration of the ventricular deflections. It may occur in a variety of supraventricular arrhythmias such as atrial and AV junctional premature systoles, AV junctional escape beats and rhythms, paroxysmal supraventricular tachycardias, and atrial fibrillation. Ventricular aberration is not confined to ectopic supraventricular beats but may be seen in sinus beats as well (e.g., capture beats and those occurring as a result of the retrograde concealed conduction of ventricular extrasystoles).

The conditions that determine aberrant ventricular conduction of supraventricular impulses are (1) the length of the cycle (R-R interval) preceding the ectopic beat; (2) the degree of prematurity of the impulse

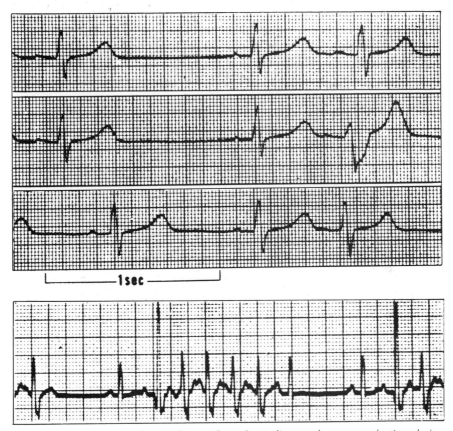

Fig. 24-30 The relation of preceding cycle and coupling to aberrant conduction during incomplete recovery. The upper three strips are from the X lead of a vector system of one patient, which roughly corresponds to lead I, and the last strip is lead I of another patient. The QRS which follows the atrial premature systole at the end of the first strip varies only slightly from the QRS of sinus origin. The atrial premature beat at the end of the second strip is conducted aberrantly to the ventricles, presumably because it occurs earlier (shorter coupling) during incomplete recovery. The preceding cycles in the first two strips are about the same. The atrial premature systole at the end of the third strip is conducted more normally than the atrial premature systole in the second strip, even though it occurs earlier. The explanation is the shorter preceding cycle, which speeds recovery after the sinus beat that precedes the atrial premature systole. In the last strip are runs of atrial premature systoles with abnormal QRS complexes, also explained by aberrant conduction during incomplete recovery. The beat after the long pause is probably of sinus origin. The onset of the subsequent run of tachycardia with a P wave identifies the focus of the tachycardia as supraventricular (probably reentrant). The eighth QRS complex is normal, whereas the third QRS is not, even though the eighth QRS occurs earlier in the cycle. The explanation is the much shorter cycle preceding the eighth QRS. The third and tenth QRS complexes differ from the aberrant QRS complexes which follow them; presumably they are more aberrant because of the much longer cycle preceding each. In both cases the configuration of QRS during aberrant conduction resembles that of right bundle branch block. (*From A. D. Kistin, Problems in the Differentiation of Ventricular Arrhythmia from Supraventricular Arrhythmia with Abnormal QRS, Progr. Cardiovsc. Dis., 9: 1, 1966. Used by permission.*)

VENTRICULAR ABERRATION vs. ECTOPY: MORPHOLOGIC CLUES

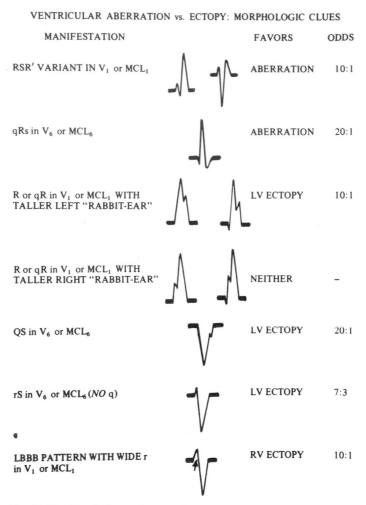

MANIFESTATION	FAVORS	ODDS
RSR' VARIANT IN V₁ or MCL₁	ABERRATION	10:1
qRs in V₆ or MCL₆	ABERRATION	20:1
R or qR in V₁ or MCL₁ WITH TALLER LEFT "RABBIT-EAR"	LV ECTOPY	10:1
R or qR in V₁ or MCL₁ WITH TALLER RIGHT "RABBIT-EAR"	NEITHER	–
QS in V₆ or MCL₆	LV ECTOPY	20:1
rS in V₆ or MCL₆ (NO q)	LV ECTOPY	7:3
LBBB PATTERN WITH WIDE r in V₁ or MCL₁	RV ECTOPY	10:1

Fig. 24-31   Morphologic clues to the differential diagnosis between aberrant ventricular conduction and ventricular ectopy. Discussed in text. (*From H. J. L. Marriott, "Workshop in Electrocardiography," Tampa Tracings, Oldsmar, Fla., 1972. Used by permission.*)

(coupling interval); (3) the speed of AV conduction; and (4) the state of recovery of excitability in the specialized ventricular conduction system.

Aberrant ventricular conduction is most likely to occur when the preceding cycle length is long, since a direct relationship exists between cycle length and refractoriness in the His-Purkinje system: the greater the preceding R-R interval, the longer the refractory period, and vice versa. Thus a long R-R interval preceding a premature supraventricular beat favors aberration, whereas a shorter interval may cause aberration to disappear. In general, the more premature the supraventricular beat, the greater the tendency for aberration to occur. Rapid AV conduction enhances the possibility of aberration, because the ectopic impulse is then delivered to the conducting system while it is still refractory. However, very early premature beats may be conducted so slowly through the AV node that they arrive at the His-Purkinje system at a time when the conduction system is no longer refractory.

The QRS pattern which results from aberrant ventricular conduction is most commonly that of right bundle branch block (over 80 percent of cases). Next in frequency are the patterns of left bundle branch block, left anterior fascicular block, combined right bundle branch block and left anterior fascicular block, right bundle branch block with left posterior fascicular block, and left posterior fascicular block. All these types of aberration may appear in the same individual, and right bundle branch block and left bundle branch block patterns may alternate. The QRS duration rarely exceeds 0.12 s in the right bundle branch block pattern of aberration and 0.14 s in left bundle branch block aberration. Parenthetically, it is worth noting that ventricular premature systoles frequently exhibit wider QRS complexes.

The frequency with which the various patterns of ventricular aberration occur, as outlined in the preceding paragraph, is attributed to differences in the refractory periods of the respective fascicles. Normally, the refractory period of the right bundle branch is longer than that of the left, and that of the anterior fascicle of the left branch longer than that of the posterior fascicle. Aberrant ventricular conduction is probably a normal phenomenon when an impulse reaches the ventricles within 0.04 s of the preceding ventricular complex. When the refractory period of the ventricular conduction system is prolonged by disease, aberrancy may occur at very slow heart rates. Ventricular aberration can occur in both normal and abnormal hearts and per se is not a sign of heart disease.

Aberrant ventricular conduction should be diagnosed in supraventricular arrhythmia when abnormal QRS complexes not due to intraventricular block are preceded by premature ectopic P waves to which they are related. This rule applies to both premature systoles and ectopic tachycardias. During paroxysms of supraventricular tachycardia with aberrant ventricular conduction, the QRS complex of the first ectopic beat often shows a greater degree of aberration than other beats in the run. This is because the sinus cycle which precedes it is longer than the ectopic cycle.

Clues to the diagnosis of aberrant ventricular conduction may be found in the morphologic characteristics of the QRS complexes. The following features favor aberration: an RSR' complex in lead V_1 (or MCL_1) in which the R' is taller than the R, a qRs complex in lead V_6 (or MCL_6), an initial vector is an anomalous beat that is identical with that of conducted sinus beats in the same lead, a relationship to preceding atrial beats, and a resemblance to previous known aberrancy. The diagnosis of aberrant ventricular conduction in atrial fibrillation is discussed in the section on atrial fibrillation, later in this chapter.

Differentiation between aberrantly conducted beats and ventricular ectopic beats from the morphologic characteristics of the beats may be difficult or even impossible, particularly because conducted beats may be quite bizarre in their appearance. Moreover, bundle branch block and fascicular rhythms frequently show relatively narrow QRS complexes with features suggesting aberrancy. The differential diagnosis between ventricular ectopy and aberrant ventricular conduction is considered in the next section.

Aberrant Atrial Conduction (Fig. 24-9)

Sometimes the first P wave or the first few P waves of the sinus beats which follow an atrial premature systole (or less often, an AV junctional or ventricular extrasystole) may have a different configuration from the other sinus P waves in the record. This phenomenon has been termed *aberrant atrial conduction*. However, it can also be explained by a shift in the pacemaker to another site in the SA node or to an ectopic focus in the atria.

ABERRANT VENTRICULAR CONDUCTION VS. VENTRICULAR ECTOPY (FIG. 24-31)

The differential diagnosis between aberrant ventricular conduction and ventricular ectopy is frequently difficult and sometimes impossible.
    The morphologic characteristics of the beats may provide a clue.

1   The diagnosis of aberrant ventricular conduction is favored by the following features:
a   A triphasic RSR' pattern in lead V_1 (or MCL_1) in which the R' deflection is taller than the R wave. Usually, but not always, the initial vector of the anomalous complex is identical to that of normally conducted beats.
b   A qRs pattern in lead V_6 (or MCL_6).
c   A definite relationship between preceding atrial activity and the anomalous beat.
d   A resemblance of the abnormal complexes to the conducted beats in the same lead.
e   Morphology similar to previous known aberrancy.
f   A QRS duration of 0.12 s or less in right bundle branch aberrancy and of 0.14 s or less when the pattern is that of left bundle branch block.
g   Variable coupling of the anomalous beat to the preceding conducted beat.
h   Long-short cycle sequences.
2   The diagnosis of ventricular ectopy is favored by the following features:
a   A monophasic or diphasic QRS morphology in lead V_1 (or MCL_1), particularly if the initial vector is dissimilar to that of the conducted

beats.   With a notched R or qR complex in lead V_1 (MCL_1), R exceeds R' in voltage.

b   A QS or rS pattern in lead V_6 (or MCL_6).

c   A QRS complex located at or near the apex of the T wave.

d   A left bundle branch block pattern in the precordial leads, with a wide r wave in lead V_1 (or MCL_1).

e   Absence of a relationship to preceding atrial activity.

f   Morphology identical to previously known ventricular ectopic beats.

g   Fixed coupling, although this is sometimes variable.

h   Long-short cycle sequences (rule of bigeminy) but with fixed coupling (vs. aberrantly conducted beats).

i   Abnormally wide QRS complexes (greater than 0.12 s in left ventricular ectopic beats and more than 0.14 s when the beats are right ventricular in origin).

Comments   With all these criteria, it may still be impossible to differentiate between aberrant ventricular conduction and beats of ventricular origin. This is particularly true when the ventricular impulses arise from the bundle branch system or the fascicles.   Such beats frequently display narrow QRS complexes with features of aberration and do not particularly resemble ventricular beats.   This problem is considered elsewhere in this chapter.

The differential diagnosis between aberrant ventricular conduction and ventricular ectopy in atrial fibrillation is discussed in the section on atrial fibrillation.   The differential diagnosis of tachycardias with abnormal QRS complexes is also discussed later in this chapter.

His bundle electrography may be of assistance in differentiating between aberrant ventricular conduction and ventricular ectopy when there are no technical problems and accessory conduction pathways (as in the W-P-W syndrome) do not exist.   Conducted beats with abnormal QRS complexes, whether due to aberration or to preexisting intraventricular block, show H spikes preceding the QRS complexes at *normal or prolonged* H-V intervals. On the other hand, with ventricular ectopic beats, the H deflections follow the onset of the QRS complexes.   When they occur within the ventricular potentials they may not be visible, but those which follow the QRS complexes are generally recognizable.   The sequence of ventricular complex-H deflection-atrial complex is characteristic of ventricular ectopic activity. In fascicular rhythms with relatively narrow QRS complexes, the ventricular potentials are preceded by H deflections with short H-V intervals, although the H potential sometimes appears shortly after the onset of the ventricular complex.

ECTOPIC TACHYCARDIAS

Ectopic tachycardias are described by their site of origin (atrial, ventricular, etc.), the type of rhythm (tachycardia, fibrillation, etc.), and their mode of onset and termination (paroxysmal or nonparoxysmal).

Nonparoxysmal Tachycardia

The term *nonparoxysmal tachycardia* refers to a rapid ectopic rhythm with a gradual onset and slow termination. The rate usually does not exceed 140 per minute. Nonparoxysmal tachycardias are most often supraventricular in origin. The atrial variety is commonly associated with digitalis therapy and potassium depletion. The AV junctional variety is caused by digitalis excess, inferior myocardial infarction, rheumatic fever, myocarditis, or cardiac surgery and may be associated with retrograde atrial activation or AV dissociation. Nonparoxysmal ventricular tachycardia (idioventricular tachycardia) occurs frequently in acute myocardial infarction, but is also sometimes caused by digitalis toxicity.

Paroxysmal Tachycardia

The term *paroxysmal tachycardia* refers to an ectopic rhythm of supraventricular or ventricular origin which begins and ends abruptly. The rate usually exceeds 140 per minute. Paroxysmal tachycardias are usually continuous, but they may be recurrent or repetitive. Every effort should be made to differentiate supraventricular from ventricular tachycardias because of the different clinical, therapeutic, and prognostic implications of each group.

The term *supraventricular tachycardia,* in a generic sense, refers to all supraventricular tachyarrhythmias, regardless of origin or mode of appearance. If the site of origin of a supraventricular tachycardia is unknown, the rhythm should be classified as a supraventricular tachycardia of undetermined origin.

Special Varieties of Paroxysmal Tachycardia

Repetitive Paroxysmal Tachycardia (Fig. 24-32)   This is a type of paroxysmal tachycardia in which short paroxysms separated by sinus beats recur constantly over a period of months or years. It is generally found in otherwise healthy children and adults. Repetitive atrial tachycardia is the most frequent variety, but repetitive atrial flutter and repetitive AV junctional or ventricular tachycardia also occur. The paroxysmal state is of variable duration and often subsides spontaneously. It responds poorly, if at all, to digitalis or quinidine therapy.

Bidirectional Tachycardia (Fig. 24-33)   Bidirectional tachycardia is a rapid regular rhythm, usually 140 to 180 beats per minute, in which there are alternating rightward and leftward axis shifts in the frontal plane with a right bundle branch block pattern in lead I. In the frontal plane, the axes of the two types of beats are approximately -60 to $-80°$ and $+120°$. Bidirectional tachycardias are most often due to digitalis intoxication in

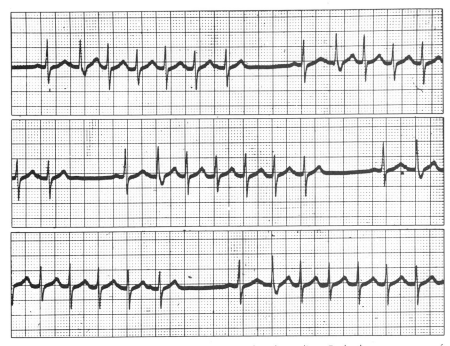

Fig. 24-32 Repetitive supraventricular paroxysmal tachycardia. Each short paroxysm of tachycardia is initiated by a premature aberrant P wave. There is aberration of the first ventricular beat in each run of tachycardia. The electrocardiogram is a continuous strip of lead II.

the presence of previous heart disease and are associated with a grave prognosis. Various mechanisms have been proposed to explain the electrocardiographic pattern. Rosenbaum and his associates have suggested that bidirectional tachycardia is a supraventricular arrhythmia with permanent aberrant conduction in the right bundle branch and alternating aberrant conduction in the two divisions of the left bundle branch. The supraventricular origin of bidirectional tachycardia has been confirmed in one case by His bundle electrocardiography. Another mechanism, also confirmed by His bundle recordings in a small number of patients, indicates that bidirectional tachycardia may result from an ectopic focus in the left ventricle. This accounts for the permanent pattern of right bundle branch

Fig. 24-33 Bidirectional tachycardia due to digitalis intoxication.

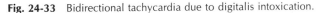
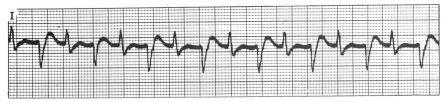

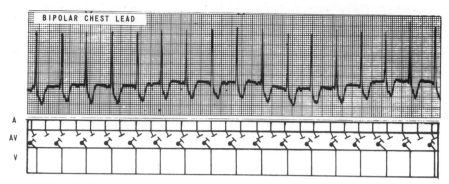

Fig. 24-34 Simultaneous automatic paroxysmal atrial and AV junctional tachycardias due to digitalis toxicity. There is complete AV dissociation. The atrial rate is 214 per minute; the ventricular rate is 125 per minute.

block. However, it is still unknown whether the alternating rightward and leftward axis shifts are the result of alternating routes of ventricular depolarization by a single ectopic left ventricular focus or of alternating discharge of two separate left ventricular foci.

Double or Simultaneous Tachycardias (Figs. 24-34, 24-35, 24-60) Double tachycardia refers to the simultaneous occurrence of two independent paroxysmal tachyarrhythmias, one controlling the atria and the other the ventricles. Although dual rhythm is a feature of parasystole, parasystolic rhythms are not considered double tachycardias in the usual sense of the term.

Fig. 24-35 Double tachycardia with complete AV dissociation. There is an automatic paroxysmal atrial tachycardia at a rate of 176 per minute and an automatic AV junctional tachycardia at a rate of 120 per minute.

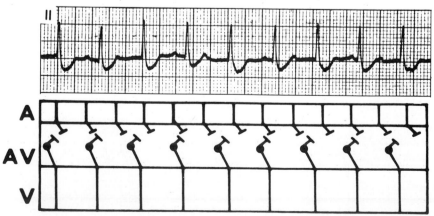

Posttachycardia Syndrome

Paroxysmal tachycardias are often associated with S-T segment and T wave changes. Sometimes these abnormalities may persist for hours or days after the tachycardia has stopped, even in normal hearts. The persistence of these S-T-T changes is referred to as the *posttachycardia syndrome*. Failure to recognize the relation of a tachycardia to these transitory changes may lead to an erroneous diagnosis of organic heart disease.

SINUS MECHANISMS

Sinus rhythms originate in the SA node. The distinction between normal sinus rhythm, sinus bradycardia, and sinus tachycardia is arbitrary and is based on the heart rate.

Normal Sinus Rhythm (Fig. 24-36)

1 A regular rhythm at a rate of 60 to 100 per minute. The duration of the cycle lengths does not vary by more than 10 percent.
2 The P waves have normal contours.
3 The P waves are upright in leads I (except in dextrocardia) and II, the left precordial leads, and usually lead aVF but are inverted in lead aVR. The configuration of the P waves is constant in each lead.
4 Each P wave is followed by a QRST complex unless the ventricles are refractory or AV block is present.
5 The P-R interval is 0.12 s or more.

Sinus Tachycardia

1 A regular sinus rhythm.
2 The rate is above 100 per minute.

Sinus Bradycardia

1 A regular sinus rhythm.
2 The rate is below 60 per minute.

Fig. 24-36 Normal sinus rhythm at a rate of 79 per minute. Sinus bradycardia and sinus tachycardia would have similar appearances, but the rates would be different.

LEAD II

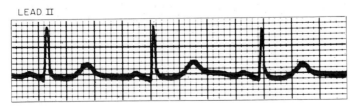

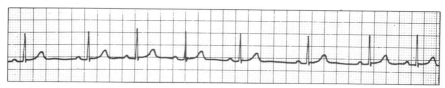

Fig. 24-37   Phasic sinus arrhythmia.

Clinical Significance   Sinus tachycardia occurs frequently in healthy persons and in a variety of disease states.   Sinus bradycardia is usually due to vagotonia.   It occurs in healthy adults, particularly in well-trained athletes, and is often seen in old age.   Sinus bradycardia is a common finding in patients with sinus node dysfunction.

Sinus Arrhythmia (Fig. 24-37)

Sinus arrhythmia is due to the irregular discharge of a single pacemaker within the SA node or to wandering of the pacemaker within the SA node.

1   An irregular sinus rhythm at a rate of less than 100 per minute, in which the cycle lengths vary by 10 percent or more.
2   There are two types:
a   *Phasic,* in which the heart rate increases during inspiration and decreases during expiration.
b   *Nonphasic,* in which the heart rate bears no relation to the respiratory cycle.

Ventriculophasic sinus arrhythmia (Fig. 24-38) is a form of nonphasic sinus arrhythmia in which atrial cycles containing ventricular complexes are shorter than those in which they are absent.   Ventriculophasic sinus arrhythmia usually occurs in advanced AV block or in association with ventricular premature systoles.

Clinical Significance   Phasic sinus arrhythmia is a frequent normal finding, particularly in children and young adults.   Nonphasic sinus arrhythmia is

Fig. 24-38   Ventriculophasic sinus arrhythmia in a patient with complete AV block.   The atrial cycles containing ventricular complexes are shorter than the other atrial cycles.   The configuration of the QRS complexes is normal because the ventricular pacemaker is located in the AV junction above the bifurcation of the common bundle.

Lead II

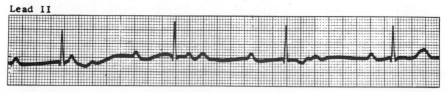

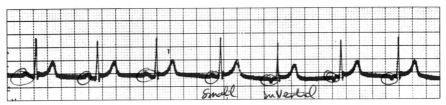

Small   inverted

Fig. 24-39   Wandering pacemaker between the SA node and the AV junction.

less frequent and is usually found in older persons, more commonly in the presence than in the absence of heart disease.   Phasic sinus arrhythmia is attributed to fluctuations in vagal tone.

Wandering Pacemaker (Figs. 24-29, 24-39)

There is a progressive shift of the pacemaker from beat to beat, either within the SA node or from the SA node to the AV junction and back again. Wandering pacemaker is a variant of sinus arrhythmia and has the same significance.   The heart rate is less than 100 per minute.

Within the SA Node

1   There are minor changes in the form of the P wave in a lead without its becoming retrograde.
2   The P-R interval varies but is always 0.12 s or more.

Between the SA Node and the AV Junction

1   There are successive changes in the form of the P wave in a lead, of minor to major degree.   It eventually becomes retrograde.   When the pacemaker is in the AV junction, the P wave may precede, coincide with, or follow the QRS complex.
2   The P-R intervals vary from 0.12 s or more to 0.10 s or less.
3   Atrial fusion beats may occur in the transition from a sinus to an AV junctional rhythm.

Sinus Arrest or Pause (Figs. 24-40, 24-176)

1   The SA node fails to initiate an impulse at the expected time or times.
2   The resulting pause is not an exact multiple of the cycle length (in contrast to SA block).
3   P waves and QRST complexes are absent during the pause except for the occasional occurrence of escape beats.

Clinical Significance   Sinus arrest may be the result of reflex vagal stimulation, carotid sinus pressure, or the use of such drugs as quinidine and

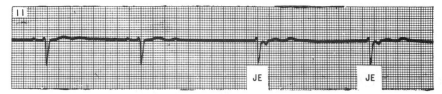

Fig. 24-40 Sinus arrest.   After two normal beats, a sinus impulse fails to appear.   During the pause, two AV junctional escape beats (JE) occur.   Each junctional beat is followed by a retrograde P wave.

reserpine.   Sinus pauses are usually terminated by the resumption of sinus rhythm or by the escape of an ectopic pacemaker.   It is not always possible to distinguish sinus arrest from SA block.   The former is attributed to failure of impulse formation; the latter, to block of the sinus impulse.

Sinoventricular Rhythm (Sinoventricular Conduction)

Sinoventricular rhythm is the transmission of the impulse from the SA node to the ventricles via the atrial internodal tracts and the specialized AV junctional and ventricular conduction pathways without activation of the atrial muscle.   This rare arrhythmia is most commonly associated with marked hyperpotassemia.   The failure of atrial activation apparently results from a specific inexcitability of the atrial musculature produced by hyperpotassmia.   The diagnosis may be suspected when absence of P waves is associated with the abnormal QRST complexes of hyperpotassemia.   The heart rate can be altered by any of the maneuvers which accelerate or slow normal sinus rhythm.

Sinus Node Dysfunction (Sick Sinus Syndrome, Bradycardia-Tachycardia Syndrome)

Sinus node dysfunction is primarily a disease of the elderly, although it can occur in younger individuals.   About one-half of the cases are associated with coronary artery disease; approximately one-third are idiopathic; the remainder are related to a variety of cardiac disorders.

Descriptions of sinus node dysfunction appear in the literature most often under the terms *sick sinus syndrome* and the *bradycardia-tachycardia (brady-tachy) syndrome.*

Electrocardiographic Features   Malfunction of the SA node may be manifested in a number of ways:

1   Drug-resistant, persistent, severe, and sometimes unexpected sinus bradycardia—usually the earliest and most frequent sign.   At times, the sinus slowing may alternate with episodes of supraventricular tachyarrhythmias; hence the designation bradycardia-tachycardia syndrome.
2   Periods of SA block, not related to drug therapy.

3   Short or long periods of sinus arrest with or without the supervention of escape rhythms, especially after premature systoles. Asystolic intervals, if sufficiently prolonged, may lead to cerebral symptoms or cardiac arrest and sudden death.
4   Failure of the heart to resume sinus rhythm following cardioversion of tachyarrhythmias.
5   Atrial fibrillation with a slow ventricular response (unrelated to digitalis or other drugs) due to concomitant AV nodal disease.
6   The bradycardia-tachycardia syndrome. Periods of sinus bradycardia alternate with rapid ectopic supraventricular rhythms such as paroxysmal atrial tachycardia, atrial fibrillation, and atrial flutter. Although these tachyarrhythmias tend to be self-limited and of short duration, SA nodal function is often so depressed at their termination that periods of asystole sufficient to cause lightheadedness, syncope, or cerebral symptoms may occur.
7   Disturbances in AV and intraventricular conduction.
8   AV junctional escape rhythms whether or not associated with stable or unstable sinus activity.
9   Carotid sinus syncope.

Tests for Sinus Node Dysfunction

1   *Ambulatory electrocardiographic monitoring.* The Holter device may be helpful in detecting periods of asystole or AV block as well as alternating episodes of bradycardia and tachycardia.
2   Procedures to determine the responsiveness of the SA node to autonomic nervous system influences:
a   *Isometric exercise.* This procedure accelerates the heart rate by sympathetic stimulation in normal persons. In patients with the sick sinus syndrome, although the heart rate may increase, the increment is minimal.
b   *Carotid sinus massage.* A period of sinus arrest following gentle right-sided carotid massage which lasts longer than three seconds is suggestive of inappropriate sinus responsiveness and sinus node disease.
c   *Valsalva maneuver.* In patients with the sick sinus syndrome, the Valsalva maneuver causes the expected drop in blood pressure but fails to elicit the appropriate chronotropic response.
d   *Atropine.* The administration of 0.5 to 1.0 mg of atropine intravenously causes a 50 percent increase in heart rate above control values in healthy persons but has little effect (less than 25 percent increase in heart rate) in patients whose sinus node is diseased.
3   Determination of sinoatrial and sinus node recovery times. When prolonged, these tests support the diagnosis.
4   His bundle electrocardiography may provide information about the status of intraventricular and AV conduction.
5   The tentative diagnosis of the sick sinus syndrome can be made in an appropriate clinical setting if the tests outlined above are abnormal.

ATRIAL MECHANISMS

The mechanism of atrial tachycardia has long been debated. Recent studies have established that both automaticity and macroreentry can cause this arrhythmia. Most paroxysmal supraventricular tachycardias without AV block are due to reentry, but ectopic automatic atrial tachycardias also occur. Atrial paroxysmal tachycardia with block due to digitalis intoxication is probably caused by enhanced activity of an ectopic pacemaker. This may also be true of multifocal atrial tachycardia. The mechanisms of atrial flutter and fibrillation, in spite of exhaustive studies, are still subject to a great deal of controversy. Some authorities subscribe to the view that atrial premature beats, atrial tachycardia, atrial flutter, and atrial fibrillation result from the single or repetitive discharge of atrial pacemakers and that the chief differentiating feature in these rhythms is the heart rate. Support of this concept is based on experimental data and on the frequently observed transition from atrial premature systoles to atrial tachycardia, flutter, and fibrillation in the same patient. The reverse progression has also been noted. This is the unitary theory of atrial arrhythmias. Contrary views are based on the clinical differences between these arrhythmias and their different responses to pharmacologic agents. Many still hold that a circus movement is the explanation of atrial flutter, but reentry in a small area low in the atrium cannot be excluded. With respect to the mechanism of atrial fibrillation, there is also divergence of opinion. This arrhythmia has been attributed to unifocal ectopic impulse formation, multifocal ectopic impulse formation, microreentry, and combinations of these mechanisms. Atrial premature beats which occur during the atrial vulnerable period may induce atrial fibrillation.

Atrial Premature Systoles
(Figs. 24-8A, 24-9, 24-11, 24-12, 24-13A and C)

See under Premature Systoles in this chapter.

Atrial Rhythm (Figs. 24-92 to 24-94)

Atrial rhythm is regular rhythm, usually between 50 and 80 per minute, which arises as an escape rhythm when the SA node defaults. The appearance of the P wave is commonly retrograde in contour, like that of low atrial premature systoles. However, if the P wave polarity is normal, the differentiation from sinus rhythm may be difficult unless previous tracings are available for comparison or unless the onset of atrial rhythm occurs after a sinus pause. The P-R interval is usually within the normal range. Isolated atrial escape beats may also occur.

No definite criteria are available for differentiating inferior atrial rhythms with retrograde P waves in leads II, III, and aVF (e.g., so-called "coronary sinus" or "left atrial" rhythm) from AV junctional rhythms in the presence of a normal P-R interval. (See section, Mechanisms of Disputed Origin.)

Atrial Paroxysmal Tachycardia

Two forms of atrial paroxysmal tachycardia can be recognized, one due to reentry (now termed *reentrant paroxysmal supraventricular tachycardia* by most authorities); and the other to enhanced automaticity of an ectopic focus. The reentrant type is by far the more common of the two. It occurs at all ages and, although often associated with organic heart disease, is frequently seen in healthy persons. Automatic ectopic atrial tachycardia is usually associated with rheumatic or other type of organic heart disease, chronic obstructive pulmonary disease, digitalis excess, and metabolic or electrolyte abnormalities. It may rarely occur in the healthy persons.

The problem of reentrant and automatic supraventricular tachycardias is discussed in detail later in this chapter. The next section deals with automatic ectopic atrial paroxysmal tachycardia.

Automatic Ectopic Atrial Paroxysmal Tachycardia
(Figs. 24-34, 24-35, 24-41, 24-43 to 24-45)

1   The onset of the tachycardia is spontaneous and is not related to any initiating event such as premature atrial or ventricular extrasystoles (either spontaneous or induced). Its occurrence is independent of intraatrial or AV nodal conduction delay.
2   The P wave of the initiating atrial premature systole is identical to subsequent P waves during the tachycardia but is different from the sinus P wave.
3   The P-R interval is rate-related.
4   There is a rapid rhythm at a rate usually between 140 and 250 per minute, but occasionally slower.
5   Although the rhythm is regular, it may be irregular, particularly at the onset, during the "warm-up" period.
6   The tachycardia has a premature onset and its termination is followed by a pause. There is often deceleration of the rate before termination.
7   The QRS interval is 0.10 s or less, unless prolonged as a result of intraventricular block or aberrant ventricular conduction.
8   The ventricles usually respond to each atrial beat (1:1 AV conduction), but there may be varying degrees of AV block. AV block may exist without affecting the rate of the tachycardia.
9   Vagal maneuvers or vagomimetic drugs do not affect or terminate the tachycardia, although they may produce AV block.
10   The tachycardia cannot be terminated by atrial or ventricular stimulation.
11   Electrophysiologic studies may be helpful in distinguishing between

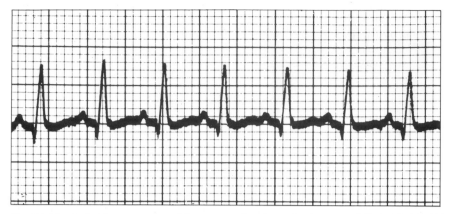

Fig. 24-41 Probable automatic atrial paroxysmal tachycardia at a rate of 187 with 1:1 AV conduction. Lead I. The P waves are uniform and upright, and the P-R interval is 0.12 s.

automatic and reentrant supraventricular tachycardia. The reader is also referred to the section on Paroxysmal Supraventricular Tachycardia later in this chapter for additional information.

Atrial Paroxysmal Tachycardia with Block (PAT with Block)

A significant proportion of cases of this arrhythmia are due to variable combinations of digitalis excess and potassium depletion. Enhanced automaticity is probably the mechanism of this arrhythmia. This variety (Fig. 24-46) is characterized by the following features:

1 The atrial rate varies between 150 and 250 per minute, but in three-fourths of the cases it is below 190 per minute. In one-half of the cases the rhythm is regular; in the other half it is irregular.

Fig. 24-42 Paroxysmal supraventricular tachycardia, probably reentrant, with aberrant ventricular conduction. The paroxysmal tachycardia, at a rate of 166 per minute, is initiated by an upright, premature, ectopic P wave, P′, with a prolonged P′-R interval. This establishes the supraventricular origin of the arrhythmia. During the tachycardia, the QRS complexes show a right bundle branch block pattern typical of aberrant ventricular conduction. The tachycardia is terminated by a pause. After the pause, a sinus beat and an ectopic P′ wave follow in succession.

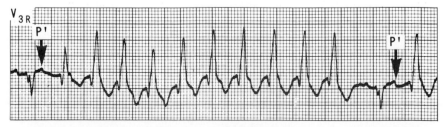

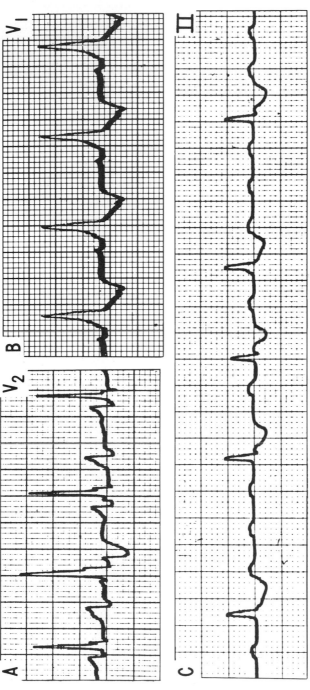

Fig. 24-43 Atrial paroxysmal tachycardia with block. (A) The atrial rate is 158 per minute. There is a Wenckebach phenomenon with 3:2 AV conduction followed by 2:1 AV conduction. From a patient with mitral stenosis and congestive heart failure. The tachycardia was not due to digitalis and was subsequently abolished by its use. (B) The atrial rate is 166 per minute. Alternate P waves, seen as notches on the S-T segments, are dropped, which indicates 2:1 AV conduction. The QRS complexes are abnormally wide because of preexisting right bundle branch block. Here too, digitalis intoxication was not the cause of the atrial tachycardia. (C) The atrial rate is 214 per minute. Conduction ratios vary between 2:1 and 4:1. From a patient with severe emphysema and cor pulmonale who was receiving digitalis. The serum potassium was normal. The tachycardia was probably caused by a combination of respiratory failure and digitalis excess.

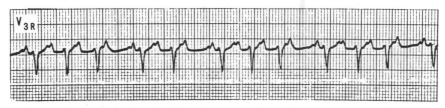

Fig. 24-44   Atrial paroxysmal tachycardia (167 per minute) probably automatic, with Type I AV block.   There are 4:3 and 3:2 Wenckebach periods.   The arrhythmia in this patient was not due to digitalis toxicity.

2   The P′ waves are often diminutive and differ in contour from sinus P waves.   They are generally upright in leads II, III, and aVF.   Sometimes they are visible only in the right precordial leads.   The baseline between the P waves is isoelectric, not mobile as in atrial flutter.
3   Although 1:1 AV conduction may occur, the usual form of the arrhythmia is associated with second-degree AV block, generally with 2:1 AV conduction but occasionally with the Wenckebach phenomenon.   More rarely, advanced degrees of AV block may occur.   The block may be increased temporarily by carotid sinus pressure or vagal stimulation.
4   The arrhythmia responds to the administration of potassium salts and to the omission of digitalis and diuretics.
5   Some cases of this arrhythmia appear to be nonparoxysmal rather than paroxysmal in nature.

Atrial paroxysmal tachycardia with block unrelated to digitalis excess and hypopotassemia may occur in coronary heart disease, diffuse pulmonary disease, and rheumatic heart disease.   In these instances, the administration of digitalis may be beneficial.

Fig. 24-45   Automatic atrial paroxysmal tachycardia.   During supraventricular tachycardia (SVT) of uncertain mechanism, carotid sinus pressure (CSP, arrow) is applied.   The diagnosis of automaticity is revealed as AV block appears, and the P waves continue at a rate of 160 per minute.   (*From M. E. Josephson and J. A. Kastor, Supraventricular Tachycardia: Mechanisms and Management, Ann. Intern. Med., 87: 346, 1977.   Used by permission.*)

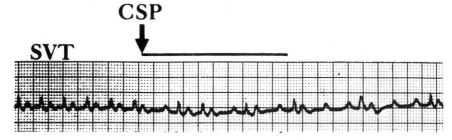

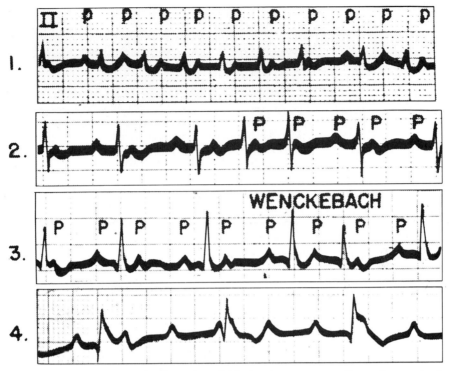

Fig. 24-46 Atrial paroxysmal tachycardia with block in four patients. All recordings are lead II. There is predominantly 1:1 atrioventricular response in strip 1; variable ventricular response, principally 2:1, in strips 2 and 3; and complete heart block in strip 4. (*From B. Lown, F. Marcus, and H. D. Levine, Digitalis and Atrial Tachycardia with Block: A Year's Experience, New Engl. J. Med., 260: 301, 1959. Used by permission.*)

Multifocal (Chaotic) Atrial Tachycardia (Figs. 24-47, 24-48)

Multifocal atrial tachycardia is usually seen in association with acute and chronic pulmonary disease complicated by cor pulmonale. It is not caused by digitalis toxicity. The mechanism is probably enhanced automatically.

1 The atrial rate exceeds 100 per minute.
2 There are discrete P' waves of varying morphology from at least three different foci.
3 The P'-P' intervals are irregular.
4 There is an isoelectric baseline between P' waves.
5 The ratio of atrial to ventricular beats is 1:1, except when the rate is rapid or AV block is present.

Multifocal atrial tachycardia may be mistaken for sinus arrhythmia or a wandering pacemaker, but in these conditions the atrial rate is 100 per minute or less. Atrial flutter is distinguished from it by the regularity of the

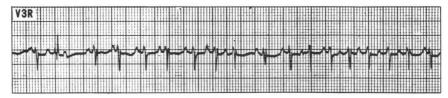

Fig. 24-47 Multifocal atrial tachycardia, untreated, in a patient with emphysema and cor pulmonale. There is an irregular atrial tachycardia at a rate of about 220 per minute. There is 1:1 AV conduction except at the beginning of the strip, where a 3:2 Wenckebach phenomenon is noted. The P waves are discrete and show variable morphology. The second ventricular complex shows aberrant ventricular conduction. Some degree of ventricular aberration is also present in other conducted beats.

F waves, the absence of an isoelectric baseline, the sawtooth morphology, and the rarity of a 1:1 AV response. Atrial fibrillation can be differentiated by the indistinct morphology of the f waves and the undulation of the baseline.

Atrial Flutter (Figs. 24-49 to 24-53)

Atrial flutter is almost invariably associated with organic heart disease. Its greatest incidence is in rheumatic heart disease, but it is also observed in arteriosclerotic and hypertensive heart disease. Sometimes it is associated with the W-P-W syndrome, hyperthyroidism, or an atrial septal defect.

Fig. 24-48 Multifocal atrial tachycardia. The tracings are not continuous but were taken from a longer recording. The morphology of the P′ waves is variable. The P′-P′ intervals are irregular. AV conduction varies from beat to beat. Although the ST-T changes are the result of digitalis effect, the arrhythmia was not produced by digitalis toxicity.

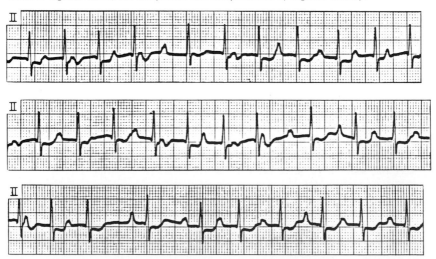

LEAD II

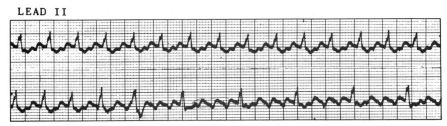

Fig. 24-49 *Upper tracing:* Atrial flutter simulating paroxysmal supraventricular tachycardia. *Lower tracing:* Following the application of carotid sinus pressure, the flutter mechanism becomes apparent.

Based on studies following open heart surgery, two types of atrial flutter have been identified. Type I or classical atrial flutter is characterized by a rate of approximately 240 to 340 beats per minute and can be influenced or terminated by rapid atrial pacing from sites high in the right atrium. Type II atrial flutter is characterized by a more rapid rate of about 340 to 433 beats per minute and by unresponsiveness to rapid atrial pacing.

In a very small number of cases, recurrent bouts of paroxysmal atrial flutter and fibrillation may occur in middle-aged healthy men over a period of years. Permanent atrial dysrhythmia does not develop. The arrhythmia has been attributed to vagal hypertonia.

1   The normal P waves are absent and are replaced by uniform, regular oscillations, namely, F waves, which usually occur at a rate of between 250 and 350 per minute, but occasionally at a slower rate. These F waves characteristically have a sawtooth appearance and are seen best in leads II, III, aVF, and V_1. The F wave can be regarded as an inverted "P" wave followed by an upright "Tp" wave.

Fig. 24-50 (A) Atrial flutter, untreated, showing 2:1 AV conduction. (B) Atrial flutter with complete AV block. The F waves are not related to the QRS complexes. The ventricular rate is 24 per minute and the flutter rate 200 per minute. It could be argued that this is atrial tachycardia rather than flutter. However, previous records from this patient showed flutter at a similar rate but with typical sawtooth morphology.

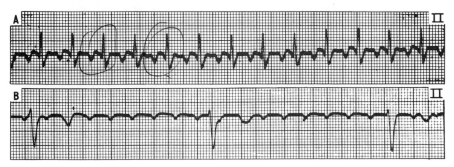

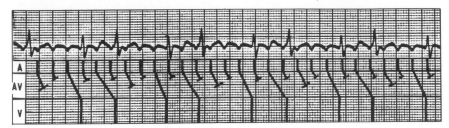

Fig 24-51 Atrial flutter with alternating 2:1 and 4:1 AV conduction. There is a 3:2 Wenckebach phenomenon in the lower AV junction involving alternate conducted beats. See text for additional information concerning AV conduction in atrial flutter.

Fig. 24-52 Atrial flutter with 1:1 AV conduction. (*A*) Admission electrocardiogram showing a regular tachycardia with wide QRST complexes at a rate of 300 per minute. Note the resemblance to ventricular flutter (Fig. 24-108). (*B*) Tracing recorded after the intravenous administration of 0.5 mg digoxin.

Atrial flutter at a rate of 300 per minute is now apparent. The ventricular response has slowed, but many of the QRS complexes in lead aVR show some degree of aberration. In retrospect, therefore, *A* shows atrial flutter with a 1:1 ventricular response and abnormal QRST complexes due to aberrant ventricular conduction. (*From M. R. Bilitch, "A Manual of Cardiac Arrhythmias," Little, Brown, Boston, 1971. Used by permission.*)

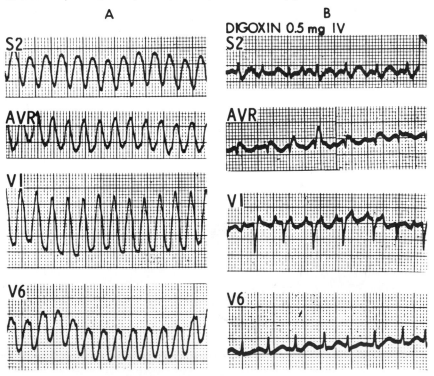

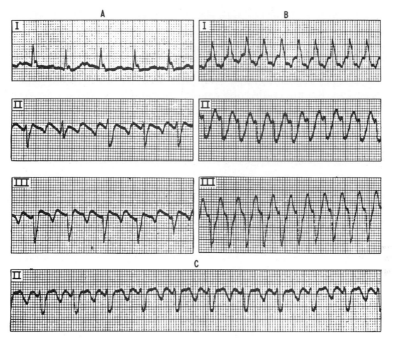

Fig. 24-53 Atrial flutter. A, B, and C are tracings from a patient with chronic atrial flutter. In A, untreated, the atrial flutter rate is 214 per minute. There is predominant 2:1 AV conduction and coexisting intraventricular block. B, recorded during an episode of rapid heart action, shows the ventricular rate to be precisely 214 per minute, which indicates 1:1 AV conduction. Intraventricular block persists. Without knowledge of A, the arrhythmia in B could be mistaken for supraventricular tachycardia with abnormal QRS complexes or for ventricular tachycardia. In order to increase the degree of AV block, 0.25 mg ouabain was administered intravenously. Tracing C was recorded 10 min later. Atrial flutter is still present at a rate of 214 per minute, but 2:1 AV conduction has been restored.

2 The ventricular rhythm and rate depend on the atrial rate, the ratio of atrial to ventricular beats, and the state of AV conduction.

a Most commonly, there is 2:1 AV conduction or 4:1 AV conduction or a basic 2:1 AV conduction alternating with 4:1 or other AV conduction ratios.

b Less commonly, there is 3:1, 5:1, or 6:1 AV conduction.

c Rarely, there is 1:1 AV conduction.

d Often the conduction ratios change in the same tracing, which results in an irregular ventricular rhythm.

3 The contour of the conducted ventricular beats in atrial flutter may be normal or abnormal. Abnormal QRST complexes result from either intraventricular block, ventricular preexcitation, or aberrant ventricular conduction.

4 Complete AV dissociation in atrial flutter may be caused by complete AV block. The ventricular rhythm is then regular, its rate is slow (25 to 40 per minute), and the F waves bear no fixed temporal relationship to the QRS complexes.

5 Less often, complete AV dissociation in atrial flutter may be caused by an independent but simultaneously occurring paroxysmal AV junctional or ventricular tachycardia. Here too, the F waves are unrelated to the QRS complexes, but the ventricular rate is rapid and the QRST complexes possess the characteristics common to ectopic tachycardias of similar origin.

6 Carotid sinus pressure has little effect on the atrial rate, but slows the ventricular response by increasing the degree of AV block.

Atrioventricular Conduction in Atrial Flutter   Since the refractory period of the AV junction is longer than that of the atria, all the atrial impulses cannot be conducted to the ventricles. In the untreated patient, there is usually 2:1 AV conduction. This is not due to block but to physiologic interference in the AV junction. Atrioventricular conduction ratios greater than 2:1 are indicative of AV block.

When the ventricular response is regular, the F-R interval is constant, whereas when it is irregular, the F-R interval varies. The F-R interval represents the AV conduction time in atrial flutter and is consistently prolonged. The usual range is between 0.26 and 0.46 s when the AV conduction ratio is 2:1. The prolongation is the result of concealed conduction of the nonconducted atrial impulse into the AV junction.

To explain the mechanism of AV conduction in atrial flutter with conduction ratios greater than 2:1, it is necessary to postulate the existence of two regions of block in the AV junction. All flutter impulses are assumed to penetrate for some distance into the upper portion of the AV junction, but only alternate impulses are transmitted to the lower portion. In the lower portion, another region of block may cause some of the arriving impulses to be dropped in a sequence that is generally in accord with the structure of the Wenckebach period. Thus, interference with halving of the atrial rate occurs at the upper level of the AV junction, and block usually with the Wenckebach phenomenon at the lower level.

Concealed conduction in the lower AV junction may be responsible for odd conduction ratios (e.g., 3:1) or alternation of F-R intervals.

The maximum ventricular rate in atrial flutter with 1:1 conduction is about 300 per minute in the adult. With 2:1 AV conduction, the maximum possible ventricular rate is 175 per minute (half of 350 per minute, the maximum flutter rate).

Atrial Fibrillation (Figs. 24-54 to 24-67)

Next to premature systoles, atrial fibrillation is the most frequently occurring cardiac arrhythmia. Although found most commonly in association with heart disease, usually arteriosclerotic or rheumatic, atrial fibrillation may

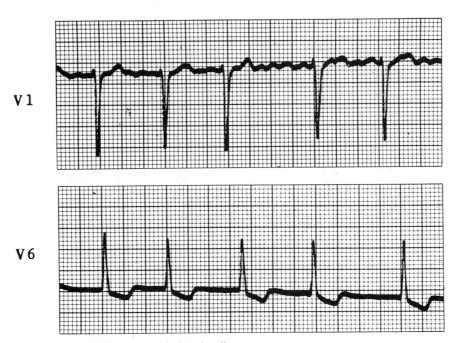

Fig. 24-54   Atrial fibrillation with digitalis effect.

occur in normal hearts and in association with hyperthyroidism.   Atrial fibrillation, once established, is usually chronic.   Occasionally, it is paroxysmal and transitory.

1   The P waves are absent and are replaced by small, irregular oscillations of variable amplitude and duration, i.e., the f waves, which occur at a rate of 350 to 600 per minute.

2   The ventricular rhythm is totally irregular, and its rate varies.

3   The contour of the conducted ventricular beats may be normal or abnormal.   Abnormal QRST complexes result from coexisting intraventricular block, aberrant ventricular conduction, or ventricular preexcitation.

4   When the ventricular rhythm is regular, AV dissociation is present.

a   In complete AV block, the ventricular rhythm is slow and regular, usually at a rate of 25 to 40 per minute.

b   In advanced, incomplete AV block, the ventricular rate is slow, its rhythm often slightly irregular, and escape beats or rhythms are observed commonly.

c   Sometimes, when advanced AV block is associated with atrial fibrillation, the AV junctional pacemaker may accelerate, which results in a rapid, regular ventricular rhythm at a rate of 65 to 130 per minute (nonparox-

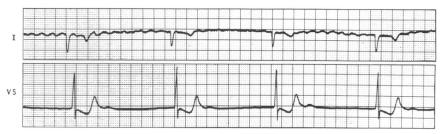

Fig. 24-55 Complete AV block in atrial fibrillation due to digitalis. The ventricular rate is 32. The ventricular pacemaker is located in the AV junction above the bifurcation of the common bundle.

ysmal AV junctional tachycardia). This is usually caused by digitalis excess.

d Rarely, complete AV dissociation in atrial fibrillation may be caused by an independent but simultaneously occurring paroxysmal AV junctional or ventricular tachycardia.

5 Anomalous beats occur frequently in atrial fibrillation. Late anomalous beats are escape beats, but those which occur early represent either aberrant ventricular conduction of the transmitted impulse or ventricular ectopic beats. It is important to differentiate between aberrant ventricular conduction and ventricular premature systoles, because the clinical significance of each is different. Aberrant ventricular conduction is relatively unimportant, but it may indicate a need for increased dosage of digitalis. Ventricular premature systoles, on the other hand, may be the result of digitalis toxicity and may require withdrawal of the drug. Differentiation between the two is sometimes possible, but it may be difficult or even impossible.

a The diagnosis of aberrant ventricular conduction of transmitted impulses is favored by

    i Variable coupling intervals with little tendency to bigeminy

    ii A triphasic (right bundle branch block) QRS morphology in lead V_1, particularly when associated with an initial vector that is identical with that of the normally conducted beats

Fig. 24-56 Atrial fibrillation with a solitary AV junctional escape beat (the fifth ventricular complex). The configuration of the escape beat basically resembles that of the conducted beats but is aberrant. Aberration of AV junctional escape beats is common.

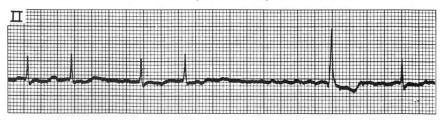

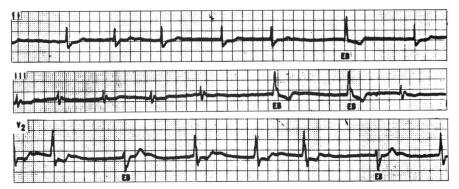

Fig. 24-57 Atrial fibrillation with a slow ventricular response and pauses terminated by escape beats (EB). The escape interval is 1.48 s.

    iii   Short cycles, preceded by long cycles, terminating the anomalous beats (to some extent, also true of ventricular extrasystoles—the *rule of bigeminy*)

    iv   Absence of substantial pauses following the anomalous beats

b   The diagnosis of ventricular ectopy is favored by

    i   Fixed coupling intervals (although coupling is sometimes variable in extrasystoles)

    ii   A monophasic or diphasic QRS morphology in lead V_1, particularly if the initial vector is dissimilar to that of the conducted beats

    iii   A left bundle branch block pattern

    iv   Short cycles preceding the cycles of the anomalous beats, particularly if the cycles terminated by anomalous beats are longer than the preceding cycle

    v   The occurrence of anomalous beats at a time when cycle-sequence comparisons indicate that aberration should not be expected

    vi   Undue prematurity of the anomalous beats (the cycles ended by anomalous beats are shorter than other cycles in the record)

    vii   The presence in previous or subsequent nonfibrillating records of ventricular premature systoles with a configuration identical with that of the anomalous beats

Fig. 24-58 Atrial fibrillation with conducted beats and a ventricular escape rhythm at a rate of 63 per minute. The beats labeled FB are the result of fusion between conducted impulses and ventricular escape beats. Excessive dosage of digoxin was responsible for the arrhythmia.

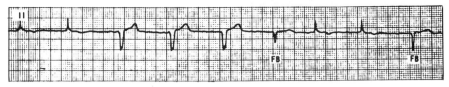

CONTINUOUS LEAD II

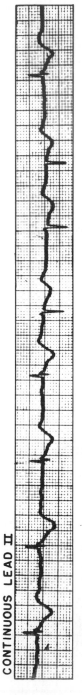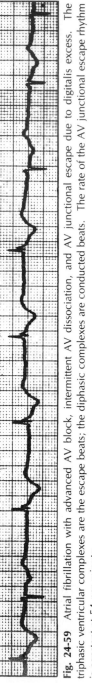

Fig. 24-59 Atrial fibrillation with advanced AV block, intermittent AV dissociation, and AV junctional escape due to digitalis excess. The triphasic ventricular complexes are the escape beats; the diphasic complexes are conducted beats. The rate of the AV junctional escape rhythm is constant at 54 per minute.

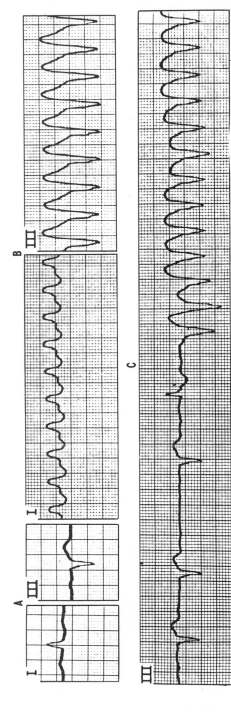

Fig. 24-60 Atrial fibrillation with AV junctional paroxysmal tachycardia. A, B, and C are tracings from the same patient. A, recorded several months before B, shows normal sinus rhythm with first-degree AV block and an intraventricular conduction defect. B, recorded during an episode of paroxysmal tachycardia, shows QRS complexes of similar contour although somewhat wider. Even though P waves are not identifiable, the tachycardia should be regarded as supraventricular because the configuration of the QRS complexes during the tachycardia is basically the same as during sinus rhythm. Following a loading dose of digoxin, the rhythm changed to atrial fibrillation, as seen in C. The first three ventricular complexes in C are conducted beats, the fourth is an ectopic beat, and the fifth initiates a bout of paroxysmal tachycardia. Since the QRS complexes of the tachycardia are similar to those in A and B, it must be concluded that the tachycardia is AV junctional in origin and probably automatic. The tachycardia disappeared after additional doses of digitalis were administered.

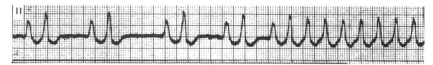

Fig. 24-61 Atrial fibrillation with ventricular extrasystoles and a run of paroxysmal ventricular tachycardia. The first four conducted beats are followed by ventricular premature systoles with fixed coupling. Following the fifth conducted beat, a ventricular extrasystole initiates a run of ventricular tachycardia.

    viii   Bigeminy with fixed coupling
    ix   Long pauses following the anomalous beats

c Aberrant beats may sometimes occur in runs, simulating ventricular tachycardia.

d Nonextrasystolic rhythms such as escape beats, parasystole, and idioventricular rhythms must be differentiated from both ventricular premature beats and aberrantly conducted beats.

e His bundle recordings can be used to differentiate between ventricular ectopic and aberrantly conducted beats. If the beat is preceded by an H deflection with an H-V time equal to or longer than normally conducted ventricular beats, it is aberrant. However, if no H spike precedes the QRS complex of if the H-V time is shorter than the conducted beats, the beat is ventricular in origin.

Fig. 24-62 Atrial fibrillation, left bundle branch block, and right ventricular paroxysmal tachycardia. The upper strip and the first portion of the middle strip show atrial fibrillation with an irregular ventricular response, exhibiting a left bundle branch block pattern. (Note the narrow R waves.) In the middle of the second strip, there is an abrupt onset of an absolutely regular rhythm with a left bundle branch block pattern but with broad R waves indicative of a right ventricular tachycardia. (*From H. J. L. Marriott, "Workshop in Electrocardiography," Tampa Tracings, Oldsmar, Fla., 1970. Used by permission.*)

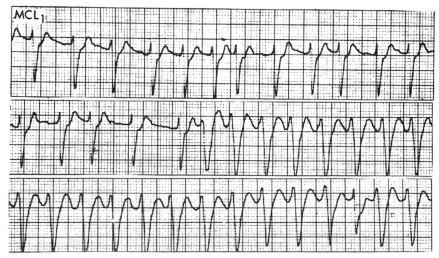

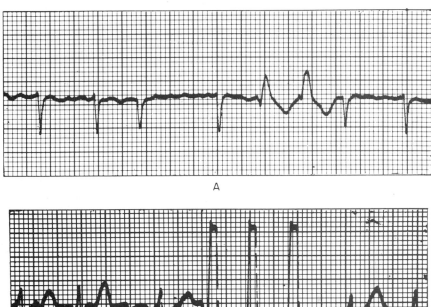

A

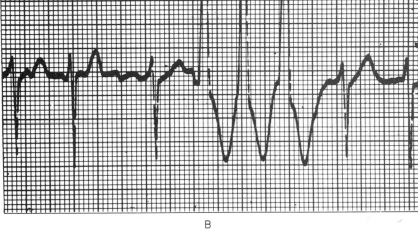

B

Fig. 24-63   (A) Lead V$_1$. Aberrant ventricular conduction in atrial fibrillation. The aberrant beats terminate a short cycle preceded by a longer cycle. The anomalous beats show a triphasic RBBB contour with an initial vector identical with that of the conducted beats. A compensatory pause does not follow the aberrant beats. (B) Lead V$_2$ from a different patient with atrial fibrillation. The three anomalous beats show a monophasic contour. The cycle preceding the first anomalous beat is slightly longer than the other cycles, and the pause following the last beat is not significant. The record illustrates the difficulty in differentiating between aberration and ectopy. On the basis of morphology and the constancy of the interectopic intervals, the anomalous complexes are probably ventricular ectopic beats.

6   Diagnostic importance has been attached to fibrillatory f wave size. Coarse fibrillatory waves (measuring 0.5 mm or more from trough to peak) in lead V$_1$ are said to be more common in rheumatic heart disease and fine fibrillatory waves more common in arteriosclerotic heart disease. However, there is sufficient variation in both types of heart disease so that fibrillatory wave size is useless as a criterion for differentiating between the two. In hyperthyroidism both wave sizes occur, but the

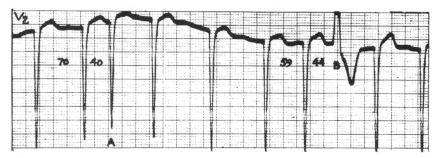

Fig. 24-64 The value of cycle-sequence comparison in the differentiation between ventricular aberrancy and ectopy in atrial fibrillation. Beat B ends a cycle of 44 (hundredths of a second) preceded by a cycle of 59. If beat B is aberrant, then beat A, which ends a shorter cycle (40) preceded by a longer one (70), should also be aberrant. However, since A is not aberrant, beat B is presumably a ventricular ectopic beat. (*From H. J. L. Marriott and I. A. Sandler, Criteria, Old and New, for Differentiating between Ectopic Ventricular Beats and Aberrant Ventricular Conduction in the Presence of Atrial Fibrillation, Progr. Cardiovasc. Dis., 9: 18, 1966. Used by permission.*)

fine variety is seen more frequently. Coarse waves have also been reported in congenital heart disease with right atrial or biatrial enlargement.

An excellent correlation exists between the amplitude of fibrillatory waves and the P terminal force during sinus rhythm. The finding of

Fig. 24-65 (*A*) Aberrant ventricular conduction in atrial fibrillation. The four anomalous beats fulfill the usual criteria for aberration: a lengthened preceding cycle, a right bundle branch block pattern with an initial vector identical with that of the flanking conducted beats, and absence of a pause following the last beat. (*B*) Atrial fibrillation with bifocal ventricular premature systoles, variable coupling, and extrasystolic bigeminy in lead II, resulting from digitalis intoxication.

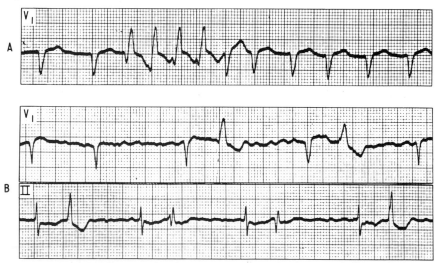

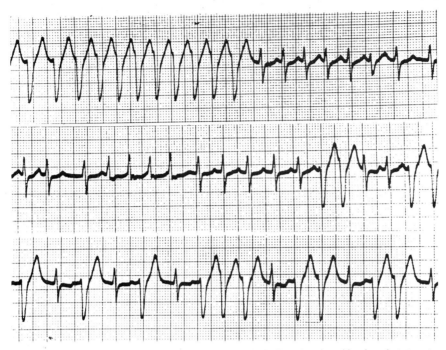

Fig. 24-66 Aberrant ventricular conduction in atrial fibrillation induced by the administration of procainamide. The first eleven ventricular complexes in the top strip are aberrantly conducted and could easily be mistaken for a run of ventricular tachycardia. Similar anomalous beats can be seen in the middle and lower tracings. In the middle strip, the fourth through the seventh ventricular complexes show a different pattern of aberrant ventricular conduction.

coarse fibrillatory waves (1.0 mm or greater) is considered indicative of left atrial hypertrophy or strain.

Atrial Standstill (Fig. 17-4)

1 Atrial complexes are absent in all electrocardiographic leads.
2 The ventricles are under the control of an idioventricular pacemaker.

NEWER CONCEPTS

Reentrant Paroxysmal Supraventricular Tachycardia

Paroxysmal supraventricular tachycardia (PSVT) is the term used by many electrocardiographers to designate arrhythmias that were formerly called atrial and AV junctional paroxysmal tachycardia (PAT and PJT, respectively).

PSVT may be caused by one of three mechanisms: reentry, enhanced automaticity, and triggered activity.

The most common mechanism is reentry, in which the impulse is continuously propagated within a closed circuit. The reentry circuit may involve the SA node, the atria, or the AV node, either alone or in combination with an accessory bypass tract.

For reentry to occur there must be longitudinal dissociation into two pathways, each with different refractory periods and conduction velocities, and a common final pathway linking the two pathways.

The provocative stimulus for reentrant PSVT is an approximately timed impulse which is blocked in the retrograde limb and conducted down the antegrade limb.   If conduction is slowed sufficiently in the antegrade limb, excitability will have recovered in the retrograde limb and the impulse can return to its point of origin in the reentry circuit.   A return to the chamber of origin of an initial impulse is called an *echo* or *reciprocal beat*.   Continued impulse propagation in the circuit results in a rapid, sustained reentrant tachycardia.

Abnormal automaticity is a much less common type of PSVT.   Triggered activity is an automatic rhythm in which an action potential results from a delayed afterdepolarization produced by the preceding action potential. Exercise-induced arrhythmias due to digitalis excess may be related to triggered activity.

According to the data of Josephson and Seides, the mechanism of PSVT in 150 cases was as follows: AV nodal reentry, 58 percent; AV reentry by a concealed bypass tract, 30 percent; SA nodal reentry, 4 percent; intraatrial reentry, 4 percent; and automatic atrial tachycardia, 4 percent.

Organic heart disease is not uncommonly associated with AV nodal reentrant tachycardia, but the arrhythmia can occur in its absence.   PSVT utilizing a concealed accessory pathway is usually associated with a young age, absence of cardiac disease, frequent occurrence of functional bundle branch block during the tachycardia, rapid rates (often exceeding 200 per minute), the occurrence of atrial flutter, fibrillation or both, and P waves which follow the QRS complexes.   Sinus and atrial reentrance are usually associated with organic heart disease.   The most rapid rates occur in PSVT which utilizes a concealed extranodal pathway.

Types of PSVT

AV Node (Figs. 24-30, 24-42, 24-68, 24-69, 24-70)   In the common type of AV nodal reentry, the initiating impulse (usually an atrial premature beat) conducts down the slow pathway and returns up the fast pathway.   The atria are depolarized in retrograde fashion and the ventricles are depolarized via the His-Purkinje apparatus.   Usually the atria and ventricles are depolarized simultaneously so that the P waves are buried in the QRS complexes.

In a much less common type of AV nodal reentry the fast pathway serves as the antegrade limb and the slow pathway as the retrograde limb. This type of reentry does not require a critically timed premature beat for initiation.   A simple acceleration of the heart rate may start this arrhythmia. It is often incessant.   Because antegrade conduction takes place by the fast pathway and retrograde conduction by the slow pathway, the retrograde P wave is delayed and may occur in front of the next QRS complex.

Accessory Bypass Tracts (Figs. 24-70, 24-71 to 24-74)   Both overt and concealed accessory bypass tracts may participate in reentrant arrhythmias. The former is associated with ventricular preexcitation in the electrocardiogram; the latter is not, hence the designation is concealed.   Reentrant tachycardias, since they utilize the ventricles, technically are not supraventricular.   They are really AV reciprocating tachycardias.

The most common type of reentrant tachycardia in patients with AV bypass tracts is referred to as *orthodromic* reciprocating tachycardia.   The antegrade limb is the AV node and the retrograde limb is the bypass tract. Typically, the QRS is narrow (unless there is functional or underlying bundle branch block) and the P waves follow shortly after the QRS complexes.

Antidromic AV reciprocating tachycardia is much less common.   The bypass tract serves as the antegrade limb with AV node functioning as the retrograde limb.   Since the impulse travels down the bypass tract to the ventricles, the P waves precede a widened QRS complex.   During sinus rhythms, the electrocardiogram shows typical ventricular preexcitation.

Nodoventricular bypass tracts (Mahaim fibers) with PSVT show a left bundle branch block QRS morphology and may mimic ventricular tachycardia.   During sinus rhythm, typical preexcitation is seen in the electrocardiogram.

Atria   In intraatrial reentrant paroxysmal tachycardia the reentry circuit is limited to the atrium.   The ventricles are depolarized in normal fashion. The P waves precede narrow QRS complexes.   Since the pathway of atrial depolarization may vary from beat to beat, the P wave may vary in morphology.

Sinus Node (Fig. 24-75)   Sustained reentry in the SA node may result in a PSVT.   This type of tachycardia may be difficult to differentiate from sinus tachycardia.   Helpful are its abrupt onset and termination, its brief duration, and a rate of 100 to 160 beats per minute.

Organic heart disease is not uncommonly associated with AV nodal reentrant tachycardia, but the arrhythmia can occur in its absence.   PSVT utilizing a concealed accessory pathway is usually associated with a young age, absence of cardiac disease, frequent occurrence of functional bundle branch block during the tachycardia, rapid rates (often exceeding 200 per minute), the occurrence of atrial flutter, fibrillation, or both, and P waves which follow the QRS complexes.   Sinus and atrial reentrance are usually associated with organic heart disease.

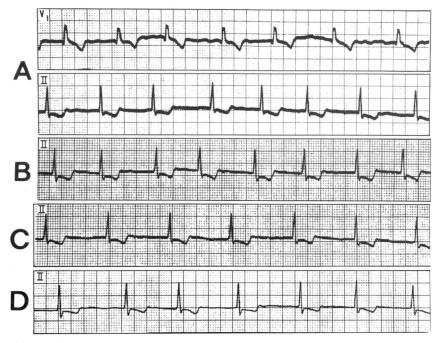

Fig. 24-67A   Atrial fibrillation with digitalis-induced nonparoxysmal AV junctional tachycardia showing exit block.   (A) Control tracing.   There is atrial fibrillation, a moderate ventricular response, and evidence of right ventricular enlargement.   Because the patient was in severe congestive heart failure, the maintenance dose of digitalis was increased.   (B) Record taken two days later shows atrial fibrillation with a regular bigeminal rhythm.   The atria and ventricles are completely dissociated.   The ladder diagram in Fig. 24-67B (strip B) reveals that the bigeminal rhythm is due to a 3:2 exit block from a nonparoxysmal AV-junctional tachycardia.   (C) Record taken the following day still shows a nonparoxysmal AV-junctional tachycardia but with 2:1 exit block.   (See Fig. 24-67B, strip C.)   (D) Record taken a few days later shows the return of the irregular irregularity of the ventricular response.   No digitalis was administered during the interval between B and D.

Electrocardiographic Criteria for the Diagnosis of Reentrant Paroxysmal Supraventricular Tachycardia (Figs. 24-30, 24-42, 24-68 to 24-75, 24-80, 24-168)

Automatic ectopic atrial paroxysmal tachycardia was considered in the section on Atrial Arrhythmias.   Automatic ectopic AV junctional tachycardia will be discussed in the section Atrioventricular Junctional Mechanisms which follows.   The criteria for the electrocardiographic diagnosis of PSVT are:

1   A rapid rhythm with a rate *usually* between 140 and 200 per minute (although occasionally it may be slightly slower or faster).

2   The tachycardia has a premature onset and its termination is followed by a pause.

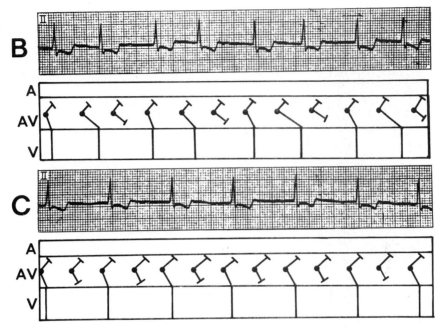

Fig. 24-67B *Tracing B*: Ladder diagram of rhythm strip B from Fig. 24-67A, showing a 3:2 Wenckebach type of exit block from the AV-junctional pacemaker (basic rate 115 per minute). *Tracing C*: Ladder diagram of rhythm strip C from Fig. 24-67A, showing 2:1 exit block from the AV-junctional pacemaker firing at the same rate as in strip B.

3   The mechanism of a tachycardia that is initiated or terminated by a premature atrial or ventricular beat is most likely to be reentry.

a   If it can be demonstrated that the initiation of the tachycardia by an atrial (or ventricular) premature systole depends on a critical degree of prolongation of the P-R interval, then reentry through the AV node or AV reentry involving a concealed bypass tract is established.   Neither SA nodal reentry, atrial reentry, nor automatic atrial tachycardia requires this critical degree of P-R prolongation for its initiation.   Both SA nodal reentry and atrial reentry are most frequently initiated by atrial premature beats.   In the atrial reentrant variety, stimulation during the atrial relative refractory period is required to initiate the tachyarrhythmia.

b   If the P wave of the initiating atrial premature systole and the subsequent P waves are identical in morphology, automatic atrial tachycardia is most likely (but atrial reentry is possible); if they are different, reentry is the most likely mechanism.

c   If an atrial premature systole initiates the tachycardia and the first atrial complex of the tachycardia is not conducted, then reentry utilizing a concealed retrograde extranodal pathway is ruled out, since depolarization of the ventricles is necessary to reach the ventricular bypass tract.   A nodal reentry is also unlikely, because it is most difficult for reentry to be sustained in the presence of block in the AV node.

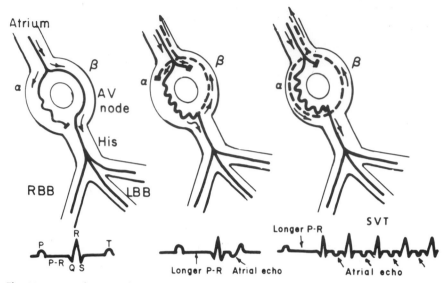

Fig. 24-68 Mechanism of AV nodal reentrant tachycardia. Each part of the figure is shown as an atrium, AV node (which is divided into alpha, or slow, and beta, or fast, pathways), His bundle, and bundle branches. In the left panel, sinus rhythm is present and the mechanism of the resulting QRS is shown. In the center panel, the response of the AV node to a single atrial premature systole, with a single atrial echo, is depicted. In the right panel, the initiation of supraventricular tachycardia with an atrial premature systole is shown. SVT = supraventricular tachycardia; RBB = right bundle branch; LBB = left bundle branch. (*From M. E. Josephson and J. A. Kastor, Supraventricular Tachycardia: Mechanisms and Management, Ann. Intern. Med., 87: 346, 1977. Used by permission.*)

4 The QRS interval is typically 0.10 s or less, unless it is prolonged because of coexisting intraventricular block or aberrant ventricular conduction. Functional bundle branch block is a feature of PSVT utilizing a concealed accessory pathway. A decrease in the rate of the tachycardia coincident with functional bundle branch block is diagnostic of this type of reentry.

5 The morphology of the P waves and the position of the P wave relative to the QRS complexes during the tachycardia when the P waves are clearly identifiable may have diagnostic significance.

a Absence of visible P waves strongly suggests AV nodal reentry, although it may occur in automatic AV junctional (His bundle) tachycardia. The presence of an extranodal bypass tract is excluded because ventricular depolarization must precede atrial depolarization in this condition; activation of these chambers cannot be simultaneous. Eccentric retrograde atrial activation (demonstrable by electrophysiologic studies) is diagnostic of a concealed bypass tract.

b Retrograde P waves with an R-P interval less than 50 percent of the R-R interval can be found in either AV nodal reentry or reentry utilizing a concealed accessory pathway. All patients with reentry via an extranodal tract exhibit this pattern.

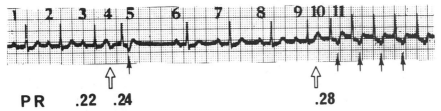

PR   .22   .24   .28

Fig. 24-69   Supraventricular tachycardia in a lead II rhythm strip.   The P waves are numbered. Atrial premature systoles (beats 4 and 10, open arrows) are associated with P-R prolongation and single (beat 5) and sustained beats (beat 11 and remaining P waves) producing an atrial echo and sustained supraventricular tachycardia, respectively.   *(From M. E. Josephson and J. A. Kastor, Supraventricular Tachycardia: Mechanisms and Management, Ann. Intern. Med., 87: 346, 1977.   Used by permission.)*

c   Retrograde P waves with an R-P interval greater than half of the R-R interval generally have AV nodal reentry of the so-called "incessant" type of PSVT.

d   P waves that are identical to the sinus P wave with a P-R interval appropriate for the rate of the tachycardia have SA nodal reentry.

e   P waves that are different from the sinus P waves (but not retrograde) with a P-R interval appropriate for the rate of the tachycardia have atrial paroxysmal tachycardia (automatic or reentrant).

f   An inverted P wave in lead I is strongly suggestive of reentry by a left-sided retrograde accessory pathway.

6   The temporal relationship between the P waves and the QRS complexes may have diagnostic significance.

a   The presence of P-R intervals appropriate for the rate of the tachycardia indicates SA nodal reentry if the P wave is identical to the sinus P wave or either automatic or reentrant atrial tachycardia if the P wave is different from the sinus P wave but is not retrograde.

b   The presence of AV or VA block or AV dissociation excludes reentry by a concealed bypass tract and can be considered diagnostic of an AV junctional origin of the tachycardia.

Fig. 24-70   Paroxysmal reentrant or reciprocating supraventricular tachycardia.   An atrial premature beat with a prolonged P'-R interval initiates a run of supraventricular tachycardia. During the paroxysm, retrograde P waves follow the QRS complexes.   The possible mechanism is AV nodal reentry or reentry utilizing a concealed accessory pathway.

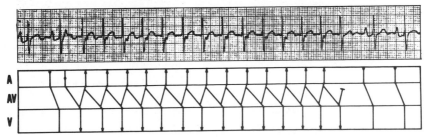

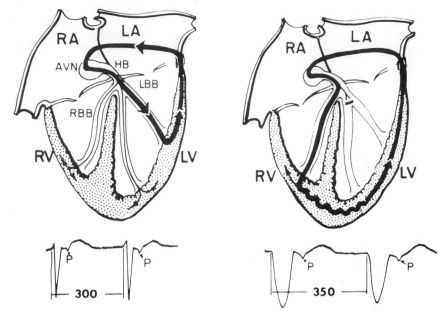

Fig. 24-71   Reentrant pathway in SVT utilizing a concealed left-sided accessory bypass tract. A schematic representation of the heart is shown with the AV conduction system.   An accessory pathway connects the left atrium and ventricle.   In the figure on the left, the electrocardiogram shows SVT with a normal QRS complex, and the tachycardia cycle length is 300 ms.   The reentrant circuit (indicated by the broad arrows) traverses the normal AV conduction system, left ventricle, accessory pathway, left atrium, and back to the AV node. In the figure on the right, left bundle branch block is present.   The cycle length has increased from 300 to 350 ms.   This increase in cycle length is caused by a longer reentrant pathway and slow intramyocardial conduction from RV to LV and insertion of the accessory pathway. RA = right atrium, LA = left atrium, RV = right ventricle, LV = left ventricle, AVN = atrioventricular node, HB = His bundle, RBB = right bundle branch, LBB = left bundle branch. (*From M. E. Josephson and S. F. Seides, "Clinical Cardiac Electrophysiology," Lea and Febiger, Philadelphia, 1979.   Used by permission.*)

c   AV block is extremely uncommon in AV nodal reentry and also excludes the participation of an accessory pathway in the mechanism of the arrhythmia.   AV block may occur in SA nodal reentry, atrial reentry, or automatic atrial tachycardia.

7   Abrupt termination of a PSVT by carotid sinus pressure or other forms of vagal stimulation suggests SA or AV nodal reentry, or reentry involving a concealed bypass tract.   The production of AV block by these maneuvers with persistence of the tachycardia, rules out the utilization of a concealed accessory pathway and makes AV nodal reentry unlikely. Abolition of PSVT by drugs (e.g., propranolol) with little or no effect on atrial tissue may help to establish SA nodal reentry.   Vagal maneuvers usually do not terminate atrial reentrant PSVT but may produce AV block in this condition.

8   Electrophysiologic studies may be of considerable help in distinguishing

between automatic and reentrant PSVT and, if the latter, in establishing the pathways of reentry. Electrophysiologic evaluation of PSVT usually includes determination of the following: the mode of initiation of the tachycardia; the requirement of participation by the atria and ventricles for its initiation and maintenance; the atrial activation sequence during the arrhythmia; the effect of bundle branch block on AV conduction and the cycle length of the dysrhythmia; the effect of atrial and ventricular stimulation during the tachycardia; and the effects of pharmacologic and physiologic maneuvers on the tachycardia.

9   The differential diagnosis of PSVT by clues from the surface electrocardiogram is listed in Table 24-1.

Fig. 24-72   Reentrant pathway in SVT utilizing a right-sided accessory pathway. A schematic representation of the heart is shown with the AV conduction system. Both panels depict the reentrant circuit during supraventricular tachycardia. RA, LA, RV, LV represent right atrium, left atrium, right ventricle, and left ventricle, respectively. AVN, HB, LBB, RBB represent AV node, His bundle, left bundle branch, and right bundle branch, respectively. K represents a right-sided Kent bundle. Two beats in lead V₁ during supraventricular tachycardia are shown below the heart schema. The cycle length is noted, as are the retrograde P waves (arrows and the letter P). In Panel a, the tachycardia occurs as usual down the normal pathway and up the accessory pathway to complete the reentrant circuit. The tachycardia has a normal QRS, cycle length of 350 ms and retrograde P waves closely following the QRS. In Panel b, functional right bundle branch block occurs. The impulse must conduct through the left bundle branch system, then slowly through muscular tissue until it reaches the distal end of the accessory pathway to complete the circuit. This produces a longer cycle length of about 400 ms with right bundle branch block in V₁ and a longer interval from the QRS to the retrograde P wave. (From M. E. Josephson and J. A. Kastor: Supraventricular Tachycardia: Mechanisms and Management, Ann. Intern. Med., 87: 346, 1977. Used by permission.)

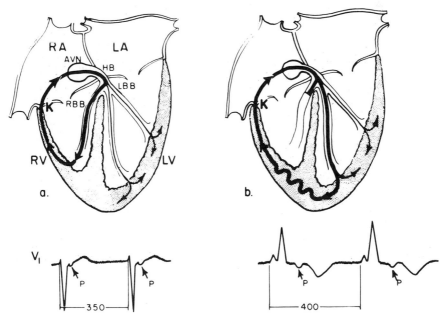

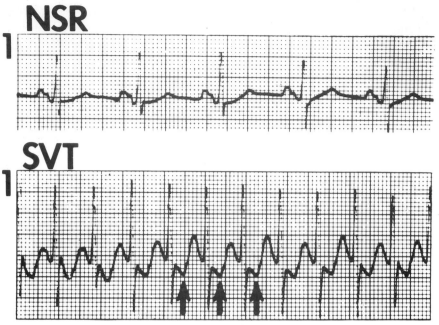

Fig. 24-73 Analysis of retrograde P waves during SVT utilizing a concealed accessory pathway. ECG lead I is shown during normal sinus rhythm and SVT in a patient with a concealed left-sided accessory pathway. During NSR, intraatrial conduction defect is present; during SVT, note the inverted P waves following the QRS complex (arrows). The R-P interval is less than 50 percent of the R-R interval. *(From L. N. Horowitz and M. E. Josephson, Diagnosis and Evaluation of Concealed Accessory Atrioventricular Pathways, Practical Cardiology, 6: 129, 1980. Used by permission.)*

Reentrant vs. Automatic Ectopic Supraventricular Tachycardias

1 In PSVT due to enhanced automaticity and rapid ectopic firing, the initial as well as the subsequent atrial depolarizations demonstrate identical P wave morphology (Figs. 24-41, 24-44) unless the tachycardia is multifocal. In reentrant PSVT, the P wave morphology (when visible) is retrograde except for the initiating extrasystole, which is upright if atrial in origin (Figs. 24-30, 24-42, 24-70). Ventricular premature systoles may also initiate this arrhythmia.

2 In automatic PSVT, the initiating beat arises late in the atrial cycle and does not exhibit either prolonged intraatrial or AV nodal conduction, whereas in reentrant PSVT the initial beat appears early in the atrial cycle and is associated with AV nodal conduction delay.

3 The atrial cycle length in reentrant PSVT is a direct linear function of AV nodal conduction. This means that when the AV refractory period lengthens, the tachycardia slows. In automatic PSVT no such relationship exists; in fact, shorter atrial cycles (more rapid rates) are accompanied by longer A-H intervals.

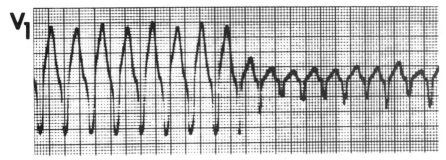

Fig. 24-74 Effect of functional bundle branch block on tachycardia rate in SVT utilizing a concealed accessory pathway. ECG lead V_1 is shown during SVT. On the left, functional left bundle branch block is present, and the tachycardia rate is 185 beats per minute. On the right the functional bundle branch block ends spontaneously and the QRS is normal. Note that coincident with this normalization of the QRS complex during SVT, the tachycardia rate increases to 215 beats per minute. *(From L. N. Horowitz and M. E. Josephson, Diagnosis and Evaluation of Concealed Accessory Atrioventricular Pathways, Practical Cardiology, 6:129, 1980. Used by permission.)*

4 Automatic PSVT demonstrates progressive shortening of the initial atrial cycles, typical of the warm-up phase of an automatic pacemaker. No such warm-up phenomena is seen in reentrant PSVT. Rather, the initial atrial cycles oscillate around the eventual cycle length of the PSVT.

5 Reentrant PSVT may be induced by atrial (or sometimes ventricular) extrastimuli or cessation of rapid atrial pacing, and terminated by timed atrial (or ventricular) extrastimuli. Automatic PSVT is not induced by atrial extrastimuli or atrial pacing nor is it terminated by atrial premature depolarizations. Atrial extrastimuli introduced during automatic PSVT result only in resetting the atrial cycle. Atrial overdrive pacing either fails to interrupt it or suppress it, the duration of suppression being related to the duration of rapid pacing.

Fig. 24-75 SA nodal reentrant tachycardia. The left and right panels show lead III during normal sinus rhythm (NSR) and supraventricular tachycardia (SVT). It is virtually impossible to distinguish SVT from ST because the P waves are identical to the sinus P waves. *(From M. E. Josephson and J. A. Kastor, Supraventricular Tachycardia: Mechanism and Management, Ann. Intern. Med., 87: 346, 1977. Used by permission.)*

NSR   **SVT**

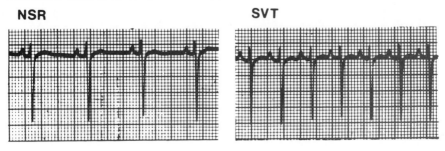

TABLE 24-1   DIFFERENTIATION OF PSVT BY CLUES FROM THE SURFACE ECG

Classification	Duration of QRS Complex	Rate (beats/min)	Configuration of P Wave in Leads II, III	Comments
AV nodal reentrant tachycardia	Narrow	140–200	Inverted; usually not seen in ECG	May terminate with CSM
Atypical AV nodal reentrant tachycardia	Narrow	100–150	Inverted; appears late with long R-P interval	May terminate with CSM
Orthodromic AV reciprocating tachycardia	Narrow	150–240	Inverted; appears after QRS complex, with short R-P interval	AV block excludes this diagnosis
Antidromic AV reciprocating tachycardia	Wide	150–240	Inverted; precedes QRS complex with short P-R interval	AV block excludes this diagnosis
Nodoventricular bypass tract (Mahaim)	Wide, LBBB	140–200	P wave location and morphology variable	Normal PR with delta wave during sinus rhythm
Intraatrial reentrant tachycardia	Narrow	100–150	P wave precedes QRS: morphology may vary from beat to beat	CSM may induce AV block without termination of tachycardia
Automatic atrial tachycardia	Narrow	100–180	P wave precedes QRS; upright or inverted P waves	Onset with premature atrial beat late in diastole. Gradual increase in rate (warm up)
Paroxysmal reciprocating sinus tachycardia	Narrow	100–160	P wave precedes QRS; same morphology as in sinus rhythm	Differentiation from sinus tachycardia by abrupt onset and termination

Abbreviations: AV = atrioventricular, CSM = carotid sinus massage, LBBB = left bundle branch block.
Source: F. Morady, and M. M. Scheinman, *Paroxysmal Supraventricular Tachycardia, Modern Concepts of Cardiovascular Disease,* 51: 107, 1982. Used **by** permission of the American Heart Association, Inc.

6 Abrupt termination of a supraventricular tachycardia by carotid massage, vagal maneuvers, or cholinergic stimuli favors a reentrant mechanism. In automatic tachycardias, such interventions may produce temporary slowing of the heart rate or a pause, followed by resumption of the tachycardia at its inherent rate of discharge.

7 Attention to the P wave morphology, the position of the P waves with respect to the QRS complexes, and the temporal relationship between the P waves and QRS complexes may provide diagnostic clues, as indicated in the preceding section.

ATRIOVENTRICULAR JUNCTIONAL MECHANISMS

Atrioventricular junctional rhythms were formerly called AV nodal rhythms, on the assumption that they originate in the AV node. Since it has been demonstrated that spontaneous diastolic depolarization characteristic of pacemaker cells does not occur in the main body (N region) of the AV, it is inappropriate to regard such rhythms as AV nodal. It is worth emphasizing, however, that pacemaker activity has been demonstrated in low atrial foci, the ostium of the coronary sinus, the bundle of His, the NH portion of the AV node, and possibly in its AN region, and that rhythms due to enhanced automaticity may therefore arise in one or more of these areas. The term *AV junctional rhythms* is more accurate for describing rhythms which arise in that portion of the AV conduction system extending from the atrial approaches to the AV node to the bifurcation of the bundle of His.

AV nodal (now termed AV junctional) rhythms were originally classified in accordance with the presumed site of origin within the node as *upper, middle,* and *lower* nodal rhythms.

In upper nodal rhythm (retrograde P wave in front of the QRS complex), it was assumed that atrial contraction preceded ventricular contraction; in middle nodal rhythm (retrograde P wave within the QRS complex), that the chambers contracted simultaneously; and, in lower nodal rhythm (retrograde P wave following the QRS complex), that atrial contraction followed ventricular contraction. Although useful descriptively, this classification is inaccurate, because electrophysiologic studies have demonstrated that the electrocardiographic criteria used to define the site of AV rhythms may be erroneous. Also, these criteria do not take into account variations in antegrade and retrograde conduction times. For example, prolongation of antegrade conduction may cause the P wave to precede the QRS complex even though the site of impulse formation is low in the AV junction; or delayed retrograde conduction may cause the P wave to follow the QRS deflection even when the pacemaker site is high in the AV junctional tissues.

Hoffman and Cranefield have suggested that atrioventricular rhythms with long P-R intervals arise either in the coronary sinus or in the bundle of His, with slow forward conduction to the ventricles. *Upper AV rhythms* with short P-R intervals are believed to arise in the coronary sinus, with slow retrograde conduction to the atria. *Middle AV rhythms* are thought to arise in the NH region of the AV node, and *lower AV rhythms* in the bundle of His. Studies by Damato and Lau suggest that in so-called lower and middle nodal rhythms the pacemaker is within the His bundle, and that so-called upper nodal rhythms represent either a coronary sinus or inferior left atrial rhythm.

The terms upper, middle, and lower AV junctional rhythms are still retained by some writers as a convenient method of expressing the relationship of the P waves to the QRS complexes, even though the original meaning is no longer applicable.

The presence of inverted P waves in leads II, III, and aVF and upright P waves in lead aVR has alway been considered an essential criterion for the diagnosis of AV junctional rhythms. The axis of the P wave in the frontal plane in these rhythms is generally between $-60°$ and $-80°$. The configuration of the P waves in the precordial leads is quite variable. Inverted P waves may be seen in some, all, or none of the precordial leads. However, it has been reported that the polarity of the P waves is not a reliable criterion for the diagnosis of AV junctional rhythms. Experimentally produced atrial activation in dogs suggests that rhythms from the area of the coronary sinus or AV node may be characterized by upright P waves in the inferior leads. Waldo and his associates, studying AV dissociation during open-heart surgery, have described junctional P waves which were diphasic $(-, +)$ or predominantly positive in leads II, III, and aVF. In these cases, the initial negative component of the P wave was often masked in the T wave, giving the impression in surface leads that AV junctional P waves were antegrade in contour. Although these experimental observations cannot be denied, the apparent rarity of this phenomenon in clinical practice does not justify abandoning the requirement of P wave inversion in leads II, III, and aVF for the diagnosis of AV junctional rhythms.

The AV junction may be the site of disturbances in impulse formation or impulse conduction, or both. Underlying such conditions as AV dissociation with or without AV block, double regions of block, unidirectional block, reciprocal beating of the atria or ventricles, concealed conduction, AV block, alternation of AV conduction, and AV junctional parasystole are physiologic or pathologic alterations in the capacity of the AV junctional tissues to conduct or initiate impulses.

In AV junctional rhythms, the atria may be depolarized in retrograde fashion, the atria and ventricles may beat independently (AV dissociation), or complex arrhythmias may occur because of the interplay of such mechanisms as concealed conduction and AV block.

The occurrence of ventricular fusion beats sometimes seen in what seem to be AV junctional rhythms with AV dissociation is difficult to explain, because hypothetically, ventricular fusion beats can occur only when two separate impulses activate the ventricles simultaneously, and at least one of these must arise below the bifurcation of the common bundle. How then can two impulses of supraventricular origin, as in AV junctional rhythms with AV dissociation, cause ventricular fusion beats? It has been suggested that this is possible if the atrial impulse descends through the AV conduction system and the AV junctional impulse reaches the ventricles by a different pathway, perhaps by the paraspecific fibers of Mahaim. Theoretically, two impulses could not use the same AV conduction pathway simultaneously, because interference in the AV junction would result in the mutual extinction of the impulses. Fusion could occur if it can be proved, as postulated by Sherf and James, that sinus and AV junctional impulses reach the ventricles through at least two separate longitudinally dissociated pathways in the bundle of His. This hypothesis is as yet unsupported by experimental evidence. Therefore, unless the atrial and AV junctional impulses are conducted to the ventricles by different pathways, the occurrence of ventricular fusion beats in AV junctional rhythms cannot be explained.

His bundle recordings have shown that many so-called AV junctional rhythms with "aberrant ventricular conduction" arise in the bundle branches, the fascicles, or the Purkinje system and therefore are really ventricular in origin. This supports the view that, in the absence of accessory pathways, ventricular fusion beats between supraventricular and ectopic impulses can occur only when the latter are ventricular in origin.

AV junctional rhythms may be associated with abnormalities of antegrade conduction, retrograde conduction, or both. First-degree antegrade or retrograde block cannot be diagnosed with certainty from surface leads. First-degree forward block may be suspected if the P'-R interval in a junctional rhythm is normal or prolonged. Retrograde second-degree block is usually of the Type I (Wenckebach) variety. Type II retrograde block is observed less commonly. Antegrade Wenckebach periods occur not infrequently, but Type II antegrade block is rare. The coexistence of both antegrade and retrograde conduction disturbances, especially if complicated by concealed conduction or discharge, may give rise to complex arrhythmias. Exit block may sometimes occur in AV junctional rhythms and tachycardias.

Atrioventricular Junctional Premature Systole
(Figs. 24-8B, 24-13B, 24-15A and B, 24-40)

See under Premature Systoles in this chapter.

Atrioventricular Junctional Rhythm
(Figs. 24-38, 24-54, 24-59, 24-76, 24-79, 24-164B, 24-167)

Atrioventricular junctional rhythm is usually a transitory escape rhythm observed under conditions in which the SA node is depressed. However, it may also occur during complete AV block.

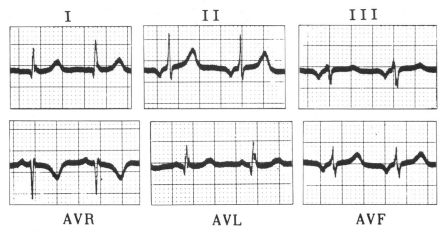

Fig. 24-76 Upper AV junctional rhythm. Retrograde P waves precede the QRS complexes by short P-R intervals in leads II, III, and aVF.

1 There is a slow, regular rhythm at a rate of 35 to 60 per minute.
2 The P' waves occur before, during, or after the QRS complexes.
3 The P' waves have abnormal contour.
4 The P' waves are retrograde (inverted in leads II, III, and aVF and upright in lead aVR).
5 The P'-R interval is from less than 0.12 s to negative.
6 The QRS complexes are of essentially normal outline and duration, but aberration is common.
7 Atrioventricular junctional rhythms are sometimes classified, purely for descriptive purposes, into three types:
a Upper AV junctional rhythm (Fig. 24-69): retrograde P' waves are followed by QRS complexes at P'-R intervals from 0.02 to 0.12 s.
b Middle AV junctional rhythm (Fig. 24-70): P' waves are not visible because they are superimposed on the QRS complexes.
c Lower AV junctional rhythm (Fig. 24-71): retrograde P' waves follow the QRS complexes at R-P intervals of from 0.02 to 0.20 s.
8 In rare instances, double junctional rhythms may occur.

AV junctional rhythm with no visible P waves cannot always be distinguished from atrial fibrillation with complete AV block or from sinus rhythm with a prolonged P-R interval and with the P wave superimposed on the preceding T wave.

Automatic Ectopic AV Junctional (His Bundle) Paroxysmal Tachycardia (Figs. 24-60, 24-81, 24-82, 24-87, 24-177)

1 The basic features which characterize all automatic rhythms are also applicable to this arrhythmia.

2   The onset of the tachycardia is spontaneous and is not related to initiating prerequisites such as critical rates or coupling intervals.

3   The arrhythmia is initiated by a premature beat (of AV junctional origin) without conduction delay.   This beat and all subsequent beats are identical in morphology.

4   The rhythm is rapid at a rate usually between 140 and 250 per minute.

5   A "warm up" period with slight initial irregularity of rhythm is common at the onset.   The rhythm thereafter is perfectly regular.

6   As already indicated, the tachycardia has a premature onset.   Its termination is followed by a pause.

7   The QRS interval is 0.10 s or less unless prolonged as a result of intraventricular block or aberrant ventricular conduction.

8   The tachycardia cannot be initiated or terminated by atrial or ventricular stimulation.

9   AV block, AV dissociation, or retrograde AV conduction defects may occur without affecting the tachycardia.

10   Vagal maneuvers or vagomimetic drugs do not affect or terminate the tachycardia.

11   Electrophysiologic studies may be helpful in the differentiation between automatic and reentrant tachycardia.   Automatic ectopic AV junctional paroxysmal tachycardia is an extremely uncommon arrhythmia, unlike the nonparoxysmal variety, which is fairly common.

Comments   Although in automatic AV junctional paroxysmal tachycardias the AV junctional pacemaker usually controls both the atria and ventricles, AV dissociation may occur so that the atria and ventricles beat independently.   AV junctional tachycardia with AV dissociation may occur in association with normal sinus rhythm, sinus bradycardia, atrial flutter, atrial fibrillation, and a second AV junctional rhythm characterized by retrograde P waves beating independently.   The occurrence of an AV junctional tachycardia with another supraventricular arrhythmia is considered a double tachycardia (Fig. 24-34).   When AV dissociation is present, ventricular capture or fusion beats may be seen on rare occasions.

An AV junctional tachycardia with abnormally wide QRS complexes may be indistinguishable from ventricular tachycardia if the atrial and ventricular rhythms are dissociated.   Similarly, it may be impossible to diagnose a continuous tachycardia with abnormal QRS complexes with a 1:1 relationship between the QRS complexes and P waves if the onset is not recorded or if additional information is not available.   The tachycardia may be atrial in origin, or it may be AV junctional or ventricular in origin with 1:1 retrograde atrial activation.   Although the configuration of the P wave may suggest retrograde conduction from an AV junctional or ventricular focus, a low atrial focus cannot be excluded.   A brief QRS-P' interval may suggest an AV junctional origin, but the P' wave might just as well be from an atrial focus whose ventricular activation is represented by the next QRS complex. The P' waves may also be the result of retrograde activation from a ventricular focus, represented by the second preceding QRS complexes. If a tachycardia with abnormal QRS complexes is initiated by a QRS complex with retrograde conduction to the atria, determination of the QRS-P' interval in the first or subsequent beats may be helpful in deciding whether the tachycardia is AV junctional or ventricular. A QRS-P' interval of 0.10 s or less is probably diagnostic of AV junctional tachycardia. Longer QRS-P' intervals may occur either in ventricular tachycardia or in AV junctional tachycardia with delayed retrograde conduction to the atria.

The use of His bundle recordings has been useful in the diagnosis of AV junctional rhythms. The presence of H potentials with normal or prolonged H-V intervals preceding either narrow or wide QRS complexes suggest that the ventricular complexes arise in or above the bundle of His. Also, the findings of retrograde P waves either in front of or following the QRS deflections suggest an AV junctional rhythm. Additional confirmation can be obtained by simultaneous recordings of bipolar atrial electrograms from both the high and the low right atrial regions. A progression of atrial conduction in caudocephalic direction indicates retrograde atrial conduction. In AV dissociation, the AV junctional beats are preceded by H deflections at normal or prolonged H-V intervals but are unrelated to atrial activity. All conducted beats and all AV junctional beats in atrial fibrillation are preceded by H deflections.

Nonparoxysmal AV Junctional Tachycardia (Figs. 24-34, 24-35, 24-67, 24-83 to 24-90, 24-142, 24-152, 24-153)

1 This is a tachycardia due to enhanced automaticity of the AV junctional tissues without the abrupt onset or termination characteristic of paroxysmal tachycardia.

2 It is most commonly caused by digitalis excess, inferior myocardial infarction, or acute rheumatic fever, but it may occur in myocarditis or following cardiac surgery.

3 Although a nonparoxysmal AV junctional tachycardia may cause retrograde activation of the atria, it usually leads to AV dissociation.

4 The rate of the tachycardia is between 65 and 130 per minute.

5 The rate may be slowed transiently by carotid sinus pressure, and it may be accelerated by exercise, inhalation of amyl nitrite, etc. Sometimes carotid sinus pressure or drugs may induce transient exit block in the ectopic focus, or exit block may occur spontaneously.

6 Nonparoxysmal AV junctional tachycardia is a common manifestation of digitalis excess in patients with atrial fibrillation.

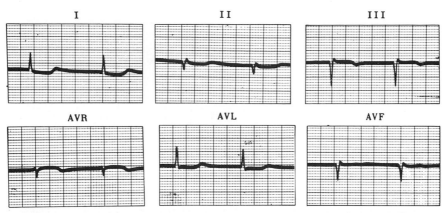

Fig. 24-77   Middle AV junctional rhythm.   P waves cannot be identified, since they are buried in the QRS complexes.   Atrial fibrillation is ruled out, since the baseline shows no oscillations.

Fig. 24-78   Lower AV junctional rhythm.   Retrograde P waves follow QRS complexes.   They are best seen in leads II, III, and aVF.

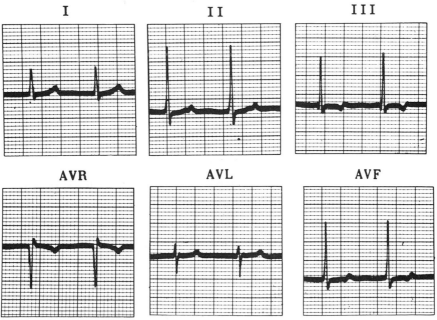

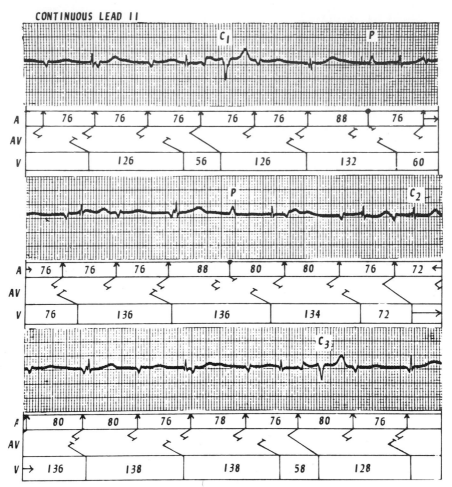

Fig. 24-79 Double AV junctional rhythm. There is incomplete dissociation between two AV junctional pacemakers. The upper pacemaker is responsible for the retrograde P waves; the lower pacemaker, for the ventricular complexes. At times, there is concealed discharge of the upper pacemaker. Sinus or atrial escape beats (P) and ventricular capture beats (C_1, C_2, and C_3) are interspersed in the record. Interestingly, capture occurs only during the supernormal phase of conduction. The time intervals are shown in hundredths of a second.

Atrioventricular Junctional Escape (Figs. 24-40, 24-57, 24-58)

See under Escape Beats in this chapter.

MECHANISMS OF DISPUTED ORIGIN

"Coronary Nodal" Rhythm (Fig. 24-91) (Short P-R, Normal QRS)

"Coronary nodal" rhythm is the term applied by some authorities to a rhythm characterized by normal P waves, short P-R intervals, and normal QRS complexes.

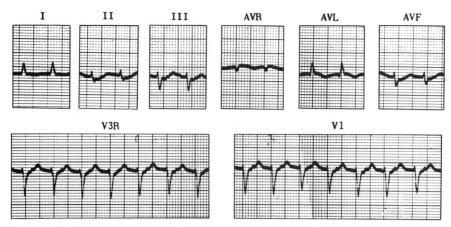

Fig. 24-80 PSVT at a rate of 150. The QRS complexes are followed by retrograde waves after an R-P interval of 0.12 s. The mechanism of the tachycardia is not apparent, but it is probably reentrant rather than automatic.

1 The P waves have normal contours.
2 The P waves are upright in leads I and II and are inverted in lead aVR.
3 The P-R interval is between 0.02 and 0.10 s but usually closer to 0.10 s.
4 No delta waves are present in the QRS complexes.

    The electrocardiographic pattern of "coronary nodal" rhythm has been reproduced by pacing a number of different sites in the right atrium. Under these circumstances, the term "coronary nodal" rhythm is inaccurate, since this rhythm can represent either an ectopic atrial rhythm arising from an atrial focus or a sinus rhythm with bypass of the AV node.

    So-called "coronary nodal" rhythm appears to be related to the Lown-Ganong-Levine syndrome (see Chap. 12).

Fig. 24-81 AV junctional paroxysmal tachycardia at a rate of 167 per minute with AV dissociation (dissociation by usurpation). The configuration of the QRS complexes is the same as was present in a previous tracing during sinus rhythm. The atrial mechanism is a sinus rhythm at a rate of 65 per minute. The presence of AV dissociation suggests an automatic rhythm, but reentry cannot be excluded entirely.

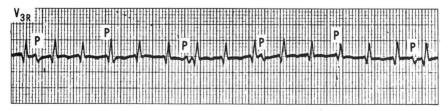

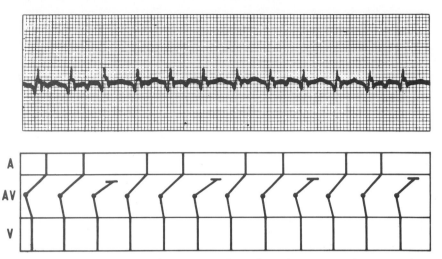

Fig. 24-82   Lead II.   Paroxysmal supraventricular tachycardia at a rate of 188 per minute with a 3:2 Wenckebach phenomenon of retrograde conduction.   From a patient with inferior myocardial infarction.   An automatic rhythm, as shown in the ladder diagram, is assumed but cannot be confirmed without electrophysiologic studies.

"Coronary Sinus" Rhythm (Fig. 24-95)

"Coronary sinus" rhythm is the term applied by some writers to a rhythm characterized by retrograde P waves and P-R intervals of 0.12 s or more. This rhythm may be interpreted alternatively as an AV junctional rhythm with delayed antegrade conduction to the ventricles.

1   The P waves are inverted in leads II, III, and aVF.
2   The P-R interval is 0.12 s or more.

   In "coronary sinus" rhythm, the impulse was originally believed to arise low in the atrium in the vicinity of the coronary sinus.   It has been produced experimentally in humans by pacing the heart with a catheter placed in the coronary sinus, but it has also been produced by stimulation of other sites located low in either the right or left atrium.   This suggests that the combination of retrograde P waves with normal P-R intervals represents an inferior atrial or AV junctional rhythm.
   "Coronary sinus" rhythm probably occurs more often in health than in disease.   One of the characteristic features of this rhythm is its instability. Transitions between sinus, "coronary sinus," and AV junctional rhythms occur frequently.

"Left Atrial" Rhythm (Figs. 24-93, 24-94)

The diagnosis of "left atrial" rhythm is based primarily on vectorial analysis of the P wave in the standard electrocardiogram, a practice which is not

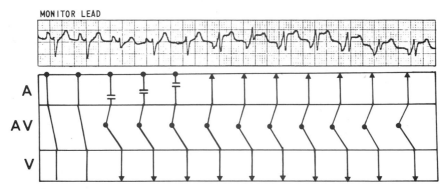

Fig. 24-83 Nonparoxysmal AV junctional tachycardia. After two sinus beats, an AV junctional tachycardia at a rate of 107 per minute takes over control of the heart. The third, fourth, and fifth P waves are atrial fusion beats.

without significant limitations. "Left atrial" rhythms are suspected of arising from specialized conduction fibers in the left atrium. These rhythms, according to published reports, are characterized by retrograde P waves in the inferior limb leads in association with approximately normal P-R intervals. Additional criteria for the diagnosis of "left atrial" rhythm include negative P waves in lead I (provided other causes are excluded), dome-

Fig. 24-84 Nonparoxysmal AV junctional tachycardia at a rate of 115. Retrograde P waves precede the QRS complexes by a P'-R interval of 0.08 s.

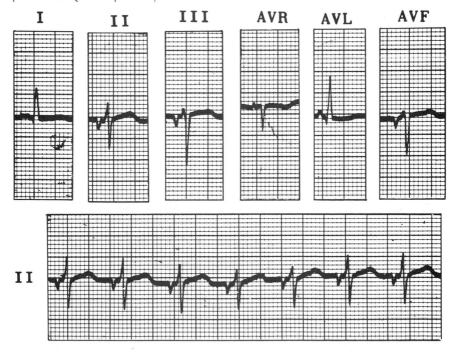

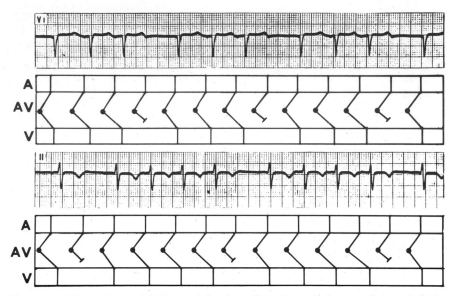

Fig. 24-85   Nonparoxysmal AV junctional tachycardia with atypical antegrade Wenckebach periods.   The R-R intervals tend to shorten progressively (although not invariably) and are followed by pauses.   The conduction ratio is 4:3 in lead V_1 and 5:4 in lead II.   Retrograde conduction is preserved at a constant rate in both tracings.   Because retrograde conduction is unaltered and antegrade conduction displays Wenckebach periodicity, the P'-R intervals increase in successive beats.   The P waves are retrograde in contour in lead II.

and-dart P waves in lead V_1, and inversion of the P waves in lead V_6 or all the precordial leads.

The existence of "left atrial" rhythm as an electrocardiographic entity has been challenged.   Atrial pacing studies by MacLean and his coworkers in patients following open-heart surgery have revealed that P wave polarity and morphology as well as the P-R interval are of limited usefulness in localizing the origin of atrial rhythms.   A negative P wave was recorded in lead I only when the left atrium was paced near the left pulmonary veins.   However, the P wave was not invariably negative in this lead in

Fig. 24-86   Nonparoxysmal AV junctional tachycardia (rate 120 per minute) with complete AV dissociation.   Antegrade Weckebach periods with 3:2 conduction ratios are responsible for the bigeminal rhythm.   The atrial mechanism is sinus bradycardia.

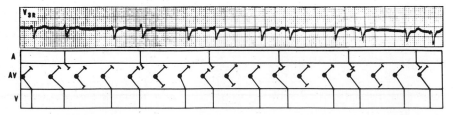

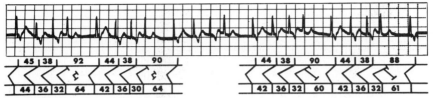

Fig. 24-87   Antegrade and retrograde Wenckebach periods in a probably automatic paroxysmal AV junctional tachycardia.   In the two diagrams, alternative interpretations of the pauses are indicated.   At the left, a continuous regular AV junctional tachycardia is assumed with a 5:4 response of the ventricles, a 5:3 response of the atria, and concealed conduction of the fourth retrograde impulse in each group.   At the right, the pauses are attributed to concealed reentry of the junctional impulse periodically disturbing the regularity of the ectopic firing.   (*From A. Pick and R. Langendorf, Approaches to the Diagnosis of Complex AV Junctional Mechanisms, in L. S. Dreifus and W. Likoff, eds., "Mechanisms and Therapy of Cardiac Arrhythmias," Grune & Stratton, New York, 1966.   Used by permission.*)

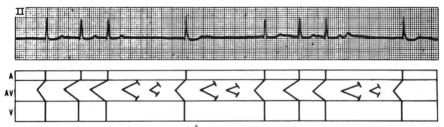

Fig. 24-88   Nonparoxysmal AV junctional tachycardia with exit block and with a Wenckebach phenomenon of both antegrade and retrograde conduction.   The rate of the AV junctional pacemaker is 115 per minute.   The arrhythmia was a consequence of digitalis excess.

Fig. 24-89   Nonparoxysmal AV junctional tachycardia due to digitalis excess in a patient with atrial fibrillation.   The ventricular rate is 125.   The S-T segment changes are characteristic of digitalis effect.

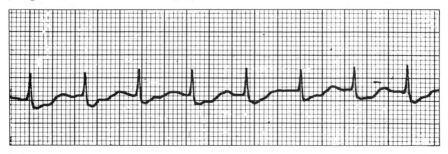

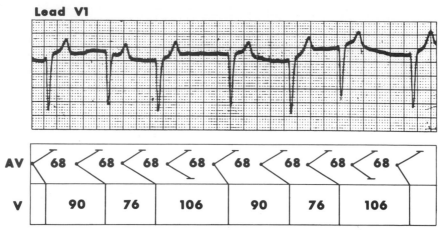

Fig. 24-90 Nonparoxysmal AV junctional tachycardia in atrial fibrillation with complete AV dissociation and a Wenckebach type of exit block due to digitalis intoxication. The atria are fibrillating and are dissociated from the ventricles because of AV block. At first glance, there appears to be the usual irregular ventricular response found in atrial fibrillation. However, closer scrutiny discloses an allorhythmia with periods of shortening of the R-R intervals separated by pauses. The cycle lengths are recorded in hundredths of a second. (*Modified after J. A. Kastor and P. M. Yurchak, Ann. Internal Med.,* 67: 1050, 1967. *Used by permission.*)

left atrial rhythms. A positive bifid (dome-and-dart) P wave in lead V_1 was recorded only with left atrial pacing near the inferior pulmonary veins and coronary sinus. However, other investigators have produced similar P waves by pacing the right atrium. A bifid positive P wave need not be present in lead V_1 during left atrial pacing. Negative P waves in lead V_6 or all the precordial leads were recorded with pacing from inferior sites in either the right or left atrium. Negative P waves in the right precordial leads were produced by pacing both left superior and right inferior atrial sites. Retrograde P waves in leads II, III, and aVF were produced by pacing either the right or left atrium, but only from an inferior focus. No definite criteria are available for differentiating inferior atrial rhythms (with inverted P waves in the inferior leads) from AV junctional rhythms in the presence of a normal P-R interval.

Beder and his associates, in an invasive electrophysiologic study of *spontaneous* left atrial rhythm, have concluded that the necessary criteria for the diagnosis of this arrhythmia are negative P waves in lead I and isoelectric or negative P waves in lead V_6. The finding of "dome-and-dart" P waves in lead V_1 is an additional useful and definitive criterion but is not present in each case.

VENTRICULAR MECHANISMS

According to Kistin, there are only two ventricular arrhythmias that can be diagnosed with certainty from the surface electrocardiogram: one is ven-

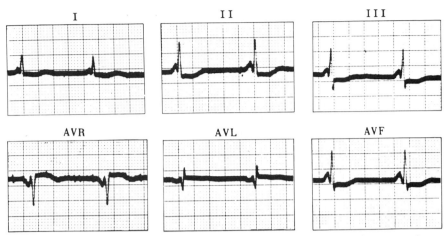

Fig. 24-91 "Coronary nodal" rhythm.   Normal P waves followed by normal QRS complexes after short P-R intervals.

tricular fibrillation, which is distinctive in its appearance; the other is an arrhythmia produced by an artificial ventricular pacemaker. All the electrocardiographic manifestations of ventricular arrhythmias except ventricular fibrillation, under some circumstances, may be simulated by supraventricular arrhythmia. Therefore, Kistin has stated, with the two exceptions noted above, it is not possible from conventional leads to prove beyond a doubt that an arrhythmia is ventricular in origin. However, by electrophysiologic techniques, including His bundle recordings and atrial pacing, it is sometimes possible to establish the diagnosis of ventricular arrhythmia with certainty.

Several mechanisms have been proposed to explain the genesis of ventricular arrhythmias. Among the many theories proposed, the two that are most widely accepted are reentry and enhanced automaticity of an ectopic focus.

Most present-day electrophysiologists believe that coupled ventricular premature systoles are reentrant in origin. Some are undoubtedly automatic (e.g., parasystolic beats and possibly multifocal ventricular premature beats

Fig. 24-92 "Coronary sinus" rhythm.   Retrograde P waves are followed by normal QRS complexes after a P-R interval of 0.16 s. Alternative diagnoses for this electrocardiogram are AV junctional rhythm with first-degree AV block or inferior atrial rhythm.

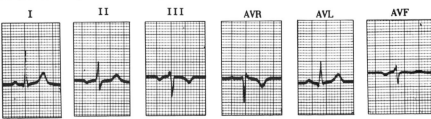

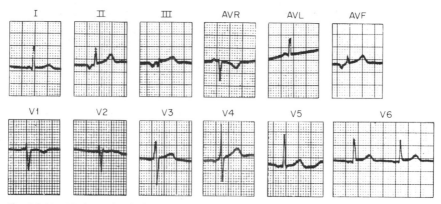

Fig. 24-93   "Left atrial" rhythm.   Retrograde P waves are present in leads II, III , and aVF, at a P'-R interval of 0.12 s.   The P' wave is diphasic (− , +) in lead I and inverted in lead V₆.   The P wave morphology in lead V₁ is not too distinct but suggests a dome-and-dart contour.   Since the P wave in lead I is not entirely negative the diagnosis of inferior atrial rhythm seems more appropriate.

and tachycardias).   However, it should be emphasized that neither of the two theories concerning the genesis of premature contractions has been proved to the exclusion of the other.

Ventricular rhythms that are considered the result of enhanced automaticity of latent pacemakers are idioventricular, bundle branch, and fascicular rhythms.

With respect to ventricular tachycardia, the chronic recurrent variety appears to be based on a reentry mechanism.   In the human heart, possible pathways for sustained reentry leading to ventricular tachycardia consist of the bundle branches, Purkinje fibers with or without adjacent ventricular myocardium, infarcted or fibrotic ventricular tissue, and various combinations of these pathways.   The weight of electrophysiologic evidence supports the hypothesis that the underlying mechanism of most cases of ventricular tachycardia is reentry, since the arrhythmia can be initiated and terminated by programmed ventricular stimulation.   Ventricular rhythms that cannot be induced or terminated by this procedure are thought to be caused by enhanced automaticity.

Patients at greater risk of developing paroxysmal ventricular tachycardia are those with severe myocardial disease (e.g., acute myocardial infarction) and prolonged Q-T intervals, especially if induced by hypopotassemia or drugs.

Abnormal focal automaticity is believed to be the mechanism of accelerated ventricular rhythm, ventricular parasystolic tachycardia, and the following ventricular paroxysmal tachycardias: those seen early in acute myocardial infarction, recurrent ventricular tachycardia in the long Q-T interval syndromes unrelated to drug or electrolyte abnormalities, and those induced by exercise.

Recurrent sustained ventricular tachycardia often presents a difficult therapeutic problem. Under such circumstances, electrophysiologic studies, including the determination of the effects of ventricular pacing, the use of pharmacologic testing techniques, and endocardial electrode catheter mapping, may assist in the selection of either drug or surgical treatment for the management of the arrhythmias.

The role of triggered activity in the genesis of ventricular tachycardia is unknown.

Ventricular Premature Systoles (Figs. 5-42, 24-8C, 24-13F, 24-15C and D, 24-16 to 24-28, 24-31, 24-60, 24-61, 24-63, 24-64)

See under Premature Systoles in this chapter.

Ventricular Escape (Figs. 24-56, 24-57, 24-58, 24-176)

See under Escape Beats in this chapter.

Ventricular or Idioventricular Rhythm (Figs. 24-164A to 24-166)

Ventricular or idioventricular rhythm is essentially a series of escape beats. It is seen most commonly in AV dissociation due to advanced or complete AV block. Less commonly, it may follow sinus arrest or SA block when the AV junction fails to produce escape beats or rhythms.

1   Ventricular or idioventricular rhythm is a regular rhythm at a rate usually between 25 and 40 per minute but occasionally faster (50 to 55 per minute) in children or in response to drugs.

Fig. 24-94 True "left atrial" rhythm. There are retrograde P waves in leads II, III, and aVF, at a P'-R interval of 0.16 s. The P' waves are also inverted in lead I and all the precordial leads.

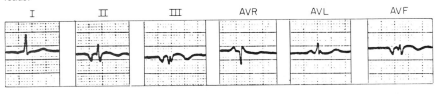

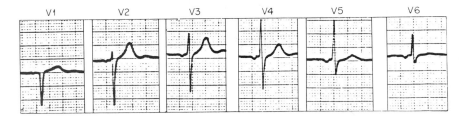

2 AV dissociation is usually present. The atrial mechanism is commonly a sinus rhythm, but atrial tachycardia, flutter, or fibrillation may occur or there may be atrial standstill. The atrial deflections have no fixed relationship to the ventricular complexes.

3 The ventricular pacemaker is situated below the region of the block. A ventricular rhythm arising in the right bundle branch shows the pattern of incomplete left bundle branch block. When the pacemaker site is in the left bundle branch, the QRS pattern is that of incomplete right bundle branch block. Rhythms arising in the anterior or posterior fascicle of the left bundle branch exhibit the pattern of incomplete right bundle branch block with left posterior fascicular block and left anterior fascicular block, respectively. Ventricular rhythms arising more distally in the Purkinje plexus of the left ventricular myocardium display the pattern of right bundle branch block and those of right ventricular origin the pattern of left bundle branch block.

It is worth emphasizing that an AV junctional rhythm conducting with abnormal QRST complexes because of coexisting intraventricular block is indistinguishable in surface leads from an idioventricular rhythm.

Ventricular Tachycardia

Four types of ventricular tachycardia can be recognized: idioventricular, paroxysmal (extrasystolic), polymorphous, and parasystolic.

Accelerated Ventricular (Idioventricular) Rhythm or
Idioventricular Tachycardia (Fig. 24-95)

Idioventricular tachycardia is essentially an accelerated ventricular rhythm. This arrhythmia occurs in from 9 to 23 percent of patients with acute myocardial infarction but may also be found in digitalis intoxication, rheumatic and other types of heart disease, and cardiomyopathy, and even in individuals without heart disease. In myocardial infarction, it is generally regarded as a benign arrhythmia. However, accelerated idioventricular rhythm frequently coexists with paroxysmal tachycardia in the early phase of myocardial infarction. The exact relationship between the two is unclear. The two arrhythmias can precede or follow each other or occur in haphazard order.

1 There is a slow regular rhythm at a rate of between 60 and 100 per minute.

2 The tachycardia is of brief duration, most runs consisting of only 4 to 30 beats.

3 The QRST complexes are wide and bizzare.

4 The tachycardia is usually initiated by a late diastolic ventricular premature systole which fuses with the conducted sinus beat. It may

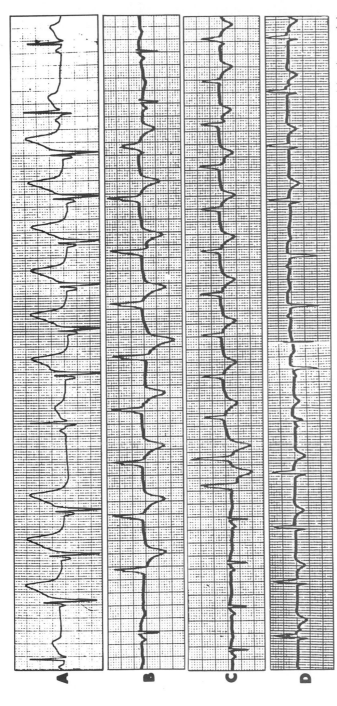

Fig. 24-95 Accelerated ventricular or idioventricular rhythm (idioventricular tachycardia). (A) Monitor lead. The first and last beats of the tracing are conducted sinus impulses. The second run of idioventricular tachycardia is initiated by a ventricular fusion beat. The final beat of the second run is also a fusion beat. (B) Monitor lead. A nine-beat run of idioventricular tachycardia beginning as an escape rhythm. The last beat of the tachycardia is a ventricular fusion beat. (C) Monitor lead. Idioventricular tachycardia initiated by two premature systoles. The QRS complexes of the tachycardia, although aberrant, are of normal duration, which suggests that the ectopic focus may be AV junctional or fascicular in origin. (D) Lead V$_{3R}$. Separate tracings from the same patient. The left-side strip shows the end of a run of tachycardia. The fifth ventricular complex is a fusion beat. The right-side strip shows escape of an accelerated ventricular pacemaker, possibly located in the AV junction or one of the fascicles because of the normal QRS duration. A, B, C, and D are from four different patients with acute myocardial infarction. Notches on the S-T segments of some of the beats in B, C, and D are probably P waves.

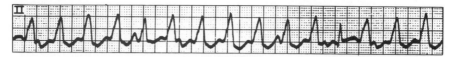

Fig. 24-96 Relatively slow paroxysmal ventricular tachycardia, at a rate of 128 per minute, dissociated from a sinus rhythm at a rate of about 75 per minute. The twelfth ventricular complex is a ventricular capture, and its pattern is that of inferior myocardial infarction. The fifth and tenth QRS complexes are ventricular fusion beats (Dressler beats).

also be the result of idioventricular escape when the sinus pacemaker slows.

5 Ventricular capture and fusion beats occur commonly.

6 It is generally accepted that the vast majority of idioventricular tachycardias with abnormal QRS complexes are ventricular and, more precisely, fascicular in origin. In acute anterior myocardial infarction, they arise in the anterior fascicle of the left bundle branch; in inferior infarcts, in its posterior fascicle. Recordings of His bundle electrograms together with analysis of the QRS configuration permit fairly precise localization of the site of origin of an idioventricular tachycardia. This is discussed further under Fascicular Beats and Rhythms later in this chapter.

7 Accelerated idioventricular rhythm is frequently accompanied by AV dissociation.

8 Some tachycardias which appear to be idioventricular in origin may actually represent a paroxysmal ventricular tachycardia whose apparent rate is slow because of exit block from a more rapidly firing focus.

Ventricular Paroxysmal Tachycardia
(Figs. 24-61, 24-62, 24-96, 24-98 to 24-102,
24-105, 24-106, 24-154, 24-183, 24-189)

Ventricular paroxysmal tachycardia, with few exceptions, occurs in the presence of organic heart disease. It is most commonly associated with

Fig. 24-97 A paroxysm of polymorphous ventricular tachycardia initiated by a ventricular premature systole interrupting the T wave of the preceding sinus beat. At the beginning of the tracing, a ventricular premature systole also interrupts the T wave of the preceding sinus beat but fails to induce ventricular tachycardia. Ventricular extrasystoles occurring during the vulnerable phase (at or near the peak of the T wave) of the preceding beat may result in ventricular tachycardia or fibrillation and sudden death. From a patient with acute myocardial infarction.

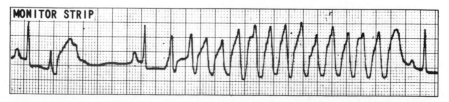

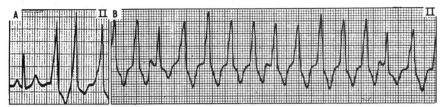

Fig. 24-98 Tracings recorded at different times from a patient with recurrent paroxysmal tachycardia. In *A*, a paroxysm is initiated by an abnormal QRS complex. The tachycardia must thus be of ventricular or AV junctional origin. In *B*, there is a tachycardia with abnormal QRS complexes as in *A*. The atrial mechanism cannot be determined, but P waves are seen before the third and thirteenth ventricular complexes, which are probably, respectively, ventricular fusion and capture beats. The most likely diagnosis is ventricular tachycardia.

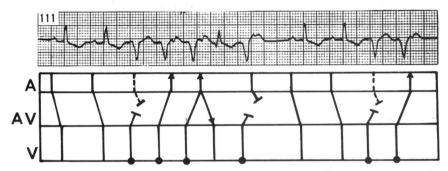

Fig. 24-99 Segment of a larger tracing from a patient with frequent ventricular extrasystoles and recurrent ventricular paroxysmal tachycardia. The three-beat burst of ventricular tachycardia at the center of the strip shows a Wenckebach phenomenon of retrograde conduction which is terminated by a reciprocal beat.

Fig. 24-100 Ventricular paroxysmal tachycardia with concordant QRS complexes in the precordial leads: all upright in *A*, all downward in *B*. (*From J. W. Hurst, ed., "The Heart,"* 3d ed. © 1974 by McGraw-Hill, Inc., New York. Used with permission of McGraw-Hill Book Company.)

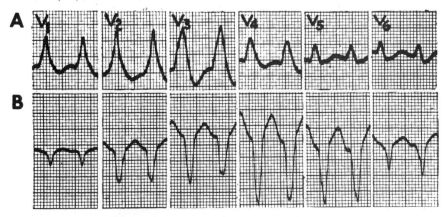

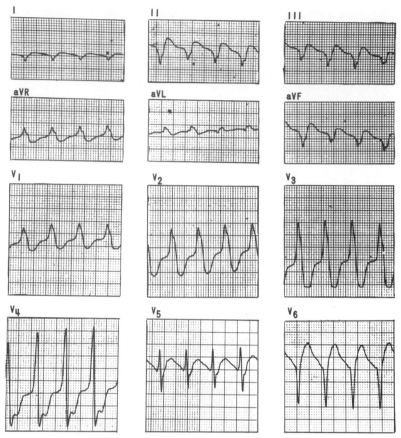

Fig. 24-101   Probable left ventricular paroxysmal tachycardia.   There are broad slurred R waves in lead V₁ and QS complexes in lead V₆ which strongly suggest left ventricular ectopy. The marked superior axis in the limb leads also suggest ventricular arrhythmia, since this is an uncommon axis for conducted beats.   The atrial mechanism cannot be identified.

acute myocardial infarction, but it may occur in arteriosclerotic or hypertensive heart disease, or both, in the absence of infarction.   Digitalis, quinidine, or procainamide toxicity, on occasion, may be the cause of this arrhythmia.

1   There is a rapid, regular or slightly irregular rhythm at a rate usually between 140 and 200 beats per minute, but occasionally slightly slower or faster.
2   The tachycardia has a premature onset, and its termination is followed by a pause.
3   The tachycardia is often initiated by a ventricular extrasystole which interrupts the T wave of the preceding beat during its vulnerable period. This is called the R on T phenomenon.

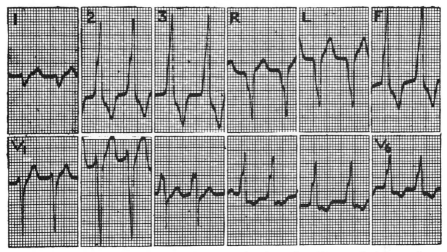

Fig. 24-102 Probable right ventricular paroxysmal tachycardia. The ventricular complexes show a left bundle branch block pattern with broad R waves in leads V_1 and V_2 and right axis deviation in the limb leads—findings which would be unusual in supraventricular arrhythmia. (*From H. J. L. Marriott, "Workshop in Electrocardiography," Tampa Tracings, Oldsmar, Fla., 1972. Used by permission.*)

4 The QRST complexes are bizarre and have the characteristics of ventricular premature systoles. There is often slight irregularity in the appearance of successive beats. The QRS intervals are 0.12 s or more.

5 Marriott has emphasized that certain morphologic characteristics favor the diagnosis of ventricular ectopy (over ventricular aberration) in a tachycardia with abnormal, wide QRS complexes (Fig. 24-31). These features are listed below:

a A monophasic or diphasic QRS complex in lead V_1 or MCL_1.

b A qR, RR', or qRR' pattern in lead V_1 or MCL_1, with R greater than R', quite common in left ventricular ectopy.

c A QS or rS complex in lead V_6 or MCL_6, also seen frequently in left ventricular ectopic rhythms.

d QRS complexes that are completely positive (preexcitation excluded) or completely negative in all the precordial leads.

e The occurrence of the deepest QS complex in lead V_4 or V_5 rather than in V_1 to V_3 when the QRS pattern is that of left bundle branch block.

f A QRS axis in the frontal plane that is directed abnormally leftward, or rightward and superiorly toward the axis of lead aVR (an uncommon axis for conducted beats).

g A pattern of right ventricular tachycardia (similar to right ventricular extrasystoles found in normal persons) consisting of (1) a left bundle branch block pattern in the left precordial leads; (2) tall and broad R waves in leads V_1 to V_3; and (3) usually, right axis deviation in the limb leads. However, endocardial mapping studies have indicated that

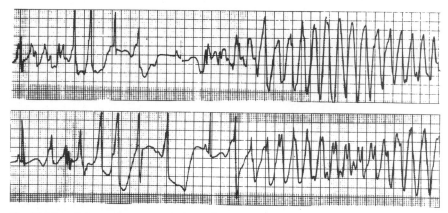

Fig. 24-103 Polymorphous ventricular tachycardia. These are short bursts of tachycardia with wide QRS complexes of varying morphology.

although ventricular tachycardias with a right bundle branch block pattern may arise in the right ventricle the origin is more frequently in a left ventricular aneurysm involving the septum or in the septum itself.

h A change (within a single lead) in the direction of the QRS complexes from positive to negative in progressive beats (called by Marriott the "swinging pattern").

6 Atrial activity may or may not be recognizable in the standard electro-cardiogram. When the P waves cannot be seen in conventional leads, simultaneously recorded right atrial, esophageal, or transsternal leads may identify the atrial mechanism. The atrial and ventricular rhythms are dissociated in about half of the cases. The atrial mechanism is then usually a sinus rhythm; less often, it is atrial tachycardia, flutter, or fibrillation. Retrograde activation of the atria occurs in the remaining cases and may be associated with varying degrees of retrograde AV block. However, it is unusual for the first or even the second beat of the paroxysm to be conducted retrogradely to the atria.

7 The two most reliable criteria for the diagnosis of ventricular tachycardia are the occurrence of ventricular capture (or reciprocal) beats with QRS durations shorter than those of the ectopic beats and, especially, the occurrence of ventricular fusion beats (Dressler beats) between the impulses of the supraventricular and ventricular pacemakers. However,

Fig. 24-104 Polymorphous ventricular tachycardia or torsades de pointes with changes in the polarity of the QRS complexes in progressive beats, also demonstrating the R on T phenomenon. (*From H. J. L. Marriott, "Workshop in Electrocardiography," Tampa Tracings, Oldsmar, Florida, 1972. Used by permission.*)

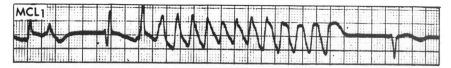

neither finding is absolutely pathognomonic of ventricular tachycardia, because such beats may occur in AV junctional tachycardias or other arrhythmias. Ventricular capture and fusion beats usually do not occur in ventricular tachycardia unless the ventricular rate is below 150 per minute. Even at slow rates, they are not common findings in ventricular tachycardia. Therefore absence of capture or fusion beats should not be regarded as a sign pointing against the diagnosis of ventricular tachycardia.

8 Vagal stimulation or carotid sinus pressure, with rare exceptions, has no effect on the tachycardia.

9 Recording of the His bundle electrogram can establish the diagnosis of ventricular tachycardia (in the absence of the preexcitation syndrome) provided the technique is satisfactory. In such recordings, the presence of short H-V intervals preceding the QRS complexes or the absence of H potentials suggests that the QRS complexes are ventricular in origin. The sequence of ventricular complex-H potential-atrial complex is especially characteristic of ventricular tachycardia.

Polymorphous Ventricular Tachycardia—Torsades de Pointes
(Figs. 24-97, 24-103, 24-104)

1 Unusual forms of ventricular tachyarrhythmias have been described with increasing frequency, employing such terms as paroxysmal ventricular fibrillation, atypical ventricular tachycardia, ventricular fibrillo-flutter, torsades de pointes, etc. Sclarovsky and his coworkers have suggested that the best descriptive term for these arrhythmias is polymorphous ventricular tachycardia, since the cardinal feature of these dysrhythmias is polymorphism of the QRS complexes.

2 Torsades de pointes is a form of polymorphous ventricular tachycardia first described by Dessertenne in 1966. As in other polymorphous ventricular tachycardias, changing R-R intervals, alternations in the QRS configuration and electrical axis, and a rapid, irregular ventricular rhythm are present.

3 The diagnosis of torsades de pointes is based on the following features:

a Phasic variation in the polarity of the QRS complexes. The complexes seem to twist or spiral around the isoelectric line over runs of usually 5 to 20 beats.

b The arrhythmia is frequently initiated by a ventricular premature systole occurring late in diastole on a prolonged T-U wave.

c There is often spontaneous termination of the arrhythmia although it occasionally degenerates into ventricular fibrillation.

d The heart rate is usually between 150 and 250 beats per minute, with varying R-R intervals a common observation.

e The arrhythmia is usually, but apparently not invariably, associated with prolongation of the Q-T interval.

f Torsades de pointes has been described in association with congenital prolonged Q-T interval syndromes, electrolyte disturbances, drug therapy (notably class I antiarrhythmic agents and psychotropic drugs), intrinsic myocardial disease, bradyarrhythmias, SA nodal dysfunction, advanced AV block, liquid protein diets, central nervous system disease, and autonomic imbalances.

3 Recognition of polymorphous ventricular tachycardia is important because of the therapeutic implications.

The arrhythmias associated with a *prolonged Q-T interval* may have a potentially fatal outcome if drugs that delay repolarization are employed (e.g., class I antiarrhythmic agents). These drugs must be avoided. Isoproterenol and bretylium may be effective. While defibrillation may be essential for prolonged episodes, because of the tendency of the tachycardia to recur, electrical cardioversion alone is not useful. The best immediate treatment is overdrive atrial pacing unless the presence of AV block requires ventricular pacing. On a long-term basis, sympathetic block is often efficacious.

Polymorphous ventricular tachycardias with a *normal Q-T interval* are reported to respond to conventional antiarrhythmic therapy (e.g., class I antiarrhythmic agents).

4 Although the mechanism is not established, it seems likely that reentry is the probable mechanism responsible for the occurrence of polymorphous ventricular tachycardia.

Ventricular Parasystolic Tachycardia (Fig. 24-107)

Ventricular parasystolic tachycardia is a rare arrhythmia. Its onset is with a premature systole, but the interectopic intervals between paroxysms of tachycardia are simple multiples of the ectopic cycle length. This indicates that the tachycardia continues between paroxysms but is not manifest because of exit block.

Ventricular Flutter and Fibrillation (Figs. 24-108, 24-109)

1 These are rapid, irregular rhythms with changing, wide, bizarre QRS complexes.
2 When the rhythm is fairly regular and the complexes are fairly uniform without an isoelectric interval, the arrhythmia is called *ventricular flutter*.
3 When the rhythm is quite irregular and the complexes are very bizarre in contour, the arrhythmia is called *ventricular fibrillation*.

FASCICULAR BEATS AND RHYTHMS
(FIGS. 24-111 to 24-115)

Electrocardiographers have long been puzzled by the seemingly paradoxical occurrence of beats (usually premature) with narrow QRS complexes in

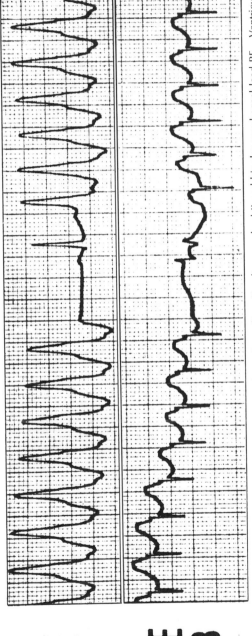

Fig. 24-105 Retrograde conduction to the atria in ventricular tachycardia. Simultaneous lead II and bipolar esophageal lead BE. Ventricular tachycardia with 1:1 VA conduction. One sinus beat interrupts the tachycardia. The retrograde P waves in the BE lead are the large, spiked, downward deflections after each small rounded QRS complex. The sinus P wave is smaller, diphasic, with a larger upward component. (*From A. D. Kistin, Retrograde Conduction to the Atria in Ventricular Tachycardia, Circulation, 24: 236, 1961. Used by permission of the American Heart Association, Inc.*)

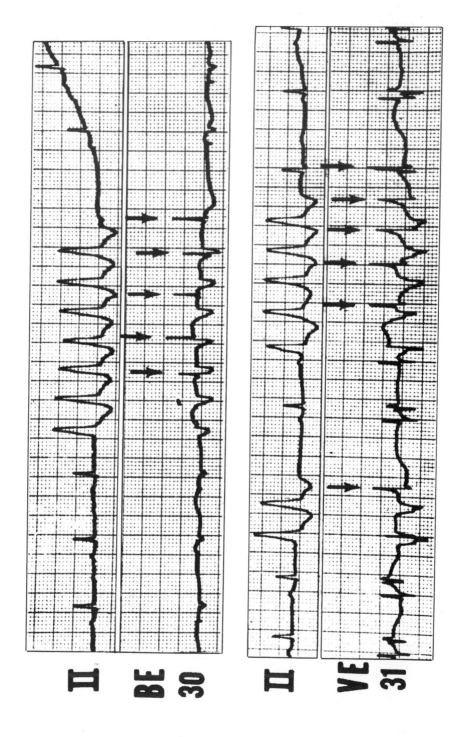

the presence of bundle branch block (Fig. 24-110).   The most common mechanism responsible for the unexpected normalization of the QRS complex in ventricular conduction defects is fusion of a conducted beat with a late diastolic ventricular extrasystole of opposite configuration. Other mechanisms which may produce the same phenomenon are super-normal conduction and intermittent bilateral bundle branch block.   Recently it has been demonstrated that such narrow beats may arise in the bundle branches or the fascicles of the specialized ventricular conduction system. Such ectopic impulses may proceed slowly through the ventricle on the affected side and, at the same time, ascend retrogradely through the bundle of His and down the other bundle at a normal rate of speed.   The slow conduction down the shorter pathway of the involved bundle may be equaled by the faster conduction along the longer path of the other bundle, resulting in almost simultaneous activation of the two ventricles and the disappearance of the bundle branch block pattern in that beat.

Ventricular rhythms can arise proximally in the bundle branches, the fascicles of the left bundle branch, or the more peripheral ramifications of the Purkinje network.   It has always been a problem to determine whether narrow ectopic QRS complexes (less than 0.12 s in duration) with slightly different morphologies from those of the sinus beats are AV junctional in origin (with aberration) or arise within the ventricles.   Most such beats are not more than 0.02 s wider than sinus beats.   His bundle recordings have shown that such beats and rhythms (which occur commonly in patients with acute myocardial infarction or digitalis intoxication) are frequently the result of impulse formation within the proximal infra-Hisian portion of the ventricular conduction system.   It is also theoretically possible for some of

Fig. 24-106   Retrograde conduction to the atria in ventricular tachycardia.   Simultaneous lead II and bipolar esophageal lead above.   Simultaneous lead II and V esophageal lead below.   Retrograde P waves are marked by arrows.   *Top:* Ventricular tachycardia with VA conduction, Wenckebach phenomenon.   The second, third, fifth, sixth, and seventh ectopic beats are followed by retrograde conduction.   There is no VA conduction after the first ectopic beat because of interference with sinus beat.   Wenckebach phenomenon, VA conduction times (in seconds): second ectopic beat 0.30; third, 0.35; fourth, blocked; fifth, 0.24; sixth, 0.32; seventh, 0.36.   The last retrograde P wave is apparent in lead II.   *Bottom:* Retrograde conduction after the second of two ventricular premature systoles near the beginning, then ventricular tachycardia with 1:1 VA conduction starting with the second ectopic beat, and a reciprocal beat at the end.   The normal QRS in lead II after the last ectopic beat is preceded by a retrograde P wave.   The VE lead shows that still another retrograde P wave is superimposed on the reciprocal QRS, as if the reciprocal impulse on its way to the ventricle turned back to the atrium again.   The reciprocal beat with normal QRS and thus normal conduction is suggestive evidence that the ectopic focus that initiates the tachycardia is ventricular rather than AV junctional.   The interval from the preceding ectopic beat is longer than the intervals between ectopic systoles, so the evidence is not conclusive; the longer interval conceivably allows for recovery from a refractory phase.   The pause after the reciprocal beat is ended by an AV junctional escape beat, its QRS occurring right after a sinus P wave.   (*From A. D. Kistin, Retrograde Conduction to the Atria in Ventricular Tachycardia, Circulation, 24: 236, 1961.   Used by permission of the American Heart Association, Inc.*)

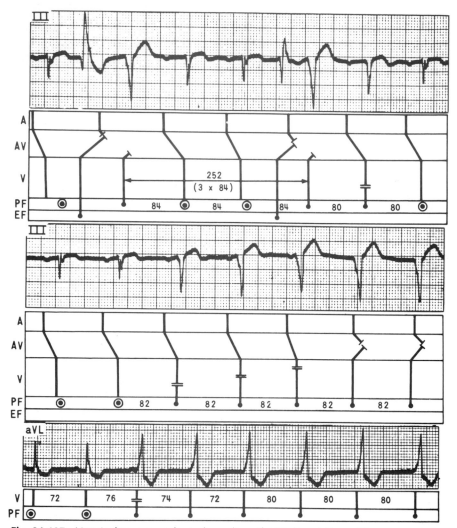

Fig. 24-107 Ventricular parasystolic tachycardia with AV dissociation. PF = parasystolic focus; EF = extrasystolic focus. The numbers at the V level are the R-R intervals in hundredths of a second. There are two separate recordings of lead III and one of lead aVL. *Upper tracing*: The second and sixth ventricular beats are ventricular extrasystoles. The third and seventh beats are identical with the last two beats of the middle strip. The interval between the parasystolic beats in the upper tracing is a simple multiple of the interectopic interval of the parasystolic beats in the two lower strips. The P-R interval of the conducted sinus impulses following the parasystolic beats in the upper tracing is prolonged because of retrograde concealed conduction. Some of the parasystolic beats, shown as circled dots, fail to activate the ventricles because of refractoriness from previous stimulation. *Middle tracing*: The third, fourth, and fifth ventricular complexes are fusion beats. *Lower tracing*: The parasystolic focus becomes the dominant ventricular pacemaker, beating at a rate of about 75 per minute. There is also isorhythmic AV dissociation. An alternate explanation, supported by some authorities, is that the ventricular rate is only 75 per minute because of a 2:1 exit block from the parasystolic center. The rate of the parasystolic tachycardia would thus be 150 per minute. These same authorities feel that most, if not all, cases of ventricular parasystole actually represent a form of ventricular tachycardia with exit block.

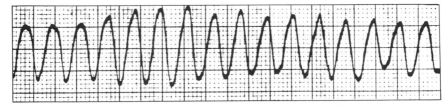

Fig. 24-108   Ventricular flutter.   There is a zigzag pattern without differentiation between the QRS complexes, S-T segments, and T waves.   Atrial flutter with aberrant ventricular conduction may mimic this pattern.   (See Fig. 24-52.)

these beats to originate in the ventricular septum equidistant from both bundle branches, in the AV junction with conduction to the ventricles via preferential pathways, within the pathways themselves, or in the AV junction with aberration due either to incomplete recovery or to phase 4 depolarization of the conducting fascicles.   These possibilities seem unlikely in the light of current knowledge.

Beats arising in the bundle of His or elsewhere in the AV junction show H-V intervals similar to those recorded in sinus beats.   They have normal QRS contours provided they do not occur too early in the cycle. If premature, they may show aberrant ventricular conduction.   The H-V intervals of bundle branch or fascicular beats or rhythms, on the other hand, are shorter than normal.   Sometimes the H deflection is actually inscribed shortly after the onset of ventricular depolarization.   It is important to realize that in these beats the H-V or V-H intervals reflect not the conduction time from the ectopic site to the His bundle but instead the differences in arrival of excitation at the common bundle retrogradely and at the ventricles antegradely.

Ectopic impulse formation in the bundle branches or the fascicles of the left bundle may produce isolated beats, slow rhythms, or tachycardias. According to Rosenbaum and his coworkers, beats arising in the proximal right bundle branch show the pattern of incomplete left bundle branch block.   Extrasystoles or rhythms arising in the posterior fascicle of the left bundle produce the pattern of incomplete right bundle branch block with some degree of left anterior fascicular block, and those arising from the

Fig. 24-109   Ventricular fibrillation.

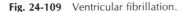
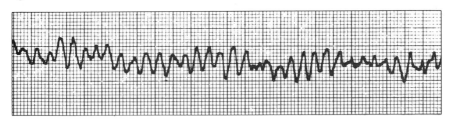

CONTINUOUS LEAD V₃ᵣ

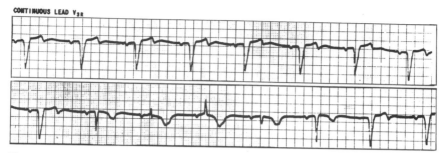

Fig. 24-110   Narrow QRS complexes in the presence of bundle branch block.   The upper tracing shows 2:1 AV block and left bundle branch block.   In the lower tracing, the second through the sixth QRS complexes are fusion beats.   The most likely explanation is intermittent bilateral bundle branch block.   The varying contour of the fusion beats can be attributed to a gradual decline and recovery of conduction through one of the bundle branches.   An alternate explanation is the transient simultaneous discharge of an ectopic focus located below the site of the block in the left bundle branch.

Fig. 24-111A   Narrow ventricular ectopic beats.   In a patient with complete AV dissociation, a ventricular pacemaker arising from the posterior fascicle of the left bundle branch produces the pattern of incomplete right bundle branch block with left anterior fascicular block.   The QRS interval is 0.10 s, just 0.01 s longer than that of the sinus beats shown in Fig. 24-111B. (*From M. B. Rosenbaum, Classification of Ventricular Extrasystoles According to Form, J. Electrocardiol., 2: 289, 1969.   Used by permission.*)

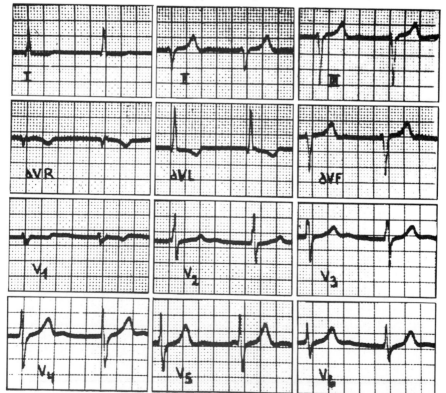

anterior fascicle, the pattern of incomplete right bundle branch block with some degree of left posterior fascicular block.   Beats showing the pattern of *pure* incomplete right bundle branch block or *pure* left anterior fascicular block have not been reported, although, on theoretical grounds, they should occur.   According to Rosenbaum et al., the failure to find such beats supports his contention that the anterior and posterior divisions are already delineated within the main left bundle branch itself.   It likewise fits their concept of the origin of the left bundle branch from the bundle of His.   Beats showing the pattern of pure left posterior fascicular block are assumed to originate at the ''pseudobifurcation'' of the bundle of His into the right bundle branch and the anterior division of the left bundle branch.   A beat arising at this site activates the anterosuperior portion of the left ventricle and the right ventricle almost simultaneously.   The pure left posterior fascicular block patterns results because the posteroinferior region of the left ventricle is activated with some delay.

The common occurrence of ventricular fusion beats in rhythms with relatively narrow but somewhat aberrant QRS complexes is one of the strongest arguments favoring the ventricular rather than AV junctional origin

Fig. 24-111B   Same patient as in Fig. 24-111A during normal sinus rhythm.   The QRS duration is 0.09 s and the electrical axis is normal.   (*From M. B. Rosenbaum, Classification of Ventricular Extrasystoles According to Form, J. Electrocardiol., 2: 289, 1969.   Used by permission.*)

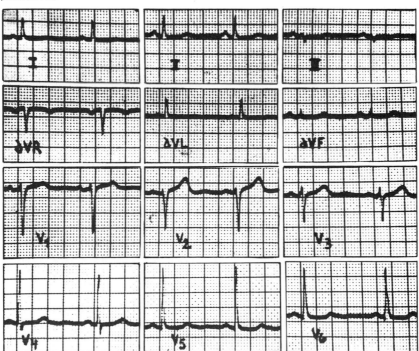

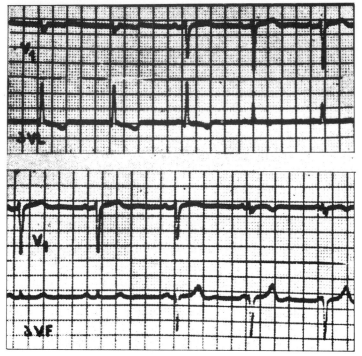

Fig. 24-111C Same patient as in Figs. 24-111A and B. There is fusion (the third beat in each strip of the simultaneously recorded leads) between the sinoatrial and fascicular beats. In the fusion beats, the pattern of incomplete right bundle branch block is canceled out, but that of left anterior fascicular block remains. (*From M. B. Rosenbaum, Classification of Ventricular Extrasystoles According to Form, J. Electrocardiol., 2: 289, 1969. Used by permission.*)

of these arrhythmias. The few studies performed on the retrograde conduction times of such narrow ectopic beats also supports this hypothesis.

Thus analysis of the configuration of the QRS complexes, in conjunction with His bundle recordings, makes it possible to establish the diagnosis of fascicular rhythms.

ATRIOVENTRICULAR DISSOCIATION

In AV dissociation, different pacemakers control the atria and ventricles so that they beat independently. The physiologic basis for AV dissociation is interference, block, or a combination of both.

Terminology

The term *AV dissociation* should be employed only in a generic sense to indicate independent beating of the atria and ventricles regardless of cause.

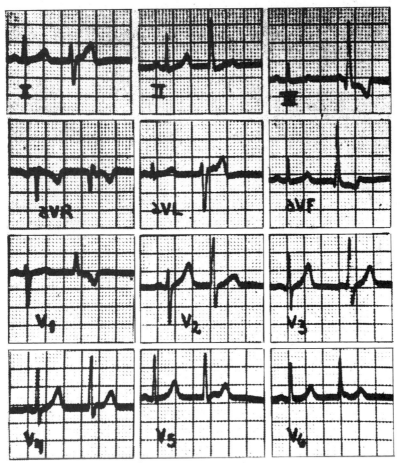

Fig. 24-112 Narrow ventricular ectopic beats produced by a parasystolic focus located in the anterior fascicle of the left bundle branch. The second beat in each lead is parasystolic and shows the pattern of incomplete right bundle branch block with left posterior fascicular block. (*From M. B. Rosenbaum, Classification of Ventricular Extrasystoles According to Form, J. Electrocardiol., 2: 289, 1969. Used by permission.*)

AV dissociation is never a primary disturbance of rhythm; it is always the result of a more basic disorder.

The terms *complete AV dissociation* and *complete AV block* are not synonymous. Block is but one of the causes of AV dissociation.

The term AV dissociation has also been used as a synonym for the arrhythmia first called *interference dissociation* by Mobitz and later changed by Scherf to *AV dissociation with interference*. In a quasi-specific sense, the term interference dissociation, or AV dissociation with interference, is applied to a dysrhythmia in which, because of slowing of the atrial pacemaker, acceleration of the ventricular pacemaker, or both, the atria and ventricles beat independently. Inherent in this definition are two

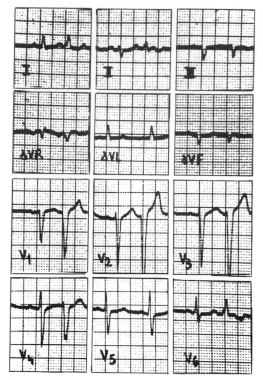

Fig. 24-113   Narrow ventricular extrasystolic beats.   The second beat in each lead shows the pattern of incomplete left bundle branch block, which indicates that they originate in the proximal portion of the right bundle branch.   (*From M. B. Rosenbaum, Classification of Ventricular Extrasystoles According to Form, J. Electrocardiol., 2: 289, 1969.   Used by permission.*)

assumptions: (1) that antegrade conduction is always possible unless the ventricles are refractory, permitting ventricular captures by atrial impulses; and (2) that retrograde conduction is impaired except for the rare occurrence of atrial captures by retrograde ventricular impulses.

Interference

The use of the term *interference* in connection with AV dissociation has engendered much controversy.

The term *interference* has been used in four different senses:

1   The term has been applied to the interruption of the regular rhythm of the ventricular pacemaker by conducted beats (ventricular captures). Thus, when atrial impulses are conducted to the ventricles, the atrial rhythm *interferes* with the ventricular rhythm by producing early capture beats.

2   The term has also been used to designate the delayed occurrence of

the ventricular beat following a ventricular capture.   Thus, when the atrial impulse descends through the AV junction, it discharges the ectopic pacemaker, which delays the appearance of the next ventricular impulse.   The timetable of ventricular activity is thereby *interfered* with.

3   The term has been used to denote the mutual extinction of two excitation waves that meet in any portion of the heart.   This may occur in the atria, the ventricles, or the atrioventricular junction.   Simultaneous activation of the atria by two impulses of different origin produces an atrial fusion beat.   A ventricular fusion beat results from a similar process taking place in the ventricles.   Collision of opposing impulses in the AV junction causes the beats to become dissociated.

4   The term has also been employed to indicate a state of physiologic refractoriness in a portion of the heart, resulting from previous impulse stimulation.   For example, when the AV junction discharges its impulse before the sinus impulse arrives, the latter finds the AV junctional tissues refractory.   The refractory junctional tissues thus *interfere* with the conduction of the normal sinus impulse through the AV junction.

Thus, the term interference has been used in two main connotations: to indicate a disturbance in rhythm, as described in the first two paragraphs, or to denote a disturbance in conduction, as outlined in the last two paragraphs.   In the first sense, the property of interference is vested in the conducted beats; in the second sense, it is vested in all beats but the conducted ones.   Because of this, the term interference should not be used without defining the sense in which it is employed.

Fig. 24-114   Narrow ventricular ectopic beats produced by a parasystolic focus located in the proximal infra Hisian portion of the conduction system.   The ectopic beats, which are only 0.09 s in duration, are nevertheless 0.03 s wider than the normally conducted impulses. The interectopic interval is 0.96 s.   The parasystolic focus fires the ventricles unless they are refractory from previous stimulation or because of exit block (represented by the circled dot). The ventricular complex labeled FB is a ventricular fusion beat.   The altered configuration of the parasystolic beats (even though narrow), together with the presence of a fusion beat, is a weighty argument in favor of their ventricular origin.   V = ventricles, PF = parasystolic focus.

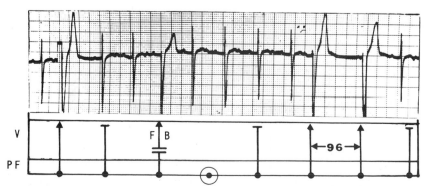

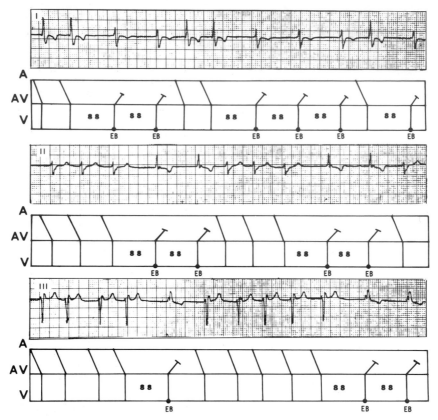

Fig. 24-115   Fascicular rhythm.   The atrial mechanism is atrial fibrillation.   The conducted beats show the pattern of right bundle branch block with left anterior fascicular block (axis −45°).   Periodically, when the degree of AV block increases, a ventricular pacemaker escapes (escape interval = 0.88 s).   The configuration of the escape beats is different from that of the conducted beats.   The pattern of the ventricular rhythm is that of right bundle branch block with left posterior fascicular block (axis +105°).   Upon analysis, it can only be concluded that the escaping pacemaker must be located in the anterior fascicle of the left bundle branch.   Conclusive proof of the ventricular origin of the escape rhythm can be established only by His bundle recordings.

The terms *block* and *interference* are not synonymous.   Interference, as used in this text, is a physiologic event and refers to the stoppage or delay in the conduction of a stimulus because of normal refractoriness in the conducting tissues.   Block is a pathologic event and refers to the stoppage or delay in the conduction of a stimulus because of abnormal prolongation of the refractory period.

Etiology

Many conditions may cause AV dissociation, but the most frequent causes are digitalis excess, coronary heart disease (especially inferior myocardial infarction), and acute rheumatic fever. It may also result from vagal stimulation or may occur in response to such drugs as quinidine, procainamide, atropine, and salicylates.

Mechanism (Figs. 24-116, 24-117)

Atrioventricular dissociation may result from slowing of the primary pacemaker (dissociation by default), acceleration of a subsidiary or latent pacemaker (dissociation by usurpation), AV block, or varying combinations of the above.

Atrioventricular dissociation usually develops when the rate of the atrial pacemaker is slower than that of a subsidiary pacemaker.

When the atrial impulse is delayed because of sinus slowing, sinus arrest, SA block, or a premature beat, a subsidiary pacemaker in the AV junction or the ventricles may escape. When escape is repetitive, the subsidiary pacemaker gains control of the ventricles. Retrograde impulses from this pacemaker are conducted back toward the atria. If the atria are activated by the sinus impulse before the arrival of the ascending ventricular

Fig. 24-116 Mechanisms of AV dissociation. (*A*) The strips are continuous. The bradycardic phase of sinus arrhythmia permits an AV junctional pacemaker to escape (at a rate of 46 per minute) and produce AV dissociation (dissociation by default). (*B*) AV dissociation due to digitalis intoxication. After two normally conducted beats slight sinus slowing permits an excitable AV junctional pacemaker to escape (at a rate of about 78 per minute). Toward the end of the tracing, the SA node recaptures the ventricles for two beats before AV dissociation returns (dissociation by default and usurpation). (*C*) Enhanced automaticity of an AV junctional pacemaker (caused by acute rheumatic fever), together with sinus slowing, produces transient AV dissociation (dissociation by default and usurpation). When the sinus node accelerates (toward the end of the tracing), the ventricles are recaptured (the last two beats in the record). (*D*) While the sinus rate remains constant, transient acceleration of an AV junctional pacemaker produces transient AV dissociation (dissociation by usurpation). At the end of the strip, the emerging P waves recapture the ventricles with aberrant conduction. (*From H. J. L. Marriott and M. M. Menendez, A-V Dissociation Revisited, Progr. Cardiovasc. Dis., 8: 522, 1966. Used by permission.*)

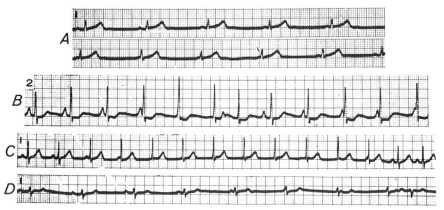

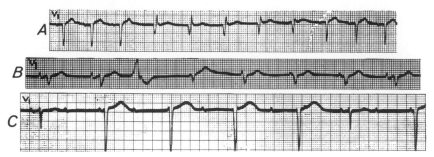

Fig. 24-117 Mechanisms of AV dissociation.   (A) After three normally conducted sinus beats, a pause resulting from a nonconducted atrial premature systole (superimposed on the T wave of the third sinus beat) permits a ventricular pacemaker to escape for several beats (dissociation by default).   (B) The postextrasystolic pause following a ventricular premature beat permits an AV junctional pacemaker to escape for four cycles (dissociation by default.).   (C) The long pause following a dropped beat in 2:1 AV block permits a ventricular pacemaker to escape at a rate of 42 per minute (dissocation due to AV block).   When the R-P interval lengthens sufficiently, the ventricles are recaptured.   (*From H. J. L. Marriott and M. M. Menendez: A-V Dissociation Revisited, Progr. Cardiovasc. Dis., 8: 522, 1966.   Used by permission.*)

impulse, retrograde conduction is prevented by interference, and the atria and ventricles will beat independently.   This is dissociation by default. On the other hand, enhanced automaticity may cause an ectopic pacemaker located below the atria to fire repetitively and result in AV dissociation. This is dissociation by usurpation.   AV dissociation also results when the ventricles are controlled by an artificial pacemaker firing independently of the atrial mechanism.

Atrioventricular block, as well as interference, may be responsible for AV dissociation.   When this happens, complex arrhythmias sometimes result.   Complete AV block, of course, implies complete AV dissociation, and in this connection, use of the term *AV dissociation* is superfluous.

Varieties

The types of AV dissociation depend not only on the rate and regularity of the pacemakers but also on the presence or absence of either antegrade or retrograde block.

Complete AV dissociation, which may be persistent or intermittent, is characterized by complete failure of atrial impulses to be conducted to the ventricles and vice versa.

In *incomplete AV dissociation,* some atrial impulses may be conducted to the ventricles when the AV node is not refractory, which will result in ventricular captures.   Similarly, retrograde conduction of ventricular impulses may lead to atrial captures.

Marriott objects to the terms *complete* and *incomplete*.   He prefers the terms *continuous* and *discontinuous,* or better still, *AV dissociation with or without capture beats.*

The term *isorhythmic* AV dissociation is applied to that type of AV dissociation in which, *fortuitously*, the atrial and ventricular rhythms occur at approximately the same rate.

The term *synchronization* refers to isorhythmic AV dissociation due to *coordinated* beating of the atrial and ventricular pacemakers. *Accrochage* means a brief period of synchronization.

Waldo and his associates believe that isorhythmic dissociation, in the majority of cases, results from the retrograde capture of the atria by an AV junctional rhythm. The P wave in leads II, III, and aVF is diphasic ($-$, $+$) during the period of synchronization, with the initial negative portion of the P wave or the entire P wave often buried within the QRS complexes. In their opinion, the only period of true dissociation occurs in the transition between sinus rhythm and AV junctional rhythm. It has been the author's experience, as well as that of others, that the transition from antegrade to retrograde P waves (or vice versa) in AV junctional rhythms with AV dissociation is usually apparent (Fig. 24-118).

Levy and Edelstein in their study of isorhythmic AV dissociation found two patterns. In one group, the P wave fluctuated cyclically back and forth across the QRS complex. They believe that this type of synchronization represents a biologic feedback control system. In the second group, in which the P wave was in a fairly constant position relative to the QRS complex, the mechanism could not be determined.

Salient Features

1 The atria and ventricles are controlled by separate pacemakers.
2 The ventricular rhythm is regular and is more rapid than the atrial rate unless AV block is present.
3 The P waves bear no fixed temporal relationship to the QRS complexes.
4 Both ventricular and atrial capture and fusion beats may occur and produce irregularity in the rhythm.

Capture Beats (Figs. 24-79, 24-95, 24-96, 24-98, 24-116 to 24-120, 24-122, 24-129, 24-148, 24-149)

Capture beats are always early beats. The contour of the capture beats may be of help in determining the site of the ventricular pacemaker. If the configuration of both the ectopic and the capture beats is identical, the ventricular pacemaker is situated above the bifurcation of the bundle of His. If the contour of the ectopic beats is normal but the configuration of the capture beats is abnormal, the ventricular pacemaker is supraventricular but the capture beats are bizarre because of aberrant ventricular conduction (Fig. 24-129). If the ectopic beats are wide and bizarre but the capture beats are essentially normal, the ventricular pacemaker is located either in the ventricles or in the AV junction.

LEAD II - CONTINUOUS

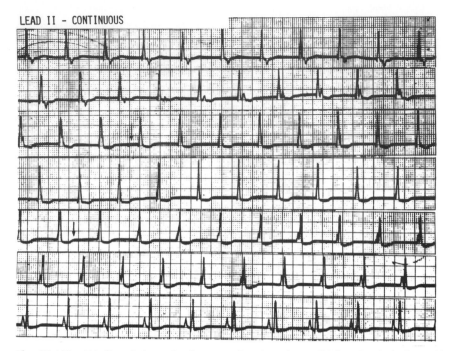

Fig. 24-118   AV dissociation.   In the top strip, there is an AV junctional rhythm with dependent activation of the atria.   In the second strip, the SA node accelerates and competes with the AV junctional pacemaker for control of the atria.   The second through the fifth P waves in this strip are atrial fusion beats.   The sinus node then assumes complete control of the atria, but the ventricles remain under the control of the AV junctional pacemaker.   This results in AV dissociation.   During the period between the arrows in the third, fourth, and fifth strips, the dissociation is isorhythmic, with the P waves hidden within the QRS complexes. However, continuing acceleration of the SA node causes the P waves to emerge in front of the QRS complexes.   Finally, in the bottom strip, normal sinus rhythm is restored.

Fusion Beats (Figs. 24-95, 24-96, 24-98, 24-107, 24-118)

Fusion beats, like capture beats, go hand in hand with AV dissociation. They may be regarded either as incompletely captured beats or as partially dissociated beats.   The reader is referred to a previous section in this chapter for additional information about fusion beats.

Atrioventricular Dissociation Due Primarily to Interference

Atrioventricular Dissociation in Sinus Rhythms

Incomplete AV Dissociation (Interference Dissociation, AV Dissociation with Interference) (Figs. 24-8F, 24-79, 24-116, 24-120)

1   Different pacemakers control the atria and ventricles so that they beat independently.   The former are under the control of the SA node, the latter under the control of a pacemaker in the AV junction (or, rarely, in the ventricles).

2 The ventricular rhythm is regular and is usually more rapid than the atrial rate but may be equal to it (contrary to the situation in advanced or complete AV block), so that the AV node is ordinarily refractory when sinus impulses reach it.   The atrial rhythm is irregular when sinus arrhythmia is the atrial mechanism.   The ventricular rate is usually less than 150 per minute.

3 The P waves are of normal contour and bear no fixed temporal relationship to the QRS complexes.

4 Occasionally or frequently sinus impulses arrive at the AV node when it is not refractory and cause ventricular beats (ventricular captures). Each ventricular capture is preceded by a normal P wave with a P-R interval of 0.12 s or more.   The P-R interval of the captured beats is

Fig. 24-119 Incomplete AV dissociation with capture beats.   The atria and ventricles beat independently.   The former are regulated by the SA node, the latter by a pacemaker in the AV junction.   The atrial rate is 60 per minute; the ventricular rate is 63 per minute.   The P waves are of normal contour and bear no fixed relationship to the QRS complexes. Occasionally, sinus impulses arrive at the AV node when it is not refractory and cause ventricular captures.   Thus the dissociation is incomplete.   The sixth ventricular beat in both the second and fourth rows is a ventricular capture.   The electrocardiogram is a continuous recording of lead II.

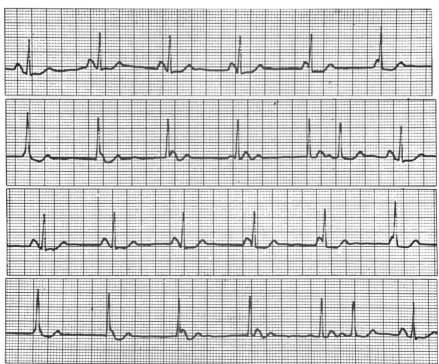

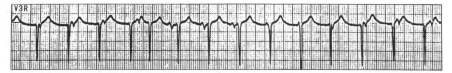

Fig. 24-120   Incomplete AV dissociation with a ventricular capture beat.   The atria and ventricles beat independently.   The sinus rate is 83 per minute, and the ventricular rate is 88 per minute.   The fifth ventricular complex is the captured beat.

inversely proportional to the preceding R-P interval and vice versa (R-P/P-R reciprocity).   Retrograde conduction of ventricular impulses may occur occasionally and lead to atrial captures.

Complete AV Dissociation

The findings are the same as listed under Incomplete AV Dissociation, above, except that atrial or ventricular captures do not occur.

Atrioventricular Dissociation Due Primarily to Block

Atrioventricular Dissociation in Atrial Flutter (Fig. 24-50B)

1   P waves are absent.
2   F waves are present.
3   The F waves bear no fixed relationship to the QRS complexes.
4   The ventricular rhythm is slow and regular.

Atrioventricular Dissociation in Atrial Fibrillation (Figs. 24-55, 24-59, 24-67A, 24-89, 24-90, 24-153)

1   The P waves are absent.
2   There are f waves present.
3   The ventricular rhythm is slow and regular, but may be moderately rapid in the presence of a nonparaoxysmal AV junctional tachycardia.

Atrioventricular Dissociation in Advanced or Complete AV Block (Figs. 24-67, 24-89, 24-90, 24-117C, 24-121, 24-122, 24-148, 24-164 to 24-167)

Second-degree AV block is characterized by failure of at least some supraventricular impulses to reach the ventricles.   The block beat results in a pause which may enable an AV junctional or ventricular pacemaker to escape.   If the escape interval is equal to or shorter than the conduction interval, dissociation between the superventricular and escape rhythms will occur.   At other times, second-degree AV block is associated with acceleration of an AV junctional or ventricular pacemaker.   More persistent AV dissociation is likely under this circumstance.

Two-to-one AV block can lead to dissociation between the atria and ventricles if the escaping ventricular rate is more than half the atrial rate.

Conducted sinus beats may alternate with escape beats to produce a form of escape-capture bigeminy when the alternate sinus beats in 2:1 AV block are not conducted.   The sequence is then P wave, QRS complex, nonconducted P wave, escape beat.

Concealed and supernormal conduction may interrupt the dominant ventricular rhythm with both shorter and longer cycles.   In advanced AV block, capture may take place only during the supernormal phase of conduction.

Complete AV block, of course, implies complete AV dissociation.

Atrioventricular Dissociation in Ectopic Tachycardias
(Figs. 24-34, 24-35, 24-59, 24-81, 24-90, 24-96, 24-98, 24-142, 24-153)

Atrioventricular junctional or ventricular tachycardias may result in AV dissociation (dissociation by usurpation).   The atrial mechanism may be a sinus rhythm or an ectopic atrial arrhythmia.

GROUP BEATING (BIGEMINY, TRIGEMINY, AND QUADRIGEMINY)
(FIGS. 24-10, 24-11B, 24-15C, 24-17, 24-19, 24-20, 24-50, 24-123,
24-124, 24-130, 24-131, 24-132, 24-155)

Group beating, such as bigeminy, trigeminy, or quadrigeminy, is usually the result of coupling of extrasystoles (which may be of any type) to the conducted sinus beats.   Premature beats may thus occur regularly every second, third, or fourth beat, respectively.

Fig. 24-121   Intermittent AV dissociation due to AV block.   The long pauses following dropped beats in 2:1 AV block permit isolated escape beats to occur.   However, starting with the middle strip, a slow escape rhythm (at a rate of 44 per minute) controls the ventricles for six consecutive beats.

CONTINUOUS LEAD V$_{3R}$

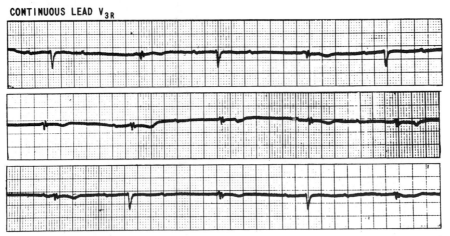

CONTINUOUS LEAD II

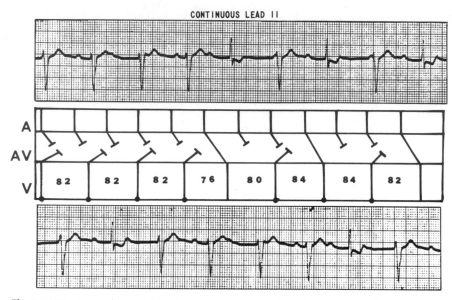

Fig. 24-122   Incomplete AV dissociation due to AV block, with frequent ventricular captures and an idioventricular or nonparoxysmal AV junctional tachycardia.   The atrial mechanism is a sinus tachycardia at a rate of 107 per minute.   The ventricular mechanism is an idioventricular (fascicular?) tachycardia at a rate of 73 per minute, or alternatively (not shown), an AV junctional rhythm with aberrant ventricular conduction.   First-degree AV block is present, since the P-R interval of the captured beats is prolonged.   The failure of most of the P waves to be conducted may be indicative of concomitant second-degree AV block.   The fifth, seventh, ninth, eleventh, and sixteenth ventricular complexes are captures.   The contour of these beats is essentially normal.   The P-R interval of the captures is inversely proportional to the preceding R-P interval (R-P/P-R reciprocity).   The numbers at the V level are the R-R intervals in hundredths of a second.

Langendorf et al. have shown that the appearance of ventricular premature systoles with fixed coupling, their continuation in the form of bigeminy, and the termination of the latter, all depend on the cycle length of the beat to which the extrasystole is coupled.   Lengthening of the ventricular cycle favors the appearance of ventricular premature systoles. This is the *rule of bigeminy*.

Although group beating is usually extrasystolic, it may be due to reciprocal rhythm, an escape-capture sequence, exit block, the Wenckebach type of SA or AV block, and other causes.   Fortuitous pairing of ventricular beats in atrial fibrillation may simulate extrasystolic bigeminy.

Schamroth and Marriott have reported that extrasystolic bigeminy or trigeminy may exist in a *concealed* form (Figs. 24-123, 24-124), possibly because of an exit block surrounding the ectopic focus.   Concealed bigeminy is recognized when only odd numbers of sinus beats intervene between consecutive extrasystoles.   This is expressed by the formula $2n + 1$, where *n* equals zero or any positive integer.   Concealed trigeminy is diagnosed when the number of sinus beats between the extrasystoles is invariably two in excess of a multiple of 3.   This is expressed by the formula, $3n + 2$, in which n is any whole number.

RECIPROCAL RHYTHM (FIGS. 24-125 to 24-131)

Reciprocal rhythm is an arrhythmia which occurs when an impulse arising in the SA node, atria, AV junction, or ventricles activates the chamber in which it originates but during its passage through the AV junction reverses its direction and enters a different pathway, which enables it to return to and activate the chamber in which it arose.   Therefore there must be at least two pathways within the AV junction in order for reciprocal rhythm to occur.

Reciprocal beats and rhythms are well-known examples of reentrant arrhythmias.   The physiologic basis of reentry was discussed earlier in this chapter and is also explained in Fig. 24-125.   Besides reciprocal rhythm, other arrhythmias that are considered reentrant include paroxysmal supraventricular tachycardia, supraventricular tachycardias in the W-P-W syndrome, coupled premature beats, and at least some paroxysmal ventricular tachycardias.

Reciprocal beats and rhythms may be initiated by impulses of atrial, AV junctional, or ventricular origin.   The reentrant beat is called a *reciprocal beat* or an *echo*.   The site in the AV junction at which the impulse turns

Fig. 24-123 Concealed bigeminy.   Only odd numbers of sinus beats intervene between consecutive extrasystoles, according to the formula $2n + 1$, where n equals zero or any positive whole number.

CONTINUOUS LEAD II

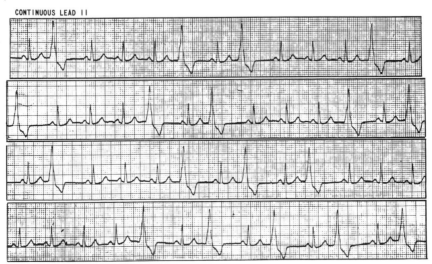

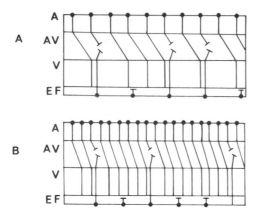

Fig. 24-124 Ladder diagram illustrating concealed bigeminy (A) and concealed trigeminy (B). EF = ectopic focus.

around is called the *reflecting level*. When there is more than one reflecting level, the impulse may alternatively ascend and descend (or vice versa) in the AV junction and activate both the atria and ventricles. This type of rhythm is called a *reciprocating* or *reentrant* rhythm.

Reciprocal beats arising from premature systoles are called *return extrasystoles*. Thus there may be atrial, AV junctional, or ventricular extrasystoles. A reciprocal rhythm originating from a sinus beat, in which antegrade conduction to the ventricles is followed by retrograde conduction to the atria, is sometimes termed *reversed reciprocal rhythm*.

Atrial Reciprocal Beats

Reciprocal rhythm of atrial origin is characterized by a P (or P')-QRS-P' sequence. The initial P wave is usually sinoatrial but is occasionally an atrial extrasystole. The QRS complex is the result of normal AV conduction to the ventricle. The P-R interval of the initiating beat must be relatively long in order for reentry to occur. The returning P' deflection, the atrial echo, is retrograde in contour and hence is inverted in the inferior limb leads. An inverse relationship exists between the R-P and P-R intervals (R-P: P-R reciprocity).

Spontaneously or electrically induced atrial premature systoles may induce a reentrant paroxysmal supraventricular tachycardia if the beats echo repeatedly.

AV Junctional Reciprocal Beats

This is the most frequent type of reciprocal beating. It is a common occurrence in AV junctional rhythms, especially when there is a Wenckebach phenomenon of retrograde VA conduction. The site of origin of such rhythms is in the NH region of the AV node or the bundle of His.

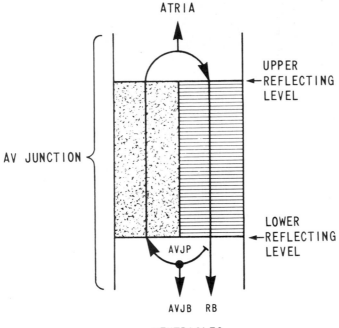

ATRIA

UPPER
REFLECTING
LEVEL

AV JUNCTION

LOWER
REFLECTING
LEVEL

AVJP

AVJB   RB

VENTRICLES

Fig. 24-125   Mechanism of reciprocal rhythm of AV junctional origin.   Functional longitudinal dissociation of the AV junctional tissues is hypothesized.   The fibers on the right side of the diagram (horizontal lines) are assumed to be completely refractory so that an AV junctional impulse is blocked from entering these fibers.   The fibers on the left side of the diagram (stippled) are partially refractory but permit slow retrograde conduction of the AV junctional impulse.   By the time this impulse reaches the atria, the right-side fibers have recovered from their refractoriness.   The AV junctional impulse turns around at the upper reflecting level and reenters these fibers.   Antegrade conduction is then completed and results in a reciprocal beat.   In the electrocardiogram, this is manifested by a retrograde P wave sandwiched between two ventricular beats.   When there are two reflecting levels in the AV junction, not only may the ascending junctional impulse reenter the antegrade pathway, but the descending impulse may reenter the retrograde pathway, so that a reciprocating rhythm is formed.   In the diagram, AVJP represents the AV junctional pacemaker; AVJB, the AV junctional beat; and RB, the reciprocal beat.   See also Fig. 24-126.

Fig. 24-126   (A) Return extrasystoles: (1) AV junctional return extrasystole; (2) ventricular return extrasystole; (3) atrial return extrasystole.   (B) Reciprocating rhythm.

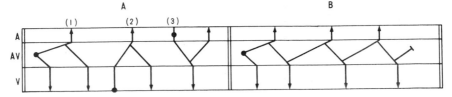

A   B

(1)   (2)   (3)

A

AV

V

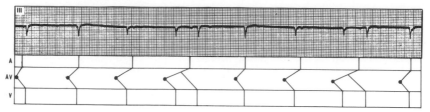

Fig. 24-127 Reciprocal beats in an AV junctional rhythm with a Wenckebach phenomenon of retrograde conduction.

Reciprocal rhythms of AV junctional origin exhibit a QRS-P'-QRS sequence. The initiating QRS complex results from normal forward conduction to the ventricles from the AV junctional focus. The P' wave, representing retrograde atrial activation, is inverted in the inferior limb leads. The second QRS complex, the AV junctional echo, is the result of antegrade reactivation of the ventricles. It is usually normal in contour but may be aberrant. The R-P interval must be relatively long (0.20 s or more) in order for reentry to occur. Reciprocal rhythms arising in the AV junction show R-P:P-R reciprocity: the longer the R-P interval, the shorter the subsequent P-R, and vice versa.

It has long been debated whether the atrium is a necessary link in AV junctional reciprocal rhythms. The problem is still unsolved. Evidence suggests that although the atrium usually comprises a portion of the pathway, this is not invariably the rule.

Sustained reentry of AV junctional beats can lead to reentrant paroxysmal supraventricular tachycardia.

Ventricular Reciprocal Beats

Reciprocal rhythm of ventricular origin is uncommon. The diagnosis should be considered in ventricular extrasystoles that are interpolated or associated with retrograde activation of the atria. Reciprocal beats are sometimes seen in ventricular tachycardias (Figs. 24-99, 24-106) and paced ventricular beats (Fig. 24-191).

Reciprocal rhythms arising in the ventricles shows a QRS-P'-QRS

Fig. 24-128 Reciprocal beats in an AV junctional rhythm with retrograde Wenckebach conduction.

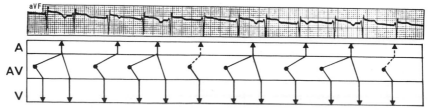

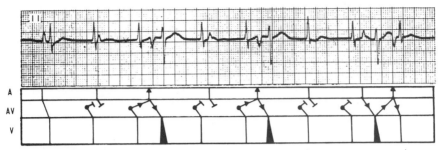

Fig. 24-129 A complex arrhythmia showing intermittent AV dissociation, retrograde conduction of some AV junctional beats resulting in echo beats, and a solitary capture beat. At the end of the strip, the capture beat is followed in turn by retrograde conduction to the atria (reversed reciprocal rhythm) and an echo beat. All the reciprocal beats except the last and the capture beat show aberrant ventricular conduction.

sequence. The initial QRS complex is a ventricular ectopic beat and hence is wide and bizarre in appearance. The P' wave reflects retrograde atrial activation and thus is inverted in leads II, III, and aVF. The second QRS complex, the ventricular echo, is the result of antegrade reactivation of the ventricles. Usually the echo beat exhibits a normal contour, but it may be aberrant. The R-P' interval in ventricular reciprocal rhythm, in contrast to atrial or AV junctional reciprocity, is usually relatively short. To make the diagnosis of ventricular reciprocal rhythm with certainty, the P' wave must be clearly identifiable as retrograde in contour and it must be premature with respect to the oncoming sinus beat.

Reciprocal beats may be difficult to differentiate from the capture beats of AV dissociation. In AV dissociation, the P-P intervals are usually regular and the P wave of the capture beats is of sinus origin, whereas in reciprocal

Fig. 24-130 Reciprocal rhythm. There is an AV junctional rhythm with a Wenkebach type of retrograde conduction, reciprocal beats, and trigeminy. The first beat in the tracing is not preceded or followed by a P wave. The P wave is presumably buried in the QRS complex. The second beat, however, is followed by a retrograde P wave, which indicates that the R-P interval of this beat has become longer. The retrograde P wave, in turn, is succeeded by a reciprocal beat. The interval between the second and third ventricular complexes is 0.37 s. The entire sequence is then repeated.

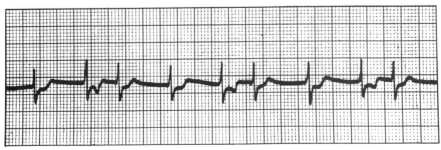

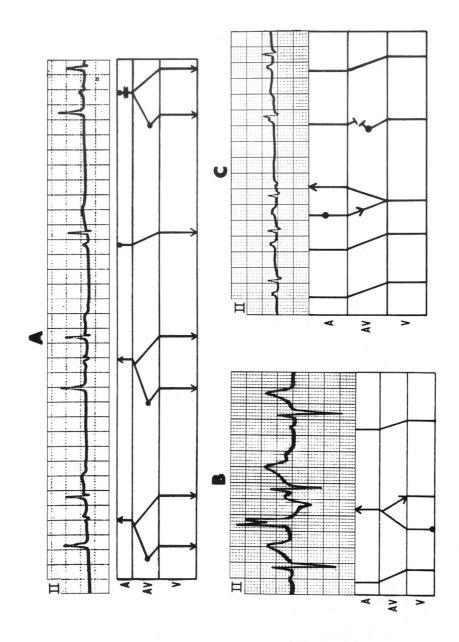

beats, the P-P intervals are irregular and the P waves are retrograde in contour.

Pseudoreciprocal rhythm (Fig. 24-132) is the term applied to the pairing of an AV junctional escape beat with a conducted sinus or atrial beat. The illusion of reciprocity is created because the P wave is flanked by two ventricular complexes. However, in pseudoreciprocal rhythm the P wave is antegrade in contour, whereas in reciprocal rhythm it is retrograde. A more descriptive term for pseudoreciprocal rhythm is *escape-capture sequence* or, if repetitive, *escape-capture bigeminy*. Pseudoreciprocal rhythm has also been called "reversed" bigeminy.

PARASYSTOLE (FIGS. 24-107, 24-114, 24-133 to 24-138)

Definition

Parasystole is an arrhythmia resulting from the presence of two (or rarely more) independently discharging pacemakers within the heart, one of which is "protected" from the impulses of the other, each of which is competing for control of the atria, the ventricles, or both. One pacemaker is usually located in the SA node, the other in an ectopic focus most often located in the ventricles, less often in the AV junction, and least often in the atria.

Parasystolic rhythms are designated as ventricular, AV junctional, or atrial, depending on the location of the ectopic focus.

Mechanism

Dual rhythm in parasystole is possible because the ectopic pacemaker is shielded from the impulses of the primary pacemaker. No disturbance in AV conduction is involved in the protective mechanism. The protection results rather from a block situated in the immediate vicinity of the ectopic pacemaker. This block, called *entrance* or *protection block,* is unidirectional. Oncoming impulses are prevented from entering and discharging the parasystolic center, but outgoing impulses are unimpeded in their

Fig. 24-131 Examples of reciprocal rhythm. (A) Atrioventricular junctional rhythm with reciprocal beats. Each of the two couples at the beginning of the tracing consists of an AV junctional beat followed in turn by a retrograde P wave and a reciprocal beat. This is reciprocal bigeminy. The fifth ventricular complex is a conducted sinus beat. In the last couplet, an atrial fusion beat is sandwiched between the two ventricular complexes. (B) Ventricular return extrasystole. The second beat is a ventricular premature systole. It is followed by a retrograde P wave which is reconducted to the ventricles, which results in a return extrasystole. (C) Atrial return extrasystole. The first two P-QRST complexes are sinoatrial in origin. The third beat is a conducted atrial premature systole. The retrograde P wave which follows the QRS complex of the premature beat is the atrial return extrasystole (or, alternatively, a second atrial premature systole from a different focus). The fourth ventricular complex is an AV junctional escape beat, and the fifth a conducted sinus impulse.

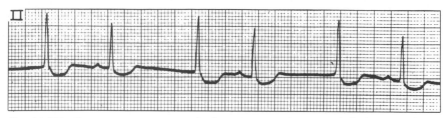

Fig. 24-132 Escape-capture ("reversed") bigeminy (pseudoreciprocal rhythm). Each AV junctional escape beat is paired with a conducted sinus impulse. The P wave is sandwiched between the two ventricular complexes of each couplet. However, in contrast to reciprocal rhythm, in which the P wave is retrograde, the P wave in pseudoreciprocal rhythm is upright.

passage through the blocked region. The ectopic focus is thus able to discharge regularly.

In parasystole, it is assumed that all parasystolic impulses will reach and activate the myocardium unless it is refractory, which will result in the appearance of ectopic beats. When the myocardium is refractory from previous stimulation, parasystolic impulses, of course, will not activate it. Discharge of the parasystolic center is then concealed. When simultaneous stimulation of one of the cardiac chambers by impulses from both pace-makers occurs, fusion beats are recorded.

Parasystolic rhythms may be faster or slower than the basic rhythm of the heart.

Rapidly firing parasystolic centers may produce ectopic tachycardias, varying degrees of AV dissociation, and other complex arrhythmias.

Slowly discharging parasystolic foci generally produce premature beats interspersed between the beats of the dominant rhythm. Since the temporal relationship of the two rhythms is different, the electrocardiogram will show variable coupling, pauses of different duration, interpolation, and fusion beats.

Sometimes, in parasystole, the ectopic focus fails to stimulate the myocardium even though the latter is in a nonrefractory state. To explain this phenomenon, it is necessary to postulate the existence of another region of unidirectional block which prevents the outward spread of impulses arising in the ectopic focus. This type of abnormal unidirectional con-duction is called *exit block*. Exit block is assumed to exist whenever, in the presence of a nonrefractory state of the myocardium, the rate of the ectopic rhythm is slower than the calculated rate of discharge of the parasystolic center. Exit block may occur in regular or irregular ratios.

Both entrance and exit blocks may be intermittent. If the entrance block is dissipated, the ectopic pacemaker will be continously discharged by the sinus impulses, and parasystole will disappear until the protection block is reestablished. This is probably the mechanism of intermittent parasystole. An important characteristic of intermittent parasystole is the constant coupling of the first ectopic beat to the preceding sinus beat. On

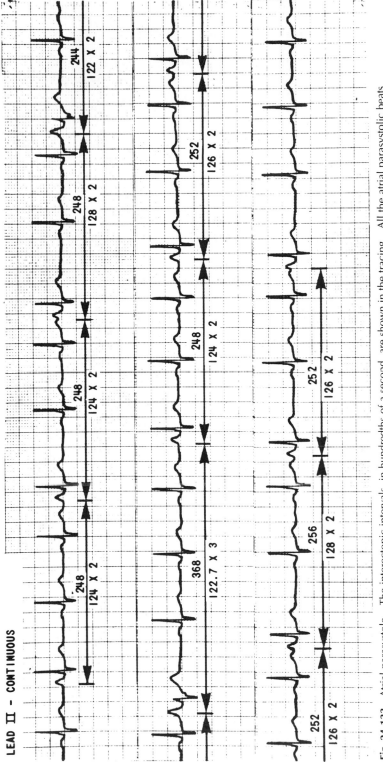

Fig. 24-133 Atrial parasystole. The interectopic intervals, in hundredths of a second, are shown in the tracing. All the atrial parasystolic beats are conducted.

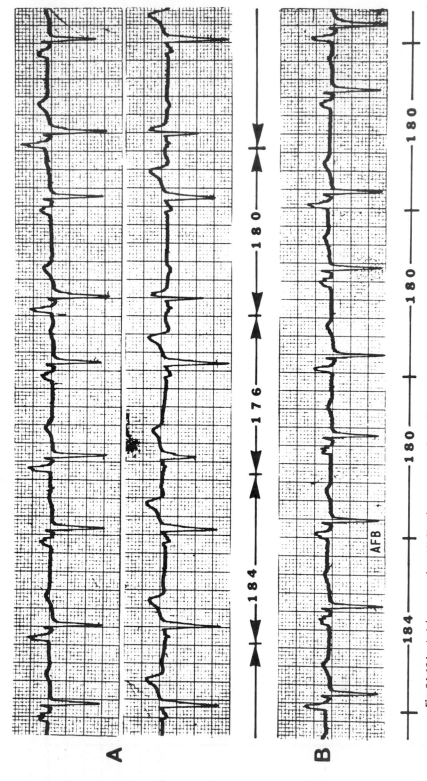

Fig. 24-134 Atrial parasystole. (A) Simultaneous recording of leads II (upper strip) and V₁ (lower strip). The second, third, and fourth parasystolic beats show a slight degree of aberrant ventricular conduction. (B) Lead II. The third P wave is an atrial fusion beat (AFB). The interectopic intervals are shown in hundredths of a second.

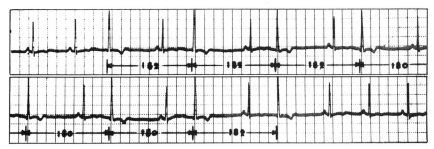

Fig. 24-135 AV junctional parasystole.   The time intervals are shown in hundredths of a second.   (*From E. K. Y. Chung, Parasystole, Progr. Cardiovasc. Dis.*, 11: 64, 1968.   *Used by permission.*)

the other hand, if the exit block surrounding a rapidly discharging parasystolic focus is released, the ectopic center may gain control of the heart until such time as the exit block returns.   Some forms of paroxysmal tachycardia may result from this mechanism.

Diagnosis

The diagnosis of parasystole is dependent on proof of the coexistence of two independently discharging pacemakers within the heart.

The diagnosis is based on three electrocardiographic features: (1) varying coupling intervals, (2) constant short interectopic intervals, and (3) the presence of fusion beats.

Varying Coupling Intervals Since the basic and parasystolic rhythms discharge independently and asynchronously, parasystolic beats will occur at different times in the cardiac cycle, which results in variable coupling, pauses of different duration, and interpolation.   Parasystole should be suspected whenever the coupling intervals of premature beats of similar configuration vary by more than 0.06 s.   Fixed coupling is rare in parasystolic rhythms but may occur when the rates of the basic and parasystolic rhythms are numerically related or if the parasystolic rhythm is rapid and dominant. Fixed coupling of parasystolic beats may also occur if normally subthreshold parasystolic impulses become threshold only during the supernormal phase of the cardiac cycle.   Ordinarily, parasystolic beats do not discharge the sinus pacemaker, especially when the parasystolic focus is in the ventricles, because decremental conduction or interference in the AV junction prevents retrograde activation of the atria and the SA node.   However, a parasystolic impulse may depolarize the sinus pacemaker when the focus is in the atria or the AV junction or if retrograde atrial activation takes place from a ventricular focus.   Depolarization of the sinus node may lead to reversed coupling in which the interval between the parasystolic and sinus beats is fixed.   The sinus cycle is then dependent on the parasystolic beat.   The

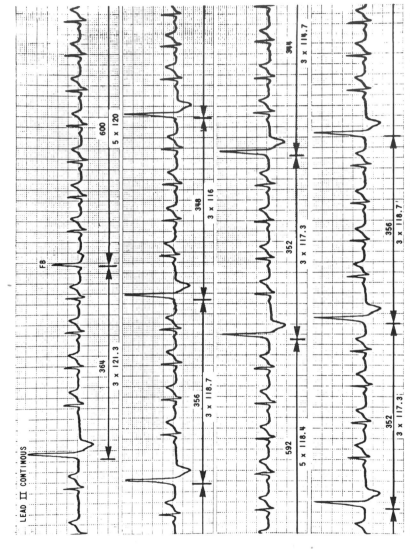

Fig. 24-136 Ventricular parasystole. The interectopic intervals, in hundredths of a second, are shown in the tracing. The beat labeled FB is a ventricular fusion beat.

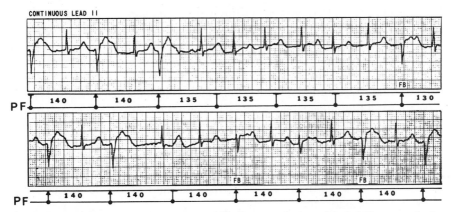

Fig. 24-137 Ventricular parasystole in atrial fibrillation. The beats labeled FB are ventricular fusion beats. The interectopic intervals are shown in hundredths of a second. PF = parasystolic focus.

relationship between the sinus and parasystolic impulse will remain fixed as long as both cycle lengths remain constant.

As a general rule, parasystolic beats rarely become manifest in the early portion of the cardiac cycle—in the vulnerable zone, at the end of the T wave, or in the U wave.

Constant Interectopic Intervals In parasystole, the intervals between ectopic beats are equal or are simple multiples having a common denominator. Constancy of the shortest interectopic intervals indicates that the ectopic focus produces impulses regularly and is independent of the primary pacemaker. Sinus rhythm is the basic mechanism of the heart in most cases of parasystole. Atrial fibrillation, flutter, or tachycardia occur much less frequently.

There is no uniform agreement concerning acceptable variation in the duration of the shortest interectopic intervals. Precisely constant interectopic intervals are rare. The majority of cases show variations ranging

Fig. 24-138 Ventricular parasystole in atrial flutter. The beats labeled FB are ventricular fusion beats. The parasystolic focus fires the ventricles unless they are refractory from previous stimulation or because of exit block (represented by circled dots). The interectopic interval is 0.43 s.

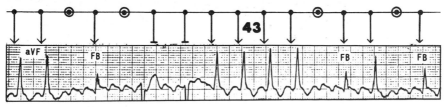

between 0.04 and 0.12 s; a lesser number exhibit variations between 0.13 and 0.27 s; and in a few, variations of less than 0.02 s are demonstrable.

Fusion Beats   Fusion or combination beats occur when impulses from the parasystolic and primary pacemakers stimulate the heart simultaneously.

Ventricular fusion beats are common in ventricular parasystole but are rare in AV junctional parasystole.   They are most apt to occur when the basic rhythm is rapid or irregular, as in sinus tachycardia or atrial fibrillation.

Atrial fusion beats are less frequent than ventricular fusion beats.   The mechanism is simultaneous activation of the atria by ectopic atrial and sinus impulses.   In AV junctional parasystole and rarely in ventricular parasystole, atrial combination beats may be the result of fusion between sinus and retrograde atrial impulses.

Fusion beats are not pathognomic of parasystole and may be found in other conditions as well, including ventricular tachycardia, advanced AV block, and incomplete AV dissociation.   The absence of fusion beats does not exclude the diagnosis of parasystole.

Other Electrocardiographic Findings

1   Parasystolic rates may range between 20 and 400 per minute, but rates between 20 and 50 per minute are most common.
2   Aberrant ventricular conduction is seen frequently in both atrial and AV junctional parasystole.
3   Aberration of postectopic sinus impulses may occur in atrial parasystole. This is probably the result of aberrant intraatrial conduction, although it can be explained by wandering of the pacemaker within the SA node.
4   Parasystolic rhythms may originate from multiple ectopic foci or may even be initiated by artificial pacemakers.   A ventricular parasystolic center may produce ventricular tachycardia.
5   The electrocardiogram is generally abnormal in parasystole.   The abnormalities most commonly encountered include left ventricular enlargement, myocardial infarction, bundle branch block, AV block, atrial enlargement, and ventricular preexcitation.

Differential Diagnosis

Parasystole is distinguished from ordinary premature systoles by the presence of varying coupling intervals and constant interectopic intervals.

Atrial parasystole should be distinguished from atrial dissociation.   The differential diagnosis is discussed in the section in this chapter on atrial dissociation.

Clinical Significance

1   The frequency of the various types of parasystole in the series collected by Chung is approximately as follows: ventricular, 60 percent; AV

junctional, 20 percent; and atrial, 20 percent. Instances of double ventricular parasystole or combined atrial and ventricular parasystole are rare.

2   Parasystole is twice as frequent in males as in females.
3   The majority of cases are associated with organic heart disease, chiefly arteriosclerotic and/or hypertensive heart disease, often with congestive heart failure as well. However, about 15 percent of cases occur in normal persons.
4   The peak incidence is in the fifth to seventh decades. Sixty-five percent of patients are over 60 years of age.
5   Carotid sinus stimulation may slow, abolish, or even provoke ventricular parasystole and occasionally affect atrial or AV junctional parasystole in similar fashion. Exercise may evoke similar effects.
6   There appears to be no direct relationship between digitalis and para-systole. Many cases of parasystole disappear after digitalization for congestive failure with improvement of the cardiac status. The occur-rence of parasystole in digitalized or digitalis-intoxicated individuals is probably coincidental.
7   Quinidine or procainamide may abolish the arrhythmia.
8   The prognosis of individuals with parasystole is influenced by status of the underlying heart disease. Some 15 percent of patients with heart disease who develop parasystole die within several months of the onset of this arrhythmia.
9   Parasystole may coexist with other cardiac arrhythmias, including extrasystoles, atrial tachyarrhythmias, and AV junctional tachycardias.

ATRIAL DISSOCIATION

In atrial dissociation there are two independent atrial rhythms, one sinus and the other ectopic. It is assumed that the ectopic focus controls either part or all of the atrium because of intraatrial block, so that none of the sinus beats can interfere with the ectopic rhythm and vice versa.

1   There are two independent atrial rhythms, one sinus and the other ectopic.
2   The ectopic atrial impulse is not conducted to the ventricles.
3   The ectopic P waves are small and bizarre or have a fibrillatory or fluttering character.
4   The interectopic interval is usually variable and not fixed.

ATRIAL DISSOCIATION VERSUS ATRIAL PARASYSTOLE

Atrial dissociation is distinguished from atrial parasystole by the failure of the ectopic impulses to be conducted to the ventricles and by the presence of small aberrant P waves or fibrillatory waves, a more variable interectopic interval, and a constant association with advanced cardiac disease.

ELECTRICAL ALTERNANS (FIG. 24-139)

1   Electrical alternans is a rare electrocardiographic phenomenon. In the overwhelming majority of cases it is indicative of organic heart disease. Electrical alternans is a grave prognostic sign in slow sinus rhythms. It is usually of no significance when it occurs in rapid sinus or ectopic tachycardias or in a few normal beats following premature systoles.

2   Electrical alternans is characterized by alternating changes in the amplitude or configuration of the P, QRS, or T complexes (or any combination of these), provided the complexes originate from one pacemaker.

3   Alternating ratios in electrical alternans are expressed numerically. Thus 2:1 alternans means that for every two beats there is one alternation; 3:1 alternans means that for every three beats, there is one alternation; etc. The most common alternating ratio is 2:1. The other ratios are seen only rarely.

4   The most common form of electrical alternans involves the QRS complexes alone (ventricular electrical alternans). Its three most common causes are pericardial effusion, severe myocardial disease, and tachycardia.

5   Total electrical alternans of the heart involving both the atrial and ventricular complexes is most frequently associated with pericardial effusion and tamponade. The most common causes of pericardial effusion that can cause total alternans are malignancy, tuberculosis, and systemic lupus erythematosus.

6   The mechanism of electrical alternans is unknown. It has been attributed to anatomic alternation of the cardiac position, alternation of cardiac output, and alternating prolongation of the refractory phase of the heart.

CONCEALED CONDUCTION (FIGS. 24-11, 24-18, 24-140 to 24-145, 24-147, 24-148, 24-157)

Concealed conduction is the term applied to the phenomenon of partial penetration of atrial, AV junctional, or ventricular impulses into any of the specialized conduction tissues of the heart. Concealed conduction is not recorded by the electrocardiogram. It is revealed only by its aftereffects on subsequent impulse formation or conduction.

Originally, concealed conduction referred to the incomplete penetration of antegrade or retrograde impulses into the AV junction. However, concealed conduction may occur within the bundle branches.

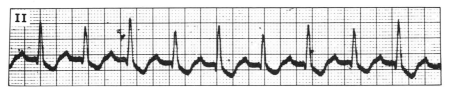

Fig. 24-139 Electrical alternans. There is variation in the amplitude of alternate ventricular beats.

Concealed conduction into the AV junction may be manifest in a number of ways: (1) by delayed transmission of the subsequent impulse, (2) by complete blockage of the subsequent impulse, (3) by repetitive partial penetration of subsequent impulses (repetitive concealed conduction), (4) by inhibition of the regular action of a subsidiary pacemaker (concealed discharge), and (5) by enhancement rather than inhibition of subsequent impulse conduction through the creation of a supernormal phase of conduction.

Concealed conduction in the bundle branches may result in aberrant ventricular conduction or the development of unexpected bundle branch block.

Concealed discharge is regarded as a form of concealed conduction. For example, concealed discharge of an AV junctional beat may delay or block the passage of the subsequent impulse through the AV junction on its way to the ventricles and so produce pseudo AV block (Figs. 24-141, 24-157).

Concealment of Atrial Premature Beats (Figs. 24-141, 24-142)

Concealed conduction of an atrial premature beat may delay or block the conduction of a subsequent sinus or atrial premature beat by establishing a new refractory period. On occasion, it may displace an ectopic AV junctional pacemaker by discharging it prematurely.

Concealment of Sinus Beats (Fig. 24-143)

Sinus beats may rarely penetrate the AV junction and affect the conduction of a subsequent sinus impulse. This phenomenon generally occurs in the presence of AV block with AV dissociation.

Concealment of AV Junctional Premature Beats (Figs. 24-144, 24-157)

The concealed discharge of AV junctional beats may produce a variety of manifestations: prolongation of the P-R interval, pseudo-Type I or pseudo-Type II AV block, simulation of supernormal conduction, variation of junctional escape intervals, postponed compensatory pauses, and concealed AV junctional discharge with reciprocation.

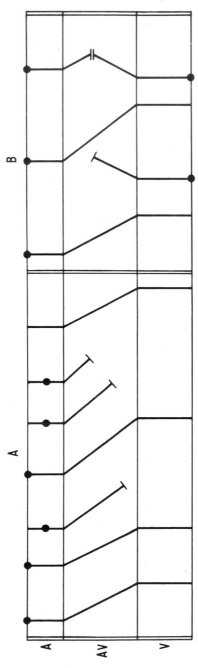

Fig. 24-140 Schematic representation of concealed conduction. (A) Two sinus beats are followed by a nonconducted atrial premature systole, which, however, penetrates for a distance into the AV junction and renders it partially refractory. The P-R interval of the following sinus beat, therefore, is prolonged because of concealed conduction of the ectopic atrial impulse. The sinus beat, in turn, is followed by two atrial premature systoles. The concealed partial penetration of the AV junction by the first extrasystole produces complete refractoriness, so that the second extrasystole is not conducted. (B) A sinus beat is followed by a ventricular extrasystole. Retrograde concealed conduction from the extrasystole renders the AV junction partially refractory. Accordingly, the P-R interval of the subsequent sinus beat is prolonged. The last beat is also a ventriuclar premature systole, which is dissociated from the oncoming sinus impulse by simple interference in the AV junction.

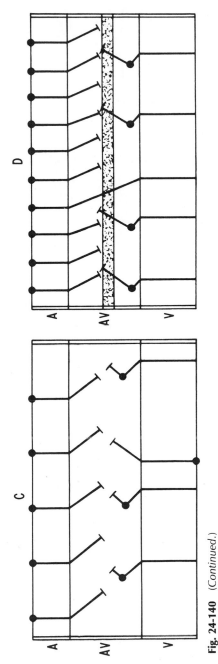

Fig. 24-140 (*Continued.*)

(*C*) There is AV dissociation due to advanced AV block, with the ventricular pacemaker located in the AV junction. Retrograde concealed conduction of a ventricular premature beat (the third ventricular complex) discharges the AV junctional pacemaker and delays the appearance of the next AV junctional beat. (*D*) Supernormal conduction induced by retrograde concealed conduction. There is advanced AV block. In the AV level, the stippled zone represents an area of unidirectional block traversed by all retrograde impulses. Antegrade conduction is blocked but is sometimes possible during a transient supernormal phase of conduction. The second AV junctional beat, reaching the region of unidirectional block immediately after the arrival of the sinus impulse, induces a transient state of supernormality in the blocked region and this permits the succeeding sinus impulse to capture the ventricles.

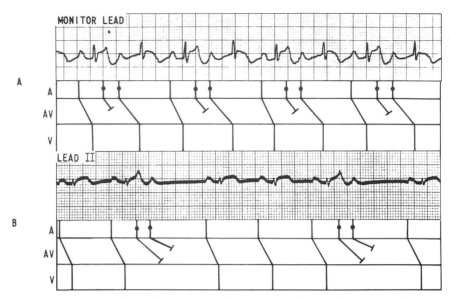

Fig. 24-141 Concealed conduction. *A* and *B* were recorded at different times from the same patient. In *A*, each P-QRST complex is followed by two atrial premature systoles. The first ectopic beat is not conducted but penetrates the AV junction and makes it partially refractory. Because of the refractoriness of the AV junction, the second ectopic P wave is conducted at a prolonged P-R interval. In *B*, each run of sinus beats is followed by two atrial premature systoles, neither of which is conducted. It is assumed that the first ectopic beat enters the AV junction, as in *A*, but makes it completely refractory to the passage of the second ectopic impulse.

Concealment of Ventricular Premature Beats (Figs. 24-18, 24-145)

Prolongation of the P-R interval in the sinus beat following an interpolated ventricular extrasystole is a common example concealed conduction. Retrograde conduction of the ectopic impulse induces partial refractoriness in the AV junction, so that conduction of the subsequent sinus impulse is delayed, with attendant prolongation of the P-R interval.

Retrograde concealed conduction of a ventricular premature beat in AV dissociation due to advanced AV block may discharge the AV junctional pacemaker which controls the ventricles. When this happens, the appearance of the next AV junctional beat is delayed.

Other Examples of Concealed Conduction

Concealed conduction of atrial impulses can explain the irregularity of the ventricular response in atrial fibrillation. This apparently results from the varying depth and frequency of penetration of the atrial impulse into the AV junction. The shorter R-R intervals in atrial fibrillation are associated with less AV junctional concealment, whereas the longer intervals are due to increased concealment.   Clinical observation supports the role of concealment in determining the rate and irregularity of the ventricular response in atrial fibrillation.   For example, when atrial flutter converts spontaneously to atrial fibrillation, the ventricular response becomes slower and more irregular.   Variation in the escape intervals seen in patients with atrial fibrillation can be explained by concealed discharge of the junctional pacemaker.

Concealed conduction explains alternation of AV conduction time in some cases of flutter and the odd conduction ratios sometimes observed in this condition.

In sinus rhythms, a sudden prolongation of cycle length following an atrial premature systole may produce persistent aberration by repetitive concealed conduction of the impulse from one bundle branch to the other. Concealed penetration of a bundle branch can also explain unexpected aberrancy in some cases of atrial fibrillation.

Runs of aberrantly conducted complexes (Ashman phenomenon) are seen not uncommonly in atrial fibrillation.   Usually the anomalous beats display the pattern of right bundle branch block.   The persistence of aberrancy under this circumstance is attributed to concealed conduction into the right bundle branch of the impulse conducted through the left bundle.

Concealment may actually enhance rather than inhibit subsequent

Fig. 24-142   Concealed conduction in AV dissociation.   The ventricular mechanism is an AV junctional tachycardia.   The second sinus beat in lead aVL is conducted to the AV junction, thereby discharging and resetting the AV junctional pacemaker.   The pause between the fifth and sixth ventricular beats in lead III is the result of the same mechanism.   The next-to-last ventricular complex in lead aVL and the second, eighth, and last ventricular beats in lead aVF are capture beats.   (*From E. N. Moore, S. B. Knoebel, and J. F. Spear, Concealed Conduction, Am. J. Cardiol., 28: 406, 1971.   Used by permission.*)

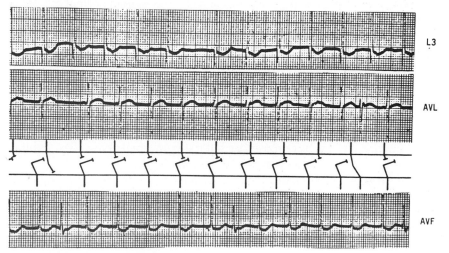

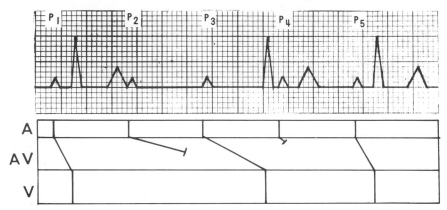

Fig. 24-143 Concealed conduction of a sinus impulse. Incomplete penetration of P_2 into the AV junction causes prolongation of the P-R interval of the subsequent sinus beat (P_3). P_4 is not conducted. Both P_1 and P_5 are conducted normally.

impulse conduction through the creation of a supernormal phase. For example, during advanced AV block, retrograde conduction of a ventricular premature systole may produce a transient state of supernormality in the blocked region by "peeling back" the refractory period. This permits the succeeding sinus impulse to be conducted and to capture the ventricles.

SUPERNORMAL CONDUCTION (FIGS. 24-79, 24-140D, 24-146 TO 24-150)

Supernormal conduction (see also page 411) is the term applied to a paradoxical improvement of conduction in depressed hearts. The term itself is a misnomer, because conduction is not faster than normal but better than could be anticipated under the circumstances. In other words, there is temporary improvement in the depressed state of conductivity.

By and large, supernormal conduction occurs clinically when AV conduction is depressed. During AV block, there is sometimes a supernormal or enhanced phase of conduction during the absolute or relative refractory periods, in which a stimulus elicits either a totally unexpected response or a response that is greater than could be anticipated considering the state of recovery form the preceding impulse. The supernormal phase of conduction is not to be confused with the supernormal phase of excitability occurring *after* the refactory period in normal hearts.

The Wedensky effect and Wedensky facilitation (Fig. 24-150), originally described in nerve-muscle preparations, are closely related to, or are specific forms of, the supernormal phase. The Wedensky effect refers to the occurrence of a relatively long period of lowered threshold excitability initiated by a maximum stimulus which permits subsequent subthreshold

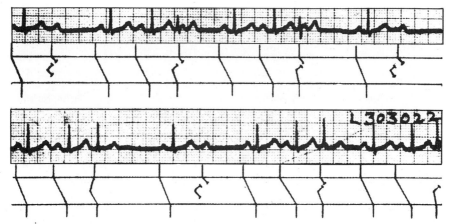

Fig. 24-144 Concealed His bundle extrasystoles producing pseudo-Mobitz Type II AV block. *(From E. N. Moore, S. B. Knoebel, and J. F. Spear, Concealed Conduction, Am. J. Cardiol., 28: 406, 1971. Used by permission.)*

stimuli to be propagated. Wedensky facilitation refers to the enhanced excitability of tissue beyond a blocked zone initiated by a stimulus which itself is not conducted through the region of block. The enhancement is believed to be brought about by a lowering of the threshold, so that a subthreshold stimulus temporarily becomes threshold. Clinically, the unexpected occurrence of a conducted sinus impulse immediately after escape or ventricular paced beats in advanced AV block is attributed to Wedensky facilitation. Sustained conduction of subsequent sinus beats is ascribed to the Wedensky effect. However, the same phenomenon can be explained by retrograde concealed AV conduction of the ventricular impulse followed by repetitive supernormal antegrade AV conduction.

Fig. 24-145 Concealed conduction of ventricular premature systoles. The second ventricular complex is a ventricular extrasystole. Retrograde concealed conduction of this beat produces partial refractoriness in the AV junction, so that the P-R interval of the succeeding sinus beat is prolonged. The sixth ventricular complex is also a ventricular extrasystole. Retrograde concealed conduction of this beat produces complete refractoriness in the AV junction, so that the next sinus impulse is dropped. Shifting of the atrial pacemaker is also seen in the record.

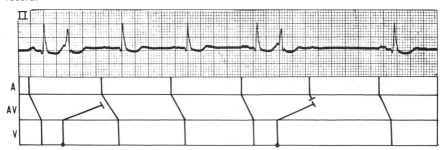

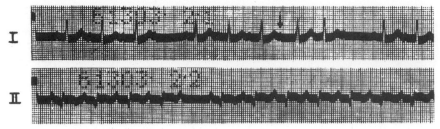

Fig. 24-146   Supernormal AV conduction in second-degree AV block.   Lead II, recorded from a patient with recent inferior myocardial infarction, shows the characteristic features of Type I second-degree AV block.   At the start of lead I, three of the four consecutive sinus impulses are conducted, the last P-R interval of this group measuring 0.28 s.   However, in this next group, the fourth P wave (indicated by the arrow) is conducted with an extraordinary long P-R interval (0.34 s), followed by another conducted P wave with an unexpectedly shorter P-R interval (0.28 s), and finally by a sixth P wave which is blocked.   Analysis of the tracings reveals that all P waves occurring 0.40 to 0.46 s after a QRS complex are conducted, but those occurring 0.38 s after a QRS deflection are blocked.   However, one P wave (indicated by the arrow), occurring earliest (0.30 s) after a QRS complex, is conducted with a relatively short P-R interval of 0.28 s.   Thus, during a short period early in the cycle, the AV junction, paradoxically, is not only responsive but transmits an impulse at a faster than anticipated rate of speed.   This represents supernormal AV conduction.   (*From A. Pick, R. Langendorf, and L. N. Katz, The Supernormal Phase of Atrioventricular Conduction, Circulation, 26: 388, 1962.   Used by permission of the American Heart Association, Inc.*)

The following have been cited as classic examples of supernormal conduction: paradoxical shortening of the P-R interval in the course of a Wenckebach period; occasional supernormal forward conduction induced by a retrograde impulse (e.g., AV junctional or ventricular escape beat), forward conduction induced by one retrograde impulse and then maintained for some time by repetitive supernormal forward conduction; and alternation of P-R intervals.

Fig. 24-147   Unidirectional AV block causing incomplete AV dissociation with atrial and ventricular captures, the latter due to a supernormal phase of AV conduction.   Retrograde concealed conduction of the fourth and sixth ventricular complexes (which are AV junctional in origin) creates a transient supernormal phase of antegrade conduction following each beat.   During this interval, the oncoming sinus impulses capture the ventricles.   All other sinus impulses, coming either too early or too late, are blocked.   The third AV junctional impulse captures the atria because it follows the sinus impulse after a sufficiently long interval, which permits the AV junctional tissues to recover.   (*From A. Pick, R. Langendorf, and L. N. Katz, The Supernormal Phase of Atrioventricular Conduction, Circulation, 26: 388, 1962.   Used by permission of the American Heart Association, Inc.*)

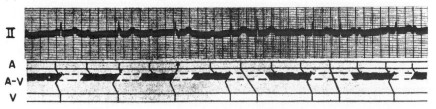

There is considerable evidence that although supernormality is a fundamental property of specialized atrial fibers and of the His-Purkinje system, it is not a property of the AV node under normal or pathologic circumstances.   Therefore, the term supernormal as applied to AV conduction disturbances is purely descriptive.

Investigators have revealed that many cases of so-called supernormal AV conduction are more apparent than real.   The use of His bundle recordings and programmed premature atrial and ventricular depolarizations have provided alternative explanations for "supernormal" conduction. Thus, sudden shortening of the P-R intervals during the Wenckebach phenomenon has been demonstrated to be a result of manifest or concealed reentry within the AV node.   A gap phenomenon in which later atrial

Fig. 24-148   Unidirectional AV block causing incomplete AV dissociation with single and paired ventricular captures during a supernormal phase induced by retrograde concealed conduction.   The three tracings are consecutive portions of lead III.   The first two strips overlap, in that the last P-QRST complex of the upper strip is reproduced as the first such complex in the middle strip.   In the diagrams, the area between the broken horizontal lines represents a region of unidirectional block traversed by all retrograde (AV junctional) impulses. Passage of some forward (sinus) impulses (producing ventricular captures) occurs only when there is a transient state of supernormality.   The numbers under A are P-P intervals; those under V, R-R intervals; and those under AV, R-P intervals.   The R-P intervals after ventricular captures are bracketed.   The time intervals are given in hundredths of a second.   (*From A. Pick, R. Langendorf, and L. N. Katz, The Supernormal Phase of Atrioventricular Conduction, Circulation, 26: 388, 1962.   Used by permission of the American Heart Asssociation, Inc.*)

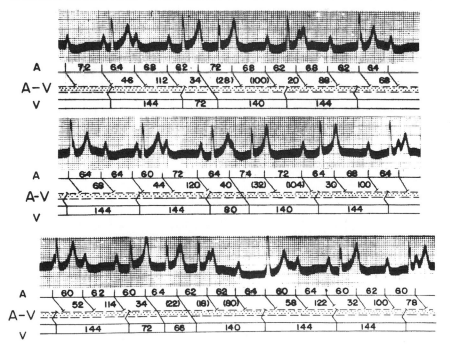

CONTINUOUS LEAD II

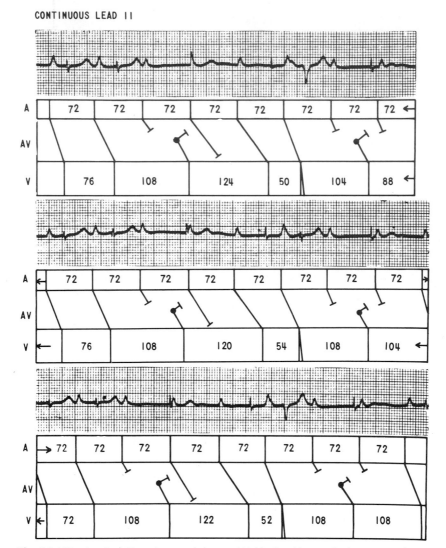

Fig. 24-149 Atypical Type I second-degree AV block with ventricular capture beats. A supernormal phase of AV conduction is postulated to account for capture of the ventricles at critically short R-P intervals. The ventricular capture beats are aberrantly conducted. In the tracings, the ventricular complexes with the longest R-R intervals (120 to 124 hundredths of a second) may not be conducted (as shown) but instead could be escape beats, with the discharge of the subsidiary pacemaker postponed by the concealed antegrade AV conduction.

premature beats are blocked whereas earlier ones are conducted has generally been regarded as a manifestation of supernormality. However, His bundle recordings have revealed the true nature of this phenomenon. At a given R-P interval, AV conduction fails within the His-Purkinje system because this system has the longest effective refractory period. At shorter

R-P intervals, AV conduction resumes because the atrial impulse encounters sufficient AV nodal delay to permit its arrival within the His-Purkinje system after the latter has repolarized more completely. A similar mechanism can explain some cases of apparent supernormal intraventricular conduction: for example, late atrial premature beats may result in aberration, whereas earlier impulses conduct normally because of a delay within the AV node or the His-Purkinje fibers. AV nodal supernormality may result from "peeling back" of the nodal refractory period by ventricular beats. Infranodal 2:1 AV block may be converted to 1:1 conduction if a premature ventricular impulse shortens the effective refractory period of the His-Purkinje system. In advanced AV block with ventriculophasic sinus arrhythmia, the late appearance of vagally induced delay at the AV node may permit some early atrial beats to be conducted, simulating supernormality. Supernormality has also been invoked in cases of alternation of AV conduction because the P-R interval is shortest in beats with the shortest R-P interval. This phenomenon is best explained by longitudinal dissociation of the AV node into two pathways with nonuniformity of conduction in the pathways. Supernormal conduction has also been explained by other physiologic mechanisms: shortening of refractoriness by changes in the preceding cycle length, the Wenckebach phenomenon in the bundle branches, bradycardia-dependent block, and summation.

24-150 The Wedensky phenomena. There is advanced AV block. In the top strip, only those sinus impulses which immediately follow the AV junctional escape beats are conducted (Wedensky facilitation). In the middle strip, the seven sinus beats which follow the initial escape beat are conducted (Wedensky effect). The last ventricular complex in this strip and the first two in the bottom strip are probably escape beats arising from another focus, because their configuration is different. The P wave following the last escape beat in the record is also conducted. These findings can also be explained by retrograde concealed conduction of the escape beats, followed by single or repetitive supernormal conduction.

CONTINUOUS LEAD II

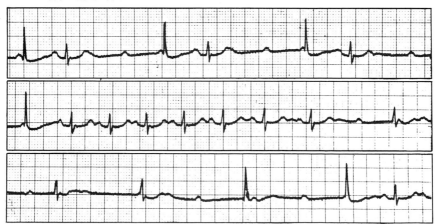

Supernormal conduction may involve the His-Purkinje system. Correction of an intraventricular conduction defect may be seen with atrial or AV junctional premature beats and in atrial fibrillation. Normalization of the QRS complex produced by an atrial premature systole can be attributed to supernormality if the P-R interval is not prolonged beyond the control value. Similar correction of a bundle branch block pattern by an AV junctional extrasystole can be ascribed to supernormality provided that bilateral bundle branch block can be excluded. In atrial fibrillation with bundle branch block, the occurrence of "normalized" QRS complexes in random fashion suggests supernormal conduction. However, fusion between ipsilateral ventricular premature systoles and the conducted beats must be excluded as the cause of the narrow beats. Unexplained normalization of a bundle branch block pattern may also result from a Wenckebach phenomenon in the bundle branches.

EXIT BLOCK (FIGS. 24-67B and C, 24-85 to 24-89, 24-90, 24-107, 24-114, 24-138, 24-151, 24-155)

Exit block is the failure of an impulse arising in an ectopic pacemaker, spontaneous or artificial, to be conducted to and to depolarize the adjacent nonrefractory myocardium. Exit block occurs commonly in parasystole but may also be found in paroxysmal and nonparoxysmal AV junctional tachycardias, ventricular tachycardias, and more rarely in atrial tachysystole, concealed bigeminy and trigeminy, and idioventricular rhythms. Exit block from the SA node, by convention, is termed SA block.

Exit block may be transient or intermittent. Sudden intermittence of propagation, comparable to Mobitz Type II AV block, can be assumed when a simple numerical relationship exists between long and short interectopic intervals. A gradual delay culminating in failure of impulse formation analogous to Type I AV block (Wenckebach periodicity) can be postulated from the arrangement of the interectopic cycles.

The diagnosis of Mobitz Type II exit block from an ectopic focus is simple when the long interectopic intervals are an exact multiple of the shorter interectopic cycles. Thus, in an ectopic tachycardia, halving of the rate is an example of 2:1 exit block. Ratios other than 2:1 may be found in this type of exit block (e.g., 3:1, 4:1, etc.)

The diagnosis of Type I exit block may be suspected when progressive shortening of the ectopic cycles is followed by a pause typical of Wenckebach periodicity.

ATRIOVENTRICULAR BLOCK

Although the term *block* has been applied to any conduction disturbance within the heart, by convention the term *heart block* is used to designate AV block.

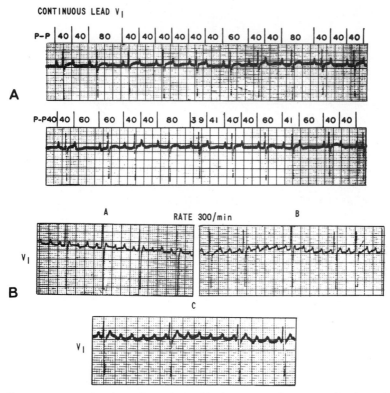

Fig. 24-151 Atrial tachycardia with exit block. (A) Atrial paroxysmal tachycardia with AV block. The average atrial cycle measures 0.40 s, corresponding to a rate of 150 per minute. There are pauses in atrial activity which measure either 0.60 or 0.80 s. Their common denominator is 0.20 s. (B) Tracings A, B, and C represent three attacks of atrial tachyarrhythmia which ocurred within 19 days. In A and C, an isoelectric baseline is seen between the atrial waves fitting the description of atrial paroxysmal tachycardia. In B, the atrial waves have a sawtooth appearance which suggests atrial flutter. The atrial rate was 300 per minute in A, B, and C. It is assumed that in A the pauses, each of which was a multiple of 0.20 s, were due to exit block. On the basis of B, however, it is postulated that the actual atrial rate was 300 per minute, that is, double the manifest rate. B also illustrates the difficulty in differentiating between paroxysmal atrial tachycardia and atrial flutter (From W. Dressler, S. Jonas, and R. Javier, Paroxysmal Atrial Tachycardia with Exit Block, Circulation, 34: 752, 1966. Used by permission of the American Heart Association, Inc.)

General Considerations   AV block may be divided into two major categories: incomplete and complete. Incomplete AV block includes first-degree, second-degree, and advanced or high-grade AV block. Complete heart block refers to third-degree AV block.

The following classification is preferred by the author: first-degree AV block, second-degree AV block (subdivided into Mobitz Type I and Type II), two-to-one AV block, advanced or high-grade AV block, and third-degree or complete heart block.

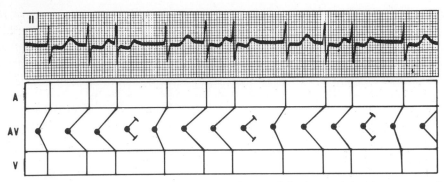

Fig. 24-152 Exit block. Antegrade and retrograde Wenckebach periods in a nonparoxysmal AV junctional tachycardia with a basic rate of 133 per minute.

Fig. 24-153 Exit block. There is atrial fibrillation, complete AV dissociation, and a nonparoxysmal AV junctional tachycardia with Type II exit block.

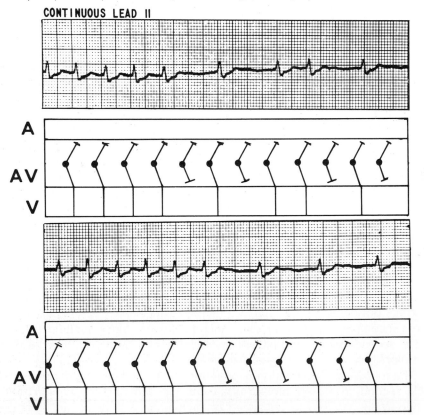

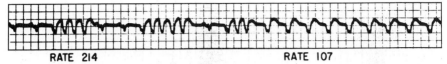

RATE 214   RATE 107

Fig. 24-154 Repetitive ventricular paroxysmal tachycardia with 2:1 exit block (Type II). (*From A. Pick, R. Langendorf, and J. Jedlicka, Exit Block, Cardiovasc. Clin., 5(3): 113, 1973. Used by permission.*)

Incomplete AV Block

First-degree AV Block (Fig. 24-156)   First-degree AV block is the most common AV conduction disorder. It has been found in approximately 0.5 to 2 percent of apparently healthy individuals, particularly in elderly persons. However, most cases are due to organic heart disease, especially chronic coronary artery disease, myocardial infarction, myocarditis, acute rheumatic fever, and certain congenital defects (e.g., patent ductus arteriosus, atrial septal defect, and Ebstein's anomaly). First-degree AV block may also result from the administration of digitalis, propranolol, quinidine, procainamide, or other drugs and from hyperpotassemia.

Atropine, exercise, and isoproterenol tend to shorten prolonged P-R intervals in both normal and diseased hearts. The P-R interval tends to shorten as the heart rate accelerates. With atrial pacing, however, the P-R interval is lengthened as the pacing rate increases whether heart disease is present or not.

Fig. 24-155 Continuous ventricular bigeminy with exit block. A bigeminal rhythm follows three sinus beats. The ventricular cycles alternate between 0.92 and 0.76 s. Because the QRS complexes are abnormal, it is assumed that they are ventricular in origin. It is further postulated that the ectopic focus fires regularly, with a cycle length of 0.56 s $\left(\dfrac{92 + 76}{3} = 56\right)$. Propagation of every second impulse is slowed and that of every third impulse is blocked, resulting in a 3:2 Wenckebach type of second-degree exit block. Another explanation for the arrhythmia (not shown) is that the rate of the ventricular pacemaker is slower, the cycle length being 0.84 s $\left(\dfrac{92 + 76}{2} = 84\right)$. Under this circumstance, first-degree intraventricular block of alternate beats is regarded as the cause of the ventricular bigeminy. EF = ectopic focus.

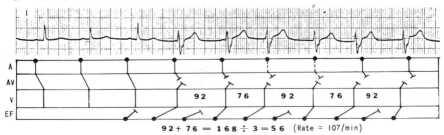

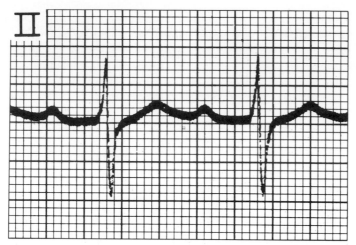

Fig. 24-156 First-degree AV block. The P-R interval is 0.32 s.

First-degree heart block associated with normal QRS complexes is due to AV nodal delay in 85 to 90 percent or more of cases. Occasionally, prolonged P-R intervals are due to intraatrial block, block within the bundle of His, delayed conduction in the His-Purkinje system, or a combination of AV nodal and His-Purkinje conduction delay. When first-degree AV block is due to infranodal block, the QRS is widened and the H-V time is prolonged.

In rare instances, revealed only by His bundle electrography, conduction delays may be observed with normal P-R intervals and normal QRS complexes. The delay may result from lesions in the bundle of His above its bifurcation or from intraatrial block.

The criteria for the diagnosis of first-degree block are listed below.

1 The P-R interval exceeds the maximum normal value (0.20 s in adults and 0.17 s in children).
2 All P waves are followed by QRST complexes.
3 Most cases of first-degree AV block have P-R intervals ranging between 0.21 and 0.35 s, but intervals as long as 0.8 s or 1.0 s have been reported.

Second-degree AV Block This is a form of AV block in which one or more P waves are not followed by QRST complexes. The atrial rate is faster than the ventricular rate.

Second-degree AV block may be associated with first-degree AV block or may occur in its absence.

Second-degree AV block is customarily classified into two types: Type I (also known as the common type, Wenckebach phenomenon, or Mobitz Type I) and Type II (the uncommon type, Mobitz Type II).

Type I second-degree AV block is considered to be due to prolongation of the absolute and relatively refractory periods in the AV junction.

Type II second-degree AV block is believed to be due to an abnormal prolongation of the absolute refractory period in the AV junction with little or no change in the relative refractory period.

Concealed, premature, nonpropagated His bundle extrasystoles may mimic Type II AV block. Rosen and his coworkers have documented this with His bundle recordings (Fig. 24-157), although the existence of these extrasystoles has long been suspected by electrocardiographers from their analysis of surface tracings (Fig. 24-144). Concealed His bundle extrasystoles may have essentially the same significance as Mobitz Type II block, because they are almost invariably associated with severe disease of the bundle of His.

Acute inferior infarction is often associated with the Wenckebach phenomenon. Since occlusion of the right coronary artery is generally responsible for inferior infarction and this artery supplies the AV node in about 90 percent of cases, it is to be expected that ischemia of the node can lead to first-degree AV block, the Wenckebach phenomenon, or both. The situation is different in the case of anteroseptal infarction; Mobitz Type II AV block and complete AV block occur more frequently than in inferior

Fig. 24-157 Pseudo AV block secondary to concealed His bundle premature depolarizations. *Upper tracing:* Lead II, showing sudden P-R prolongation of the second P wave. The seventh P wave is blocked without preceding P-R prolongation, suggesting Type II second-degree AV block. *Lower tracing:* Simultaneous lead II (ECG) and His bundle electrogram (HBE). A nonpropagated premature His bundle depolarization (H′) causes the following P wave to be blocked. The preceding P-R intervals are normal and constant. The ECG resembles Type II second-degree AV block. *(From K. M. Rosen, S. H. Rahimtoola, and R. M. Gunnar, Pseudo A-V Block Secondary to Premature His Bundle Depolarizations, Circulation, 42: 367, 1970. Used by permission of the American Heart Association, Inc.)*

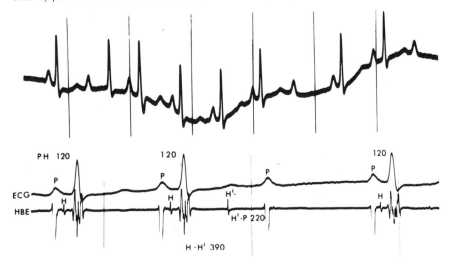

infarction, because the destructive changes produced by the infarct often involve the bundle of His, the bundle branches, or both, as well as the ventricular myocardium.

Mobitz Type I (Figs. 24-158 to 24-160)

This form of second-degree AV block is often a transitory phenomenon. It may be caused by digitalis excess, toxicity from antiarrhythmic drugs, acute (especially inferior) myocardial infarction, acute rheumatic fever, myocarditis, and acute infectious diseases.

In classic Mobitz Type I second-degree AV block, there is progressive prolongation of the P-R interval in successive beats until a P wave is nonconducted.

Type I second-degree block is localized in the AV node in about 75 percent of cases and in the His-Purkinje system in the remainder. When

Fig. 24-158 Schematic representtion of the classic Wenckebach type of AV block. The symbols A, A-V, and V refer, respectively, to the rhythm of the atria, atrioventricular conduction, and the ventricular rhythm. The numbers corresponding to the letter A represent the cycle length, expressed in seconds, of a normal pacemaker discharging at a rate of 100. The numbers superimposed on the diagonal lines opposite the symbol A-V refer to the duration of AV conduction, and those corresponding to V represent the ventricular cycle length. These also are expressed in seconds.

There is progressive lengthening of the P-R interval of each conducted beat. The maximum increment in the P-R interval occurs between the first and second beats. The increment in the P-R interval then becomes less with subsequent beats. The ventricular cycle lengths progressively shorten until the pause, after which the sequence is repeated. In the diagram, the pause results from complete blocking of the fifth sinus beat so that there is 5:4 AV block.

Quite characteristic of the Wenckebach period is the fact that the pause (cycle 4) is shorter than any two consecutive short cycles, and the cycle (cycle 5) following the pause is shorter than the one preceding it (cycle 3).

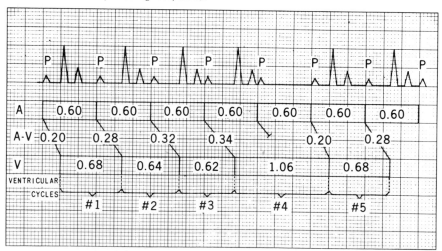

LEAD II

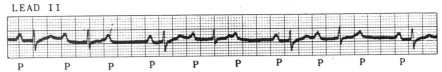

P   P   P   P   P   P   P   P   P   P

Fig. 24-159 Wenckebach type of second-degree AV block with a 3:2 AV conduction ratio. There is normal sinus rhythm at a rate of 94. The P-R interval of the first beat is 0.24 s; the P-R interval of the second, 0.36 s; the third beat is dropped. Following the pause, the sequence is repeated.

compared to nodal block, infranodal block is characterized by a more frequent association with bundle branch block and a lesser increase in the P-R interval from the first to the last conducted beat in the Wenckebach sequence. These features are not reliable enough to base the differentiation between nodal and infranodal block solely on the findings in surface leads.

The structure of the typical AV nodal Wenckebach period (Wenckebach phenomenon) is diagnostic:

1   A pause follows a series of progressively shorter ventricular cycles (R-R intervals).
2   The first ventricular cycle following the pause is longer than the one preceding it.
3   The duration of the pause is shorter than any two consecutive short ventricular cycles.

Usually there is progressive lengthening of the R-R interval of each conducted beat. The maximum increment in P-R interval characteristically occurs between the first and second beats of the period. With each successive beat the increment in the P-R interval becomes less so that the ventricular cycles (R-R intervals) shorten proportionately. Eventually a beat is dropped and is followed by a pause. The duration of the pause containing the nonconducted P wave is usually equal to twice the P-P interval less the sum of the increments of P-R prolongation.

Most cases of Type I second-degree AV block, however, do not follow this classic pattern, especially when conduction ratios are 4:3 or greater. The greatest increment in the P-R interval may be observed with the last

Fig. 24-160 Wenckebach type of second-degree AV block with a 7:6 AV conduction ratio.

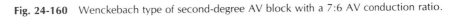

V3R

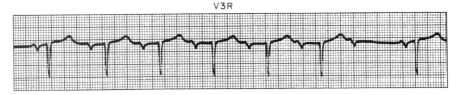

conducted P wave.   Sometimes little or no change may be seen for several beats during the cycle.   Another variant is the termination of the sequence by an escape beat, an echo beat, a reciprocating tachycardia, or another arrhythmia.   Moreover, the P-R intervals may be variable and may appear quite haphazard when there is marked sinus arrhythmia.

The Wenckebach phenomenon may rarely be caused by delay within the bundle of His itself.   This is recognized in the His bundle electrogram by the presence of split H potentials (H and H').   As the P-R interval increases, the H-H' time increases; the nonconducted P wave is followed by an H but not an H' deflection.

Because typical Wenckebach periods are the exception rather than the rule, the traditional concept that Type I AV block is synonymous with the classic Wenckebach phenomenon is no longer tenable.   Barold and Friedberg's definition of Type I AV block as "the intermittent failure of AV conduction of a single beat (known not to be of Type II) associated with inconstant AV conduction" appears more appropriate.

Mobitz Type II(Figs. 11-33, 24-161, 24-163)

Mobitz Type II second-degree AV block (the uncommon type) occurs less commonly than Type I.   According to Narula, a bundle branch block pattern is associated in about 65 percent of cases.   Mobitz Type II block is almost always the result of conduction delay in the His-Purkinje system.

The basic criterion for the diagnosis is the dropping of a ventricular beat (blocked P wave) intermittently in the presence of a constant, normal or prolonged P-R interval.   Most authorities require that the P-R intervals of *all* beats (provided there are at least two consecutive conducted P waves) before and after a single dropped beat not be measurably different.   Some investigators also accept the diagnosis if the first, or the first and second, P-R intervals after the pause are slightly shorter (less than 20 ms) than the other P-R intervals.   Those who adhere to a more strict definition believe that a short P-R interval after a pause represents either an escape beat or some type of infranodal block.

Type II second-degree AV block is almost always associated with organic heart disease, often with a high incidence of congestive heart

Fig. 24-161   Type II second-degree AV block.   In the middle of the tracing, there are five successive sinus beats.   The fifth P wave is dropped.   The P-R interval of the conducted beats is constant at 0.18 s.

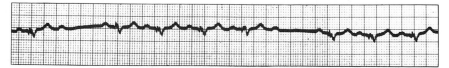

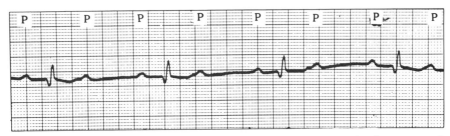

Fig. 24-162 Two-to-one AV block. Alternate ventricular beats are dropped. The P-R interval of the conducted beats is 0.32 s.

failure, symptoms of light-headedness, dizziness, fatigue and syncope, and Stokes-Adams attacks.

Two-to-One AV Block (Figs. 11-30, 24-121, 24-162, 24-167)

This type of AV block may be a transient phase in either Type I or Type II AV block or it may be permanent. Unless an opportunity to observe the P-R intervals presents itself during periods of changing conduction ratios, it is not possible from surface leads to determine whether 2:1 AV block represents Type I or Type II AV block. For example, a change in the conduction ratio from 2:1 to 3:2 with a constant P-R interval indicates Type II AV block, whereas a changing P-R interval suggests Wenckebach periodicity.

    Like other types of AV block, 2:1 AV block may result from lesions of the AV node, the bundle of His, or the His-Purkinje system. Narula has reported localization of the block in the AV node in 35 percent, in the His-Purkinje system in 50 percent, and in the bundle of His in 15 percent of

Fig. 24-163 Advanced AV block. The first and second P waves are conducted at a constant P-R interval of 0.18 s. The third P wave is dropped, and the fourth is conducted. Then the AV conduction ratio becomes 3:1. The P-R interval of all the conducted beats is constant. This is basically an advanced form of Mobitz Type II second-degree AV block.

CONTINUOUS LEAD II

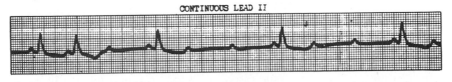

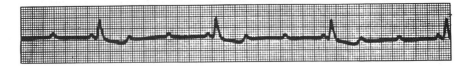

cases. According to Damato and other investigators, a fixed 2:1 AV block in the presence of normal QRS complexes is almost always due to AV nodal block. However, in 2:1 block with a bundle branch block pattern, the site of block is found within the His-Purkinje system somewhat more commmonly than in the AV node.

From a diagnostic standpoint, in 2:1 AV block alternate ventricular beats are dropped, so that there are two atrial beats for every ventricular beat. Conducted P waves have a constant normal or prolonged P-R interval.

Advanced (High-Grade) AV Block (Fig. 24-163)

High degrees of AV block may be due to mechanisms similar to that responsible for Type I or Type II AV block. Advanced AV block may be associated with intermittent or continuous incomplete or complete AV dissociation. Concealed conduction may be responsible for dropped ventricular beats in some cases.

The clinical significance of advanced AV block is similar to that of complete AV block.

The atrial rate is faster than the ventricular rate. Two or more successive P waves are blocked.

Dropped beats may occur in definite ratio of atrial to ventricular response (e.g., 3:1 or 4:1) in the presence of a constant normal or prolonged P-R interval.

Complete AV Block

Third-Degree AV Block (Figs. 11-26B, 24-38, 24-164A and B to 24-167) Complete heart block may result from involvement of the AV node, the bundle of His, or the His-Purkinje system. According to Narula, complete heart block is localized distal to the H potential in 68 percent of cases and more proximally in the remainder (16 percent in the AV node and 16 percent within the bundle of His).

Permanent complete AV block is almost always associated with either primary or secondary lesions of the conduction system. It may be found in many conditions, including coronary artery disease (notably myocardial infarction), hypertension, cardiomyopathy, rheumatic heart disease, aortic valvular disease, and less frequently other disorders (e.g., syphilis, infective endocarditis, connective tissue disease, tumors, trauma, myocarditis). In addition, sclerosis of the left side of the cardiac skeleton is an important type of primary heart block. Complete heart block may occasionally be a complication of cardiac surgery.

One of the most common types of chronic heart block is variously called primary heart block, idiopathic sclerosis of the left side of the cardiac

CONTINUOUS LEAD II

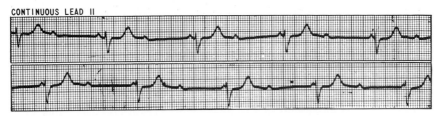

Fig. 24-164A Complete AV block. The atrial mechanism is a normal sinus rhythm at a rate of 75. The P waves bear no temporal relationship to the QRS complexes. The ventricular pacemaker is located below the bifurcation of the bundle of His. The ventricular rate is 38.

skeleton, idiopathic bundle branch block fibrosis, or sclerodegenerative disease of the bundle branches. Davies (quoted by Lev and Bharati) found the following incidence in 100 cases: idiopathic bilateral bundle branch fibrosis (a sclerodegenerative process, also termed *Lenegre's disease*), 46; ischemia coronary artery disease, 15; cardiomyopathy, 13; calcific valve disease, 8; myocarditis, 4; connective tissue disease, 3; amyloidosis, 3; transfusion siderosis, 3; congenital heart block, 3; and gumma of the interventricular septum, 2. Others have reported similar findings.

Complete AV block may be due to intoxication by drugs (such as digitalis, quinidine, or procainamide), electrolyte abnormalities, and acute infectious disease (acute rheumatic fever, diphtheria, etc.).

Congenital heart block may occur as an isolated abnormality but is frequently associated with other congenital anomalies, notably atrial septal defects, complete or corrected transposition of the great vessels, and ventricular septal defects. Congenital heart block may be the result of a lack of connection between the atria and the AV node, discontinuity between the AV node and the bundle of His, or discontinuity within the bundle itself or in an aberrant bundle of His.

In coronary artery disease, complete AV block may be acute or chronic. The acute form is associated with acute myocardial infarction. The mechanism in inferior infarction is usually ischemia of the AV node, but occasionally it may be the result of infarction of the approaches to the AV node or focal necrosis of the node and bundle branches. In such cases, His bundle recordings have revealed the block to be localized to

Fig. 24-164B Complete AV block. The atrial mechanism is a sinus rhythm at a rate of 100. The ventricular pacemaker is located in the AV junction above the bifurcation of the common bundle. The ventricular rate is 42.

LEAD II

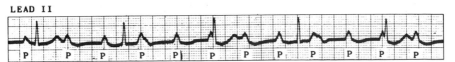

II

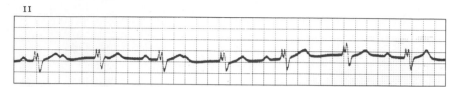

Fig. 24-165 Complete or advanced AV block. The atrial mechanism is a sinus rhythm at a rate of 83. The ventricular pacemaker is probably located below the bifurcation of the bundle of His, because the ventricular complexes are wide and aberrant. The ventricular rate is 54, which indicates acceleration of the ventricular pacemaker and raises the possibility that the block, although advanced, may not be complete.

the AV node or the bundle of His. On the other hand, in anteroseptal infarction, complete AV block results from destructive lesions of the bundle of His and the bundle branches. His bundle electrograms accordingly show the block to be located below the common bundle. In chronic artery disease, ischemia, together with fibrosis and calcification of the summit of the ventricular septum (sclerosis of the left side of the cardiac skeleton, or Lev's disease), is responsible for the occurrence of complete AV block.

Bilateral bundle branch block and trifascicular block, rather than block in the AV node or bundle of His, are the most common causes of complete AV block.

When complete AV block is due to a lesion of the AV node, the atrial impulses are blocked within the node. The escape pacemaker is generally located in the bundle of His, so that each QRS complex is preceded by an H deflection. Usually the QRS complexes and the H-V times are the same as existed prior to the occurrence of the block. Such AV junctional pacemakers usually beat at a rate of 40 to 60 per minute, but they may accelerate in response to exercise or the administration of atropine. Complete AV block due to involvement of the His bundle itself is characterized by nonconducted atrial beats followed by H deflections. However, the escaping ventricular complexes, whether normal or abnormal in configuration, are preceded by H' potentials at normal or prolonged H'-V intervals. In these instances, the pacemaker site is believed to be located within the bundle of His but distal to the site of the block. Ventricular pacemakers of this type may show no response to exercise or atropine. When complete AV block is caused by lesions of the bundle branches and fascicles, the ventricular pacemaker is located in the His-Purkinje system. Its rate of discharge is usually less than 40 per minute and is rarely responsive to exercise or atropine. In His bundle recordings, the nonconducted atrial impulses are followed by H deflections, but the abnormally wide and bizarre QRS complexes produced by the ventricular pacemaker are not preceded by H potentials.

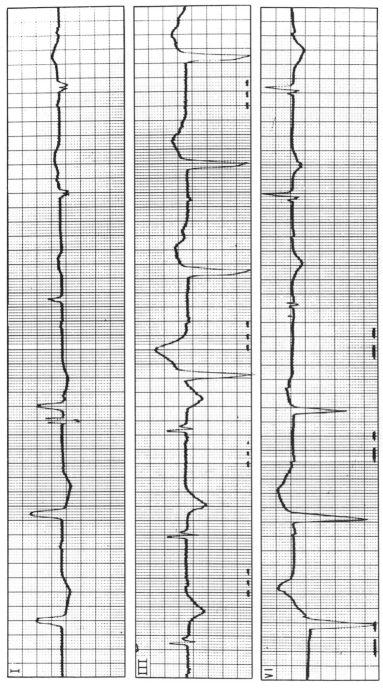

Fig. 24-166 Complete AV block. There are two idioventricular pacemakers competing for ventricular activation. Their rates are similar but uneven and so permit one or the other to escape. Occasionally impulses from both pacemakers stimulate the ventricles simultaneously, which results in fusion beats. The third and fourth beats in leads I and V₁ are fusion beats. In lead III, a sequence of right ventricular beats is initiated by the premature discharge of the right ventricular focus, which transiently suppresses impulse formation in the left ventricular focus.

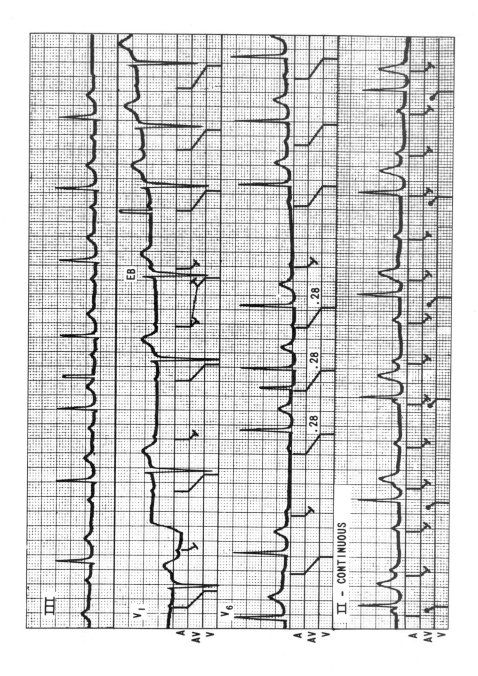

Criteria for Diagnosis

1   Independent pacemakers control the atria and ventricles. Complete AV dissociation is thus present.

2   The atrial rhythm may be of sinus origin, but atrial standstill or any other rhythm of supraventricular origin may be present. At sinus rates of 60 to 100 per minute, the occurrence of AV block usually represents pathologic abnormality of the AV conduction system. On the other hand, varying degrees of AV block may be seen in atrial tachyarrhythmias. This type of block should be regarded as primarily physiologic unless the ventricular rate is 40 or less.

3   The ventricular mechanism is an AV junctional or ventricular rhythm. When the rhythm is ventricular in origin, the heart rate is usually between 25 and 40 per minute but may be more rapid in response to drugs. The rate tends to be somewhat faster with AV junctional pacemakers. When the pacemaker is located in the AV junction or in the bundle of His, the QRS complexes have essentially normal contours. When it is located below the bifurcation of the common bundle in the His-Purkinje system, the QRS complexes are wide and aberrant. An AV junctional pacemaker conducting with a bundle branch block pattern produces QRS complexes which may be indistinguishable from those resulting from a lower ventricular pacemaker.

4   The atrial rate is faster than the ventricular rate (in contrast to AV dissociation due to interference), unless atrial standstill is present.

5   The atrial and ventricular complexes bear no fixed temporal relationship to each other.

6   Irregularity of the ventricular rate in complete AV block is usually caused by ventricular premature systoles or by two pacemakers competing for control of the ventricles.

7   The mechanism of Stokes-Adams attacks observed in complete AV block is ventricular asystole (most frequent) or ventricular tachyarrhythmia (tachycardia or fibrillation); either of these mechanisms may be followed by the other.

8   Retrograde AV conduction is seen on rare occasions in the presence of completely blocked antegrade AV conduction. It is manifested by the occurrence of retrograde P waves following the QRS complexes.

9   The diagnosis of bundle branch block in the presence of complete AV block usually cannot be made, because a rhythm arising in or above

Fig. 24-167   An unusual example of first-degree, second-degree, and third-degree AV block in the same tracing. Lead III shows first-degree AV block with a P-R interval of 0.28 s. In lead V₁ there is 2:1 AV block involving the first four P waves. The beat EB is either an escape beat or the second conducted beat of a Wenckebach period. In the middle of lead V₆ there is Type II second-degree AV block with a constant P-R interval but with a 4:3 AV conduction ratio. Lead II is part of a continuous strip showing complete AV block with no ventricles under the control of an AV junctional pacemaker.

the common bundle, with abnormal QRST complexes resulting from coexisting intraventricular block is indistinguishable from an idioventricular rhythm of lower ventricular origin.

10 AV block associated with an accelerated ventricular pacemaker should not be classified as *complete* even if complete AV dissociation appears to be present.

SINOATRIAL BLOCK

Sinoatrial block is a rare condition. Its most common cause is increased vagal tone in response to digitalis, but it may also occur during acute infection, hyperpotassemia, or as a result of the administration of quinidine or other drugs.   Sinoatrial block may sometimes be due to organic disease of the SA node.

Sinoatrial block, like AV block, may be classified into three types: first-degree, second-degree, and third-degree.

First-Degree SA Block

Prolongation of the conduction time from the SA node to the atrial muscle is not ordinarily recognizable, because the electrocardiogram does not record activity of the SA node.   According to Schamroth, it is sometimes possible to diagnose first-degree SA block when second-degree SA block occurs concomitantly, if the pause (resulting from the dropped beat) is shorter than two P-P intervals.   This indicates that the returning sinus P wave is conducted from the SA node to the atria with an improved or normal SA conduction time.

Second-Degree SA Block

Type I (Wenckebach) SA Block (Figs. 24-168 to 24-170)

1 The P-P intervals preceding a pause progressively shorten.
2 The P-P interval following the pause is longer than the one preceding it.
3 The duration of the pause is less than the sum of any two consecutive short cycles.

Type II SA Block (Figs. 24-171, 24-172)

1 The SA node fails to initiate an impulse at the expected time or times.
2 The resulting pause equals two or more cycle lengths.
3 P waves and QRST complexes are absent during the pauses except for the occasional presence of escape beats.

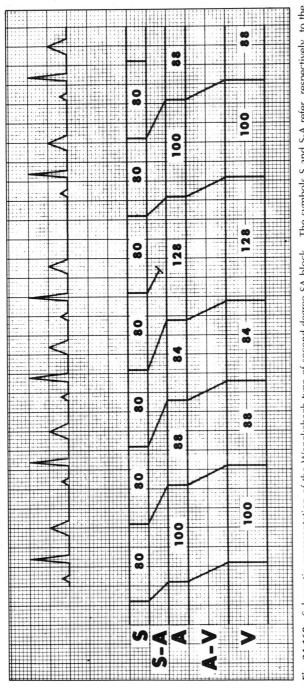

Fig. 24-168 Schematic representation of the Wenckebach type of second-degree SA block. The symbols S and S-A refer, respectively, to the discharge of the SA node and SA conduction to the atria. The numbers corresponding to the letter S represent the sinoatrial cycle length, expressed in hundredths of a second. The numbers corresponding to the letters A and V refer to the respective cycle lengths of the atria and ventricles. There is progressive lengthening of the SA conduction time. The maximum increment in the SA interval occurs between the first and second SA impulses. The increment in the SA interval then becomes less with subsequent beats, so that the P-P intervals shorten proportionately. The fifth S-A impulse is not conducted and is followed by a pause. The pause is less than any two consecutive short cycles, and the cycle following the pause is longer than the one preceding it. This is an example of 5:4 SA block.

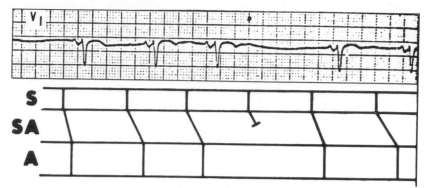

Fig. 24-169   Type I (Wenckebach) 4:3 SA block.

Two-to-One Block (Fig. 24-173)

1   Every second SA beat is dropped.
2   The heart rate doubles suddenly, either spontaneously following exercise or after the administration of atropine.   Abrupt halving of the heart rate has the same significance.

Third-Degree SA Block

Atrial standstill is present.

THE WENCKEBACH PHENOMENON

The Wenckebach phenomenon is most commonly associated with antegrade AV nodal block, but it may be involved in retrograde VA block, exit block, SA block, and conduction in the bundle branches (Fig. 24-174).

The Wenckebach phenomenon most frequently exists in atypical form. (See section on Type I second-degree AV block.)   There may be unexpected changes in the P-R or R-R intervals.   In some cases, concealed conduction

Fig. 24-170   Type I (Wenckebach) SA block with 4:3 and 2:1 conduction ratios.

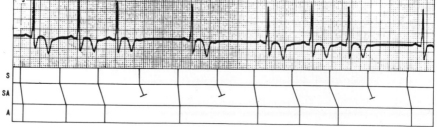

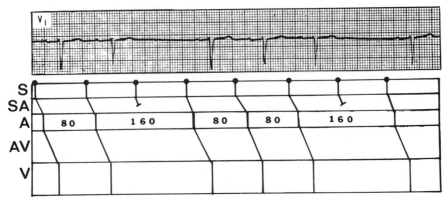

Fig. 24-171 Type II SA block. The pauses equal two cycle lengths. The time intervals are shown in hundredths of a second.

may result in the dropping of more than one beat in the Wenckebach sequence. Other variations may also be observed.

DIFFERENTIAL DIAGNOSIS OF SUPRAVENTRICULAR TACHYCARDIA

1   The supraventricular origin of a paroxysmal tachycardia is established if the QRS complexes have essentially normal contour and duration. There are exceptions, which fortunately are relatively uncommon. These are tachycardias in which the QRS complexes, although less than 0.12 s in duration, show slightly different morphologies from those of the sinus beats. It has always been a problem to determine whether such tachycardias are AV junctional in origin (with aberration) or arise within the ventricles. His bundle records have shown that many of these arrhythmias arise within the proximal infra-Hisian portion of the ventricular conduction system. By analysis of the configuration of the

Fig. 24-172 SA block with irregular dropped beats. The tracings are not continuous but are from the same patient. The SA node fails to initiate an impulse at the expected time. The resulting pause equals two cycle lengths.

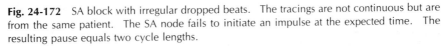

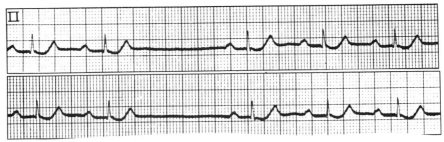

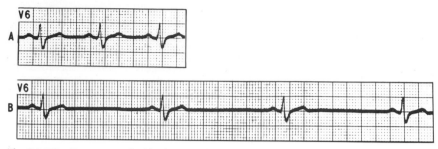

Fig. 24-173   Two-to-one SA block.   *A* and *B* are separate portions of a continuous recording from the same patient.   In *A*, there is normal sinus rhythm.   In *B*, the heart rate halved spontaneously and abruptly, indicating the presence of 2:1 SA block.

QRS complexes and the use of His bundle electrography, it is usually possible to differentiate these rhythms from supraventricular arrhythmias. (See under Fascicular Beats and Rhythms, earlier in this chapter.)

Supraventricular tachycardia may be associated with abnormal QRS complexes because of intraventricular block, aberrant ventricular conduction, conduction by a pathway different from normal, or conduction by way of an accessory pathway in ventricular preexcitation.   Such tachycardias must be distinguished from ventricular tachycardia.   This differential diagnosis is discussed separately on page 584.

2   Electrophysiologic studies have established that the overwhelming majority of paroxysmal supraventricular tachycardias are reentrant.   The differentiation between reentrant and automatic tachycardias is discussed earlier in this chapter.

3   The differential diagnosis between automatic atrial paroxysmal tachycardia, atrial paroxysmal tachycardia with block, multifocal atrial tachycardia, and atrial flutter may be found in the descriptions of these arrhythmias.   Atrial fibrillation is usually distinguished with ease from other supraventricular arrhythmias by the presence of f waves, the undulation of the baseline, and the irregular ventricular response.

4   During a continuous tachycardia with retrograde P waves in leads II, III, and aVF and a P-R interval of 0.12 s or more, it may be impossible to determine whether the tachycardia is atrial, AV junctional or reentrant (Fig. 24-175A and B).

5   Atrial flutter with 1:1 or 2:1 AV conduction may be indistinguishable from other paroxysmal supraventricular tachycardias (see Fig. 24-48).

6   A rapid sinus tachycardia may likewise simulate other supraventricular paroxysmal tachycardias.

7   When P waves are not identifiable or their origin cannot be determined, the tachycardia is classified as a supraventricular paroxysmal tachycardia of undetermined origin (Fig. 24-176).

8   The use of carotid sinus massage or other forms of vagal stimulation while the electrocardiogram is recorded is sometimes helpful in deter-

mining the origin or nature of a tachycardia.   Abrupt termination of a
supraventricular tachycardia by carotid massage, vagal maneuvers, or
cholinergic stimuli favors a reentrant mechanism.   In ectopic, automatic
tachycardia, such interventions tend to produce temporary slowing of
the heart rate or a pause, followed by resumption of the tachycardia at
its inherent rate of discharge.   In atrial flutter, carotid sinus massage
temporarily slows the ventricular response and may thus reveal the atrial
mechanism.   The flutter rate is unchanged or even accelerated by this
maneuver.   In sinus tachycardia, carotid sinus stimulation usually
produces gradual, transient slowing of the heart rate, often accompanied
by a change in the morphology of the P wave, indicating a downward
displacement of the atrial pacemaker.   Sometimes sinus tachycardia is
unaffected by vagal stimulation.

9   Exercise has little or no effect on automatic atrial or AV junctional

Fig. 24-174   The Wenckebach phenomenon is left bundle branch block.   There is sinus
tachycardia at a rate of 118.   The P-R interval is 0.18 s.   Intraventricular conduction varies
in a regularly recurring manner in groups of three: The *first beat of the sequence* (the second
and fifth QRS complexes in each lead) shows relatively normal intraventricular conduction.
The QRS duration is 0.10 s.   The prominent Q waves in leads II, III, and aVF suggest old
inferior myocardial infarction.   Small Q waves are present in leads V_5 and V_6.   The *second
beat of the sequence* (the third QRS complex in each lead) shows the pattern of incomplete
left bundle block.   The QRS interval measures 0.11 s.   The initial Q waves in leads V_5 and
V_6 are no longer present.   The beginning of the QRS complex in these leads is slurred.
Secondary S-T segment and T wave changes are present.   The *third beat of the sequence* (the
first and fourth beats in each lead) shows the typical pattern of complete left bundle branch
block.   (*From H. D. Friedberg and L. Schamroth, The Wenckebach Phenomenon in Left
Bundle Block, Am. J. Cardiol., 24: 591, 1969.   Used by permission.*)

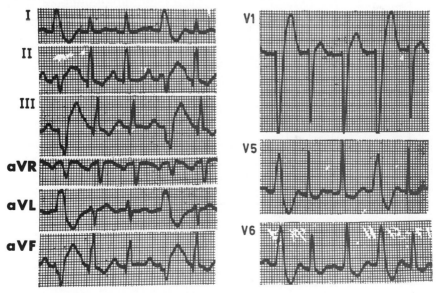

paroxysmal tachycardia. In sinus tachycardia, it may either have no effect or may accelerate the heart rate slightly. In atrial flutter with an irregular ventricular response, exercise may not only accelerate the heart rate but may cause the rhythm to become regular. This usually represents a change from a variable block to a 2:1 AV response. In atrial fibrillation, the heart rate usually becomes more rapid after exercise but remains irregular.

DIFFERENTIAL DIAGNOSIS OF SUPRAVENTRICULAR TACHYCARDIA WITH ABNORMALLY WIDE QRS COMPLEXES AND VENTRICULAR TACHYCARDIA

All the electrocardiographic manifestations of ventricular arrhythmias, with the exception of ventricular fibrillation, may under some conditions be simulated by supraventricular arrhythmias.

Fig. 24-175A Possible mechanisms of a continuous supraventricular tachycardia with retrograde P waves in lead II. (*A*) Atrial tachycardia. (*B*) AV junctional tachycardia with delayed antegrade activation of the ventricles. (*C*) AV junctional tachycardia with delayed retrograde activation of the atria. (*D*) Reentrant or reciprocating tachycardia. A recording of the onset of the tachycardia is helpful in differential diagnosis. See Fig. 24-175B.

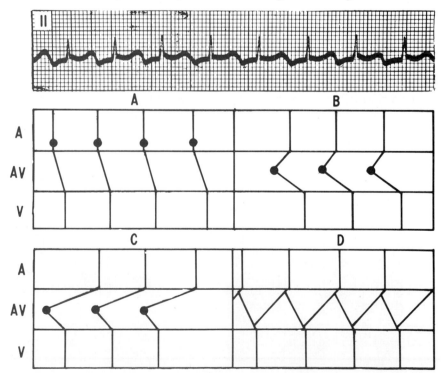

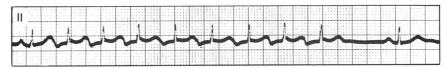

Fig. 24-175B   Same tracing as in Fig. 24-175A.   The tachycardia begins with a retrograde P wave.   The P'-R interval is normal.   The P' waves are uniform in contour throughout the tracing.   The most likely diagnosis is an (inferior) atrial tachycardia (A), although possibilities B, C, and D in Fig. 24-175A cannot be completely excluded.

It is often possible to prove that an arrhythmia with abnormally wide QRS complexes is supraventricular in origin if appropriate data are available.

It is rarely possible to prove beyond a doubt that an arrhythmia is ventricular, except for ventricular fibrillation, which is distinctive, and except for an arrhythmia known to be produced by artificial ventricular stimulation.

Onset of the Tachycardia

The site of origin of a tachycardia can often be determined if its onset is recorded.   Localization then may be possible from the appearance of the first premature beat.

Fig. 24-176   Paroxysmal supraventricular tachycardia terminated by carotid sinus massage. At the end of the tachycardia there is a sinus pause, a ventricular escape beat, and the eventual resumption of sinus rhythm after periods of sinus arrest.   The fourth ventricular complex in the second strip is the escape beat.   The tachycardia is probably reentrant.

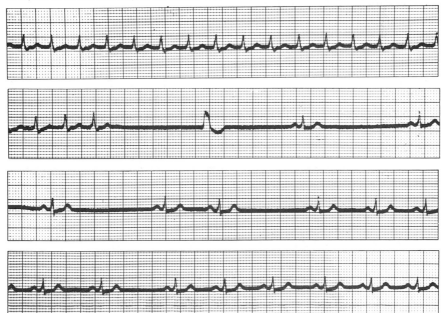

The supraventricular origin of a tachycardia is established if it begins with an ectopic, premature P wave, regardless of the contour and duration of the QRS complexes.

Arrhythmia initiated by wide, bizarre QRST complexes may be of either ventricular or AV junctional origin (see Figs. 24-105, 24-106, 24-108). If, in such a tachycardia, there is retrograde conduction to the atria, the relationship of the QRS complex to the retrograde P wave may be established and the QRS-P' interval may be measured in the first or in subsequent suitable beats. For this purpose, it is necessary to record an esophageal or right atrial lead simultaneously with at least one other lead. If the QRS-P' interval is 0.10 s or less in such leads, then the tachycardia is probably AV junctional, because such a QRS-P' interval is too brief to be explained by conduction from a ventricular focus. If the QRS-P' interval is greater than 0.10 s, or if it is similar to the P-R interval in the presence of normal AV conduction, the tachycardia may be ventricular. However, prolongation of the QRS-P' interval may also occur in AV junctional tachycardia with delayed retrograde conduction to the atria. It should be noted that in ventricular tachycardia with retrograde conduction to the atria, the first, and sometimes the first and second, beats of the tachycardia may not be conducted back to the atria because of interference by the sinus impulse in the AV junction.

Both supraventricular and ventricular arrhythmias may be precipitated by premature systoles (Fig. 24-177).

The tachycardia which results when a premature beat interrupts the T wave of the preceding beat during the vulnerable period is considered ventricular in origin (see Fig. 24-97).

The progression of a tachycardia with abnormal QRS complexes to ventricular flutter and fibrillation indicates that the tachycardia is probably ventricular in origin.

Termination of the Tachycardia

Study of the mode of termination of the tachycardia may be of some assistance in differential diagnosis. Supraventricular tachycardias usually discharge the SA node, so that after the termination of the arrhythmia the intrinsic sinus rate tends to be slower than it was previously. Thus sinus bradycardia after the offset of a paroxysmal tachycardia is an argument against ventricular tachycardia unless retrograde 1:1 conduction has been present. However, other factors, such as sympathetic tone, may alter the sinus rate after cessation of a tachycardia.

Configuration of the Ventricular Complexes

Tachycardias with abnormally wide QRS complexes may be supraventricular or ventricular in origin. The configuration, duration, and axis of the

Continuous strip V1

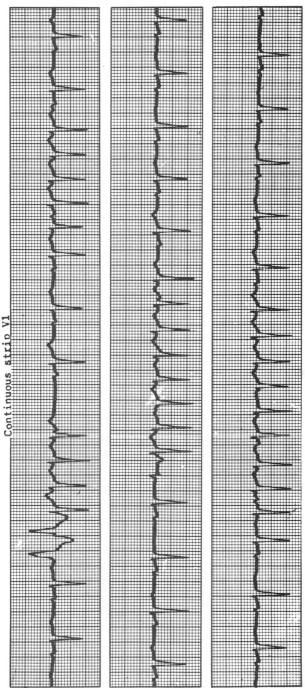

Fig. 24-177 Recurrent paroxysmal supraventricular tachycardia. Two paroxysms of tachycardia are noted in the top tracing. The first bout is initiated by a pair of ventricular (?) extrasystoles; the second run, by a premature AV junctional beat. In the middle tracing, the tachycardia is initiated by an aberrant beat whose origin cannot be determined. In the bottom tracing, the tachycardia is again initiated by a premature AV junctional beat. During each run of the tachycardia, the atria and ventricles are dissociated. The sinus rate is 83 per minute; that of the tachycardia is 187 per minute, but its rhythm is slightly irregular. The initiation of the paroxysms of tachycardia in the two upper strips by premature beats favors a reentrant mechanism. However, the presence of AV dissociation suggests an automatic mechanism. Electrophysiologic studies and the response to drug therapy would be necessary to determine the mechanism precisely.

ventricular complexes per se cannot absolutely differentiate between them but may provide some diagnostic clues. (1) The morphologic features which may be helpful in differential diagnosis are discussed in the sections, Aberrant Ventricular Conduction vs. Ventricular Ectopy and Ventricular Tachycardia. (2) A QRS interval greater than 0.14 s strongly favors ventricular tachycardia. Supraventricular tachycardias with aberrant conduction are usually about 0.12 s in duration. A QRS width between 0.12 and 0.14 s is compatible with either arrhythmia. (3) Abnormal left axis deviation or a rightward, superior axis in the frontal plane favors the diagnosis of ventricular tachycardia.

Supraventricular tachycardia may be associated with abnormal QRS complexes because of aberrant conduction during incomplete recovery, because of coexisting intraventricular block, or, in ventricular preexcitation, because of the availability of dual pathways for AV conduction.

The diagnosis of supraventricular tachycardia with preexisting intraventricular block can be established if electrocardiograms prior or subsequent to the tachycardia show the presence of an intraventricular conduction defect during sinus rhythm (Fig. 24-180). The diagnosis can also be made if during carotid sinus pressure there are ventricular beats related to the atrial beats or if the tachycardia is terminated.

Aberrant ventricular conduction of supraventricular impulses tends to show the pattern of right bundle branch block or to preserve the essential features of the preexisting ventricular complexes. The diagnosis is aided by finding atrial complexes which are related to the ventricular beats and by the finding of a gradual transition between aberrant and normal ventricular complexes. (See also section, Aberrant Ventricular Conduction vs. Ventricular Ectopy.)

Aberrant ventricular conduction during atrial fibrillation is easily mistaken for ventricular tachycardia. The differentiation between aberrant ventricular conduction and ventricular ectopy in atrial fibrillation is discussed in greater detail in the section on atrial fibrillation earlier in this chapter. Also, measurement of the cycle length of the anomalous beats may provide a clue. The interectopic interval in ventricular tachycardia usually does not vary by more than 0.01 to 0.04 s, whereas in atrial fibrillation with aberrant conduction the rhythm is usually more irregular, with cycle length varying as much as 0.08 to 0.10 s.

The diagnosis of preexcitation in the presence of supraventricular tachycardias, including atrial tachycardia, fibrillation, and flutter, is aided by finding transitional complexes or alternate runs of normal and anomalous conduction during the tachycardia, or both. The presence of typical preexcitation complexes during sinus rhythm likewise establishes the diagnosis.

Bidirectional tachycardias pose still another problem. It has been suggested that this arrhythmia is supraventricular, with permanent aberrant conduction in the right bundle branch and alternating aberrant conduction in the two divisions of the left bundle branch.   The supraventricular origin of bidirectional tachycardia has been confirmed in one case studied with His bundle recordings.   However, in a small number of patients, it has been established by His bundle electrocardiography that bidirectional tachycardia may be ventricular in origin. (See section on bidirectional tachycardia earlier in this chapter.)

Identification of the Atrial Mechanism

Identification of the atrial mechanism is fundamental to the analysis of any arrhythmia.

The supraventricular origin of a tachycardia is established if it can be demonstrated that the ventricular beats are the result of atrial activity, regardless of the configuration of the QRS complexes.

In tachycardia with abnormal QRS complexes, the presence of AV dissociation is almost diagnostic of ventricular tachycardia, but it may rarely occur in supraventricular tachycardia.   Unfortunately, AV dissociation occurs in only 50 percent of cases of ventricular tachycardia; the remainder show retrograde VA conduction (Figs. 24-105, 24-106).   Retrograde VA conduction may also occur in AV junctional tachycardia (Fig. 24-178).   Identification of the atrial mechanism may be possible only by the use of intraatrial leads.

With an intraatrial lead, in the presence of retrograde atrial conduction it is sometimes possible to distinguish between AV junctional and ventricular tachycardias if the onset is recorded and the QRS-P' interval is measured. A QRS-P' interval of 0.10 s or less is virtually diagnostic of an AV junctional tachycardia, but a longer QRS-P' interval can occur in both conditions. However, it may be impossible to diagnose a continuous tachycardia with abnormal QRS complexes with a 1:1 relationship between the QRS complexes and P waves if the onset is not recorded or if additional information is not available.   The tachycardia may be atrial in origin, or it may be AV junctional or ventricular with 1:1 retrograde atrial activation. Although the configuration of the P wave may suggest retrograde conduction from an AV junctional site, a low atrial focus cannot be excluded.   A brief QRS-P' interval may suggest an AV junctional origin, but the P' wave might just as well arise in an atrial focus whose ventricular activation is represented by the next QRS complex, or the P' wave may be the result of retrograde activation from a ventricular pacemaker, represented by the second preceding QRS complex.

During a continuous tachycardia with abnormal QRS complexes, right atrial leads may show more P waves than QRS complexes, occurring in a relationship that establishes the supraventricular origin of the tachycardia. Sometimes vagal stimulation or carotid sinus pressure must be employed to elicit this relationship.   On the other hand, if there are more QRS

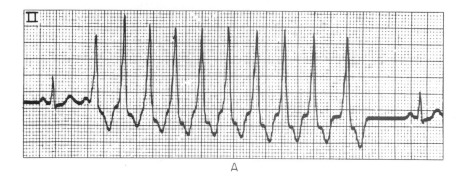

A

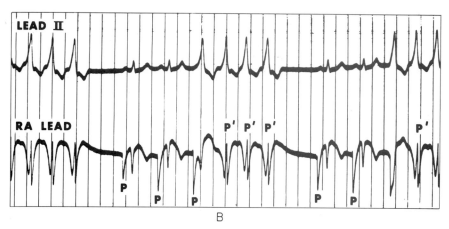

B

Fig. 24-178 *(A)* Paroxysmal tachycardia with abnormal QRS complexes in a patient with recurrent bouts of tachycardia. The tachycardia is initiated late in diastole (following the sinus P wave) by an abnormal QRS complex. Thus the tachycardia must be of either ventricular or AV junctional origin. Atrial activity during the tachycardia is not identifiable. Ventricular fusion or capture beats are not present, nor were they recorded during other episodes of tachycardia. A right atrial lead was later recorded simultaneously with lead II during another bout of tachycardia. That recording, shown in *B*, established the AV junctional origin of the tachycardia.

(B) Simultaneous recording of lead II and a right atrial lead during another bout of tachycardia from the patient described in *A*. Retrograde P waves, labeled P′, are seen within each QRS complex of the tachycardia except in the third beat from the end. There is no VA conduction after this ectopic beat because of interference with the sinus beat. The QRS-P′ interval is less than 0.10 s, which indicates that the tachycardia is AV junctional rather than ventricular in origin. In the right atrial lead, the sinus P waves are inverted and the retrograde P waves are upright. Each vertical time line is 0.20 s.

complexes than P waves, it is likely that the tachycardia is either AV junctional or ventricular in origin, with intermittent retrograde block. As mentioned previously, a completely independent atrial rhythm, of sinus or ectopic origin, may occur with either AV junctional or ventricular tachycardia.

Carotid Sinus Massage and Vagal Stimulation

Vagal stimulation by carotid sinus massage or by the use of drugs is a most useful maneuver.

If a tachycardia is slowed or terminated by this procedure, its supraventricular origin is established.

On the other hand, if a tachycardia is unaffected by cholinergic stimuli, its origin cannot be determined, since many supraventricular and all ventricular tachycardias are unaffected by vagal stimulation.

In a supraventricular tachycardia with abnormal QRS complexes, vagal stimulation, by increasing the degree of AV block, may reveal not only the atrial mechanism, as in atrial tachycardia or flutter (Figs. 24-49, 24-179), but also the relationship between the atrial and ventricular beats.

The termination of a ventricular tachycardia by carotid massage has been reported but is quite rare.

The supraventricular origin of a paroxysmal tachycardia is established if during carotid sinus pressure or other modes of vagal stimulation the ventricular beats are shown to be the result of atrial activity (Fig. 24-180). This rule is valid regardless of the contour or duration of the QRS complexes.

Comparison of the QRS Complexes during and in the Absence of Tachycardia

A tachycardia with abnormal QRS complexes is considered supraventricular if the configuration of the QRS complexes during the tachycardia is the same as that found during conduction from a known supraventricular focus before or after the tachycardia (Figs. 24-60, 24-180).

Rate of the Tachycardia

A tachycardia with abnormal QRS complexes is regarded as probably supraventricular in origin if the rate of the abnormal QRS complexes is

Fig. 24-179   The value of carotid sinus massage in revealing the origin of a tachycardia.   At the beginning of the tracing, there is a tachycardia with wide QRS complexes at a rate of 120 per minute.   The atrial mechanism cannot be identified.   Following the application of carotid sinus pressure in the middle of the tracing, the atrial mechanism is shown to be atrial flutter. There is thus atrial flutter at a rate of 240 per minute with 2:1 AV conduction.   The abnormal QRS complexes are the result of intraventricular block.

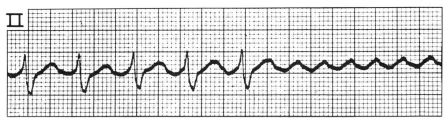

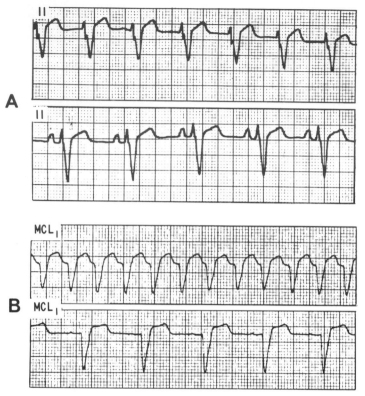

Fig. 24-180   Supraventricular tachycardia with preexisting intraventricular block.   (A) *Upper strip:* There is a tachycardia with abnormal QRS complexes.   P waves are not visible.   It cannot be determined whether the tachycardia is ventricular or AV junctional with preexisting block or aberration.   *Lower strip:* Same patient as in the upper strip but during normal sinus rhythm.   The QRS complexes are identical to those present during the tachycardia, which indicates that the tachycardia in the upper strip is AV junctional in origin.   (B) *Upper strip:* There is a tachycardia with abnormal QRS complexes.   The differential diagnosis is the same as in *A*.   *Lower strip:* Same patient as in the upper strip but during normal sinus rhythm restored by carotid sinus massage.   The QRS complexes are identical to those present during the tachycardia, which establishes that the tachycardia in the upper strip is supraventricular in origin.

identical with the rate during a known supraventricular rhythm (Figs. 24-181, 24-182).

The most frequent rate in ventricular tachycardia is 130 to 170 per minute.   Rates above 170 per minute, particularly if associated with a right bundle branch block QRS morphology, favor the diagnosis of supraventricular tachycardia with aberrant ventricular conduction.

Comparison of Ectopic Beats with Those during Tachycardia

The presence of isolated ectopic beats before, during, or after the tachycardia whose QRS configuration is like that of the QRS during the arrhythmia may help in differential diagnosis if the criteria for supraventricular or ventricular origin can be established for the isolated beats (Fig. 24-183). Otherwise this finding is of little value, because supraventricular premature beats, like ventricular premature beats, may have abnormal QRS contours.

Duration of the First Ectopic Cycle Following a Capture

The duration of the first ectopic cycle following a capture in a tachycardia may be helpful in differentiating between supraventricular and ventricular tachycardia.

Shortening of this cycle compared with the interectopic interval suggests that the ectopic beat as well as the preceding capture beat must have traveled over the same pathway. Such a pathway can be located only above the bifurcation of the bundle of His. Thus shortening of the ectopic cycle following a capture is indicative of the supraventricular origin of the tachycardia.

However, either absence of shortening of the first ectopic cycle or its prolongation does not exclude a supraventricular origin, since the conducted impulse may have transiently depressed the discharge of the ectopic focus.

Ventricular Capture and Reciprocal Beats

The ventricular origin of a paroxysmal tachycardia with abnormal QRS complexes is suggested if, when supraventricular impulses capture the ventricles during the tachycardia, the contour of the capture beats is essentially normal but that of the ectopic beats is abnormal (see Figs. 24-96, 24-99). Although this rule is useful, it is not infallible. If the configurations of both the ectopic and capture beats are identical, the supraventricular origin of the tachycardia is established, because the ventricular pacemaker must then be located above the bifurcation of the bundle of His.

Fig. 24-181 The rate of the tachycardia with abnormal QRS complexes in the first part of the tracing is the same as the atrial rate (marked by dots) uncovered after the tachycardia ceases. This makes it likely that the tachycardia is supraventricular in origin. (*From A. D. Kistin, Problems in the Differentiation of Ventricular Arrhythmia from Supraventricular Arrhythmia with Abnormal QRS, Progr. Cardiovasc. Dis., 9: 1, 1966. Used by permission.*)

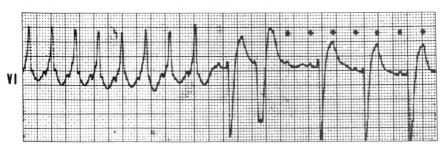

VI

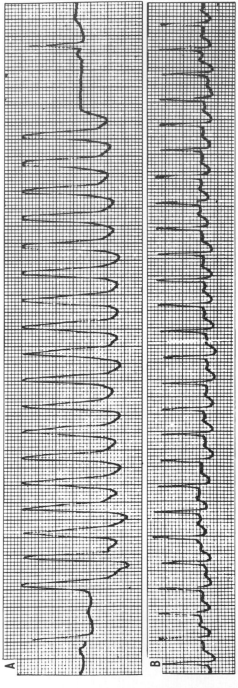

Fig. 24-182 Probable AV junctional tachycardia. A and B are monitor leads recorded at different times from the same patient. The rate of the tachycardia is the same in A and B and is 214 per minute. A unified likely interpretation is that the tachycardia is AV junctional in origin and that varying conditions of myocardial recovery favored aberrant conduction in A but not in B.

Capture beats are not decisive criteria under other (although rare) circumstances: (1) in supraventricular tachycardia, ventricular ectopic beats may simulate capture beats; (2) in supraventricular tachycardia with aberration, atrial or AV junctional beats may appear normal if discharged during the supernormal phase of conduction; and (3) in ventricular preexcitation, occasional impulse transmission over the normal AV pathway may suggest capture.

Reciprocal beats with normal configurations in a tachycardia with abnormal QRS complexes, like capture beats, are suggestive of the ventricular origin of the tachycardia (Fig. 24-99).

Fig. 24-183A   Probable left ventricular paroxysmal tachycardia.   There are qRR′ complexes in lead V₁ (with R taller than R′) and QS deflections in leads V₅ and V₆—findings which suggest left ventricular ectopy.   The axis in the limb leads points toward lead aVR, common in ventricular but uncommon in supraventricular tachycardia.   The configuration of the QRS complexes is practically the same as that of the QRS complexes in the ectopic beats recorded one year earlier (Fig. 24-183B).

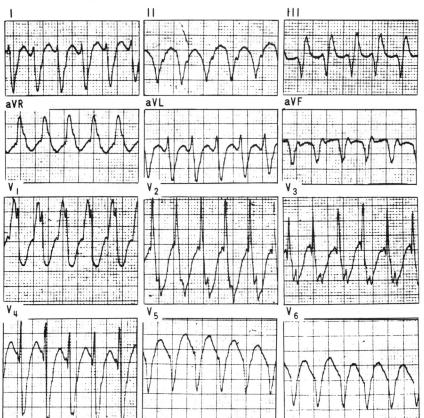

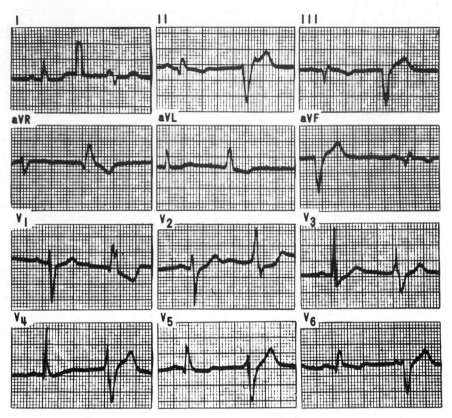

Fig. 24-183B Same patient as in Fig. 24-183A, recorded one year previously. Each sinus beat is followed by a ventricular extrasystole. In each lead, the QRS complexes of the ectopic beats are similar in configuration to those in the tachycardia (Fig. 24-183A).

Ventricular Fusion Beats

In tachycardias with abnormal QRS complexes, the occurrence of ventricular fusion beats (incomplete captures) is considered the most reliable evidence for the ventricular origin of the tachycardia (see Figs. 24-96, 24-98). Since ventricular fusion beats usually result from the simultaneous activation of the ventricles by both supraventricular and ectopic ventricular impulses, the ventricular origin of the ectopic pacemaker is assumed. However, because fusion beats, on rare occasions, may occur in supraventricular rhythms, this sign cannot be regarded as absolutely pathognomonic of ventricular tachycardia. There are other exceptions. In supraventricular tachycardias with coexisting intraventricular block, ventricular tachycardia may be simulated if aberrant ventricular conduction happens to neutralize the conduction defect temporarily, if fusion takes place between a supraventricular impulse and an ectopic ventricular impulse originating on the same side as the block, or if a supernormal phase of conduction supervenes and temporarily eliminates the block.   Fusion beats also occur in ventricular preexcitation when atrial impulses are conducted simultaneously through both the normal and accessory pathways.

Electrophysiologic Studies

His bundle recordings may be helpful or diagnostic in the differentiation between supraventricular and ventricular tachycardia.   The presence of H potentials with normal or prolonged H-V intervals preceding each ventricular complex suggests that the rhythm is supraventricular.   The absence of H potentials or the presence of short H-V intervals suggests the ventricular origin of the tachycardia.

Atrial pacing is sometimes a useful procedure in differential diagnosis. In a tachycardia with wide QRS complexes and AV dissociation, pacing the atria at a more rapid rate than that of the tachycardia may be revealing. If 1:1 conduction is restored and the QRS complexes are normalized (preexisting bundle branch block being excluded), the diagnosis is ventricular tachycardia.   Under similar circumstances, but without AV dissociation because of retrograde AV conduction, the production of normal QRS complexes by overdrive atrial pacing indicates the diagnosis of ventricular tachycardia unless a preexisting conduction defect is present.

ARTIFICIAL PACEMAKERS

Electronic pacemakers are employed primarily for the treatment of the sick sinus syndrome and heart block or other life-threatening arrhythmias but have also been used for electrophysiologic investigations.

Pacemakers consist of two major components: the pulse generator and the electrodes.   The electrodes can be inserted transvenously, to pace the right ventricular or atrial endocardium, or transthoracically, by implantation into the left ventricular myocardium, to produce left ventricular pacing. Either bipolar or unipolar electrodes are suitable for pacing.

Bipolar and Unipolar Pacing

1   Bipolar pacing causes small spikes in front of the QRST complex.
2   Unipolar pacing results in large, diphasic spikes which may sometimes obscure or mask the onset of the complex.

Atrial Pacing (Fig. 24-184B)

Beats produced by normally functioning atrial pacemakers consist of a stimulus artifact or spike followed by a P wave and its corresponding ventricular complex.

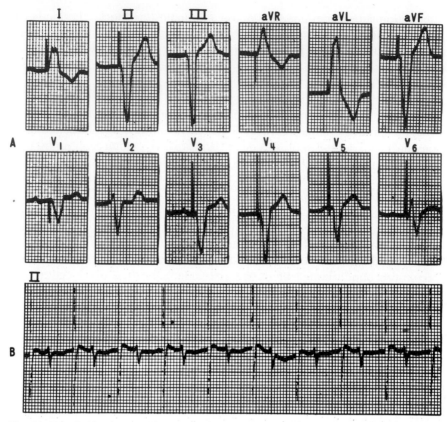

Fig. 24-184   Artificial pacemaker.   (*A*) The pacemaker electrode is located at the apex of the right ventricle.   The electrocardiogram shows the pattern of complete left bundle branch block with abnormal left axis deviation.   (*B*) The pacemaker is in the right atrium.   Each stimulus artifact is followed by a P wave and QRST complex.

Ventricular Pacing (Fig. 24-184A)

Beats produced by normally functioning ventricular pacemakers consist of a spike followed by a QRST complex.   In some patients with pacemakers, T wave inversions may develop in spontaneous beats, simulating those found in myocardial ischemia.

Right Ventricular Pacing

1   Right ventricular pacing produces the pattern of complete left bundle branch block.
2   The direction of the QRS axis is dependent on the site of stimulation.
a   Pacing from the inflow or outflow tract of the right ventricle results in a normal axis (Fig. 24-185).
b   Pacing from the outflow tract of the right ventricle directly beneath the

pulmonary valve sometimes results in a vertical axis or even right axis deviation.

c   Apical pacing causes left axis deviation (Fig 24-184A), but occasionally an $S_1S_2S_3$ pattern with negative deflections in leads V_1 and V_2 may appear.

Left Ventricular Pacing

1   Left ventricular pacing produces the pattern of complete right bundle branch block with right axis deviation (Fig. 24-186).
2   Pacing close to the apex may result in an $S_1S_2S_3$ pattern, usually (but not always) associated with a positive deflection in lead V_1.
3   Transvenous pacing with the catheter in the coronary sinus may produce the appearance of left ventricular pacing (Fig. 24-187).
4   Pacing a transvenously placed catheter that has perforated the right ventricular wall may simulate left ventricular pacing if the extruded catheter tip is in contact with the left ventricular epicardium.

Nomenclature (Tables 24-2, 24-3)

The Inter-Society Commission for Heart Disease Resources (ICHD) in 1974 proposed a three-letter code for the identification of pacemakers (Table 24-2). This code was widely adopted. It has subsequently become apparent that a five-position code would be more useful. Hence, a new code was prepared which retained the original three-position code and added two additional ones (Table 24-3). Further details may be found in the source cited for the tables.

Fig. 24-185   Electrocardiogram during pacing of the outflow tract of the right ventricle. There is a complete left bundle branch block pattern with a normal QRS axis in the extremity leads.

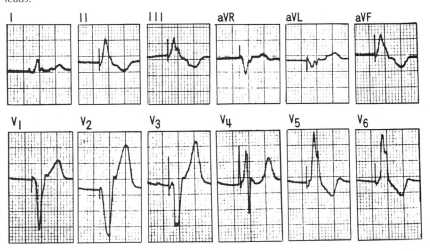

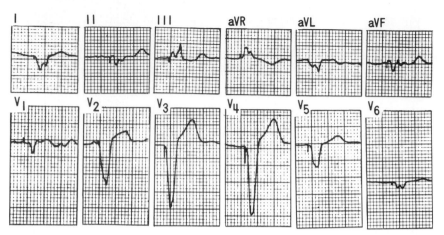

Fig. 24-186   Electrocardiogram produced by a left ventricular epicardial pacemaker implanted near the apex.   The QRS complexes are downward in all the precordial leads.   The electrical axis points rightward and superiorly in the limb leads.   The complete right bundle branch pattern produced by left ventricular pacing can be seen in lead aVR.

Examples of the revised code are listed below:

VVIP—Ventricular pacing, ventricular sensing, inhibitory mode, simple one- or two-function programmable.
VVIMP—Ventricular pacing, ventricular sensing, inhibitory mode, multi-programmable with pacing bursts for tachyarrhythmia.

Fig. 24-187   Electrocardiogram during coronary sinus pacing.   The QRS pattern is that of complete right bundle branch block.   In the limb leads, the electrical axis is directed superiorly and to the right.

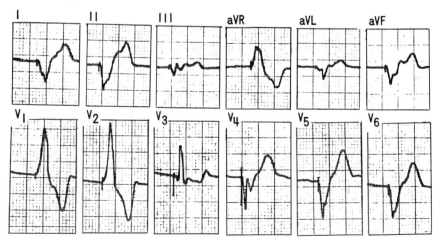

TABLE 24-2   THREE-POSITION PACEMAKER CODE (ICHD)

Position Category	I Chamber(s) Paced	II Chamber(s) Sensed	III Mode of Response(s)
Letters used	V—ventricle A—atrium D—double	V—ventricle A—atrium D—double O—none	T—triggered I—inhibited D—double* O—none

* Atrial-triggered and ventricular-inhibited
SOURCE: V. Parsonnet et al., A Revised Code for Pacemaker Identification, *Circulation*, 64: 60A, 1981. Used by permission of the American Heart Association, Inc.

Types of Pacemakers

1 *Asynchronous or fixed-rate.* These nonsynchronized pacemakers discharge continuously at a fixed rate.
2 *Ventricular-inhibited (R-wave-inhibited, or demand).* These nonsynchronized pacemakers discharge only when natural ventricular beats fail to occur for a preselected period of time.
3 *Ventricular-triggered (R-wave-synchronous, or standby).* This type of synchronized pacemaker, whose spikes are triggered by the QRS complexes, will fire automatically at a fixed rate when natural ventricular beats do not appear for a preselected interval.
4 *Atrial-triggered (P-wave-synchronous).* This type of synchronized pacemaker, whose spikes are triggered by the P waves, will fire automatically at a fixed rate if P waves or QRST complexes do not appear during a preselected period of time.
5 *AV-sequential (dual-chamber)* (Fig. 24-196). This type of pacemaker has separate electrodes for atrial sensing and pacing and for ventricular sensing and pacing. If the sinus rate exceeds the pacemaker's escape interval, the pacemaker's output is inhibited. If atrial activity fails, the pacemaker will stimulate the atrium. Should the atrial impulse be conducted to the ventricle, at a suitable P-R interval, spontaneous ventricular depolarization will take place. If the ventricle is not depolarized spontaneously, it will be paced after a preset R-R interval. (See Fig. 24-197.) In the presence of atrial fibrillation, tachycardia or flutter, sequential pacing cannot take place. Therefore, the pacemaker functions like a ventricular-inhibited pacemaker. Many such sequential units are programmable. Intense research and development of such pacemakers is in progress. Arrhythmias associated with dual-chamber pacing systems may occur as a result of asynchronous stimulation of either chamber or of the artificial bypass tract created with dual-chamber sensing and pacing. Common arrhythmias include endless loop tachycardia and the Wenckebach phenomenon. These do not imply pace-

TABLE 24-3 FIVE-POSITION PACEMAKER CODE (ICHD)

Position Category	I Chamber(s) Paced	II Chamber(s) Sensed	III Mode of Response(s)	IV Programmable Functions	V Special Tachyarrhythmia Functions
Letters used	V—ventricle	V—ventricle	T—triggered	P—programmable (rate and/or output)	B—bursts
	A—atrium D—double	A—atrium D—double O—none	I—inhibited D—double* O—none R—reverse	M—mulitprogrammable O—none	N—normal rate competition S—scanning E—external
Manufacturer's designation only	S—single chamber	S—single chamber	Optional , comma		

* Atrial-triggered and ventricular-inhibited

SOURCE: V. Parsonnet et al., A Revised Code for Pacemaker Identification, *Circulation*, 64: 60A, 1981. Used by permission of the American Heart Association, Inc.

maker malfunction. A complete discussion of dual-chamber pacing systems is beyond the scope of this text.

Asynchronous Pacemakers (Fig. 24-188)

1 Spikes are delivered to the heart at a fixed rate regardless of the intrinsic atrial or ventricular rhythms.

2 All pacemaker spikes stimulate the heart unless they occur during the absolute refractory period of the ventricle.

3 Pacemaker parasystole is a common finding in the presence of conducted beats. As with natural parasystole, the interectopic intervals are constant, coupling is variable, and fusion between conducted and paced beats occurs.

4 Ventricular extrasystoles and conducted beats are commonly interpolated between the paced beats. When they appear frequently, a dangerous rapid ventricular rate may ensue.

5 Ventricular tachycardia or fibrillation may occur if the pacemaker spike falls on the T wave of conducted or ectopic beats or if the extrasystoles interrupt the T wave of paced beats (Figs. 24-189, 24-190).

6 Noncapture or exit block may be a transitory phenomenon following pacemaker insertion but is usually a sign of pacemaker malfunction.

7 Sometimes capture will occur only when the pacing impulse arrives in the supernormal period of conductivity and not during the remainder of the cardiac cycle. This phenomenon does not indicate pacemaker malfunction.

8 In other instances, capture occurs only when the P wave immediately

Fig. 24-188 Normal operation of an asynchronous pacemaker. Spikes are delivered to the ventricles at a fixed rate. The pacemaker impulses fire the ventricles unless they are refractory as a result of previous stimulation (as occurs in spontaneous ventricular parasystole). The seventh ventricular complex in the upper strip is a fusion beat.

CONTINUOUS LEAD II

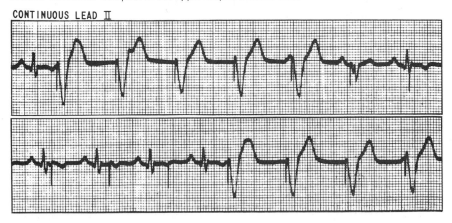

Monitor Lead

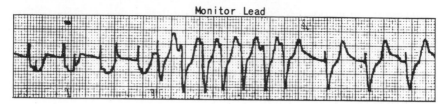

Fig. 24-189   Pacemaker-induced ventricular tachycardia.   Near the middle of the tracing, a pacemaker stimulus delivered to the T wave during the vulnerable period initiates a run of ventricular tachycardia.

precedes the pacemaker impulse.   This phenomenon is probably related to Wedensky facilitation and is also unrelated to pacemaker malfunction.

9   Depression of spontaneous impulse formation or conduction, or both, and even asystole may occur when pacemaker stimulation is stopped abruptly.   The mechanism of this phenomenon is probably similar to that involved in postectopic impulse inhibition.

10   Complete AV dissociation may be induced by artificial pacing when the sinus rate is slower than the escape rate of the pacemaker. Sometimes the dissociation may be isorhythmic.

11   Retrograde conduction (Fig. 24-191), apparent or concealed, and reciprocal rhythms occur infrequently in patients with pacemakers, since the AV block which is usually present impairs impulse transmission in both the retrograde and antegrade pathways of the conduction system.

Ventricular-inhibited Pacemakers

1   The pacemaker operates on demand, firing when the heart rate is below a predetermined level and turning off when the natural rhythm exceeds this level.

2   Since the pacemaker operates only on demand, the heart is stimulated only when necessary.   Thus competitive rhythms and stimulation during the vulnerable period are avoided.

Fig. 24-190   Ventricular fibrillation produced by a spontaneous ventricular premature systole falling on the T wave of the third paced beat.   The pacemaker continues to discharge during the fibrillatory episode.

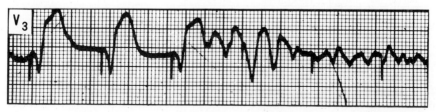

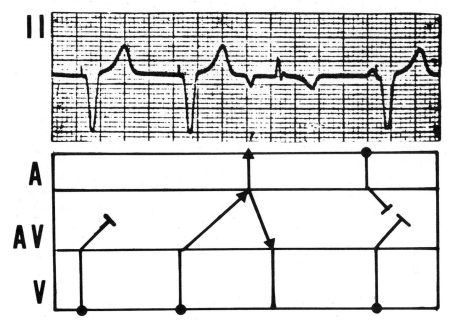

Fig. 24-191 Retrograde conduction of the second paced beat is followed in turn by a retrograde P wave and a reciprocal beat.

3 The pacemaker has a very short refractory period or none at all.

4 The pacemaker is inhibited by extrasystoles as well as conducted beats.

5 R-wave-inhibited pacemakers may show different escape and pace intervals (Fig. 24-192). The escape interval is that period from the instant an intrinsic beat is sensed until the pacemaker is discharged. The pace interval is the time between two consecutive pacemaker discharges in the absence of intervening natural beats.

6 During sinus rhythm, when the cycle length is approximately equal to the escape interval, fusion or pseudofusion beats may occur (Fig. 24-193). The former result from simultaneous activation of the ventricles by supraventricular impulses and pacemaker stimuli; the latter, from the superimposition (without fusion) of pacemaker artifacts on the QRS complexes of supraventricular beats. Neither finding is indicative of pacemaker malfunction.

7 In the presence of conducted beats at rates below the inherent discharge rate of the pacemaker, nonparasystolic escape rhythms appear.

8 Noncapture of exit block may occur, as with other types of pacemakers.

9 Arrhythmias which have counterparts in nonpaced patients may sometimes be seen. Examples include escape-capture bigeminy, pacemaker ventriculophasic sinus arrhythmia, trigeminy, and a concertina effect.

10 Demand pacemaker function during sinus rhythm may be assessed by

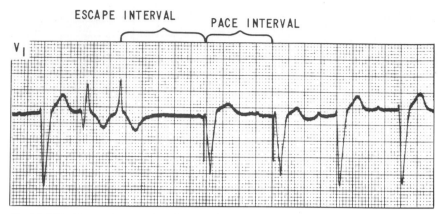

Fig. 24-192   Demand pacemaker showing different escape and pace intervals.

carotid sinus massage or by a magnet.   The latter method is preferable, because the pacemaker may fail to capture the ventricles after iatrogenic AV block induced by carotid sinus massage.

11   Demand pacemaker function during complete AV block may be assessed by testing the inhibition mechanism.   In patients with complete AV block without ventricular extrasystoles, the demand pacer controls

Fig. 24-193   Normal operation of a demand pacemaker.   During the three upper strips, the sinus cycle length is approximately equal to the discharge rate of the pacemaker.   Because of this, fusion and pseudofusion beats occur.   The second through the fifth ventricular complexes in the second strip and the first four and last two ventricular complexes in the third strip are fusion beats.   Pseudofusion is evident in the third ventricular beat in the uppermost strip.   In the bottom strip, the pacemaker has taken control of the ventricles.

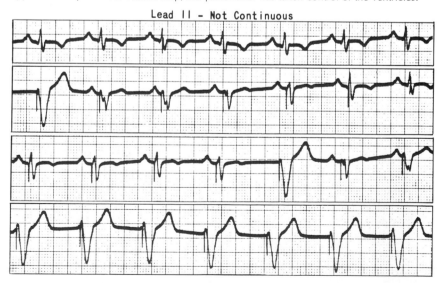

the heart completely. In these cases, it may be important to determine whether the pacemaker can sense natural QRS complexes (should they appear) and avoid competition. For this purpose, a drip of isoproterenol may be employed to enhance AV conduction or to accelerate the idioventricular rhythm.

Ventricular-triggered Pacemakers (Fig. 24-194)

1 Each QRS complex triggers a pacemaker discharge.
2 Since the QRS-to-stimulus interval is short, (usually 0.08 s), the spikes are delivered during the absolute refractory period of the ventricles and hence are unable to elicit a ventricular response.
3 The pacemaker has a built-in refractory period of 0.40 to 0.50 s, depending on the model.
4 The pacemaker does not sense QRS complexes falling in its refractory period.
5 When natural QRS complexes do not appear for a preset interval, the pacemaker discharges at a fixed rate.

Atrial-triggered Pacemakers (Fig. 24-195)

1 Atrial, or P-synchronous, pacemakers are programmed to sense the P waves and then stimulate the ventricles after an artificial P-R interval.
2 The pacemaker has a refractory period of 0.50 s, measured from the beginning of the P wave.

Fig. 24-194 Normal operation of a ventricular-triggered pacemaker. Sinus rhythm is present. Each QRS complex triggers a pacemaker discharge, which is fired during the absolute refractory period of the ventricles. The QRS-to-spike interval is 0.08 s. The large unipolar pacemaker spike appears at the end of the S wave and produces marked distortion of the S-T segment (pseudo injury pattern). In the diagram, A, A-V, and V are the conventional symbols; V-T P stands for ventricular-triggered pacemaker. The shaded areas at V and V-T P represent the refractory periods of the ventricles and the pacemaker. *(From A. Castellanos, Jr., "Pacemaker Slide Guide and Commentary," Tampa Tracings, Oldsmar, Fla., 1969. Used by permission.)*

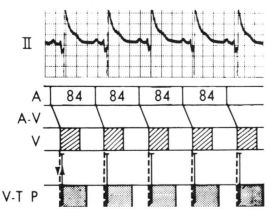

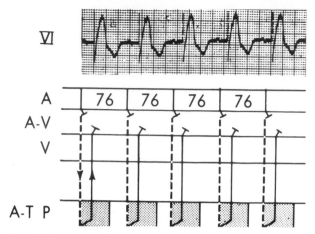

Fig. 24-195 Normal operation of an atrial-triggered pacemaker. In the diagram, A, A-V, and V are the conventional symbols; A-T P stands for atrial-triggered pacemakers. The pacemaker senses the P wave and then stimulates the ventricles after a preset artificial P-R interval. *(From A. Castellanos, Jr., "Pacemaker Slide Guide and Commentary," Tampa Tracings, Oldsmar, Fla., 1969. Used by permission.)*

3 P waves or QRS complexes falling in the refractory period of the pacer are not sensed.

4 QRS complexes appearing after the refractory period of the pacer can trigger the spikes.

5 When P waves or QRS complexes fail to appear for a preset interval, pacemaker escapes occur.

6 To prevent excessively rapid ventricular rates in response to atrial tachyarrhythmias, a blocking mechanism is incorporated in the pacemaker which prevents the ventricular rate from exceeding a fixed upper limit.

Electrocardiographic Evidence of Pacemaker Malfunction (Fig. 24-197)

1 When each pacemaker stimulus fails to elicit a cardiac response, it can be assumed that the pacemaker is failing or has failed, unless the absence of response is due to electrode movement or to competition, so that the pacemaker fires during the absolute refractory period of the ventricle.

2 Noncapture or exit block, with the aforementioned exceptions, is thus a sign of pacemaker failure. It should be remembered that noncapture immediately after pacemaker insertion may be due to elevation of the electrode threshold rather than to pacemaker malfunction.

3 Failure of a unit to sense the electrocardiographic signal from the heart either by suppression (R-wave-inhibited pacemaker) or by firing of pacing stimuli (R-wave-triggered pacemaker) is indicative of impending pacemaker failure.

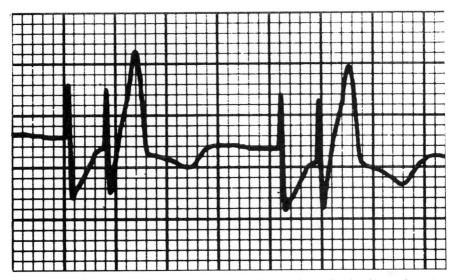

Fig. 24-196 A-V sequential pacemaker. An initial pacemaker spike depolarizes the atria, and, after a preset AV conduction time, a second pacemaker spike depolarizes the ventricles. No spontaneous beats are present.

4 A decrease in the height of the pacing artifact, measured in the three standard leads, has been said by some to be a sign of impending failure, but its reliability is questionable because of the difficulty in accurately measuring the size of the spike.

5 A decrease or increase in the rate of discharge of a generator of a few beats or even one beat per minute may indicate early pacemaker malfunction, provided the paper speed of the electrocardiograph is accurate. If the paper speed is correct, the slightest change in rate warrants further investigation for pacemaker malfunction. With specially constructed electronic counters, a change in the spike-to-spike interval of more than 10 ms may indicate early generator failure.

6 Pacemakers which unexpectedly develop very rapid rates, so-called "runaway" pacemakers, are rarely encountered nowadays because of improved pacemaker circuitry. Runaway pacemakers may cause life-

Fig. 24-197 Failure of an asynchronous pacemaker. The fifth and sixth pacemaker stimuli fail to elicit a ventricular response (noncapture or exit block), even though the ventricles are not refractory at the time.

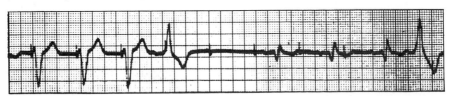

threatening tachycardias and should be disconnected from the electrodes as an emergency procedure as soon as the condition is diagnosed.

7   A detailed discussion of other methods for detecting pacemaker failure is beyond the scope of this text.

REFERENCES

Books and Symposia

Brest, A. N. (ed.) and C. Fisch (guest ed.): "Complex Electrocardiography," *Cardiovasc. Clin.*, 5 (3), 1973 and 6 (1), 1974.

Dreifus, L. and W. Likoff: "Cardiac Arrhythmias," Grune & Stratton, New York, 1973.

————: "The Mechanism and Therapy of Cardiac Arrhythmias," Grune & Stratton, New York, 1966.

Fisch, C. (guest ed.): "Symposium on Electrophysiologic Correlates of Clinical Arrhythmias," *Am. J. Cardiol.*, 28: 243–287, 371–427, 499–535, 1971.

Greenwood, R. J., and D. Finkelstein: "Sinoatrial Heart Block," Charles C Thomas, Publisher, Springfield, Ill., 1964.

Helfant, R. H., and B. J. Scherlag: "His Bundle Electrocardiography," Medcom Press, New York, 1974.

Josephson, M. E., and S. F. Seides: "Clinical Cardiac Electrophysiology: Techniques and Interpretations," Lea & Febiger, Philadelphia, 1979.

Katz, L. N., and A. Pick: "Clinical Electrocardiography: Part I. The Arrhythmias," Lea & Febiger, Philadelphia, 1956.

Marriott, H. J. L.: "Workshop in Electrocardiography," Tampa Tracings, Oldsmar, Fla., 1972.

Narula, O. S.: "His Bundle Electrocardiography and Clinical Electrophysiology," F. A. Davis, Philadelphia, 1975.

———— (ed.): "Cardiac Arrhythmias," Williams & Wilkins, Baltimore, 1979.

Pick, A., and R. Langedorf: "Intepretation of Complex Arrhythmias," Lea & Febiger, Philadelphia, 1979.

Resnekov, L. (ed.): Symposium on Cardiac Rhythm Disturbances, *Med. Clin. North Am.*, 60: 1–210, 211–386, 1976.

Samet, P., and N. El-Sharif (eds.): "Cardiac Pacing," Grune & Stratton, New York, 2d ed., 1980.

Sandoe, E., E. Flensted-Jensen, and K. H. Olesen: "Symposium on Cardiac Arrhythmias," A. B. Astra, Sweden, 1970.

Schamroth, L.: "The Disorders of Cardiac Rhythm," 2d ed., Blackwell, Oxford, 1980.

Schlant, R. C., and J. W. Hurst (eds.): "Advances in Electrocardiography," Grune & Stratton, New York, vol. 1, 1972, and vol. 2, 1976.

Zipes, D. P. (ed.): Symposium on the New Aspects of Antiarrhythmic Therapy, *Am. J. Cardiol.*, 41: 975, 1978.

Literature

Ambrust, C. A., Jr., and S. A. Levine: Paroxysmal Ventricular Tachycardia: A Study of One Hundred and Seven Cases, *Circulation,* 1: 28, 1950.

Barold, S. S., and H. D. Friedberg: Second Degree Atrioventricular Block—A Matter of Definition, *Am. J. Cardiol.,* 33: 311, 1974.

Beder, S. D., P. C. Gillet, A. Garson, Jr., and D. G. McNamara: Clinical Confirmation of ECG Criteria for Left Atrial Rhythms, *Am. Heart J.,* 103: 848, 1982.

Bellet, S., and J. Jedlicka: Sinoventricular Conduction and Its Relation to Sinoatrial Conduction, *Am. J. Cardiol.,* 24: 831, 1969.

Benchimol, A., J. E. Lasry, and F. R. Carvalho: The Ventricular Premature Contraction, Its Place in Diagnosis of Ischemic Heart Disease, *Am. Heart J.,* 65: 334, 1963.

Bernstein, L. M., L. R. Pascale, H. M. Schoolman, and E. F. Foley: Intravenous Procaine Amide as an Aid to Differentiate Auricular Flutter with Bundle Branch Block from Paroxysmal Ventricular Tachycardia, *Am. Heart J.,* 48: 82, 1954.

Besoain-Santander, M., A. Pick, and R. Langedorf: A-V Conduction in Auricular Flutter, *Circulation,* 2: 604, 1950.

Bisteni, A., G. A. Medrano, and D. Sodi-Pallares: Ventricular Premature Beats in the Diagnosis of Myocardial Infarction, *Brit. Heart J.,* 23: 521, 1961.

Bix, H. H.: Various Mechanisms in Reciprocal Rhythm, *Am. Heart J.,* 41: 448, 1951.

Bradley, S. M., and H. J. L. Marriott: Escape-Capture Bigeminy, *Am. J. Cardiol.,* 1: 640, 1958.

Castellanos, A., Jr.: The Genesis of Bidirectional Tachycardias, *Am. Heart J.,* 61: 733, 1961.

———, L. Azan, and J. M. Calvino: Simultaneous Tachycardia, *Am. Heart J.,* 59: 358, 1960.

———, J. M. Ortiz, N. Pastis, and C. Castillo: "The Electrocardiogram in Patients with Pacemakers," *Progr. Cardiovasc. Dis.,* 13: 190, 1970.

Childers, R. W.: Supernormality, *Cardiovasc. Clin.,* 5 (3): 135, 1973.

———: Usefulness of Extrasystoles in Cardiac Diagnosis and Prognosis, *Med. Clin. N. Amer.,* 50: 51, 1966.

Chung, E. K.: Pacemaker-induced Arrhythmias, *Cardiovasc. Clin.,* 6 (1): 199, 1974.

———: Parasystole, *Progr. Cardiovasc. Dis.,* 11: 64, 1968.

———, T. J. Walsh, and E. Massie: A Review of Atrial Dissociation, with Illustrative Cases and Critical Discussion, *Am. J. Med. Sci.,* 250: 72, 1965.

———, ———, and ———: Ventricular Parasystolic Tachycardia, *Brit. Heart J.,* 27: 392, 1965.

Cohen, H. C., E. G. Gozo, Jr., and A. Pick: Ventricular Tachycardia with Narrow QRS Complexes (Left Posterior Fascicular Tachycardia), *Circulation,* 45: 1035, 1972.

Cohen, J., and D. Scherf: Complete Interatrial and Intra-atrial Block (Atrial Dissociation), *Am. Heart J.,* 70: 23, 1965.

Cohen, M., and A. Castellanos, Jr.: Accelerated A-V Junctional Rhythms, *Cardiovasc. Clin.,* 5 (3): 100, 1973.

Cohen, S. I., A. Deisseroth, and H. S. Hecht: Infra-His Origin of Bidirectional Tachycardia, *Circulation,* 47: 1260, 1973.

——— and P. Voukydis: Supraventricular Origin of Bidirectional Tachycardia: Report of a Case, *Circulation,* 50: 634, 1974.

Culler, M. R., J. A. Boone, and P. C. Gazes: Fibrillatory Wave Size as a Clue to Etiological Diagnosis, *Am. Heart J.,* 66: 435, 1963.

Damato, A. N.: Cardiac Arrhythmia, in P. W. Beeson and W. McDermott (eds.): "Textbook of Medicine," 14th ed., Saunders, Philadelphia, 1975.

———— and S. H. Lau: Clinical Value of the Electrogram of the Conduction System, *Progr. Cardiovasc. Dis.,* 13: 119, 1970.

———— and ————: Concealed and Supernormal Atrioventricular Conduction, *Circulation,* 43: 967, 1971.

———— and ————: His Bundle Rhythms, *Circulation,* 40: 527, 1969.

Danzig, R., and G. Diamond: Increase in Threshold to Ventricular Activation Related to Atrial Contraction: A Possible Example of "Wedensky Inhibition," *Am. Heart J.,* 82: 531, 1971.

Denes, P., R. C. Dhingra, and K. M. Rosen: Electrophysiologic Evidence for Dual AV Nodal Pathways in Man, in O. S. Narula (ed.): "His Bundle Electrocardiography and Clinical Electrophysiology," Davis, Philadelphia, 1975.

————, L. Levy, A. Pick and K. M. Rosen: The Incidence of Typical and Atypical A-V Wenckebach Periodicity, *Am. Heart J.,* 89: 26, 1975.

———— and K. M. Rosen: His Bundle Electrograms: Clinical Applications, *Cardiovasc. Clin.,* 6: 69, 1974.

Dhingra, R. C.: His Bundle Recordings in Acquired Conduction Disease, *Arch. Intern. Med.,* 135: 397, 1975.

Dorkin, J. R.: Sinus Premature Systoles, *Am. J. Cardiol.,* 9: 804, 1962.

Dressler, W., S. Jonas, and R. Javier: Paroxysmal Atrial Tachycardia with Exit Block, *Circulation,* 34: 752, 1966.

———— and H. Roesler: The Occurrence in Paroxysmal Ventricular Tachycardia of Ventricular Complexes Transitional in Shape to Sinoauricular Beats: A Diagnostic Aid, *Am. Heart J.,* 44: 485, 1952.

Eyring, E. J., and D. H. Spodick: Coronary Nodal Rhythm, *Am. J. Cardiol.,* 5: 781, 1960.

Ferrer, M. I.: The Sick Sinus Syndrome, *Circulation,* 47: 635, 1973.

Fisch, C., and K. Greenspan: Wedensky Observations, *Circulation,* 35: 819, 1967.

————, ————, and G. J. Anderson: Exit Block, *Am. J. Cardiol.,* 28: 402, 1971.

————, D. P. Zipes, and P. L. McHenry: Electrocardiographic Manifestations of Concealed Junctional Ectopic Impulses, *Circulation,* 53: 217, 1976.

Fontaine, G., R. Frank, and Y. Grosgogeat: Torsades de Pointes—Definition and Management, *Mod. Concepts Cardiovasc. Dis.,* 51: 103, 1982.

Frankl, W. S., and L. A. Soloff: Left Atrial Rhythm: Analysis by Intra-atrial Electrocardiogram and the Vectorcardiogram, *Am. J. Cardiol.,* 22: 645, 1968.

Friedberg, H. D., and L. Schamroth: The Wenckebach Phenomenon in Left Bundle Branch Block, *Am. J. Cardiol.,* 24: 591, 1969.

Friedman, H. S., J. A. Games, and J. I. Haft: An Analysis of Wenckebach Periodicity, *J. Electrocardiol.,* 8: 307, 1975.

Gallagher, J. J., A. M. Damato, P. J. Varghese et al.: Alternative Mechanisms of Apparent Supernormal Atrioventricular Conduction, *Am. J. Cardiol.,* 31: 362, 1973.

Goldberg, L. M., J. D. Bristow, B. M. Parker, and L. Ritzmann: Paroxysmal Atrial Tachycardia with Atrioventricular Block: Its Frequent Association with Chronic Diseases, *Circulation,* 21: 499, 1960.

Goldreyer, B. N.: Sinus Node Dysfunction: A Physiologic Consideration of Arrhythmias Involving the Sinus Node, *Cardiovasc. Clin.,* 6 (3): 178, 1974.

———, J. J. Gallagher, and A. N. Damato: The Electrophysiologic Demonstration of Atrial Ectopic Tachycardia in Man, *Am. Heart J.,* 85: 205, 1973.

Goodman, R. M., and A. Pick: An Unusual Type of Intermittent AV Dissociation in Acute Rheumatic Myocarditis, *Am. Heart J.,* 61: 259, 1961.

Gouaux, J. L., and R. Ashman: Auricular Fibrillation with Aberration Simulating Ventricular Tachycardia, *Am. Heart J.,* 34: 366, 1947.

Harris, B. C., J. A. Shaver, S. Gray et al.: Left Atrial Rhythm: Experimental Production in Man, *Circulation,* 37: 1000, 1968.

Hoffman, B. F., and P. F. Cranefield: "Electrophysiolgoy of the Heart," McGraw-Hill, New York, 1960.

——— and ———: The Physiologic Basis of Cardiac Arrhythmias, *Am. J. Med.,* 37: 670, 1964.

———, ———, and A. G. Wallace: Physiologic Basis of Cardiac Arrhythmias, *Mod. Concepts Cardiovasc. Dis.,* 35: 103, 107, 1966.

Horowitz, L. N., and M. E. Josephson: Diagnosis and Evaluation of Concealed Accessory Atrioventricular Pathways, *Practical Cardiology,* 6: 129, 1980.

———, A. M. Greenspan, S. K. Spielman, and M. E. Josephson: Torsades de Pointes: Electrophysiologic Studies in Patients Without Transient Pharmacologic or Metabolic Abnormalities, *Circulation,* 63: 1120, 1981.

Hwang, W., and R. Langendorf: Auriculoventricular Nodal Escape in the Presence of Atrial Fibrillation, *Circulation,* 1: 930, 1950.

Irons, G. V., Jr., and E. S. Orgain: Digitalis induced Arrhythmias and Their Management, *Progr. Cardiovasc. Dis.,* 8: 539, 1966.

Jacobs, D. R., E. Donoso, and C. K. Friedberg: A-V Dissociation: A Relatively Frequent Arrhythmia, *Medicine,* 40: 101, 1961.

Josephson, M. E.: Paroxysmal Supraventricular Tachycardia: An Electrophysiologic Approach, *Am. J. Cardiol.,* 41: 1123, 1978.

———, L. N. Horowitz, A. Harken, and M. E. Josephson: Clinical Electrophysiology of Ventricular Tachycardia, *New Eng. J. Med.,* 304: 1004, 1981.

Kaplan, B. M., R. Langendorf, M. Lev, and A. Pick: Tachycardia-Bradycardia Syndrome (So-called "Sick Sinus Syndrome"), *Am. J. Cardiol.,* 31: 497, 1973.

Kastor, J. A.: Atrioventricular Block, *New Eng. J. Med.,* 292: 462–465, 572–574, 1975.

———: Digitalis Intoxication in Patients with Atrial Fibrillation, *Circulation,* 47: 888, 1973.

——— and B. N. Goldreyer: Reciprocal Rhythms, in L. S. Dreifus and W. Likoff (eds.), "Cardiac Arrhythmias," Grune & Stratton, New York, 1973.

——— and ———: Ventricular Origin of Bidirectional Tachycardia: Case Report of a Patient Nontoxic from Digitalis, *Circulation,* 48:897, 1973.

———, ———, E. N. Moore, and J. F. Spear: Re-entry: An Important Mechanism of Cardiac Arrhythmias, *Cardiovasc. Clin.,* 6 (1): 111, 1974.

Killip, T., and J. H. Gault: Mode of Onset of Atrial Fibrillation in Man, *Am. Heart J.,* 70: 172, 1965.

Kistin, A. D.: Mechanisms Determining Reciprocal Rhythms Initiated by Ventricular Premature Systoles, *Am. Heart J.,* 65: 162, 1963.

———: Problems in the Differentiation of Ventricular Arrhythmia from Supraventricular Arrhythmia with Abnormal QRS, *Progr. Cardiovasc. Dis.,* 9:1, 1966.

————: Retrograde Conduction to the Atria in Ventricular Tachycardia, *Circulation,* 24: 236, 1961.

———— and M. Landowne: Retrograde Conduction from Ventricular Premature Contractions, A Common Occurrence in the Human Heart, *Circulation,* 3: 738, 1951.

————, A. Tawakkol, and R. A. Massumi: Atrial Rhythm in Ventricular Tachycardia during Cardiac Catheterization, *Circulation,* 35: 10, 1967.

Knoebel, S. B., and C. Fisch: Concealed Conduction, *Cardiovasc. Clin.,* 5 (3): 21, 1973.

Lancaster, J. F., J. J. Leonard, D. F. Leon et al.: The Experimental Production of Coronary Sinus Rhythm in Man, *Am. Heart J.,* 70: 89, 1965.

Langendorf, R.: Aberrant Ventricular Conduction, *Am. Heart J.,* 41: 700, 1951.

———— and A. Pick: Approach to the Interpretation of Complex Arrhythmias, *Progr. Cardiovasc. Dis.,* 2: 706, 1960.

———— and ————: Artificial Pacing of the Heart: Its Contribution to the Understanding of Arrhythmias, *Am. J. Cardiol.,* 28: 516, 1971.

———— and ————: Concealed Conduction: Further Evaluation of a Fundamental Aspect of Propagation of the Cardiac Impulse, *Circulation,* 13: 381, 1956.

————, ————, A. Edelist, and L. N. Katz: Experimental Demonstration of Concealed AV Conduction in the Human Heart, *Circulation,* 32: 386, 1965.

————, ————, and L. N. Katz: Ventricular Response in Atrial Fibrillation: Role of Concealed Conduction in the AV Junction, *Circulation,* 32: 69, 1965.

————, ————, and M. Winternitz: Mechanisms of Intermittent Ventricular Bigeminy, *Circulation,* 11: 422, 1955.

Lau, S. H., S. I. Cohen, E. Stein et al.: P Waves and P Loops in Coronary Sinus and Left Atrial Rhythms, *Am. Heart J.,* 79: 201, 1970.

————, A. N. Damato, C. Steiner, K. M. Rosen, and G. Bobb: Isorhythmic AV Dissociation, *Circulation,* 40 (Suppl. III): 129, 1969.

Leachman, D. R., G. J. Dehmer, B. G. Ferth, et al.: Evaluation of Postextrasystolic T Wave Alterations in the Identification of Patients with Coronary Artery Disease or Left Ventricular Dysfunction, *Am. Heart J.,* 102: 658, 1981.

Lev, M., and S. Bharati: Atrioventricular and Intraventricular Conduction Disease, *Arch. Intern. Med.,* 135: 405, 1975.

Levy, M. N., D. S. Adler, and J. R. Levy: Three Variants of Concealed Bigeminy, *Circulation,* 51: 646, 1975.

———— and J. Edelstein: The Mechanisms of Synchronization in Isorhythmic A-V Dissociation: II. Clinical Studies, *Circulation,* 42: 689, 1970.

Lown, B., J. V. Temte, and W. J. Arter: Ventricular Tachyarrhythmias: Clinical Aspects, *Circulation,* 42: 1364, 1973.

————, N. F. Wyatt, and H. D. Levine: Clinical Progress: Paroxysmal Atrial Tachycardia with Block, *Circulation,* 21: 129, 1960.

Luceri, R. M., A. Castellanos, L. Zaman, and R. J. Myerburg: The Arrhythmias of Dual-Chamber Cardiac Pacemakers and Their Management, *Ann. Int. Med.,* 99: 354, 1983.

MacLean, W. A. H., R. B. Karp, N. J. Kouchoukos et al.: P Waves during Ectopic Atrial Rhythms in Man, *Circulation,* 52: 426, 1975.

Malinow, M. R., and R. Langendorf: Different Mechanisms of Fusion Beats, *Am. Heart J.,* 35: 448, 1948.

Mandel, W. J., M. M. Laks, and K. Obayashi: Sinus Node Function, *Arch. Intern. Med.,* 135: 388, 1975.

Marriott, H. J. L.: "Armchair Arrhythmias," Tampa Tracings, Oldsmar, Fla., 1966.

────── and S. M. Bradley: Main-Stem Extrasystoles, *Circulation,* 16: 544, 1957.

────── and M. M. Menendez: A-V Dissociation Revisited, *Progr. Cardiovasc. Dis.,* 8: 522, 1966.

────── and P. M. Nizet: Main-Stem Extrasystoles with Aberrant Ventricular Conduction Mimicking Ventricular Extrasystoles, *Am. J. Cardiol.,* 19: 755, 1967.

────── and H. M. Rogers: Mimics of Ventricular Tachycardia Associated with the W-P-W Syndrome, *J. Electrocardiol.,* 2: 77, 1969.

────── and I. A. Sandler: Criteria, Old and New, for Differentiating between Ectopic Ventricular Beats and Aberrant Ventricular Conduction in the Presence of Atrial Fibrillation, *Progr. Cardiovasc. Dis.,* 9: 18, 1966.

──────, A. F. Schubart, and S. M. Bradley: A-V Dissociation: A Reappraisal, *Am. J. Cardiol.,* 2: 586, 1958.

──────, N. L. Schwartz, and H. H. Bix: Ventricular Fusion Beats, *Circulation,* 26: 880, 1962.

Martinez, A.: Aberrant Ventricular Conduction in the Diagnosis of Myocardial Infarction, *Am. J. Cardiol.,* 14: 352, 1964.

Martinez-Lopez, J. I.: Clinical Differentiation Between Reentrant and Automatic Tachycardias, *Practical Cardiology,* 6: 71, 1980.

Massumi, R. A., and N. Ali: Accelerated Isorhythmic Ventricular Rhythms, *Am. J. Cardiol.,* 26: 170, 1970.

──────, G. Hilliard, A. DeMaria et al.: Paradoxic Phenomenon of Premature Beats with Narrow QRS in the Presence of Bundle-branch Block, *Circulation,* 47: 543, 1973.

──────, D. T. Mason, R. A. Fabregas et al.: Intraventricular Aberrancy versus Ventricular Ectopy, *Cardiovasc. Clin.,* 5 (3): 35, 1973.

──────, A. A. Tawakkol, and A. D. Kistin: Reevaluation of Electrocardiographic and Bedside Criteria for Diagnosis of Ventricular Tachycardia, *Circulation,* 36: 628, 1967.

Mirowski, M.: Left Atrial Rhythm. Diagnostic Criteria and Differentiation from Nodal Arrhythmias, *Am. J. Cardiol.,* 17: 203, 1966.

Moe, G. K., and C. Mendez: The Physiologic Bias of Reciprocal Rhythm, *Progr. Cardiovasc. Dis.,* 7: 461, 1966.

Morady, F., and M. M. Scheinman: Paroxysmal Supraventricular Tachycardia, *Mod. Concepts Cardiovasc. Dis.,* 51: 107, 1982.

Morris, S., and D. P. Zipes: His Bundle Electrocardiography during Bidirectional Tachycardia, *Circulation,* 48: 32, 1975.

Moss, A. J., and R. J. Davis: Brady-Tachy Syndrome, *Progr. Cardiovasc. Dis.,* 16: 439, 1974.

Narula, O. S.: Current Concepts of Atrioventricular Block, in O. S. Narula (ed.): "His Bundle Electrocardiography and Clinical Electrophysiology," Davis, Philadelphia, 1975.

──────: Wolff-Parkinson-White Syndrome: A Review, *Circulation,* 47: 872, 1973.

Norris, R. M., and C. J. Mercer: Significance of Idioventricular Rhythms in Acute Myocardial Infarction, *Progr. Cardiovasc. Dis.,* 16: 455, 1974.

Palmer, D. G.: Interruption of T Waves by Premature QRS Complexes and the Relation of This Phenomenon to Ventricular Fibrillation, *Am. Heart J.,* 63: 367, 1962.

Parkinson, J., and C. Papp: Repetitive Paroxysmal Tachycardia, *Brit. Heart J.,* 9: 241, 1947.

Parsonnet, A. E., R. Miller, A. Bernstein, and E. Klosk: Bigeminy: An Electrocardiographic Study of Bigeminal Rhythms, *Am. Heart J.,* 31: 74, 1946.

Peter, R. H.: Parasystole, *Circulation,* 8: 243, 1953.

————, J. J. Morris, Jr., and H. D. McIntosh: Relationship of Fibrillatory Waves and P Waves in the Electrocardiogram, *Circulation,* 33: 599, 1966.

Pick, A.: Aberrant Ventricular Conduction of Escaped Beats: Preferential and Accessory Pathways in the A-V Junction, *Circulation,* 13: 702, 1956.

————: A-V Dissociation: A Proposal for a Comprehensive Classification and Consistent Terminology, *Am. Heart J.,* 66: 147, 1963.

————: Mechanisms of Cardiac Arrhythmias from Hypothesis to Physiologic Fact, *Am. Heart J.,* 86: 249, 1973.

———— and P. Dominguez: Nonparoxysmal AV Nodal Tachycardia, *Circulation,* 16: 1022, 1957.

———— and L. N. Katz: Manifestations of a "Vulnerable Phase" in the Human Heart, *Circulation,* 28: 785, 1963.

———— and R. Langendorf: Differentiation of Supraventricular and Ventricular Tachycardias, *Progr. Cardiovasc. Dis.,* 2: 91, 1960.

———— and ————: The Dual Function of the A-V Junction, *Am. Heart J.,* 88: 790, 1974.

———— and ————: Recent Advances in the Differential Diagnosis of A-V Junctional Arrhythmias, *Am. Heart J.,* 76: 553, 1968.

————, ————, and J. Jedlicka: Exit Block, *Cardiovasc. Clin.,* 5 (3): 113, 1973.

————, ————, and L. N. Katz: A-V Nodal Tachycardia with Block, *Circulation,* 24: 12, 1961.

————, ————, and ————: Depression of Cardiac Pacemakers by Premature Impulses, *Am. Heart J.,* 41: 49, 1951.

————, ————, and ————: The Supernormal Phase of Atrioventricular Conduction: I. Fundamental Mechanisms, *Circulation,* 26: 388, 1962.

Rosen, K. M.: Catheter Recording of His Bundle Electrograms, *Mod. Concepts Cardiovasc. Dis.,* 42: 23, 1973.

————, S. A. Rahimtoola, and R. M. Gunnar: Pseudo A-V Block Secondary to Premature Nonpropagated His Bundle Depolarizations, *Circulation,* 42: 367, 1970.

Rosenbaum, M. B.: Classification of Ventricular Extrasystoles According to Form, *J. Electrocardiol.,* 2: 289, 1969.

————, M. V. Elizari, and J. O. Lazzari: The Mechanism of Bidirectional Tachycardia, *Am. Heart J.,* 78: 4, 1969.

————, M. S. Halpern, G. J. Nau et al.: The Mechanism of Narrow Ventricular Ectopic Beats, in E. Sandow et al. (eds.), "Symposium on Cardiac Arrhythmias," Astra, Sweden, 1970.

————, G. J. Nau, R. J. Levi et al.: Wenkebach Periods in the Bundle Branches, *Circulation,* 40: 79, 1969.

Rothfeld, E., L. R. Zucker, V. Parsonnet, and C. A. Alinsonorin: Idioventricular Rhythm in Myocardial Infarction, *Circulation,* 37: 203, 1968.

Sandler, I. A., and H. J. L. Marriott: The Differential Morphology of Anomalous Ventricular Complexes of RBBB-type in Lead V_1, *Circulation,* 21: 551, 1965.

Sano, T., and Y. Ida: The Sino-atrial Connection and Wandering Pacemaker, *J. Electrocardiol.,* 1: 147, 1968.

Schamroth, L: Genesis and Evolution of Ectopic Ventricular Rhythm, *Brit. Heart J.,* 28: 244, 1966.

————: Idioventricular Tachycardia, *J. Electrocardiol.,* 1: 205, 1968.

———— and E. Dove: The Wenckebach Phenomena in Sino-atrial Block, *Brit. Heart J.,* 28: 350, 1966.

———— and H. D. Friedberg: Wedensky Facilitation and Wedensky Effect During High Grade A-V Block in the Human Heart, *Am. J. Cardiol.,* 23: 893, 1969.

———— and H. J. L. Marriott: Concealed Ventricular Extrasystoles, *Circulation,* 27: 1043, 1963.

Scherlag, B. J., R. Lazzara, and R. H. Helfant: Differentiation of A-V Junctional Rhythms, *Circulation,* 48: 304, 1973.

Schott, A: Atrioventricular Dissociation with and without Interference, *Progr. Cardiovasc. Dis.,* 2: 444, 1960.

Sclarovsky, S., B. Strasberg, R. F. Lwin, and J. Agmon: Polymorphous Ventricular Tachycardia: Clinical Features and Treatment, *Am. J. Cardiol.,* 44: 339, 1979.

Sherf, L., and T. N. James: The Mechanisms of Aberration in Late Atrioventricular Junctional Beats, *Am. J. Cardiol.,* 29: 529, 1972.

———— and ————: A New Look at Some Old Questions in Clinical Electrocardiography, *Henry Ford Hosp. Med. Bull.,* 14: 265, 1966.

Shine, K. I., J. A. Kastor, and P. M. Yurchak: Multifocal Atrial Tachycardia, *New Engl. J. Med.,* 279: 344, 1968.

Simon, A. J., and R. Langendorf: Intraventricular Block with Ectopic Beats Approaching Normal QRS Duration, *Am. Heart J.,* 27: 345, 1944.

Skoulas, A., and L. Horlick: The Atrial F-wave in Various Types of Heart Disease and Its Response to Treatment, *Am. J. Cardiol.,* 14: 174, 1964.

Smirk, F. H., and D. G. Palmer: A Myocardial Syndrome with Particular Reference to the Occurrence of Sudden Death and of Premature Systoles Interrupting Antecedent T Waves, *Am. J. Cardiol.,* 6: 620, 1960.

Smith, W. M., and J. J. Gallagher: Les Torsades de Pointes: An Unusual Ventricular Arrhythmia, *Ann. Intern. Med.,* 93: 578, 1980.

Soffer, J., L. S. Dreifus, and E. L. Michelson: Polymorphous Ventricular Tachycardia Asssociated with Normal and Long Q-T Intervals, *Am. J. Cardiol.,* 49: 2021, 1982.

Soloff, L. A.: Ventricular Premature Beats Diagnostic of Myocardial Disease, *Am. J. Med. Sci.,* 242: 315, 1961.

Steffens, T. G., and L. S. Gettes: Parasystole, *Cardiovasc. Clin.,* 6 (1): 99, 1974.

Stock, J. P. P.: Repetitive Paroxysmal Ventricular Tachycardia, *Brit. Heart J.,* 24: 297, 1962.

Surawicz, B., and K. C. Lasseter: Effect of Drugs on the Electrocardiogram, *Progr. Cardiovasc. Dis.,* 13: 26, 1970.

Talbott, S., and L. S. Dreifus: Characteristics of Ventricular Extrasystoles and Their Prognostic Importance, *Chest,* 67: 665, 1975.

Thurmany, M., and J. G. Janney: The Diagnostic Importance of Fibrillatory Wave Size, *Circulation,* 25: 991, 1962.

Waldo, A. L., K. J. Vitikainen, P. D. Harris, J. R. Malm, and B. F. Hoffman: The Mechanism of Synchronization in Isorhythmic A-V Dissociation, *Circulation,* 38: 880, 1968.

————, ————, G. A. Kaiser et al.: The P Wave and P-R Interval: Effects of the Site of Origin of Atrial Depolarization, *Circulation,* 42: 653, 1970.

Walsh, T. J.: Ventricular Aberration of AV Nodal Escape Beats: Comments Concerning the Mechanism of Aberration, *Am. J. Cardiol.,* 10: 217, 1962.

Watanabe, Y., and L. S. Dreifus: Inhomogeneous Conduction in the AV Node: A Model for Reentry, *Am. Heart J.,* 70: 505, 1965.

Wellens, H. J. J., F. W. H. Bär, and K. I. Lie: The Value of the Electrocardiogram in the Differential Diagnosis of a Tachycardia with a Widened QRS Complex, *Am J. Med.,* 64: 27, 1978.

Wit, A. L., and P. L. Friedman: Basis for Ventricular Arrhythmias Accompanying Myocardial Infarction, *Arch. Intern. Med.,* 135: 459, 1975.

Zipes, D. P., H. R. Besch, Jr., and A. M. Watanabe: Role of the Slow Current in Electrophysiology, *Circulation,* 51: 761, 1975.

CHAPTER 25

TABULAR OUTLINE OF THE DIFFERENTIAL DIAGNOSIS OF VARIOUS ELECTROCARDIOGRAPHIC ABNORMALITIES

ABNORMAL Q WAVE

Lead I

1　Myocardial infarction (anterolateral or superior)
2　Dextrocardia or dextroversion
3　Conditions simulating myocardial infarction (see text under differential diagnosis of myocardial infarction, Chap. 13)
4　Reversal of right- and left-arm leads

Lead aVL

1　Same as lead I
2　In aVL alone
a　Normal (usually P and T inverted)
b　Superior myocardial infarction

Leads aVF and III

1　Normal
2　Myocardial infarction
3　Acute or chronic cor pulmonale
4　Right ventricular enlargement
5　Preexcitation
6　Other conditions simulating myocardial infarction (see text)

Precordial Leads

1 Myocardial infarction
2 Myocardial infarction with bundle branch block
3 Right ventricular enlargement
4 Acute cor pulmonale
5 Preexcitation
6 Left ventricular enlargement
7 Other conditions simulating myocardial infarction (see text)

QS DEFLECTION

Lead aVF, Usually with QS Deflection in Lead III, Rarely in Lead II

1 Normal variant (uncommon)
2 Inferior myocardial infarction with or without left anterior fascicular block
3 Chronic obstructive pulmonary disease
4 Preexcitation
5 Left bundle branch block
6 Other conditions simulating myocardial infarction (see text)

Precordial Leads

1 Normal variant (confined to V_1 or V_1 and V_2)
2 Left ventricular enlargement
3 Left bundle branch block
4 Myocardial infarction
5 Emphysema
6 Right ventricular enlargement (cor pulmonale)
7 Other conditions simulating myocardial infarction (see text)

QRS COMPLEX

High Voltage in Precordial Leads

1 Normal
2 Left ventricular enlargement
3 Right ventricular enlargement
4 Bundle branch block
5 Strictly posterior myocardial infarction
6 Preexcitation

Low Voltage

1 Normal
2 Nonspecific abnormality—anemia, diffuse myocardial damage, myxe-dema, pericardial or pleural effusion, obesity, malnutrition, emphysema

Tall and/or Broad R Wave in V_1

1 Normal
2 Right ventricular enlargement
3 Strictly posterior myocardial infarction
4 Preexcitation
5 Right bundle branch block
6 Congenital dextroversion
7 Idiopathic hypertrophic subaortic stenosis
8 Duchenne muscular dystrophy
9 Chronic constrictive pericarditis (rarely)

Poor R Wave Progression in Right Precordial Leads

1 Normal variant
2 Anteroseptal infarction or fibrosis
3 Left ventricular enlargement
4 Right ventricular enlargement
5 Emphysema with or without cor pulmonale
6 Left bundle branch block
7 Diffuse myocardial disease
8 Localized myocardial disease
9 Idiopathic hypertrophic aortic stenosis
10 Left anterior fascicular block
11 Mitral valve prolapse syndrome

RSR' Complex in V_1 with Normal QRS Interval

1 Normal
2 $S_1S_2S_3$ syndrome
3 Right ventricular enlargement
4 Left anterior fascicular block
5 Strictly posterior myocardial infarction
6 Acute cor pulmonale
7 Chronic obstructive pulmonary disease with or without cor pulmonale
8 Incomplete right bundle branch block

RSR′ Complexes in V_1 with Prolonged QRS Interval

1 Uncomplicated right bundle branch block
2 Right bundle branch block with left anterior fascicular block
3 Right bundle branch block with left posterior fascicular block
4 Right bundle branch block with right ventricular enlargement
5 Right bundle branch block with myocardial infarction

Prolonged QRS Interval

1 Right bundle branch block
2 Left bundle branch block
3 Diffuse or indeterminate type of intraventricular block
4 Preexcitation
5 Myocardial infarction
6 Myocardial infarction plus bundle branch block
7 Nonspecific intraventricular block
8 Electrolyte abnormalities
9 Ventricular rhythms
10 Drugs (e.g., quinidine, procainamide)
11 Left ventricular enlargement
12 Aberrant ventricular conduction
13 Hypothermia

S-T SEGMENT

Depressed in Direction Opposite to Main QRS Deflection

1 Nonspecific abnormality
2 Digitalis effect
3 Bundle branch block
4 Left ventricular strain
5 Right ventricular strain
6 Electrolyte abnormality
7 Subendocardial anoxemia (angina pectoris, coronary insufficiency, subendocardial infarction)
8 Tachycardia
9 Reciprocal changes
10 Mitral valve prolapse syndrome

Elevated in Same Direction as Main QRS Deflection

1 Normal variant (early repolarization)
2 Myocardial infarction with subepicardial injury
3 Prinzmetal's angina

4 Pericarditis
5 Ventricular aneurysm
6 Hyperpotassemia

Elevated in Direction Opposite to Main QRS Deflection

1 Normal (early repolarization)
2 Myocardial infarction
3 Pericarditis
4 Ventricular aneurysm
5 Bundle branch block
6 Reciprocal changes

Q-T INTERVAL

Prolonged

1 Hypocalcemia
2 Hypopotassemia (sometimes)
3 Left ventricular enlargement
4 Myocardial infarction
5 Myocarditis
6 Diffuse myocardial disease
7 Cerebral disease (subarachnoid hemorrhage)
8 Drugs (quinidine)
9 Hypothermia
10 Heritable anomaly
11 Ventricular conduction defects
12 Complete heart block
13 Mitral valve prolapse syndrome

Shortened

1 Hypercalcemia
2 Digitalis

T WAVES

High Voltage in Precordial Leads

1 Normal
2 Nonspecific abnormality
3 Hyperpotassemia
4 Acute subendocardial ischemia in anterior myocardial infarction

5 Reciprocal effect in strictly posterior myocardial infarction
6 Angina pectoris
7 Left ventricular enlargement
8 Anemia

Inverted or Diphasic Instead of Normally Upright

1 Normal
2 Juvenile T wave pattern
3 Nonspecific abnormality
4 Functional abnormality
5 Myocardial ischemia, including angina pectoris and coronary insufficiency
6 Myocardial infarction
7 Myocarditis
8 Pericarditis
9 Ventricular strain
10 Acute or chronic cor pulmonale
11 Cerebral disease (subarachnoid hemorrhage)
12 Drug and electrolyte abnormalities
13 Mitral valve prolapse syndrome

Marked T Wave Inversion

1 Myocardial ischemia due to coronary artery disease
2 Right ventricular strain
3 Left ventricular strain
4 Cerebral disease (subarachnoid hemorrhage)
5 Electrolyte abnormality
6 Complete AV block
7 Vagotomy

U Wave

Tall

1 Normal
2 Bradycardia
3 Complete heart block
4 Left ventricular enlargement
5 Hypopotassemia
6 Hypomagnesemia
7 Hypercalcemia
8 Drugs
9 Mitral valve prolapse syndrome

10 Hyperthyroidism
11 Hypothermia

Negative

1 Coronary artery disease
2 Systemic hypertension
3 Aortic regurgitation
4 Mitral regurgitation

$S_1S_2S_3$ SYNDROME

1 Normal
2 Right ventricular enlargement
3 Emphysema with or without cor pulmonale
4 Myocardial infarction

RIGHT AXIS DEVIATION

1 Normal
2 Right ventricular enlargement
3 Emphysema with or without cor pulmonale
4 Acute cor pulmonale
5 Superior or anterolateral myocardial infarction
6 Left posterior fascicular block
7 Inferior infarction with left posterior fascicular block
8 Dextrocardia
9 Reversal of right and left arm leads
10 Hyperpotassemia

ABNORMAL LEFT AXIS DEVIATION

1 Normal
2 Left anterior fascicular block
3 Anterior infarction with left anterior fascicular block
4 Left ventricular enlargement with left anterior fascicular block
5 Chronic coronary artery disease with left anterior fascicular block
6 Chronic diffuse pulmonary disease (pseudo left axis deviation)
7 Diffuse myocardial disease
8 Inferior myocardial infarction
9 Inferior infarction with left anterior fascicular block

10 Certain varieties of congenital heart disease—e.g., ostium primum defects, atrioventricularis communis, tricuspid atresia, ventricular septal defects, single ventricle, endocardial fibroelastosis of the left ventricle, coarctation of the aorta, aortic stenosis, anomalous origin of the left coronary artery from the pulmonary trunk, and pulmonary AV fistula

11 Hyperpotassemia

12 Preexcitation

13 Acute cor pulmonale

14 Lev's disease

15 Some neuromuscular diseases

16 Right ventricular ectopic rhythms

APPENDIX

TABLE 1   P-R INTERVAL FOR VARIOUS AGES AND HEART RATES*
Upper limit of normal, s

Age, yr	Heart rate, beats per min				
	Below 70	71–90	91–110	111–130	Over 130
0–1.5	0.16	0.15	0.15	0.14	0.13
1.5–6	0.17	0.17	0.16	0.15	0.14
7–13	0.18	0.17	0.16	0.15	0.14
14–17	0.19	0.18	0.17	0.16	0.15
Small adults	0.20	0.19	0.18	0.17	0.16
Large adults	0.21	0.20	0.19	0.18	0.17

* P-R interval (seconds) measured in the standard lead with the tallest P.
SOURCE: Adapted from "Electrocardiographic Test Book," The American Heart Association, Inc., 1956, by permission of The American Heart Association, Inc.

TABLE 2   MEANS (M) AND STANDARD DEVIATIONS (±) OF LIMB LEADS FOR 649 MEN AND 311 WOMEN BY AGE GROUPS

	Men						Women					
	I	II	III	aVR	aVL	aVF	I	II	III	aVR	aVL	aVF
Q amplitudes:												
20–29 yr M	0.30	0.48	0.61	...	0.29	0.46	0.12	0.29	0.50	...	0.13	0.29
±	0.51	0.63	0.84	...	0.55	0.65	0.26	0.42	0.64	...	0.31	0.43
30–39 yr M	0.19	0.28	0.50	...	0.19	0.28	0.16	0.27	0.33	...	0.12	0.25
±	0.33	0.37	0.66	...	0.33	0.38	0.28	0.42	0.43	...	0.23	0.34
40–59 yr M	0.23	0.25	0.41	...	0.24	0.23	0.19	0.24	0.38	...	0.23	0.22
±	0.30	0.35	0.83	...	0.34	0.35	0.31	0.43	0.67	...	0.41	0.36
R amplitudes:												
20–29 yr M	5.68	11.68	7.11	0.61	2.03	8.75	4.84	9.88	6.01	0.47	1.89	7.56
±	2.97	3.98	4.30	0.84	2.11	4.39	2.35	3.04	3.84	0.50	1.67	3.54
30–39 yr M	5.41	9.30	5.02	0.60	2.40	6.72	5.12	8.71	4.51	0.48	2.30	6.41
±	2.52	3.37	3.64	0.83	2.20	3.65	3.12	3.43	3.41	0.62	2.49	3.30
40–59 yr M	5.97	7.50	3.21	0.47	3.37	4.71	6.16	8.09	3.59	0.39	3.32	5.33
±	2.69	3.33	3.10	0.63	2.50	3.26	2.70	3.37	3.19	0.45	2.45	3.21
S amplitudes:												
20–29 yr M	1.30	1.39	1.07	9.03	2.68	1.11	0.78	0.58	0.53	6.91	2.00	0.46
±	1.14	1.41	1.53	2.98	2.51	1.28	0.91	0.74	1.04	2.34	2.34	1.18
30–39 yr M	1.25	1.31	1.35	7.56	1.77	1.01	0.57	0.75	0.77	6.27	1.00	0.53
±	1.55	1.73	2.05	2.45	1.91	1.28	0.76	0.91	1.26	2.68	1.30	0.76
40–59 yr M	0.70	0.82	1.61	6.75	1.08	0.87	0.34	0.67	1.40	6.76	0.69	0.76
±	0.95	1.07	2.21	2.21	1.51	1.30	0.59	1.07	2.39	2.36	1.11	1.43
T amplitudes:												
20–29 yr M	2.14	2.92	0.81	−2.48	0.68	1.77	2.14	2.43	0.31	−2.20	0.99	1.34
±	0.82	1.32	0.93	0.98	0.74	1.05	0.82	0.96	0.80	0.90	0.68	0.88
30–39 yr M	2.01	2.68	0.71	−2.34	0.76	1.73	1.99	2.20	0.42	−2.10	1.16	1.37
±	0.82	1.05	1.00	0.83	0.80	0.92	0.75	0.93	0.81	0.70	0.76	0.80
40–59 yr M	1.90	2.33	0.43	−2.08	0.88	1.40	1.93	2.24	0.35	−2.01	1.04	1.32
±	0.75	0.91	0.86	0.72	0.71	0.81	0.69	0.82	0.81	0.64	0.67	0.70

	Men				Women			
	ΣQRS	QRS axis	ΣT	T axis	ΣQRS	QRS axis	ΣT	T axis
20–29 yr M	28.25	62.6	6.07	41.4	22.63	61.2	5.30	33.6
±	7.46	26.9	2.36	18.5	6.25	21.9	1.82	18.1
30–39 yr M	23.61	51.7	5.74	43.1	20.17	53.8	4.98	35.0
±	6.75	29.1	2.05	18.3	7.03	24.8	1.71	20.7
40–59 yr M	19.81	37.2	5.01	37.7	20.26	41.9	4.91	36.9
±	5.73	32.0	1.64	20.2	6.41	25.8	1.43	18.7

Note: S wave includes Q in aVR and QS in leads III, aVL, and aVF.   Sample size for men = 115 for age 20 to 29 years, 110 for age 30 to 39 years, and 424 for age 40 to 49 years.   Sample size for women = 104 for age 20 to 29 years, 65 for age 30 to 39 years, and 142 for age 40 to 59 years.   Groups 40 to 49 and 50 to 59 years of age were combined, since few significant differences were found.

SOURCE: Adapted from "Differentiation between Normal and Abnormal in Electrocardiography," by E. Simonson, M.D., The C. V. Mosby Company, St. Louis, 1961, by permission.

TABLE 3   MEANS (M) AND STANDARD DEVIATIONS (±) OF PRECORDIAL LEADS FOR HEALTHY MEN AND WOMEN BY AGE GROUPS

	Men						Women					
	V_1	V_2	V_3	V_4	V_5	V_6	V_1	V_2	V_3	V_4	V_5	V_6
Q amplitudes:												
20–29 yr M	...	...	...	0.34	0.66	0.69	...	...	...	0.11	0.26	0.35
±	...	...	...	0.70	0.84	0.70	...	...	...	0.25	0.34	0.40
30–39 yr M	...	...	...	0.15	0.40	0.45	...	...	...	0.18	0.29	0.33
±	...	...	...	0.43	0.55	0.49	...	...	...	0.65	0.62	0.54
40–59 yr M	...	...	...	0.12	0.31	0.37	...	...	...	0.16	0.28	0.33
±	...	...	...	0.31	0.47	0.45	...	...	...	0.38	0.40	0.40
R amplitudes:												
20–29 yr M	3.25	7.39	11.58	16.61	15.27	11.57	1.62	4.63	8.15	11.48	11.06	9.57
±	1.93	3.42	5.66	6.02	4.77	4.17	1.31	2.54	4.39	3.82	3.38	2.85
30–39 yr M	2.16	5.37	9.39	14.80	14.28	10.89	1.62	3.70	7.13	11.76	10.75	9.16
±	1.58	3.00	5.57	5.63	4.16	3.24	1.39	2.29	5.47	5.00	4.26	3.65
40–59 yr M	1.66	4.64	8.39	14.21	14.07	10.52	1.36	3.61	7.09	12.38	11.55	9.55
±	1.26	3.05	4.77	5.41	4.78	3.53	1.01	2.71	4.86	4.95	3.89	3.16
S amplitudes:												
20–29 yr M	11.35	17.97	10.62	6.06	2.19	0.86	7.43	12.40	6.09	2.91	1.04	0.30
±	4.85	6.01	5.40	3.78	1.69	0.95	3.70	4.75	3.57	2.30	1.17	0.50
30–39 yr M	9.15	15.23	9.99	5.67	2.30	0.81	7.56	11.32	5.11	2.37	0.83	0.31
±	3.70	5.59	4.74	2.99	2.05	1.15	3.57	4.28	2.95	1.95	0.93	0.50
40–59 yr M	8.58	12.73	9.77	6.24	2.43	0.65	7.18	9.44	5.96	2.81	1.01	0.31
±	3.62	4.67	4.25	3.42	2.02	0.86	3.20	4.08	3.49	2.22	1.32	0.73
T amplitudes:												
20–29 hr M	0.86	6.47	6.51	5.60	3.80	2.62	−0.64	3.14	3.54	3.60	2.98	2.43
±	1.75	2.73	2.69	2.50	1.81	1.69	0.94	1.89	2.20	1.59	1.18	0.99
30–39 yr M	0.74	6.24	6.34	5.35	3.72	2.51	−0.61	2.90	3.08	3.31	2.89	2.33
±	1.21	2.28	2.24	2.05	1.50	1.03	0.86	1.71	1.70	1.43	1.09	0.85
40–59 yr M	0.92	5.46	6.00	5.37	3.86	2.55	−0.24	2.96	3.40	3.45	2.85	2.28
±	1.31	2.17	2.15	2.17	1.69	1.11	0.85	1.67	1.81	1.50	1.17	0.92

Note: S wave in V_1 includes QS pattern.   Sample size for men = 115 for age 20 to 29 years, 110 for age 30 to 39 years, and 424 for age 40 to 59 years.   Sample size for women = 104 for age 20 to 29 years, 65 for age 30 to 39 years, and 142 for age 40 to 59 years.   Groups 40 to 49 and 50 to 59 years of age were combined, since few significant differences were found. SOURCE: Adapted from "Differentiation between Normal and Abnormal in Electrocardiography," by E. Simonson, M.D., The C. V. Mosby Company, St. Louis, 1961, by permission.

TABLE 4   Q WAVES
Amplitude, mm

		Limb leads					Precordial leads		
Lead	Age	No. cases	Mean	Range	Lead	Age	No. cases	Mean	Range
I	24 hr	32	0.5	0.0–0.5	V_1	24 hr	41	0.0	0.0–0.0
	0–2 yr	72	0.7	0.0–2.0		0–2 yr	72	0.0	0.0–0.0
	3–5	72	0.1	0.0–1.0		3–5	72	0.0	0.0–0.0
	6–10	72	0.2	0.0–2.0		6–10	72	0.0	0.0–0.0
	12–16	68	0.1	0.0–3.0		12–16	49	0.0	0.0–0.0
	Adults	500	0.9	0.0–4.0		Adults	121	0.0	0.0–0.0
II	24 hr	32	1.5	0.0–5.0	V_2	24 hr	41	0.0	0.0–0.0
	0–2 yr	72	1.3	0.0–3.0		0–2 yr	72	0.0	0.0–0.0
	3–5	72	0.3	0.0–2.0		3–5	72	0.0	0.0–0.0
	6–10	72	0.5	0.0–3.0		6–10	72	0.0	0.0–0.0
	12–16	68	1.2	0.0–2.5		12–16	49	0.0	0.0–0.0
	Adults	500	1.1	0.0–4.0		Adults	121	0.0	0.0–0.0
III	24 hr	32	2.5	0.5–9.0	V_3	24 hr	41	0.0	0.0–0.0
	0–2 yr	72	1.6	0.0–4.0		0–2 yr	72	0.0	0.0–0.0
	3–5	72	1.4	0.0–3.0		3–5	72	0.0	0.0–0.0
	6–10	72	0.6	0.0–3.0		6–10	72	0.4	0.0–1.0
	12–16	68	1.6	0.0–5.0		12–16	49	0.0	0.0–0.7
	Adults	500	1.4	0.0–6.0		Adults	121	0.0	0.0–0.5
aVR	24 hr	32	2.4	0.0–4.0	V_4	24 hr	41	1.3	0.0–1.5
	0–2 yr	16	1.6	0.0–10.5		0–2 yr	72	0.1	0.0–1.0
	2–4	16	2.9	0.0–10.0		3–5	72	0.3	0.0–2.5
	5–10	53	1.4	0.0–10.0		6–10	72	0.2	0.0–1.5
	11–14	15	1.0	0.0–8.0		10–15	49	0.1	0.0–2.4
	Adults	151	2.0	0.0–8.0		Adults	121	0.1	0.8–1.6
aVL	24 hr	32	1.3	0.0–2.0	V_5	24 hr	41	2.2	0.0–5.5
	0–2 yr	16	0.1	0.0–0.5		0–5 yr	72	0.8	0.0–6.0
	2–4	16	0.2	0.0–1.0		3–5	72	0.8	0.0–3.0
	5–10	53	0.1	0.0–1.0		6–10	72	0.6	0.0–4.0
	11–14	15	0.1	0.0–0.5		10–15	49	0.3	0.0–2.1
	Adults	151	0.2	0.0–3.5		Adults	121	0.5	0.0–2.1
aVF	24 hr	32	1.8	0.0–6.0	V_6	24 hr	41	1.3	0.0–2.0
	0–2 yr	16	1.2	0.0–4.0		0–2 yr	72	1.1	0.0–3.0
	2–4	16	1.3	0.0–4.0		3–5	72	0.7	0.0–2.5
	5–10	53	0.5	0.0–3.0		6–10	72	0.4	0.0–3.0
	11–14	15	0.4	0.0–2.0		10–15	49	0.5	0.0–1.7
	Adults	151	0.5	0.0–3.0		Adults	121	0.4	0.0–2.7

SOURCE: Adapted from "Electrocardiographic Test Book," The American Heart Association, Inc., 1956, by permission of The American Heart Association, Inc.

TABLE 5   R WAVES
Amplitude, mm

	Limb leads					Precordial leads			
Lead	Age	No. cases	Mean	Range	Lead	Age	No. cases	Mean	Range
I	24 hr	32	2.6	0.0–5.5	V_1	24 hr	41	16.7	3.0–23.0
	0–2 yr	72	4.2	0.0–10.0		0–2 yr	16	7.0	1.0–14.5
	3–5	72	5.0	2.0–10.0		2–4	16	7.5	2.0–14.0
	6–10	72	5.0	2.0–9.0		8–10	16	3.6	1.0–9.0
	10–15	49	4.8	1.3–11.4		11–14	15	5.1	0.5–15.5
	Adults	121	5.3	0.7–11.3		Adults	151	2.3	0.0–7.0
II	24 hr	32	5.5	1.0–21.0	V_2	24 hr	41	21.0	3.0–41.0
	0–2 yr	72	5.7	0.0–14.0		0–2 yr	16	13.0	4.5–22.0
	3–5	72	7.6	3.0–12.0		2–4	16	12.7	5.0–25.0
	6–10	72	7.2	3.0–13.0		8–10	16	7.8	2.0–14.5
	10–15	49	9.1	3.7–16.0		11–14	15	8.3	1.5–23.5
	Adults	121	7.1	1.8–16.8		Adults	151	5.9	0.0–16.0
III	24 hr	32	8.8	2.0–21.0	V_3	24 hr	41	20.0	14.0–28.0
	0–2 yr	72	5.6	1.0–11.0		0–2 yr	16	14.0	3.0–24.0
	3–5	72	5.6	2.0–10.0		2–4	16	13.4	6.0–25.0
	6–10	72	4.2	0.5–13.0		8–10	16	8.4	5.0–12.5
	10–15	49	6.0	0.7–15.8		11–14	15	9.2	3.0–22.0
	Adults	121	3.8	0.3–13.1		Adults	151	8.9	1.5–26.0
aVR	24 hr	32	3.7	0.0–9.0	V_4	24 hr	41	19.0	3.0–32.0
	0–2 yr	16	1.0	0.5–4.0		0–2 yr	16	20.0	3.5–35.0
	2–4	16	1.3	0.0–3.0		2–4	16	18.5	9.0–30.0
	8–10	16	1.2	0.5–6.0		8–10	16	14.9	4.0–30.0
	11–14	15	1.2	0.5–8.0		11–14	15	17.2	7.0–28.0
	Adults	151	0.8	0.0–5.0		Adults	151	14.2	4.0–27.0
aVL	24 hr	32	2.1	1.0–6.0	V_5	24 hr	41	12.0	4.5–21.0
	0–2 yr	16	4.0	0.5–8.0		0–2 yr	16	16.0	2.5–25.0
	2–4	16	3.1	0.5–7.0		2–4	16	18.4	10.0–26.0
	8–10	16	1.2	0.5–8.8		8–10	16	17.4	6.0–28.0
	11–14	15	1.6	0.5–6.0		11–14	15	16.4	6.0–29.0
	Adults	151	2.1	0.0–10.0		Adults	151	12.1	4.0–26.0
aVF	24 hr	32	6.6	2.0–20.0	V_6	24 hr	41	4.5	0.0–11.0
	0–2 yr	16	8.8	0.5–16.0		0–2 yr	16	12.0	2.0–20.0
	2–4	16	9.5	0.5–19.5		2–4	16	14.6	8.0–23.0
	8–10	16	8.5	3.5–14.0		8–10	16	12.5	5.0–19.1
	11–14	15	10.5	5.0–21.0		11–14	15	13.5	4.0–25.0
	Adults	151	1.3	0.0–20.0		Adults	151	9.2	4.0–22.0

SOURCE: Adapted from "Electrocardiographic Test Book," The American Heart Association, Inc., 1956, by permission of The American Heart Association, Inc.

TABLE 6   S WAVES
Amplitude, mm

		Limb leads					Precordial leads		
Lead	Age	No. cases	Mean	Range	Lead	Age	No. cases	Mean	Range
I	24 hr	32	6.3	0.0–15.0	V_1	24 hr	41	10.0	0.0–28.0
	0–2 yr	72	3.9	0.0–7.0		0–2 yr	16	4.8	0.5–14.0
	2–5	72	2.5	0.0–6.0		2–4	16	8.6	3.0–16.0
	6–10	72	1.6	0.0–3.0		8–10	16	8.6	3.0–16.0
	10–15	49	1.8	0.0–6.8		11–14	15	11.6	0.0–20.0
	Adults	121	1.0	0.0–3.6		Adults	151	8.6	2.0–25.0
II	24 hr	32	3.2	0.0–7.0	V_2	24 hr	41	22.0	1.0–42.0
	0–2 yr	72	2.7	0.0–5.0		0–2 yr	16	9.3	0.5–21.0
	2–5	72	1.6	0.0–4.0		2–4	16	16.0	8.5–30.0
	6–10	72	1.4	0.0–3.5		8–10	16	16.8	8.0–30.0
	10–15	49	1.6	0.0–4.9		11–14	15	20.8	7.0–36.0
	Adults	121	1.2	0.0–4.9		Adults	151	12.7	0.0–29.0
III	24 hr	32	2.3	0.0–3.0	V_3	24 hr	41	26.4	0.0–39.0
	0–2 yr	72	1.1	0.0–3.5		0–2 yr	16	10.2	0.5–23.0
	2–5	72	0.8	0.0–5.0		2–4	16	12.7	3.5–21.0
	6–10	72	0.7	0.0–4.0		8–10	16	16.3	8.0–27.0
	10–15	49	0.9	0.0–5.3		11–14	15	14.8	1.0–30.0
	Adults	121	1.2	0.0–5.5		Adults	151	8.8	0.0–25.0
aVR	24 hr	32	3.9	0.0–9.5	V_4	24 hr	41	23.0	0.0–42.0
	0–2 yr	16	6.3	0.0–14.0		0–2 yr	16	10.2	2.0–22.0
	2–4	16	5.9	0.0–14.0		2–4	16	9.0	0.0–20.0
	8–10	16	4.9	0.0–10.0		8–10	16	11.2	4.0–17.0
	11–14	15	8.3	0.0–17.0		11–14	15	8.0	1.0–16.0
	Adults	151	4.3	0.0–13.0		Adults	151	5.2	0.0–20.0
aVL	24 hr	32	6.6	0.0–16.0	V_5	24 hr	41	12.0	1.5–30.0
	0–2 yr	16	3.4	0.0–7.0		0–2 yr	16	6.1	1.0–13.0
	2–4	16	2.7	0.0–6.0		2–4	16	4.4	0.0–11.0
	8–10	16	3.2	0.0–7.0		8–10	16	5.7	0.5–12.0
	11–14	15	3.1	0.0–9.0		11–14	15	3.7	0.5–8.0
	Adults	151	0.4	0.0–18.0		Adults	151	1.5	0.0–6.0
aVF	24 hr	32	3.0	0.0–7.5	V_6	24 hr	41	4.5	0.0–13.0
	0–2 yr	16	0.7	0.0–2.5		0–2 yr	16	2.5	0.0–7.5
	2–4	16	2.1	0.0–14.0		2–4	16	1.6	0.5–5.0
	8–10	16	0.7	0.0–2.0		8–10	16	1.1	0.0–4.0
	11–14	15	0.8	0.0–2.5		11–14	15	0.9	0.0–2.0
	Adults	151	0.2	0.0–8.0		Adults	151	0.6	0.0–7.0

SOURCE: Adapted from "Electrocardiographic Test Book," The American Heart Association, Inc., 1956, by permission of The American Heart Association, Inc.

TABLE 7   T WAVES
Amplitude, mm

Lead	Age	No. cases	Mean	Range	Lead	Age	No. cases	Mean	Range
		Limb leads					**Precordial leads**		
I	24 hr	41	0.3	−2.0 to 3.0	V_1	24 hr	32	1.3	−4.0 to 6.0
	0–2 yr	72	2.6	0.5 to 5.0		0–2 yr	16	−2.3	−4.5 to −0.5
	3–5	72	1.7	0.0 to 4.0		2–4	16	−2.2	−5.5 to −1.0
	6–10	72	2.0	0.5 to 4.0		8–10	16	−1.7	−3.0 to 1.5
	10–15	49	2.6	1.1 to 5.0		11–14	15	−1.3	−3.5 to 0.2
	Adults	500	3.0	1.0 to 5.0		Adults	151	0.2	−4.0 to 4.0
II	24 hr	41	1.2	0.0 to 3.0	V_2	24 hr	32	1.3	−7.5 to 9.0
	0–2 yr	72	2.4	1.0 to 4.0		0–2 yr	16	−2.4	−6.0 to 0.4
	3–5	72	1.8	0.5 to 4.0		2–4	16	−2.6	−7.0 to 3.0
	6–10	72	2.1	0.5 to 5.0		8–10	16	0.0	−3.5 to 3.0
	10–15	49	3.0	0.9 to 6.5		11–14	15	0.7	−1.5 to 3.5
	Adults	500	3.8	1.0 to 6.6		Adults	151	5.5	−3.0 to 18.0
III	24 hr	41	1.0	−1.0 to 3.0	V_3	24 hr	32	−0.4	−0.7 to 4.0
	0–2 yr	72	0.2	0.0 to 3.0		0–2 yr	16	−0.7	−5.0 to 4.5
	3–5	72	0.2	0.0 to 1.5		2–4	16	−0.7	−5.0 to 5.0
	6–10	72	0.1	0.0 to 1.0		8–10	16	1.8	−2.0 to 4.5
	10–15	49	0.4	−1.9 to 3.1		11–14	15	1.7	0.0 to 5.0
	Adults	500	0.8	−1.4 to 3.4		Adults	151	5.4	−2.0 to 16.0
aVR	24 hr	41	−0.4	−3.0 to 2.0	V_4	24 hr	32	−0.6	−7.0 to 3.0
	0–2 yr	16	−2.0	−3.0 to −0.5		0–2 yr	16	1.7	−2.5 to 5.0
	2–4	16	−2.5	−5.0 to −1.5		2–4	16	2.4	0.0 to 11.0
	8–10	16	−2.0	−3.5 to −0.2		8–10	16	3.2	0.0 to 9.0
	11–14	15	−2.2	−4.0 to −1.5		11–14	15	3.3	0.0 to 7.0
	Adults	151	−2.3	−5.0 to 1.5		Adults	151	4.8	0.0 to 17.0
aVL	24 hr	41	0.1	−1.5 to 2.0	V_5	24 hr	32	1.3	−4.0 to 5.0
	0–2 yr	16	0.7	−0.5 to 2.0		0–2 yr	16	2.6	1.2 to 5.5
	2–4	16	1.4	−0.5 to 3.0		2–4	16	3.4	0.0 to 7.0
	8–10	16	0.7	−1.0 to 2.5		8–10	16	4.1	0.5 to 11.0
	11–14	15	0.8	0.5 to 2.0		11–14	15	3.1	1.0 to 5.0
	Adults	151	0.5	−4.0 to 6.0		Adults	151	3.4	0.0 to 9.0
aVF	24 hr	41	0.9	−1.0 to 3.0	V_6	24 hr	32	1.2	−3.0 to 6.0
	0–2 yr	16	1.6	0.8 to 3.5		0–2 yr	16	2.2	0.5 to 4.0
	2–4	16	1.8	−0.2 to 4.0		2–4	16	3.2	1.5 to 5.0
	8–10	16	1.4	−0.2 to 3.0		8–10	16	3.1	0.0 to 8.0
	11–14	15	1.3	0.0 to 3.5		11–14	15	2.3	1.0 to 4.0
	Adults	151	1.7	−0.5 to 5.0		Adults	151	2.4	−0.5 to 5.0

SOURCE: Adapted from "Electrocardiographic Test Book," The American Heart Association Inc., 1956, by permission of The American Heart Association, Inc.

TABLE 8 NORMAL VALUES OF CORRECTED Q-T INTERVALS FOR VARIOUS AGES

Age	No. cases	Mean	Range
0–24 hr	32	0.42	0.37–0.53
0–2 yr	16	0.40	0.37–0.42
2–4	16	0.40	0.38–0.42
8–10	16	0.41	0.39–0.42
11–14	15	0.41	0.40–0.42
Adults	48	0.38	0.35–0.44

SOURCE: Adapted from "Electrocardiographic Test Book." The American Heart Association, Inc., 1956, by permission of The American Heart Association, Inc.

TABLE 9 SQUARE ROOT TABLE FOR CORRECTING Q-T INTERVAL FOR HEART RATE

Bazett formula: $\text{Q-Tc} = \dfrac{\text{Q-T (s)}}{\sqrt{\text{R-R interval (s)}}}$

R-R	$\sqrt{\text{R-R}}$	R-R	$\sqrt{\text{R-R}}$	R-R	$\sqrt{\text{R-R}}$	R-R	$\sqrt{\text{R-R}}$
0.40	0.63	0.61	0.78	0.83	0.91	1.04	1.01
0.41	0.64	0.62	0.78	0.84	0.91	1.05	1.02
0.42	0.64	0.63	0.79	0.85	0.92	1.06	1.02
0.43	0.65	0.64	0.80	0.86	0.92	1.07	1.03
0.44	0.66	0.65	0.80	0.87	0.93	1.08	1.03
0.45	0.67	0.66	0.81	0.88	0.93	1.09	1.04
0.46	0.67	0.67	0.81	0.89	0.94	1.10	1.04
0.47	0.68	0.68	0.82	0.90	0.94	1.11	1.05
0.48	0.69	0.69	0.83	0.91	0.95	1.12	1.05
0.49	0.70	0.70	0.83	0.92	0.95	1.13	1.06
0.50	0.70	0.71	0.84	0.93	0.96	1.14	1.06
0.51	0.71	0.73	0.85	0.95	0.97	1.16	1.07
0.52	0.72	0.74	0.86	0.96	0.97	1.17	1.08
0.53	0.72	0.75	0.86	0.97	0.98	1.18	1.08
0.54	0.73	0.76	0.87	0.98	0.98	1.19	1.09
0.55	0.74	0.77	0.87	0.99	0.99	1.20	1.09
0.56	0.74	0.78	0.88	1.00	1.00	1.21	1.10
0.57	0.75	0.79	0.88	1.00	1.00	1.22	1.10
0.58	0.76	0.80	0.89	1.01	1.00	1.23	1.10
0.59	0.76	0.81	0.90	1.02	1.00	1.24	1.11
0.60	0.77	0.82	0.90	1.03	1.01		

SOURCE: Adapted from "Electrocardiographic Test Book," The American Heart Association, Inc., 1956, by permission of The American Heart Association, Inc.

TABLE 10   Q-T INTERVAL
Normal range for various heart rates and cycle lengths

| | Lepeschkin | | Ashman | | | |
| | | | Means, s | | Upper limit of normal, s | |
Heart rate, min	Cycle length (R-R interval), s	Lower limit of normal, s	Men and children	Women	Men and children	Women
40	1.50	0.42	0.45	0.46	0.49	0.50
43	1.40	0.39	0.44	0.45	0.48	0.49
46	1.30	0.38	0.43	0.44	0.47	0.48
48	1.25	0.37	0.42	0.43	0.46	0.47
50	1.20	0.36	0.41	0.43	0.45	0.46
52	1.15	0.35	0.41	0.42	0.45	0.46
55	1.10	0.34	0.40	0.41	0.44	0.45
57	1.05	0.34	0.39	0.40	0.43	0.44
60	1.00	0.33	0.39	0.40	0.42	0.43
63	0.95	0.32	0.38	0.39	0.41	0.42
67	0.90	0.31	0.37	0.38	0.40	0.41
71	0.85	0.31	0.36	0.37	0.38	0.41
75	0.80	0.30	0.35	0.36	0.38	0.39
80	0.75	0.29	0.34	0.35	0.37	0.38
86	0.70	0.28	0.33	0.34	0.36	0.37
93	0.65	0.28	0.32	0.33	0.35	0.36
100	0.60	0.27	0.31	0.32	0.34	0.35
109	0.55	0.26	0.30	0.31	0.33	0.33
120	0.50	0.25	0.28	0.29	0.31	0.32
133	0.45	0.24	0.27	0.28	0.29	0.30
150	0.40	0.23	0.25	0.26	0.28	0.28
172	0.35	0.22	0.23	0.24	0.26	0.26

SOURCE: Adapted from "Electrocardiographic Test Book," The American Heart Association, Inc., 1956, by permission of The American Heart Association, Inc.

TABLE 11 DETERMINING HEART RATE FROM CYCLE LENGTH

C.L.*	Rate	C.L.*	Rate	C.L.*	Rate	C.L.*	Rate	C.L.*	Rate
.20	300	.48	125	.74	81	1.00	60	1.30	46
.24	250	.50	120	.76	79	1.02	59	1.32	45
.26	230	.52	115	.78	77	1.04	58	1.36	44
.28	214	.54	111	.80	75	1.06	56	1.40	43
.30	200	.56	107	.82	73	1.08	55	1.44	42
.32	188	.58	103	.84	71	1.10	54	1.48	41
.34	176	.60	100	.86	70	1.14	53	1.50	40
.36	167	.62	96	.88	68	1.16	52	1.52	39
.38	158	.64	94	.90	67	1.18	51	1.56	38
.40	150	.66	91	.92	65	1.20	50	1.60	37
.42	143	.68	88	.94	64	1.22	49	1.66	36
.44	136	.70	86	.96	62	1.26	48	1.72	35
.46	130	.72	83	.98	61	1.28	47	2.00	30

* C.L. = cycle length (P-P or R-R interval) in seconds.

TABLE 12 DETERMINING HEART RATE

Count the number of vertical time lines (1 mm = 0.04 s) between R waves or P waves and refer to the table—

mm	Rate	mm	Rate	mm	Rate	mm	Rate	mm	Rate	mm	Rate
3.0	500	8.75	171	14.5	103	20.5	73	32.5	46	54	28
3.25	462	9.0	167	14.75	102	21.0	71	33.0	45	55	27
3.5	428	9.25	162	15.0	100	21.5	70	34.0	44	56	27
3.75	400	9.5	158	15.25	98	22.0	68	35.0	43	57	26
4.0	375	9.75	154	15.5	97	22.5	67	36.0	42	58	26
4.25	353	10.0	150	15.75	95	23.0	65	37.0	41	59	25
4.5	334	10.25	146	16.0	94	23.5	64	37.5	40	60	25
4.75	316	10.5	143	16.25	92	24.0	63	38.0	39	61	25
5.0	300	10.75	140	16.5	91	24.5	61	39.0	38	62	24
5.25	286	11.0	136	16.75	90	25.0	60	40	38	63	24
5.5	273	11.25	133	17.0	88	25.5	59	41	37	64	23
5.75	261	11.5	130	17.25	87	26.0	58	42	36	65	23
6.0	250	11.75	128	17.5	86	26.5	57	43	35	66	23
6.25	240	12.0	125	17.75	85	27.0	56	44	34	67	22
6.5	231	12.25	123	18.0	83	27.5	55	45	33	68	22
6.75	222	12.5	120	18.25	82	28.0	54	46	33	69	22
7.0	214	12.75	118	18.5	81	28.5	53	47	32	70	21
7.25	207	13.0	115	18.75	80	29.0	52	48	31	71	21
7.5	200	13.25	113	19.0	79	29.5	51	49	31	72	21
7.75	194	13.5	111	19.25	78	30.0	50	50	30	73	20
8.0	188	13.75	109	19.5	77	30.5	49	51	30	74	20
8.25	182	14.0	107	19.75	76	31.0	48	52	29	75	20
8.5	176	14.25	105	20.0	75	32.0	47	53	28	76	20

TABLE 13 TRIPS IN MASTER DOUBLE (3-MIN) TWO-STEP EXERCISE TEST

Weight		Trips, males and females Age, yr													
Lb	Kg	15–19	20–24	25–29	30–34	35–39	40–44	45–49	50–54	55–59	60–64	65–69	70–74	75–79
50–59	22.7–26.8	64(64)												
60–69	27.2–31.3	62(60)												
70–79	31.8–35.8	60(58)												
80–89	36.3–40.4	56(56)	58(56)	58(56)	56(54)	54(52)	54(48)	52(46)	50(44)	50(42)	48(42)	46(40)	46(38)	44(36)
90–99	40.8–44.9	56(52)	56(54)	56(52)	54(50)	54(48)	52(46)	50(44)	50(44)	48(42)	46(40)	44(38)	44(38)	42(36)
100–109	45.4–49.4	54(50)	56(52)	56(52)	54(50)	52(48)	50(46)	50(44)	48(42)	46(40)	44(38)	44(36)	42(36)	40(34)
110–119	49.9–54.0	52(46)	54(50)	54(50)	52(48)	50(46)	48(44)	48(42)	46(40)	44(38)	44(36)	42(36)	40(32)	40(32)
120–129	54.4–58.5	50(44)	52(48)	54(48)	52(46)	50(44)	48(42)	46(40)	44(38)	42(36)	42(36)	40(34)	40(32)	38(30)
130–139	59.0–63.0	48(40)	50(46)	52(46)	50(44)	48(42)	46(40)	46(38)	44(38)	42(36)	40(34)	38(32)	38(30)	36(30)
140–149	63.5–67.6	46(38)	48(44)	50(44)	48(42)	48(40)	46(38)	44(38)	42(36)	40(34)	38(32)	38(32)	36(30)	36(28)
150–159	68.0–72.1	44(34)	48(42)	48(38)	43(40)	46(38)	44(38)	42(36)	40(34)	38(32)	36(30)	36(30)	36(28)	34(26)
160–169	72.6–76.7	42(32)	46(40)	48(38)	45(38)	44(36)	44(36)	42(34)	40(32)	36(30)	36(30)	36(28)	34(26)	34(24)
170–179	77.1–81.2	40(28)	44(38)	46(36)	45(36)	44(34)	42(34)	40(32)	38(32)	36(30)	36(28)	34(26)	34(26)	32(24)
180–189	81.6–85.7	38(26)	42(36)	46(34)	44(34)	42(34)	40(32)	38(32)	38(30)	36(28)	34(28)	32(26)	32(24)	30(22)
190–199	86.2–90.3	36(24)	40(34)	44(32)	42(32)	42(32)	40(30)	38(30)	36(28)	34(26)	32(26)	30(24)	30(24)	28(22)
200–209	90.7–94.8		38(32)	42(30)	42(30)	40(30)	38(28)	36(28)	34(26)	32(26)	32(24)	30(22)	28(22)	28(20)
210–219	95.3–99.4		36(30)	42(28)	40(28)	38(28)	36(26)	34(26)	34(26)	32(24)	30(22)	28(22)	28(22)	26(20)
220–229	99.8–103.9		34(28)	40(26)	40(26)	38(26)	36(26)	34(24)	32(24)	30(22)	28(22)	26(20)	26(20)	24(18)

Source: Adapted from A. M. Master and I. Rosenfeld, N.Y. State J. Med., 61: 1850, 1961, by permission.

DIRECTIONS FOR USING TABLES 14 AND 15 FOR DETERMINING THE ELECTRICAL AXIS

1   Using the amplitudes of the deflections, calculate the algebraic sum of the positive and negative waves in lead I.   If the sum is positive, use Table 14; if negative, use Table 15.
2   Determine the algebraic sum of the positive and negative waves in lead III.
3   Plot the values obtained under the appropriate headings.   The intersection of the lead I and lead III columns is the electrical axis in degrees.

TABLE 14

Lead III Positive										Lead I Positive												
	0.0	0.5	1.0	1.5	2.0	2.5	3.0	3.5	4.0	4.5	5.0	6.0	7.0	8.0	9.0	10.0	11.0	12.0	13.0	14.0	15.0	20.0
0.0		30	30	30	30	30	30	30	30	30	30	30	30	30	30	30	30	30	30	30	30	30
0.5	90	60	49	44	41	39	38	37	36	35	35	34	33	33	33	32	32	32	32	32	32	31
1.0	90	71	60	53	49	46	44	42	41	40	39	38	37	36	35	35	34	34	34	33	33	32
1.5	90	76	67	60	55	52	49	47	45	44	43	41	39	38	38	37	36	36	36	35	35	33
2.0	90	79	71	65	60	56	53	51	49	47	46	44	42	41	40	39	38	38	37	37	36	35
2.5	90	81	74	68	64	60	57	54	52	51	49	47	45	43	42	41	40	39	39	38	38	36
3.0	90	82	76	71	67	63	60	57	55	53	52	49	47	45	44	43	42	41	40	39	39	37
3.5	90	83	78	73	69	66	63	60	58	56	54	51	49	47	46	44	43	42	42	41	40	38
4.0	90	84	79	75	71	68	65	62	60	58	56	53	51	49	47	46	45	44	43	42	42	39
4.5	90	85	80	76	73	69	67	64	62	60	58	55	53	51	49	48	47	45	44	43	43	40
5.0	90	85	81	77	74	71	68	66	64	62	60	57	55	52	51	49	48	47	46	45	44	41
6.0	90	86	82	79	76	73	71	69	67	65	63	60	57	55	53	52	50	49	48	47	46	43
7.0	90	87	83	81	78	75	73	71	69	67	65	63	60	58	56	54	53	51	50	49	48	44
8.0	90	87	84	82	79	77	75	73	71	69	68	65	62	60	58	56	55	53	52	51	50	46
9.0	90	87	85	82	80	78	76	74	73	71	69	67	64	62	60	58	57	55	54	53	52	48
10.0	90	88	85	83	81	79	77	76	74	72	71	68	66	64	62	60	58	57	56	54	53	49
11.0	90	88	86	84	82	80	78	77	75	73	72	70	67	65	63	62	60	59	57	56	55	50
12.0	90	88	86	84	82	81	79	78	76	75	73	71	69	67	65	63	61	60	59	57	56	52
13.0	90	88	86	84	83	81	80	78	77	76	74	72	70	68	66	64	63	61	60	59	58	53
14.0	90	88	87	85	83	82	80	79	78	77	75	73	71	69	67	66	64	63	61	60	59	55
15.0	90	88	87	85	84	82	81	80	78	77	76	74	72	70	68	67	65	64	62	61	60	55
20.0	90	89	88	87	85	84	83	82	81	80	79	77	76	74	72	71	70	68	67	65	65	60

TABLE 14 (continued)

Lead III Negative	0.0	0.5	1.0	1.5	2.0	2.5	3.0	3.5	4.0	4.5	5.0	6.0	7.0	8.0	9.0	10.0	11.0	12.0	13.0	14.0	15.0	20.0
0.0		30	30	30	30	30	30	30	30	30	30	30	30	30	30	30	30	30	30	30	30	30
0.5	-90	-30	0	11	16	19	21	22	23	24	25	26	26	27	27	27	28	28	28	28	28	29
1.0	-90	-60	-30	-11	0	7	11	14	16	18	19	21	22	23	24	25	25	26	26	26	27	27
1.5	-90	-71	-49	-30	-16	-7	0	5	7	11	13	16	18	20	21	22	23	23	24	24	25	26
2.0	-90	-76	-60	-44	-30	-19	-11	-5	0	4	7	11	14	16	18	19	20	21	22	22	23	25
2.5	-90	-79	-67	-53	-41	-30	-21	-14	-8	-4	0	6	9	12	14	16	17	19	20	20	21	23
3.0	-90	-81	-71	-60	-49	-39	-30	-22	-16	-11	-7	0	5	8	11	13	15	16	17	18	19	22
3.5	-90	-82	-74	-65	-55	-46	-38	-30	-23	-18	-13	-6	0	4	7	10	12	14	15	16	17	21
4.0	-90	-83	-76	-68	-60	-52	-44	-37	-30	-24	-19	-11	-5	0	4	7	9	11	13	14	15	19
4.5	-90	-84	-78	-71	-64	-56	-49	-42	-36	-30	-25	-16	-9	-4	0	3	6	8	10	12	13	18
5.0	-90	-85	-79	-73	-67	-60	-53	-47	-41	-35	-30	-21	-14	-8	-4	0	3	6	8	9	11	16
6.0	-90	-86	-81	-76	-71	-66	-60	-54	-49	-44	-39	-30	-22	-16	-11	-7	-3	0	3	5	7	13
7.0	-90	-86	-82	-78	-74	-69	-65	-60	-55	-51	-46	-38	-30	-23	-18	-13	-9	-6	-3	0	2	10
8.0	-90	-87	-83	-80	-76	-72	-68	-64	-60	-56	-52	-44	-37	-30	-24	-19	-15	-11	-8	-5	-2	7
9.0	-90	-87	-84	-81	-78	-74	-71	-67	-64	-60	-56	-49	-42	-36	-30	-25	-20	-16	-13	-9	-7	3
10.0	-90	-87	-85	-82	-79	-76	-73	-70	-67	-63	-60	-53	-47	-41	-35	-30	-25	-21	-17	-14	-11	0
11.0	-90	-88	-85	-83	-80	-77	-75	-72	-69	-66	-63	-57	-51	-45	-40	-35	-30	-26	-22	-18	-15	-3
12.0	-90	-88	-86	-83	-81	-79	-76	-74	-71	-68	-66	-60	-54	-49	-44	-39	-34	-30	-26	-22	-19	-7
13.0	-90	-88	-86	-84	-82	-80	-77	-75	-73	-70	-68	-63	-57	-52	-47	-43	-38	-34	-30	-26	-23	-10
14.0	-90	-88	-86	-84	-82	-80	-78	-76	-74	-72	-69	-65	-60	-55	-51	-46	-42	-38	-34	-30	-27	-13
15.0	-90	-88	-87	-85	-83	-81	-79	-77	-75	-73	-71	-67	-62	-58	-53	-49	-45	-41	-37	-33	-30	-16
20.0	-90	-89	-87	-86	-85	-83	-82	-81	-79	-78	-76	-73	-70	-67	-63	-60	-57	-53	-50	-47	-44	-30

Lead I Positive

SOURCE: Adapted from the "Electrocardiographic Test Book," The American Heart Association, Inc., 1956, by permission of The American Heart Association, Inc.

TABLE 15

Lead I Negative

Lead III Negative	0.0	0.5	1.0	1.5	2.0	2.5	3.0	3.5	4.0	4.5	5.0	6.0	7.0	8.0	9.0	10.0	11.0	12.0	13.0	14.0	15.0	20.0
0.0	-150	-150	-150	-150	-150	-150	-150	-150	-150	-150	-150	-150	-150	-150	-150	-150	-150	-150	-150	-150	-150	-150
0.5	-90	-120	-131	-136	-139	-141	-142	-143	-144	-145	-145	-146	-147	-147	-147	-148	-148	-148	-148	-148	-148	-149
1.0	-90	-109	-120	-127	-131	-134	-136	-138	-139	-140	-141	-142	-143	-144	-145	-145	-146	-146	-146	-147	-147	-148
1.5	-90	-104	-113	-120	-125	-128	-131	-133	-135	-136	-137	-139	-141	-142	-142	-143	-144	-144	-144	-145	-145	-147
2.0	-90	-101	-109	-115	-120	-124	-127	-129	-131	-133	-134	-136	-138	-139	-140	-141	-142	-142	-143	-143	-144	-145
2.5	-90	-99	-106	-112	-116	-120	-123	-126	-128	-129	-131	-133	-135	-137	-138	-139	-140	-141	-141	-142	-142	-144
3.0	-90	-98	-104	-109	-113	-117	-120	-123	-125	-127	-128	-131	-133	-135	-136	-137	-138	-139	-140	-141	-141	-144
3.5	-90	-97	-102	-107	-111	-114	-117	-120	-122	-124	-126	-129	-131	-133	-134	-136	-137	-138	-138	-139	-140	-143
4.0	-90	-96	-101	-105	-109	-112	-115	-118	-120	-122	-124	-127	-129	-131	-133	-134	-135	-136	-137	-138	-138	-142
4.5	-90	-95	-100	-104	-107	-111	-113	-116	-118	-120	-122	-125	-127	-129	-131	-132	-133	-135	-136	-137	-137	-141
5.0	-90	-95	-99	-103	-106	-109	-112	-114	-116	-118	-120	-123	-125	-128	-129	-131	-132	-133	-134	-135	-136	-140
6.0	-90	-94	-98	-101	-104	-107	-109	-111	-113	-115	-117	-120	-123	-125	-127	-128	-130	-131	-132	-133	-134	-139
7.0	-90	-93	-97	-99	-102	-105	-107	-109	-111	-113	-115	-117	-120	-123	-124	-126	-127	-129	-130	-131	-132	-137
8.0	-90	-93	-96	-98	-101	-103	-105	-107	-109	-111	-112	-115	-118	-120	-122	-124	-125	-127	-128	-129	-130	-136
9.0	-90	-93	-95	-97	-100	-102	-104	-106	-107	-109	-111	-113	-116	-118	-120	-122	-123	-125	-126	-127	-128	-134
10.0	-90	-92	-95	-96	-99	-101	-103	-105	-106	-108	-108	-112	-114	-116	-118	-120	-122	-123	-124	-126	-127	-132
11.0	-90	-92	-94	-96	-98	-100	-102	-103	-105	-107	-107	-110	-113	-115	-117	-118	-120	-121	-123	-124	-125	-130
12.0	-90	-92	-94	-96	-97	-99	-101	-102	-104	-105	-106	-109	-111	-113	-115	-117	-119	-120	-121	-123	-124	-128
13.0	-90	-92	-94	-95	-97	-99	-100	-102	-103	-104	-105	-108	-110	-112	-114	-116	-117	-119	-120	-121	-122	-127
14.0	-90	-92	-93	-95	-97	-98	-100	-101	-102	-103	-104	-107	-109	-111	-113	-114	-116	-117	-119	-120	-121	-125
15.0	-90	-92	-93	-95	-96	-98	-99	-100	-102	-103	-104	-106	-108	-110	-112	-113	-115	-116	-118	-119	-120	-125
20.0	-90	-91	-92	-93	-95	-96	-97	-98	-99	-100	-101	-103	-104	-106	-108	-109	-110	-112	-113	-115	-115	-102

TABLE 15 (continued)

Lead III Positive	Lead I Negative																					
	0.0	0.5	1.0	1.5	2.0	2.5	3.0	3.5	4.0	4.5	5.0	6.0	7.0	8.0	9.0	10.0	11.0	12.0	13.0	14.0	15.0	20.0
0.0		−150	−150	−150	−150	−150	−150	−150	−150	−150	−150	−150	−150	−150	−150	−150	−150	−150	−150	−150	−150	−150
0.5	90	150	180	−169	−164	−161	−159	−158	−157	−156	−155	−154	−154	−153	−153	−153	−152	−152	−152	−152	−152	−151
1.0	90	120	150	169	180	−173	−169	−166	−164	−162	−161	−159	−158	−157	−156	−155	−155	−154	−154	−154	−153	−153
1.5	90	109	131	150	164	173	180	−175	−172	−169	−167	−164	−162	−160	−159	−158	−157	−157	−156	−156	−155	−154
2.0	90	104	120	136	150	161	169	175	180	−176	−173	−169	−166	−164	−162	−161	−160	−159	−158	−158	−157	−155
2.5	90	101	113	127	139	150	159	166	172	176	180	−174	−171	−168	−166	−164	−163	−161	−160	−160	−159	−157
3.0	90	99	109	120	131	141	150	158	164	169	173	180	−175	−172	−169	−167	−165	−164	−163	−162	−161	−158
3.5	90	98	106	115	125	134	142	150	157	162	167	174	180	−176	−173	−170	−168	−166	−165	−164	−163	−159
4.0	90	97	104	112	120	128	136	143	150	156	161	169	175	180	−176	−173	−171	−169	−167	−166	−165	−161
4.5	90	96	102	109	116	124	131	138	144	150	155	164	171	176	180	−177	−174	−172	−170	−168	−167	−162
5.0	90	95	101	107	113	120	127	133	139	145	150	159	166	172	176	180	−177	−174	−172	−171	−169	−164
6.0	90	94	99	104	109	114	120	126	131	136	141	150	158	164	169	173	177	180	−177	−175	−173	−167
7.0	90	94	98	102	106	111	115	120	125	129	134	142	150	157	162	167	171	174	177	180	−178	−170
8.0	90	93	97	100	104	108	112	116	120	124	128	136	143	150	156	161	165	169	172	175	178	−173
9.0	90	93	96	99	102	106	109	113	116	120	124	131	138	144	150	155	160	164	167	171	173	−177
10.0	90	93	95	98	101	104	107	110	113	117	120	127	133	139	145	150	155	159	163	166	169	180
11.0	90	92	95	97	100	103	105	108	111	114	117	123	129	135	140	145	150	154	158	162	165	177
12.0	90	92	94	97	99	101	104	106	109	112	114	120	126	131	136	141	146	150	154	158	161	173
13.0	90	92	94	96	98	100	103	105	107	110	112	117	123	128	133	137	142	146	150	154	157	170
14.0	90	92	94	96	98	100	102	104	106	108	111	115	120	125	129	134	138	142	146	150	153	167
15.0	90	92	93	95	97	99	101	103	105	107	109	113	118	122	127	131	135	139	143	147	150	164
20.0	90	91	93	94	95	97	98	99	101	102	104	107	110	113	117	120	123	127	130	133	136	150

DIRECTIONS FOR USING TABLE 16*

1 Choose one of the following sets of axes:
a aVL and II
b aVR and III
c aVF and I
2 Using the net areas of the deflections, calculate the algebraic sum of the positive and negative waves, rounded to the nearest integer, on each lead of the set selected.   Alternatively, the net amplitudes may be utilized if the QRS complexes have similar contours and durations.   If the absolute values are too large for the table, divide the value for each lead in the set by two.
3 Use Table 16 to obtain the angle θ.   The absolute values for aVL, aVR, and aVF are listed in the side column; those for II, III, and I are listed on the top row.
4 Calculate the angle θ_{QRS} using the equations listed in the table, with due consideration for the proper sign $(+$ or $-)$.
5 Average the angle θ_{QRS} as determined for each of the three sets of leads. This probably ensures maximum accuracy.

*Note: The values for the augmented unipolar leads have been multiplied by 1.15 in the table for greater accuracy.

TABLE 16

Use side column for aVL, aVR, aVF; use top row for II, III, I

	1	2	3	4	5	6	7	8	9	10	11	12	13	14	15	16	17	18	19	20	21	22	23	24	25	26	27	28	29	30
1	41	60	69	74	77	79	81	82	83	83	84	85	85	85	86	86	86	86	87	87	87	87	87	87	87	87	88	88	88	88
2	23	41	53	60	65	69	72	74	76	77	78	79	80	81	81	82	82	83	83	83	84	84	84	85	85	85	85	85	85	86
3	16	30	41	49	55	60	64	67	69	71	73	74	75	76	77	78	79	79	80	80	81	81	81	82	82	82	83	83	83	83
4	12	23	33	41	47	53	57	60	63	65	67	69	71	72	73	74	75	76	76	77	78	78	79	79	80	80	80	81	81	81
5	10	19	28	35	41	46	51	54	57	60	62	64	66	68	69	70	71	72	73	74	75	75	76	77	77	78	78	78	79	79
6	8	16	23	30	36	41	45	49	53	55	58	60	62	64	65	67	68	69	70	71	72	73	73	74	75	75	76	76	77	77
7	7	14	20	26	32	37	41	45	48	51	54	56	58	60	62	63	65	66	67	68	69	70	71	71	72	73	73	74	74	75
8	6	12	18	23	29	33	37	41	44	47	50	53	55	57	58	60	62	63	64	65	66	67	68	69	70	71	71	72	72	73
9	6	11	16	21	26	30	34	38	41	44	47	49	51	54	55	57	59	60	61	63	64	65	66	67	68	68	69	70	70	71
10	5	10	15	19	24	28	31	35	38	41	44	46	49	51	53	54	56	57	59	60	61	62	63	64	65	66	67	68	69	69
11	5	9	13	18	22	25	29	32	35	38	41	43	46	48	50	52	53	55	56	58	59	60	61	62	63	64	65	66	66	67
12	4	8	12	16	20	23	27	30	33	36	39	41	43	45	47	49	51	53	54	55	57	58	59	60	61	62	63	64	65	65
13	4	8	11	15	18	22	25	28	31	34	36	39	41	43	45	47	49	50	52	53	55	56	57	58	59	60	61	62	63	64
14	4	7	11	14	17	20	23	26	29	32	34	37	39	41	43	45	47	48	50	51	53	54	56	57	58	60	60	61	61	62
15	3	7	10	13	16	19	22	25	28	30	33	35	37	39	41	43	45	46	48	49	51	52	54	55	57	58	59	60	60	61
16	3	6	9	12	15	18	21	23	26	29	31	33	35	37	39	41	43	44	46	47	49	50	52	53	54	55	57	57	58	58
17	3	6	9	12	14	17	20	22	25	27	30	32	34	36	38	39	41	43	44	45	47	49	50	51	52	53	54	55	56	57
18	3	6	8	11	14	16	19	21	23	26	28	30	32	34	36	38	39	41	43	44	45	47	48	49	50	51	53	54	54	55
19	3	5	8	10	13	15	18	20	22	25	27	29	31	33	34	36	38	39	41	42	44	45	46	48	49	50	51	51	52	53
20	2	5	7	10	12	15	17	19	21	23	26	28	29	31	33	35	36	38	40	41	42	44	45	46	47	49	50	51	51	52
21	2	5	7	9	12	14	16	18	20	22	24	26	28	30	31	33	35	37	38	39	41	42	44	45	45	47	48	49	50	51
22	2	5	7	9	11	14	15	18	20	22	23	25	27	29	30	32	34	35	37	38	40	41	42	43	44	45	47	48	48	50
23	2	4	6	9	11	13	15	17	19	21	23	24	26	28	29	31	32	34	36	37	39	40	41	42	43	44	45	46	47	48
24	2	4	6	8	10	12	14	16	18	20	22	23	25	26	28	30	31	33	35	36	38	39	40	41	42	43	44	45	46	47
25	2	4	6	8	10	12	14	16	17	19	21	23	24	25	27	29	30	32	34	35	37	38	39	40	41	42	43	44	45	46
26	2	4	6	8	9	11	13	15	17	18	20	22	23	25	26	28	29	31	33	34	36	37	38	39	40	41	42	43	44	45
27	2	4	6	8	9	11	13	15	16	18	20	22	23	24	25	27	28	30	32	33	35	36	37	38	39	40	41	42	43	44
28	2	3	5	7	9	11	12	14	16	17	19	21	22	23	25	26	28	29	31	32	34	35	36	37	38	39	40	41	42	42
29	2	3	5	7	9	10	12	14	15	16	18	20	21	23	24	26	27	28	30	31	33	34	35	36	37	38	39	40	41	42
30	2	3	5	7	8	10	11	13	15	16	18	19	21	22	23	25	26	28	29	30	31	33	34	35	36	37	38	39	40	41

aVL	II	θ_{QRS}
+	+	$\theta - 30$
+	−	$150 - \theta$
−	−	$150 + \theta, \theta < 30$
		$\theta - 20, \theta \geq 30$
+	−	$-30 - \theta$

aVR	III	θ_{QRS}
+	+	$210 - \theta, \theta \geq 30$
		$-150 - \theta, \theta < 30$
−	+	$30 + \theta$
+	−	$\theta - 150$
+	−	$30 - \theta$

aVF	I	θ_{QRS}
+	+	$90 - \theta$
−	+	$-90 + \theta$
−	−	$-90 - \theta$
+	−	$90 + \theta$

SOURCE: Adapted from S. Laiken, N. Laiken, R. A. O'Rourke, and J. S. Karliner, A Rapid Method for Frontal Plane Axis Determination in Scalar Electrocardiograms, *Am. Heart J.*, 85:620, 1973, by permission.

TABLE 17   MAXIMAL P, QRS, AND T VECTORS IN FRONTAL, SAGITTAL, AND HORIZONTAL PLANES TOGETHER WITH SPATIAL AMPLITUDE AND ORIENTATION*

	Maximal P vector	Maximal QRS vector	Maximal T vector
Frontal plane			
Amplitude, mV	0.18 ± 0.06	157 ± 0.42	0.36 ± 0.14
	$0.08 \rightarrow 0.31$	$0.81 \rightarrow 2.53$	$0.12 \rightarrow 0.69$
Direction, degrees	67 ± 18	41 ± 14	40 ± 20
	$22 \rightarrow 91$	$14 \rightarrow 71$	$4 \rightarrow 74$
Sagittal plane			
Amplitude, mV	0.17 ± 0.06	1.32 ± 0.45	0.36 ± 0.13
	$0.06 \rightarrow 0.31$	$0.60 \rightarrow 2.42$	$0.13 \rightarrow 0.67$
Direction, degrees	87 ± 23	48 ± 30	142 ± 23
	$54 \rightarrow 129$	$343 \rightarrow 114$	$93 \rightarrow 180$
Horizontal plane			
Amplitude, mV	0.09 ± 0.03	1.39 ± 0.36	0.40 ± 0.14
	$0.04 \rightarrow 0.14$	$0.74 \rightarrow 2.19$	$0.15 \rightarrow 0.72$
Direction, degrees	349 ± 41	327 ± 34	46 ± 19
	$285 \rightarrow 91$	$245 \rightarrow 29$	$8 \rightarrow 83$
Spatial amplitude mV	0.18 ± 0.06	1.73 ± 0.44	0.46 ± 0.16
	$0.09 \rightarrow 0.32$	$0.92 \rightarrow 2.75$	$0.18 \rightarrow 0.82$
Spatial orientation			
Azimuth, degrees	342 ± 38	331 ± 27	44 ± 19
	$277 \rightarrow 75$	$263 \rightarrow 23$	$4 \rightarrow 79$
Elevation, degrees	63 ± 17	35 ± 13	29 ± 13
	$20 \rightarrow 86$	$7 \rightarrow 60$	$2 \rightarrow 58$

* The vectors in the plane projections were obtained from XY, YZ, and XZ leads, respectively, and therefore do not represent projections of the spatial maximal vectors onto these planes. SOURCE: Adapted from H. W. Draper, C. J. Peffer, F. W. Stallmann, D. Littman, and H. V. Pipberger, The Corrected Orthogonal Electrocardiogram and Vectorcardiogram in 510 Normal Men (Frank Lead System), *Circulation*, 30:853, 1964, by permission of the American Heart Association, Inc.

TABLE 18   QUANTITATIVE ANALYSIS OF EARLY QRS VECTORS*

Instantaneous vectors	Scalar amplitude, mV			Planar direction, degrees		
	X	Y	Z	Frontal	Sagittal	Horizontal
0.01 s after	-0.04 ± 0.04	-0.03 ± 0.06	-0.11 ± 0.06	210 ± 61	189 ± 36	110 ± 34
QRS onset	$-0.14 \rightarrow 0.07$	$-0.13 \rightarrow 0.08$	$-0.25 \rightarrow 0.01$	$59 \rightarrow 330$	$79 \rightarrow 242$	$17 \rightarrow 168$
0.02 s after	0.05 ± 0.14	-0.01 ± 0.12	-0.31 ± 0.15	325 ± 87	180 ± 25	81 ± 26
QRS onset	$-0.19 \rightarrow 0.38$	$-0.25 \rightarrow 0.29$	$-0.68 \rightarrow -0.06$	$162 \rightarrow 136$	$117 \rightarrow 220$	$23 \rightarrow 124$
0.03 s after	0.56 ± 0.27	0.35 ± 0.25	-0.20 ± 0.32	29 ± 23	120 ± 40	21 ± 30
QRS onset	$0.06 \rightarrow 1.19$	$-0.06 \rightarrow 0.97$	$-0.89 \rightarrow 0.48$	$350 \rightarrow 59$	$41 \rightarrow 186$	$319 \rightarrow 79$
0.04 s after	1.05 ± 0.37	0.86 ± 0.37	0.34 ± 0.46	40 ± 16	72 ± 27	343 ± 25
QRS onset	$0.33 \rightarrow 1.79$	$0.24 \rightarrow 1.79$	$-0.59 \rightarrow 1.26$	$14 \rightarrow 66$	$28 \rightarrow 139$	$294 \rightarrow 35$
0.05 s after	0.65 ± 0.51	0.74 ± 0.47	0.77 ± 0.40	52 ± 36	42 ± 24	307 ± 28
QRS onset	$-0.27 \rightarrow 1.76$	$-0.09 \rightarrow 1.74$	$-0.01 \rightarrow 1.67$	$343 \rightarrow 147$	$351 \rightarrow 89$	$248 \rightarrow 1$

* The mean and standard deviation of each item are shown on the upper line. The second line indicates the limits of a 96-percentile range.
SOURCE: Adapted from H. W. Draper, C. J. Peffer, F. W. Stallmann, D. Littman, and H. V. Pipberger, The Corrected Orthogonal Electrocardiogram and Vectorcardiogram in 510 Normal Men (Frank Lead System), *Circulation,* 30:853, 1964, by permission of the American Heart Association, Inc.

INDEX

INDEX

A wave, 105, 106
Aberrant atrial conduction, 423, 448
Aberrant ventricular conduction, 426–431, 444–449, 462, 466–467, 474–477, 526–527, 539, 544, 560
  in atrial fibrillation, 470–477
  definition of, 444
  in parasystole, 547–548
  QRS complexes, 445–449
  ventricular ectopy and, differential diagnosis between, 446, 448–449, 470–474
Accessory AV connection, 228
Accrochage, 529
Acecainide hydrochloride, 336
Acidosis, 348
Action potentials (see Potentials, transmembrane)
Activation (see Depolarization)
Acute myocarditis, 262
African endomyocardial fibrosis, 373–374
Afterpotentials, 448
A-H time, 107
Alcoholic cardiomyopathy, 265
Alkalosis, 348
Allorhythmia, definition of, 419
Amiodarone hydrochloride, 336
Amyloidosis, 373
AN (atrionodal) region, 22, 24, 26
Anatomic axis, electrical axis and, 96–97

Aneurysm, ventricular, 258, 259
Angina, preinfarction, 308, 309
Angina pectoris, 307–308
  variant pattern of (Prinzmetal's angina), 307, 308
Angles of vectors, nomenclature of, 113
Angular measurements, 113
Anterior infarction (see Myocardial infarction, anterior)
Anteroposterior axis, 94–95
Antidepressant drugs, 334–335
Aorta, 23
  coarctation of, 392
Aortic atresia, 392
Aortic stenosis, congenital, 391
Aortic valve, 23
Aprindine hydrochloride, 336
Arrhythmias:
  atrial, 458–477
  AV junctional, 489–502
  AV ladder diagrams for, 419–421
  capture beats (see Capture beats)
  clinical classification of, 418
  conduction disturbances in (see Conduction, in arrhythmias)
  ectopic beats (see Ectopic beats)
  fibrillation (see Fibrillation)
  flutter (see Flutter)
  fusion beats (see Fusion beats)
  in myocardial infarction, 258

Arrhythmias (*Cont.*):
  physiological basis of, 403–418
    concealed conduction, 411–412
    decremental conduction, 409–410
    electrocardiogram and action potentials of cardiac cells, relationship between, 413–415
    impulse conduction, disturbances in, 408–412
    impulse formation, disturbances in, 407–408
    inhomogeneous conduction, 410–411
    normal cardiac automaticity, 405–407
    refractory period, 415–418
    supernormality, 411
    transmembrane potential of cardiac cells, 403–405
    unidirectional block, 412–413
  premature systoles (*see* Premature systoles)
  sinus, 425–426, 454–455
  supraventricular (*see* Supraventricular arrhythmias)
  terminology of, 419
  ventricular, 313, 502–514
  (*See also* Bradycardias; Tachycardias; *and specific arrhythmias*)
Ashman phenomenon, 555
Asymmetric septal hypertrophy, 276
Athletes, abnormalities in, 269–273
Atria, 22
Atrial abnormality (atrial enlargement or hypertrophy):
  combined (biatrial abnormality), 133
    vectorcardiogram in, 137
  left: diagnosis, 130–133
    in left ventricular enlargement, 148–149
    vectorcardiogram, 137
  Macruz index for diagnosis of, 133–134
  right: diagnosis, 129–130
    right ventricular enlargement, 161
    vectorcardiogram, 137
  theoretical considerations, 128–129
Atrial conduction, aberrant, 423, 448
Atrial conduction time, 59
Atrial depolarization, 21, 50–52, 59
Atrial dissociation:
  atrial parasystole distinguished from, 549–550
  atrial rhythms in, 549
Atrial echo, 430
  (*See also* Reciprocal beats and rhythms)
Atrial enlargement (*see* Atrial abnormality)
Atrial escape beats, 441–442

Atrial fibrillation, 468–477
  aberrant ventricular conduction in, 470–471, 475
  AV dissociation in, 469–470, 532
  ventricular ectopy in, 471, 474
  in W-P-W syndrome, 231, 233, 235
Atrial flutter, 464–468
  AV dissociation in, 532
  in W-P-W syndrome, 231, 235
Atrial fusion beats, 443, 499, 530, 544
Atrial hypertrophy (*see* Atrial abnormality)
Atrial infarction, 134–136
  diagnostic criteria for, 136
Atrial injury, 134–136
  diagnostic criteria for, 136
Atrial leads, 99
Atrial pacing, effect of, 107–108
Atrial parasystole, atrial dissociation distinguished from, 549–550
Atrial paroxysmal tachycardia, 459–464
  automatic ectopic, 459–460, 462
    versus PSVT, 486–489
  with block, 460–462
  multifocal (chaotic), 463–464
  (*See also* Reentrant paroxysmal supraventricular tachycardia)
Atrial premature beats, concealment of, 554
Atrial premature systoles, 421–424, 426–430, 458
  clinical significance, 424–425
Atrial reciprocal beats, 536
Atrial repolarization, 21, 52, 62–63
Atrial rhythm, 458–459
Atrial septal defect, 158, 371, 394–395
Atrial standstill, 477
Atrial tachycardia, reentrant, paroxysmal, 477–478
  (*See also* Reentrant paroxysmal supraventricular tachycardia)
Atriofascicular bypass tract, 228
Atrionodal (AN) region, 22, 24, 26
Atrioventricular (*see entries commencing with* AV)
Atropine:
  conduction affected by, 335
    W-P-W syndrome, 235
  electrocardiographic changes produced by, 334
Atypical AV nodal reentrant tachycardia, 488
Auricle, left, 23
Automatic atrial tachycardia, 488
Automatic cells, 405–406

Automatic ectopic supraventricular tachy-cardia, 459–460
  vs. reentrant paroxysmal supraventricular tachycardia, 486–489
Automaticity, normal cardiac, 405–407
AV block (heart block), 562–578
  AV dissociation due to, 527–528, 532–533
  congenital, 573
  decremental conduction as cause of, 409–410
  diagnosis of, 577–578
  first-degree, 63, 409, 563, 565–566, 576
  incomplete, 565–572
  refractory periods in various types of, 415–418
  second-degree, 563, 566–572, 576
    advanced (high-grade), 571
    Mobitz Type I, 568–570
    Mobitz Type II, 217, 564, 570–571
    2:1, 571–572
  third-degree (complete), 572–576
    acute, 573
    anatomic bases of, 572–574
    chronic, 573
    permanent, 572
  unidirectional (see Unidirectional block)
AV bundle, 22–26, 31
  electrograms (see His bundle electrograms)
  potential, 106, 107
AV conduction, 32, 33
  anomalous, 32
    in W-P-W syndrome (see Wolf-Parkin-son-White syndrome)
  in atrial flutter, 464–468
  bundle branch block and, relationship be-tween, 215
AV dissociation, 522–533
  in atrial fibrillation, 469–470, 532
  AV block as cause of, 528, 532
  capture beats and, 529, 531, 532
  complete, 528, 532
  in ectopic tachycardias, 533
  etiology, 526–527
  fusion beats and, 530
  incomplete, 528, 531
  interference: AV dissociation due primarily to, 530–532
    meanings of term, 523–526
  isorhythmic, 529
  mechanism, 527–528
  salient features of, 529
  in sinus rhythms, 530–532
AV dissociation (Cont.):
  synchronization and, 529
  terminology, 522–524
AV excitation, anomalous, 228
AV junction:
  unidirectional block and macroreentry in, 412
  wandering pacemaker between SA node and, 455
AV junctional arrhythmias, 489–502
  (See also specific arrhythmias)
AV junctional escape (see Escape beats)
AV junctional premature beats, concealment of, 554
AV junctional premature systoles, 421–423, 430–431
  clinical significance of, 425
AV junctional reciprocal beats, 538–541
AV junctional rhythms, 421, 489–492
  upper, middle, and lower, 489–490
AV junctional tachycardia:
  automatic ectopic, 492–494
  nonparoxysmal, 494
  reentrant (PSVT), 477–480
AV ladder diagrams for arrhythmias, 419–421
AV membranous septum, 23
AV nodal reentrant tachycardia, 488
AV nodal rhythms (see AV junctional rhythms)
AV node, 22–23, 26, 29, 31
  bypass tracts and, relationship between, 32
  decremental conduction in, 409–410
  (See also entries commencing with AV junctional)
AV reciprocating tachycardia, 488
Axis:
  anatomic, electrical axis and, 92
  anteroposterior, 94–95
  electrical (see Electrical axis)
  longitudinal, 94–95
  transverse, 94–95
Axis deviation, 82
  absence of, 88
  in atrial abnormality, P wave, 134
  bundle branch block and, 219–220
  left (see Left axis deviation)
  of P wave, in atrial abnormality, 134
  right (see Right axis deviation)

Bachmann's bundle, 22, 23
Basal portion of interventricular septum, 28
Bazett's formula (for Q-T interval determina-tion), 80
Beats:
  atrial premature, concealment of, 551

Beats (*Cont.*):
  AV junctional premature, concealment of, 551
  capture (*see* Capture beats)
  ectopic (*see* Ectopic beats and rhythms)
  escape, 408, 441–442
    AV junctional, 409, 441–442
  fascicular, 511–522
  fusion (or combination or summation) (*see* Fusion beats)
  group (*see* Bigeminy; Quadrigeminy; Trigeminy)
  premature, atrial, 551
    (*See also* Premature systoles)
  reciprocal (*see* Reciprocal beats and rhythms)
  sinus (*see* Sinus beats and rhythms)
  (*See also specific types of beats*)
Beta blockers, 336
BH potential (His bundle potential), 106, 107
Bidirectional tachycardia, 451
Bifascicular blocks, 206–213
  (*See also specific bifascicular blocks*)
Bigeminy, 533–535
  atrial extrasystolic, 426–430
  concealed, 534
  escape-capture, 541
  "reversed," 541
Bipolar leads, definition of, 5
Bipolar limb leads (standard extremity leads; standard limb leads), 36–38, 91
  derivation of, from FP loop, 116–117
  unipolar limb leads and, relationship between, 40–41
Block:
  atrial paroxysmal tachycardia with 460–462
  AV (*see* AV block)
  bifascicular, 206–213
    (*See also specific bifascicular blocks*)
  bilateral bundle branch block, 218–219
  bundle branch (*see* Bundle branch block)
  entrance or protection, 541, 542
  exit, 542, 562, 563
  fascicular (*see* Fascicular blocks)
  intraatrial, 133, 136
  intraventricular (*see* Intraventricular block)
  monofascicular, 198–206
    (*See also specific monofascicular blocks*)
  peri-infarction, 278
  SA (*see* SA block)
  trifascicular, 215–218
  unidirectional (*see* Unidirectional block)

Bradycardia, sinus, 453–454
Bradycardia-dependent bundle branch block, 198
Bradycardia-tachycardia syndrome, 456–457
Bundle branch:
  left, 22, 23, 25–27, 198
    anterior fascicle, 22, 25, 27
    anterior fascicular block (*see* Left anterior fascicular block)
    block (*see* Left bundle branch block)
    posterior fascicle, 22, 25, 27
    posterior fascicular block (*see* Left posterior fascicular block)
    septal fascicle, 22, 25, 198
  right, 22, 23, 25, 27
    block (*see* Right bundle branch block)
Bundle branch block:
  anatomic basis of, 178
  AV conduction and, relationship between, 215
  axis deviation and, 188, 195, 219–220
  bilateral, 178, 213–215
  bradycardia-dependent, 198
  complete, definition of, 177
  differential diagnosis of, 236
  fascicular beats and rhythms in, 514–522
  incomplete, 177, 178
  intermittent, 197–198
  left (*see* Left bundle branch block)
  lesions in conduction system and, 178
  masquerading (*see* Masquerading bundle branch block)
  myocardial infarction with (*see* Myocardial infarction, with left bundle branch block; Myocardial infarction, with right bundle branch block)
  right (*see* Right bundle branch block)
  S-T segment or vector abnormalities in, 125, 127
  trifascicular block, 218–219
Bundle of His, 22–23, 25, 27, 31
  electrograms (*see* His bundle electrograms)
  potential, 106, 107
Bundle of Kent, 23, 31, 33
Burger triangle, 36–37
"Bypass" fibers, 23
Bypass tracts, 32, 33

Calcium (*see* Hypercalcemia; Hypocalcemia)
Calcium ions, action potential and, 405
Capture beats, 442
  AV dissociation and, 529, 531
  in ventricular tachycardia, differential diagnosis, 593–595

Cardiac amyloidosis, 264, 373
Cardiac muscle fiber:
    depolarization in, 1–3
    electrophysiology of, 1–20
    polarized state in, 1, 2
    repolarization in, 3, 4
    (*See also* Cells, cardiac)
Cardiac tumors, differential diagnosis from
    myocardial infarction, 266
Cardiomyopathy, 370–374
    pseudoinfarction patterns in, 262
Cathode-tube vectorcardiography, 46–47
Cells, cardiac:
    automatic, 405–407
    nonautomatic, 406–407
    as semipermeable barrier to ionic ex-
        change, 404–405
    transmembrane potentials of, 403–405
Central nervous system lesions, differential
    diagnosis between myocardial infarction
    and, 272
Central terminal, Wilson's, 39, 40
Cerebrovascular accidents, electrocardio-
    graphic changes after, 374
Chagas' disease, 374
Chagasic myocarditis, 264
Children:
    axis deviation in (abnormal): left, 89, 364
        right, 89, 359
    normal electrocardiogram in, 382–386
    P wave and vector in, 60, 382
    P-R interval in, 63, 383
    QRS complex in, 67, 68, 383–385
    QRS-T angle in, 89, 386
    T wave in, 76, 385–386
    ventricular enlargement in: left, 144–145
        right, 154, 155, 158–161, 171
Coarctation of the aorta, 392
Combination beats (*see* Fusion beats)
Common bundle (bundle of His; AV bundle),
    22–26, 31
    electrocardiograms (*see* His bundle elec-
        trograms)
    potential, 106–107
Compensatory pauses after premature sys-
    toles, 421–423
Concealed conduction, 411–412, 550–556
    in atrial flutter, 468
    (*See also* Concealment)
Concealment:
    of atrial premature beats, 551
    of AV junctional premature beats, 551
    of sinus beats, 551
    of ventricular premature beats, 554

Concertina effect in W-P-W syndrome, 231
Conduction:
    in arrhythmias: aberrant conduction (*see*
        Aberrant atrial conduction; Aberrant
        ventricular conduction)
        combined disturbances of impulse for-
            mation and conduction, 413
        concealed conduction (*see* Concealed
            conduction)
        decremental conduction, 409–410
        disturbances, factors in, 408–409
        inhomogeneous conduction, 410–411
        local unidirectional block and micro-
            reentry, 412–413
        supernormality, 411, 556–562
        unidirectional block and macroreentry
            in the AV junction, 412
        unidirectional block without reentry, 412
    atrial, aberrant, 423, 448–449
    AV (*see* AV conduction)
    determinants of, 408–409
    drugs' effects on, 335, 336
        W-P-W syndrome, 235
    His bundle electrogram in evaluation of,
        108
    sinoventricular, 32–33, 456
    supraventricular, 429
    ventricular, defects in (*see* Ventricular con-
        duction defects)
Conduction system, anatomy and physiology
    of, 21–34
Congenital dextroversion, 276
Congenital heart disease:
    anomalous left coronary artery arising from
        pulmonary artery, 398
    anomalous pulmonary venous connection,
        396–397
    aortic atresia, 392
    aortic stenosis, 391–392
    atrial septal defect, 158, 371, 394–395
    coarctation of the aorta, 392
    dextrocardia, uncomplicated, with situs in-
        versus, 388, 389
    dextroversion, 388–389
    Ebstein's anomaly, 390–391
    endocardial cushion defects, 395–396
    idiopathic hypertrophic subaortic stenosis,
        262–263, 373, 392
    left axis deviation in, 367
    patent ductus arteriosus, 397–398
    pulmonary atresia with intact ventricular
        septum, 399
    pulmonic stenosis with intact ventricular
        septum, 157, 393

Congenital heart disease (Cont.):
  single ventricle, 399
  tetralogy of Fallot, 155, 393, 394
  transposition of the great vessels: complete,
    400–401
    congenitally corrected, 389–390
  tricuspid atresia, 399
  truncus arteriosus, 401
  ventricular septal defect, 397
Contraction, premature (see Premature sys-
    toles)
Contusion, myocardial, differential diagnosis
    between myocardial infarction and, 272,
    275
Cor pulmonale:
  acute: differential diagnosis, 165–166, 266,
    353
    pulmonary embolism and, 266, 351–353
    right axis deviation, 361
    RSR' complex in, 164–166
  chronic, 130, 354–358
    differential diagnosis, 353
    emphysema with, 354–357
Coronary artery, anomalous, left, arising from
    pulmonary artery, 398
Coronary artery disease:
  chronic, left axis deviation in, 201, 366
  exercise testing in, 309–314
Coronary insufficiency, 308–309
"Coronary nodal" rhythm, 237, 496–497
"Coronary sinus" rhythm, 498
Coronary syndrome, intermediate, 308–309
Coronary T (Pardee T) wave, 244
Coupling index, formula for, 428
Coupling interval, 421
  in parasystole, 547
Cove-plane T wave, 244
Crista pattern, 55, 93
Crista supraventricularis, 28
Crista terminalis, 23

Decremental conduction, 409–410
Deflection:
  extrinsic, 10
  intrinsic, 10, 11
  intrinsicoid (see Intrinsicoid deflection)
Delta wave in W-P-W syndrome, 231, 235–
    236
Depolarization (activation), 2, 26–29, 32–34
  atrial, 21, 50–52, 59
  definition of, 1, 3
  factors affecting repolarization and, 10–13
    subendocardial injury, 18–20
    subepicardial injury, 14–18

Depolarization (activation), (Cont.):
  impulse formation disturbances and, 407–
    408
  potentials recorded by unipolar leads during
    repolarization and, 5–6
  repolarization direction and, 10–11
  transmembrane potentials during, 403–405
    unipolar leads, recorded by, 5–6
  ventricular (see Ventricular depolarization)
Dextrocardia, 362
  uncomplicated, with situs inversions, 388,
    389
Dextroversion, 388–389
  congenital, 276
Diastolic overloading of ventricles:
  left, 142, 174
  right, 158, 173–174
Digitalis, 122, 126, 130, 328–331
  biventricular enlargement and, 170
  conduction affected by, 335
    W-P-W syndrome, 235
  electrocardiographic changes produced by,
    329–330
  hyperpotassemia masked by, 342
  in hypopotassemia and, 344
  intoxication, ventricular premature systoles
    due to, 432, 433
  theoretical considerations on, 328–329
  therapeutic effects of, 330
  toxic effects of, 331
Diltiazem hydrochloride, 336
Diphenylhydantoin (phenytoin):
  conduction affected by, 335
  electrocardiographic changes produced by,
    333
Dipole (doublet), 1–3
  equivalent cardiac, 111
  single equivalent, 3
Double tachycardia, 452
Doublet (see Dipole)
Drugs:
  antiarrhythmic, effect of newer, on ECG
    intervals and on effective refractory
    period, 335, 336
  antidepressant, 334–335
  conduction affected by, 335, 336
    W-P-W syndrome, 235
  electrocardiographic changes produced by,
    328–336
    antidepressant drugs, 334–335
    atropine, 235, 334, 335
    digitalis (see Digitalis)
    lidocaine, 235, 333, 335
    newer antiarrhythmics, 336

Drugs, electrocardiographic changes produced by (*Cont.*):
  phenothiazines, 334–335
  phenytoin (diphenylhydantoin), 333, 335
  procainamide, 235, 332–333
  propanalol, 235, 333–334
  quinidine, 235, 331–332
  sympathomimetic drugs, 334
Duchenne's muscular dystrophy, 264–265, 276, 373
  differential diagnosis between myocardial infarction and, 264
Dysrhythmias (*see* Arrhythmias)

E point, 108
Ebstein's anomaly, 390–391
Echo, atrial, 430
  (*See also* Reciprocal beats and rhythms)
Echo beat, 478
Ectopic beats and rhythms, 408, 421
  in exercise testing, 313
  (*See also* Ectopic tachycardias; Escape beats and rhythms; Premature systoles)
Ectopic tachycardias, 449–453
  AV dissociation in, 533
Ectopy, ventricular (*see* Ventricular ectopy)
Einthoven triangle hypothesis, 35
Einthoven's law, 37–38
Electrical alternans, 550
Electrical axis, 82–90
  determination of: by Einthoven triangle, 82
    QRS complex, 83–87
    spatial vectors, 85, 86, 90
    by vector analysis, 83–87
  deviation of (*see* Axis deviation)
  electrical position of heart and, relationship between, 96–100
  instantaneous, 82
  mean, 82
    estimation of, to nearest 30°, 83, 87
  modal, 82
  normal values for, 87–89
Electrical position of the heart, 94–99
Electrocardiogram:
  action potentials of cardiac cells and relationship between, 413–415
  components of (general discussion), 57–58
  definition of, 5
  derivation of, 50–56
    from vectorcardiogram, 116–118
  effect of certain drugs on, 328–336
  grid lines on, 57
  His bundle electrogram and (relationship between), 107

Electrocardiogram (*Cont.*):
  intracardiac, 101
  normal, 57–108
    in infants and children, 382–386
  standardization of, 57
  vector analysis of, by spatial vector method, 47–48
  vectorcardiogram and: derivation of electrocardiogram, 116–118
    relationship between, 48
  (*See also specific topics*)
Electrocardiograph, 4
Electrocardiography, exercise, 309–314
  graded (*see* Graded exercise tests)
  Master two-step (*see* Master two-step test)
Electrode:
  exploring (positive), 5–8
    definition of, 5
  indifferent (negative), 5
Electrode placement, errors in, Einthoven's law used in detecting, 38
Electrogram:
  definition of, 5
  His bundle (*see* His bundle electrograms)
Electrolyte abnormalities, electrocardiogram affected by, 338–349
  hyperpotassemia (*see* Hyperpotassemia)
  hypopotassemia (*see* Hypopotassemia)
Electrophysiology, basic principles of, 1–20
  (*See also* Conduction; Impulse formation; Potentials, transmembrane)
Embolism, pulmonary, and acute cor pulmonale, 266, 351–353
Emphysema (chronic obstructive pulmonary disease):
  with cor pulmonale, 354–358
  diagnostic criteria of, 355–356
  differential diagnosis between myocardial infarction and, 266
  left axis deviation in, 203, 366
  with right ventricular hypertrophy, 356–357
  RSR' pattern, in, 166
  vectorcardiogram in, 357, 358
Encainide hydrochloride, 336
Endocardial cushion defects, 395–396
Endocardial fibroelastosis, primary, 392–393
Endocardial leads, 7
Endomyocardial fibrosis, African, 373–374
Entrance block, 541, 542
Epicardial leads, 6, 7
Equivalent cardial dipole, 111
Erb's limb girdle dystrophy, 265

Escape beats and rhythms, 408, 441–442
    AV junctional, 409, 441–442, 496
Escape-capture bigeminy, 541
Escape-capture sequence, 541
Esophageal leads, 100
Ethmozin hydrochloride, 336
Exercise electrocardiography (exercise test-
    ing), 309–314
    graded exercise tests, 314–317
    maximal, 314
Exit block, 542, 562, 563
Extrasystole (see Premature systoles)
Extremity leads (see Limb leads)
Extrinsic deflections, 10

F waves, 62
f waves, 62
Fascicle:
    anterior (superior), 22, 25, 27, 198
        block (see Left anterior fascicular block)
    posterior (inferior), 22, 25, 27, 198
        block (see Left posterior fascicular block)
    septal (central or medial fascicle), 22, 25,
        198
Fascicular beats and rhythms, 514–522
Fascicular blocks:
    bi-, 206–213
    left anterior (see Left anterior fascicular
        block)
    left posterior (see Left posterior fascicular
        block)
    mono-, 198–206
    tri-, 215–218
        bilateral bundle branch block, 218–219
Fasciculoventricular connection, 228
Fibrillation:
    atrial, 468–477
        aberrant ventricular conduction, 470–
            471, 475
        AV dissociation, 469–470, 532
        ventricular ectopy, 471, 474
        W-P-W syndrome, 231, 233, 235
    ventricular, 514, 519
Fibrosis, African endomyocardial, 373–374
Flecainide acetate, 336
Flutter:
    atrial, 464–468
        AV dissociation, 532
        W-P-W syndrome, 231, 235
    ventricular, 514, 519
Frank lead system, 43, 44, 47
Friedreich's ataxia, 265, 374

Frontal plane:
    angular measurements of vectors in,
        113
    normal vectorcardiogram in, 115
    QRS loop in, 116
    vectorcardiogram displayed in, 47
Funnel chest, T wave inversion in patients
    with, 76–77
Fusion beats:
    atrial, 443, 499, 530, 544
    AV dissociation and, 530
    in parasystole, 548
    ventricular, 471, 507, 518, 520, 521, 525,
        546–548, 603, 606
        diagnosis, 443–444
        in ventricular tachycardias, differential di-
            agnosis, 596–597

Galvanometer, 3–4
Glycogen storage disease, 373
Graded exercise tests, 314–317
    clinical significance, 317
    contraindications, 315
    indications, 315
    limitations, 315
Grid lines on electrocardiogram, 59
Group beating (see Bigeminy; Quadrigeminy;
    Trigeminy)

H potential, 106, 107
Half-area vector, 112
HB potential, 106, 107
Heart block (see AV block)
Heart rate:
    calculation of, 81, 82
    in infants and children, 386
Hemopericardium, acute, 326
Hemorrhage, spontaneous subarachnoid, 374–
    376
Hexaxial reference diagram, 36–37
    electrical axis determination by, 87, 88
    electrocardiogram derived from vectorcar-
        diogram by, 116–118
His bundle (common or AV bundle), 22–26,
    31
His bundle electrograms, 103–108
    with atrial pacing, 107–108
    clinical applications of, 108
    definition of terms used in, 106–107

His bundle electrograms (*Cont.*):
electrocardiogram and, 107
in L-G-L syndrome, 236–237
normal values of, 106–107
technique for, 107
value of, 104–106
in ventricular conduction defects, 220–221
in W-P-W syndrome, 235
His bundle potential (BH potential; H potential), 106, 107
Holter monitoring, 102–103
Horizontal plane, vectorcardiogram recorded in, 47
H-V time, 107
Hypercalcemia, 345–346
Hypermagnesemia, 347–348
Hyperpotassemia, 125, 127, 338–342
differential diagnosis between myocardial infarction and, 268, 269
Hyperventilation, T wave changes induced by, 77
Hypocalcemia, 346, 347
Hypomagnesemia, 348
Hypopotassemia, 125, 127, 342–345
Hypothermia, 373

Idiopathic hypertrophic subaortic stenosis, 262, 263, 373, 391–392
Idioventricular rhythm, 421, 505–506
accelerated, 506–508
Idioventricular tachycardia, 506–508
Impulse formation, arrhythmias due to disturbances in, 407–408
combined disturbances of conduction and, 413
Infants (*see* Children)
Infarction:
atrial, 134–136
myocardial (*see* Myocardial infarction)
Inhomogeneous conduction, 410–411
Injury:
atrial, 134–136
subendocardial, 18–20, 123, 124, 126
subepicardial (*see* Subepicardial injury)
transient ischemia (*see* Ischemia, transient, and injury)
zone of, in myocardial infarct, 241–242
Interatrial conduction defect, 133
Interatrial conduction delay, 133, 136
Interatrial septum, 321

Interectopic intervals in parasystole, 547
Interference dissociation, 523–526
(*See also* AV dissociation, interference)
Internodal tracts:
anterior, 22, 23, 29–30
middle, 22, 23, 29–30
posterior, 22, 23, 29–30
Interpolated premature systoles, 421
Inter-Society Commission for Heart Disease Resources (ICHD) pacemaker identification code, 599, 601, 602
Intervals, definition of, 58
(*See also* specific intervals)
Interventricular septum, 22, 23, 27, 31, 53
Intraatrial block, 133, 136
Intraatrial reentrant tachycardia, 488
Intracardiac electrocardiogram with platinum electrode wire, 101
Intranodal bypass tract, 228
Intraventricular block:
diffuse, 198
left inferior (*see* Left posterior fascicular block)
left superior (*see* Left anterior fascicular block)
nonspecific, 198
Intraventricular conduction time, 29, 64
Intrinsic deflection, 10, 11
Intrinsicoid deflection:
measurement of, 69–70
normal values for, 69–70
in ventricular enlargement: left, 141, 143, 146, 147
right, 154, 156, 159–160
(*See also* specific abnormal conditions)
Ionic exchange, 404–405
Ischemia:
left bundle branch block with, 290, 292
repolarization affected by, 13–14
subarachnoid hemorrhage mistaken for, 374
subendocardial, and injury, 307–309
subepicardial, 307, 309
T wave abnormalities due to, 119–120
transient, and injury, 309–317
angina pectoris, 307–308
coronary insufficiency, 308–309
exercise testing, 309–314
transmural, 307, 309
zone of, in myocardial infarct, 241, 242
Ischemic depression, 312
Isoproterenol, 335
conduction affected by, in W-P-W syndrome, 235

J (junction), 52, 70
J deflection (Osborn wave), 370
J point, 111
J point depression, 312
Junctional S-T depression, 312

Kirchhoff's law, 38–39

Ladder diagrams, AV, 419–421
LB potential, 106
Lead vector, 36–37
Leads, 3–5, 9
  atrial, 100–101
  axis of, 5
  bipolar, definition of, 5
  endocardial, 7
  epicardial, 6–7
  esophageal, 100
  Holter monitoring, 102–103
  limb: bipolar (see Bipolar limb leads)
    unipolar (see Unipolar limb leads)
  for monitoring, 101–102
  orthogonal, 43
  precordial (see Precordial leads)
  transsternal, for monitoring, 101–102
  unipolar (see Unipolar leads)
  X, Y, and Z, normal, 44
Left anterior fascicular block, 177, 199
  anterior infarction, with (see Myocardial infarction, with left anterior fascicular block, anterior)
  axis deviation in, left, 201–204, 364–365
  bundle branch block with, left, 220
  bundle branch block with, right (see right bundle branch block with, below)
  diagnosis of, 201–204
    differential, between myocardial infarction and, 267–268
    between S₁ S₂ S₃ syndrome, 369
    vectorcardiographic, 221–223
  His bundle electrogram in, 220–221
  myocardial infarction and, differential diagnosis between, 267–268
  (See also Myocardial infarction, with left anterior fascicular block)
  right bundle branch block with, 183, 189, 207–208
    His bundle electrogram, 220
    masquerading bundle branch block (see Masquerading bundle branch block)
    RSR' complex, 183, 189
    trifascicular blocks, 215–218
    vectorcardiogram, 221–223

Left anterior fascicular block (*Cont.*):
  in trifascicular blocks, 215–218
  vectorcardiogram in, 221–223
  with ventricular enlargement, 202, 204
  ventricular strain with, 143
Left atrial enlargement (see Interatrial conduction defect)
"Left atrial" rhythm, 498–502
  spontaneous, 202
Left axis deviation, 88, 364–368
  abnormal, 89
    in bundle branch block, 188, 195, 219–220
    in children, 364
    differential diagnosis, 625
    in emphysema, 203
    in fascicular block, 201–204, 364–365
    in ventricular enlargement, 148, 365–366
  causes of, 364–368
Left bundle branch block, 25, 126
  with axis deviation, abnormal, 195, 219–220
  clinical significance of, 190–191
  complete: diagnosis, 193–197
    vectorcardiogram, 196–197
  diagnosis of: complete, 193–197
    differential, between myocardial infarction and left bundle branch block, 266, 303–304
    incomplete, 195
    vectorcardiographic, 196–197
  divisional, 190
  His bundle electrogram in, 220–221
  incomplete, 195
  intermittent, 197–198, 214
  myocardial infarction and, differential diagnosis between, 266, 303–304
  myocardial infarction with (see Myocardial infarction, with left bundle branch block)
  predivisional, 190
  S-T segment abnormality in, 125
  T wave or vector abnormalities in, 121
  theoretical considerations about, 189–190
  vectorcardiogram in, 196–197
  vectorelectrocardiographic criteria for, 195
  ventricular depolarization in, 191–193
  with ventricular enlargement, 148–149, 195–196
  ventricular repolarization in, 193
Left bundle potential, 106
Left posterior fascicular block, 177, 200
  axis deviation in, right, 361–362

Left posterior fascicular block (*Cont.*):
  bundle branch block with (*see* right bundle
    branch block with, *below*)
  diagnosis of, 204–206
    vectorcardiographic, 223
  His bundle electrogram in, 220–221
  myocardial infarction with (*see* Myocardial
    infarction, with left posterior fascicular
    block)
  right bundle branch block with, 206–207,
    212–213
    His bundle electrogram, 220–221
    RSR' patterns, 183
    trifascicular block, 215–218
    vectorcardiogram, 223
  in trifascicular blocks, 215–218
  vectorcardiogram in, 223
  ventricular enlargement and, right, 164
Left ventricular enlargement:
  atrial abnormality in diagnosis of, 148
  axis deviation in, 148, 365
  bundle branch block and, 148–149
    right, 149, 187–189
  in children, 144–145
  definite, 146, 147, 152
  diagnosis of: differential, 260–262, 303
    electrocardiographic, 143–149
    intrinsicoid deflection, 145, 146
    point score system, 147
    QRS voltage, 144–145
    S-T segment and T waves changes, 145–
      146
    vectorcardiographic, 149–152
  intrinsicoid deflection in, 141, 143, 145,
    146
  with left anterior fascicular block, 202,
    204
  myocardial infarction and, differential di-
    agnosis between, 260–261, 303
  myocardial infarction with, 149, 282
  possible or probable, 146, 147, 152
  pseudoinfarction patterns in, 148
  QRS complex and vector in, 140–152
  S-T segment and vector in, 142–146, 149,
    151
  ST-T abnormalities and, 149
  T wave or vector in, 141–146, 149, 152
  theoretical considerations on, 140–143
  vectorcardiogram, 149–152
  vectorelectrocardiographic criteria for, 149
  by voltage criteria, 147
  voltage criteria for diagnosis of, 147–148
L-G-L syndrome (*see* Lown-Ganong-Levine
  syndrome)

Lidocaine:
  conduction affected by, 335
    W-P-W syndrome, 235
  electrocardiographic changes produced by,
    333
Limb leads:
  bipolar (*see* Bipolar limb leads)
  reversal of right and left, 274, 275, 363
  unipolar (*see* Unipolar limb leads)
Local potentials hypothesis (semidirect lead
  hypothesis), vector concept versus, 45–
  46
Longitudinal axis, 94–95
Loop, timing of, 112
  (*See also specific loops*)
Lorcainide hydrochloride, 336
Lown-Ganong-Levine (L-G-L) syndrome:
  differential diagnosis of 236–237
  His bundle electrogram in, 236–237

Macroreentry, unidirectional block and, in
  the AV junction, 412
Macruz index for atrial enlargement diagnosis, 133–134
Magnesium, 346–348
Mahaim, paraspecific fibers of, 23, 31, 33
Masquerading bundle branch block, 178, 207–
  212
  precordial, 209, 211–212
  standard, 208–211
Master two-step test, 308, 310–314
  positive, criteria for, 312–313
  procedure for, 310–311
  standards for interpretation of, 311–312
Mexiletine hydrochloride, 336
Microreentry, local unidirectional block and,
  412–413
Midseptum, 27
Mitral valve, 22, 23, 32
Mitral valve prolapse syndrome, 275, 374–
  377
  electrocardiographic findings, 376–377
Moderator band, 23
Monitoring, leads for, 101–102
Monofascicular blocks, 198–206
  (*See also specific monofascicular blocks*)
Multifocal atrial tachycardia, 463–464
Multistage treadmill tests (*see* Graded exercise
  tests)
Muscle fiber, cardiac (*see* Cardiac muscle
  fiber)
Muscular dystrophy, Duchenne's, 373
  differential diagnosis between myocardial
    infarction and, 264

Myocardial contusion, differential diagnosis between myocardial infarction and abnormalities caused by, 272, 274

Myocardial disease:
diffuse: differential diagnosis between myocardial infarction and, 262–266
left axis deviation, 366
localized, differential diagnosis between myocardial infarction and, 266

Myocardial infarction:
acute: anterior, 135
inferior, 251
with left bundle branch block, 290–291
anterior: acute, 135
extensive, 254
with fascicular block (see with left anterior fascicular block, below)
with left bundle branch block, 291
localized, 246–250, 294–295
with pericarditis, 326
with right bundle branch block, 288–289
strictly, 246–249
anteroinferior, 254
anterolateral or lateral, 247, 250, 251, 279, 359–360
with left anterior fascicular block, 277, 279, 283–284
with pericarditis, 326
vectorcardiogram, 293–294
anteroseptal (see strictly anterior or anteroseptal, below)
apical (see localized anterior or apical, below)
arrythmias, 258
axis deviation in, 359–361
with bundle branch block (see with left bundle branch block and with right bundle branch block, below)
central nervous system lesions and, differential diagnosis between, 272
classification of, 246
cor pulmonale and, differential diagnosis between, 266, 353
diagnosis of: differential (see differential diagnosis of, below)
in pacemaker patients, 258
Q wave abnormalities, 242–244
S-T segment and T wave changes, 244–245
subendocardial infarction, 256
vectorcardiographic, 47, 293–304
diagnostic features of, in various locations, 246–256
correlation of coronary arteriographic findings with anatomic location, 256, 258

Myocardial infarction (Cont.):
diagnostic problems in, 259
diaphragmatic (see inferior or diaphragmatic, below)
differential diagnosis of, 236, 260–276
bundle branch block, left, 266
central nervous system lesions, 272
cor pulmonale, acute, 266, 353
fascicular block, left anterior, 267–268
hyperpotassemia, 268–270
myocardial contusion, 272, 274
myocardial disease, 262–266
pericarditis, 324–325
pneumothorax, 271, 273
pulmonary emphysema, 266
repolarization, early, 268–269
strictly posterior myocardial infarction, 275–276
vectorcardiographic, 303–304
ventricular hypertrophy, 165, 261–262, 303
W-P-W syndrome, 267
dorsal (see strictly posterior, below)
evolution of, 245–246
extensive anterior, 254, 360, 361
vectorcardiogram, 298
with fascicular block, 276–278
left anterior (see with left anterior fascicular block, below)
left posterior (see with left posterior fascicular block, below)
vectorcardiogram in, 278–279, 302–304
fascicular block and, differential diagnosis between, 267–268
high lateral (see superior or high lateral, below)
hyperpotassemia and, differential diagnosis between, 268–270
inferior or diaphragmatic, 247, 248, 250–253, 289–290, 366–367
acute, 251
with fascicular block, 200, 277, 279–287, 302
left axis deviation, 366–367
with left bundle branch block, 291–293, 303
old, 252
with pericarditis, 326
with right bundle branch block, 289–290
vectorcardiogram, 296–298
inferolateral, 254
vectorcardiogram, 300, 301

Myocardial infarction (*Cont.*):
  lateral (*see* anterolateral or lateral, *above*)
  with left anterior fascicular block: anterior,
      199, 276–287
    axis deviation, left, 365
    differential diagnosis, 165, 303–
      304
    RSR' complex, 165
    vectorcardiogram, 302–304
    anterolateral, 277–278, 287
    differential diagnosis of, 165, 304
    inferior, 285–287
    vectorcardiogram, 302
  left anterior fascicular block and, differ-
      ential diagnosis between, 267–268
  with left bundle branch block, 288
    acute, 290
    anterior, 291
    inferior, 291–292
    lateral wall, 291, 303
    vectorcardiogram, 303–304
  with left posterior fascicular block: inferior,
      200, 278, 282–283
    axis deviation, right, 362
    vectorcardiogram, 302
  localization of, 246
    correlation of coronary arteriographic
      findings with, 256, 258
  localized anterior or apical, 249–250
    vectorcardiogram, 294–295
  midanterior (*see* localized anterior or api-
      cal, *above*)
  myocardial contusion and, differential di-
      agnosis between, 272, 274
  myocardial disease and, differential diag-
      nosis between, 262–266
  old, inferior, 252
  pericarditis complicating, 326
  pneumothorax and, differential diagnosis
      between, 271, 273
  posterior (*see* inferior or diaphragmatic,
      above)
    strictly (*see* strictly posterior, *below*)
  posterobasal (*see* strictly posterior, *below*)
  posteroinferolateral, 255
  pseudo- (*see* Pseudoinfarction patterns)
  pulmonary emphysema and, differential di-
      agnosis between, 266
  Q wave in (*see* Q wave, in myocardial
      infarction)
  repolarization and, early, differential di-
      agnosis between, 268–269
  with right bundle branch block, 184, 287–
      288
    anterior, 288–289

Myocardial infarction, with right bundle branch
    block (*Cont.*):
    inferior, 289–290
    posterior (posterobasal), 184, 287–288
    vectorcardiogram in, 302
  right ventricular, 254–256
  S-T segment in, 244–245
  strictly anterior or anteroseptal, 246–249,
      280, 281
    with right bundle branch block: differ-
      ential diagnosis between ventricular
      hypertrophy and, 303
    with left anterior fascicular block, 280,
      283–286
    vectorcardiogram, 295
  strictly posterior, 247, 248, 253–254
    differential diagnosis, 275–276
    differential diagnosis between ventricular
      hypertrophy and, 165, 303
    with right bundle branch block, 184, 288
    RSR' complex in, 165
    vectorcardiogram, 300, 301
  subendocardial, 256
  superior or high lateral, 247, 248, 250,
      252, 359–360
    vectorcardiogram, 296
  superoanteroseptal, with fascicular block,
      281
  T wave in (*see* T wave, in myocardial
      infarction)
  theoretical considerations on, 241–242
  vectorcardiogram in, 47, 293–304
    anterolateral, 295–296
    extensive anterior, 296
    inferior, 296–299
    inferolateral, 300, 301
    with left bundle branch block, 302–303
    localized anterior, 294–295
    with right bundle branch block, 302
    strictly anterior, 294–295
    strictly posterior, 300, 301
    superior, 296, 297
  vectorelectrocardiographic criteria for, 245
  ventricular aneurysm and, 258
  with ventricular enlargement, left, 149–
      150, 281
  ventricular enlargement and, differential
      diagnosis between, 165, 260–262, 303
  W-P-W syndrome and, differential diag-
      nosis between, 267
Myocardial ischemia (*see* Ischemia)
Myocarditis, 262–264
  acute, 262
  Chagasic, 264
Myotonia atrophica, 265

Necrosis, 20
zone of, in myocardial infarct, 241
Negativity, QRS vector and distribution of, 100
Neurosurgical procedures, electrocardiographic changes after, 374
Nifedipine, 336
Nodal artery, 23
Nodal-His (NH) region, 22, 24, 26
Nodal (N) region, 22, 24, 26
Nodoventricular bypass tract, 488
Nodoventricular connection, 228
Noncompensatory pauses after premature systoles, 421–422
Nonparoxysmal tachycardia:
AV junctional, 494–496
definition of, 450
Nonphasic sinus arrhythmia, 454
Normal electrocardiogram, 57–108
in infants and children, 382–386
(See also specific topics)
Normal vectorcardiogram, 111–118
Notch, definition of, 64

O point, 111
Orthodromic AV reciprocating tachycardia, 488
Orthogonal leads, 43, 44
Osborn wave (J deflection) in hypothermia, 370
Oscilloscope, 46–47

P congenitale, 129
P loop, 111, 113, 114
in atrial enlargement, 137
normal, 138
vectors of atrial activation and, 50–52
(See also specific abnormal conditions)
P mitrale, 128, 131
P pulmonale, 128–131
P terminal force, 59, 60
P tricuspidale, 130
P wave, 21, 26, 59, 63
abnormality, 61–62
atrial abnormality, 128–133
(See also specific abnormal conditions)
axis deviation of, in atrial abnormality, 134
in children and infants, 60, 383
electrical axis of, 87
deviation, in atrial abnormality, 134
His bundle electrogram and, 106, 107
measurement of, 60, 61

P wave (Cont.):
normal values of, 60–61
vectors of atrial activation and, 50–52
P-A time, 106–107
Pacemaker cells, 406
rate of discharge of, variables affecting, 407
wandering, 455
Pacemakers, artificial (electronic), 597–610
asynchronous or fixed-rate, 601, 603–604
atrial pacing by, 597
atrial-triggered (P-wave-synchronous), 601, 607–608
AV-sequential (dual chamber), 601–603
bipolar and unipolar pacing by, 597
diagnosis of myocardial infarction in pacemaker patients, 258
malfunction of, 608–610
nomenclature, 599–602
ICHD five-position code, 602
ICHD three-position code, 601
ventricular-inhibited (R-wave-inhibited, or demand), 601, 604–607
ventricular pacing by, 598–599
ventricular-triggered (R-wave-synchronous, or standby), 601, 607
Papillary muscle, 22, 23
Paraseptal region, anterior, 27
Paraspecific fibers of Mahaim, 23, 31, 33
Parasystole, 541–549
atrial, distinguished from atrial dissociation, 548–550
clinical significance of, 548–549
definition of, 541
diagnosis of, 545–548
mechanism of, 541–545
Parasystolic tachycardia, ventricular, 514, 517, 518
Pardee T (coronary T) wave, 244
Parietal block (see Left anterior fascicular block; Left posterior fascicular block)
Paroxysmal reciprocating sinus tachycardia, 488
Paroxysmal supraventricular tachycardia (PSVT), reentrant, 477–480
automatic ectopic versus, 486–489
electrocardiographic criteria for diagnosis, 480–485
differential diagnosis by clues from surface electrocardiogram, 488
types of, 478–479
accessory bypass tracts, 479
atria, 479
AV node, 478–479
sinus node, 479

Paroxysmal tachycardia:
  atrial (*see* Atrial paroxysmal tachycardia)
  automatic ectopic AV junctional (His bun-
    dle), 492–494
    reentrant (PSVT), 477–480
  bidirectional, 450–452
  definition of, 450
  double or simultaneous, 452
  reentrant supraventricular (PSVT), 477–489
    (*See also* Reentrant paroxysmal supra-
    ventricular tachycardia)
  repetitive, 450, 451
  supraventricular (*see* Supraventricular par-
    oxysmal tachycardia)
  ventricular, 508–513
Patent ductus arteriosus, 397–398
Pause:
  after premature systole, 421–423
  sinus arrest or, 455–456
Pectus excavatum, 377
Pericardial effusion, 324
Pericarditis:
  acute, 320–324
    differential diagnosis: of early polariza-
      tion and, 325
    between myocardial infarction and, 324–
      325
    P waves, 321
    P-R segment, 323–324
    QRS complexes, 321
    S-T segment and T wave abnormalities,
      320–323
  chronic constrictive, 276, 324–325
  myocardial infarction complicated by,
    326
Peri-infarction block, 278
  anterior (*see* Left anterior fascicular block)
  inferior (*see* Left posterior fascicular block)
Pes excavatum, 275
P-H time in His bundle electrogram, 106
Phasic sinus arrhythmia, 455
Phenothiazines, 334–335
Phenytoin (diphenylhydantoin):
  conduction affect by, 335
  electrocardiographic changes produced by,
    333
Planar vectors, angular measurements of, 113
Plotting vectors, 85, 86
Pneumothorax, differential diagnosis between
    myocardial infarction and, 271, 273
Polarized state (resting state), 1, 2
  (*See also* Depolarization; Repolarization)
Polymorphous ventricular tachycardia, 512–
    514

Poor R wave progression (PRWP), 92–93,
    148, 377–381, 621
Positions of heart, electrical, 94–99
Positivity, QRS vector and distribution of, 100
Posterobasal myocardial infarction (*see* Myo-
    cardial infarction, strictly posterior)
Posterobasal region, 28
Postextrasystolic T wave change, 425, 434
Posttachycardia syndrome, 75, 453
Potassium (*see* Hyperpotassemia; Hypopotas-
    semia)
Potentials, transmembrane, 403–405
  of automatic cells, 406
  of cardiac cells, 403–405
  electrocardiogram and, 413–415
  of nonautomatic cells, 407
  recorded by unipolar leads, 5–6
  threshold, 406
P-R interval, 62–63
  abnormality, 63
  in children, 63, 383
  definition of, 26
  His bundle electrogram and, 105, 107
  measurement of, 63
  normal values of, 63
P-R segment:
  definition of, 26
  depression of, 62, 71
  displacements of S-T segment and, 71–72
  in early repolarization, 323–324
  in pericarditis, 323–324
  (*See also specific abnormal conditions*)
Precordial leads, 41–42, 91–92
  derivation of, from TP loop, 118
  electrocardiographic poor or reversed R
    wave progression in the right, 377–
    381
  QRS complexes in, 54
  vectorcardiogram and, 46
Preexcitation syndrome (*see* Wolff-Parkinson-
    White syndrome)
Premature beats, atrial, concealment of, 551
  (*See also* Premature systoles)
Premature contraction (*see* Premature sys-
    toles)
Premature systoles, 421–441
  atrial, 421–424, 426–430, 458
    clinical significance, 424–425
  AV, 491
  AV junctional, 421–423, 430–431
    clinical significance, 425
  clinical significance of, 424–425
  differential diagnosis of, 430–441
  etiology of, 424

Premature systoles (*Cont.*):
  interpolated, 421
  mechanism of, 423–424
  sinus, 425–426
  ventricular, 421–423, 431–441
    bigeminy due to digitalis intoxication, 432, 433
    clinical significance, 424–425
    compensatory pauses following, 438
    differential diagnosis, 438–441
    interpolated, 431, 433, 435
    multiform, 432–435
    site of origin, 435–437
    unifocal or multifocal origin, 432–435
Prinzmetal's angina, 307
Procainamide, 235, 332–333, 335
Progressive muscular dystrophy, electrocardiogram of, 265
Propanolol, 325, 333–335
Protection block (entrance block), 541, 542
Pseudobifurcation of bundle of His, 25
Pseudoinfarction patterns:
  in athletes, 271
  in cardiomyopathies, 262
  in left anterior fascicular block, 268
  in ventricular enlargement: left, 148
    right, 164
  (*See also* Myocardial infarction, differential diagnosis of)
Pseudoreciprocal rhythm, 541
Pseudosubepicardial injury patterns, in athletes, 272
PSVT (*see* Paroxysmal supraventricular tachycardia)
Pulmonary atresia with intact ventricular septum, 399
Pulmonary conus, 28
Pulmonary disease, chronic obstructive (*see* Emphysema)
Pulmonary embolism and acute cor pulmonale, 266, 351–354
Pulmonary stenosis, congenital, with intact ventricular septum, 157, 393
Pulmonary trunk, 23
Pulmonary valve, 23
Pulmonary veins, right, 23
Pulmonary venous connection, anomalous, 396–397
Purkinje fibers, 22, 23, 25, 27
Purkinje plexus, 25

Q wave, 63, 65–66
  abnormal, differential diagnosis, 619–620
  absent, 194, 195

Q wave (*Cont.*):
  in myocardial infarction, 242–244, 246–252, 254–255, 260, 262
    with bundle branch block, 288–293
    with fascicular block, 277–287
  in precordial leads, 93
  (*See also* QRS complex; *and specific abnormal conditions*)
qR complex in right ventricular enlargement, 153–157, 161
QRS complex, 29, 52, 63–69, 99, 100
  in aberrant ventricular conduction, 445
  abnormal, differential diagnosis, 621–622
  area enclosed by, 90
  in children, 68, 383–385
  definition of, 6
  duration of, 67
  electrical axis of: determination of, 83–87
    deviation (*see* Left axis deviation; Right axis deviation)
    mean, 88–89
  in limb leads, 91
    derivation of, from QRS loop, 117
  measurement of, 64
  nomenclature of, 63–64
  in pericarditis, 321, 324–326
  plotting mean vector for, 85, 86
  in precordial leads, 54. 91–94
    derivation of, from QRS loop, 117
  supraventricular tachycardia with abnormal, versus ventricular tachycardia, 584–597
  vector of (*see* QRS vector)
  in ventricular enlargement: left, 140–149
    right, 152–159
  voltage of, 68–69
    differential diagnosis, 620–622
    in left ventricular enlargement, 140, 144–149
    low, 69
    in right ventricular enlargement, 156–159
  (*See also specific abnormal conditions*)
QRS interval (*see* QRS complex)
QRS loop, 55, 111, 114–116
  in ventricular enlargement: left, 150–151
    right, 168–170
  (*See also specific abnormal conditions*)
QRS vector, 55, 97, 100
  in children, 383–385
  maximum, 111
  plotting mean spatial, 85, 86
  (*See also specific abnormal conditions*)

QRS-T angle, 26, 89, 116
  calculation of, 112
  in children, 89, 386
  in left ventricular enlargement, 141, 152
  (*See also specific abnormal conditions*)
QS complex, 63, 66–67
  abnormal, differential diagnosis, 620
  definition of, 7
  in precordial leads, 93
  (*See also specific abnormal conditions*)
Q-T calculator, 300–301
Q-T interval, 29, 80–81, 623
Quadrigeminy, 533–535
Quinidine, 235, 331–332

R wave:
  definition of, 6
  differential diagnoses of abnormal, 62
  poor progression of, 92–93, 148, 377–381,
    621
  in precordial leads, 91–93, 377–381
  reversed progression of, 377–381
  in right ventricular enlargement, 153–158,
    163–164
  secondary (*see* R′ wave)
  (*See also* QRS complex; *and specific ab-
    normal conditions*)
R′ wave (secondary R wave), 63
  in precordial leads, 93–94
  in right ventricular enlargement, 158, 164
  (*See also* RSR′ complex; *and specific ab-
    normal conditions*)
RB potential (right bundle potential), 106
Reciprocal beats and rhythms, 412, 430, 478,
    535–541
  atrial, 430, 536
  AV junctional, 536–538
  pseudo-, 541
  reversed, 536
  ventricular, 538–541
  in ventricular tachycardia, differential di-
    agnosis, 593–595
Reciprocating rhythm, 536
Reentrant paroxysmal supraventricular tachy-
    cardia (PSVT), 477–480
  automatic ectopic versus, 486–489
  electrocardiographic criteria for diagnosis,
    480–485
    differential diagnosis by clues from sur-
      face electrocardiogram, 488
  types of, 478–479
    atria, 479
    AV node, 478–479
    sinus node, 479

Reentry:
  in reciprocal rhythms (*see* Reciprocal beats
    and rhythms)
  unidirectional block without, 412
Reflecting level, 536
Refractory period in arrhythmias, 415–418
  effect of newer antiarrhythmic drugs on,
    335, 336
Repetitive paroxysmal tachycardia, 450, 451
Repolarization, 3, 4
  atrial, 21, 52, 62–63
  early, differential diagnosis: between myo-
    cardial infarction and, 268–269
    between pericarditis and, 325
  factors affecting depolarization and, 10–
    20
    ischemia, 13–14
    subendocardial injury, 18–20
    subepicardial injury, 14–18
    transmembrane potential during, 403–405
    unipolar leads, recorded by, 5–6
  ventricular (*see* Ventricular repolarization)
Resting state (polarized state) of cardiac mus-
    cle fiber, 1, 2
Return extrasystole (*see* Reciprocal beats and
    rhythms)
Rhythms:
  atrial, 458–459
  AV junctional (*see* AV junctional rhythms)
  "coronary nodal," 496–497
  "coronary sinus," 498
  ectopic (*see* Ectopic beats and rhythms)
  fascicular, 514–522
  "left atrial," 498–502
  sinoventricular, 456
  sinus (*see* Sinus beats and rhythms)
  ventricular or idioventricular (*see* Idioven-
    tricular rhythm)
  (*See also* Arrhythmias)
Right axis deviation, 88
  abnormal, 89, 359–363
    in children, 359
    differential diagnosis, 625
    in ventricular enlargement, 157, 160–
      161, 163, 361
  causes of, 359–363
Right bundle branch block, 87, 103–105
  clinical significance of, 180
  complete: diagnosis of, 182
    vectorcardiogram, 185–186
  His bundle electrogram in, 220
  incomplete, 184
    RSR′ pattern in, 166, 167
    vectorcardiogram, 184

Right bundle branch block (*Cont.*):
  intermittent, 197–198, 214
  with left anterior and left posterior fascicular
    blocks (trifascicular blocks), 215–
    218
  with left anterior fascicular block, 183
    His bundle electrogram, 220
    masquerading bundle branch block (*see*
      Masquerading bundle branch block)
    vectorcardiogram, 223
  with left posterior fascicular block, 183,
    206, 207, 212–213
    His bundle electrogram, 220
    vectorcardiogram, 223
  masquerading (*see* Masquerading bundle
    branch block)
  myocardial infarction with (*see* Myocardial
    infarction, with right bundle branch
    block)
  RSR' patterns in, differential diagnosis of,
    166, 183
  S-T segment in, 125
  T wave or vector in, 121
  theoretical considerations on, 178–180
  trifascicular blocks and, 215–218
    vectorcardiogram in, 185–186
    with ventricular enlargement, 187–189
  vectorcardiographic criteria for, 182
  ventricular depolarization in, 180, 181
  with ventricular enlargement: left, 149, 187
    right, 161, 183, 186, 187
    vectorcardiogram, 187–189
  ventricular repolarization in, 181–182
Right ventricular enlargement, 130, 132, 152–
    170
  atrial enlargement and, 161
  axis deviation in, right, 157, 161, 163,
    361
  with bundle branch block, right, 161, 183,
    186–187, 190
  in children, 154, 155, 158–161, 171
  definite, 162
  diagnosis of: differential, 165, 261–262,
    303
    electrocardiographic, 156–163
    point-score system, 163
    vectorcardiographic, 168–170
  emphysema with, 356–357
  with left anterior fascicular block, 204
  with left posterior fascicular block, 164
  myocardial infarction and, differential di-
    agnosis between, 165, 261–262, 303
  precordial electrocardiogram in, genesis of,
    153

Right ventricular enlargement (*Cont.*):
  probable, 162
  pseudoinfarction patterns in, 164
  QRS complex in, 152–164, 168–170
  RSR' complex in, differential diagnosis of,
    165, 166
  S-T segment in, 156, 160
  ST-T abnormalities and, primary, 168
  T wave in, 156, 160, 161, 168
  theoretical considerations on, 152–156
  vectorcardiogram in, 168–170
  vectorelectrocardiographic criteria for, 166
RS complex, definition of, 8
R/S ratio in right ventricular enlargement, 162
RSR' complex, 47, 55
  differential diagnosis of: with normal QRS
    interval, 164–166, 621
    with prolonged QRS interval, 183–184,
    622
  normal, 164, 167
  in precordial leads, 93
  (*See also specific abnormal conditions*)

S wave, 63
  in right ventricular enlargement, 161
  (*See also* QRS complex; *and specific ab-
    normal conditions*)
S' wave, 63
SA (sinoatrial) block, 578–581
  first-degree, 578
  second-degree, 578–580
  third-degree, 580
  3:2, sinus premature systoles versus, 426
SA (sinoatrial) node, 21–23, 26
  impulse formation and, 407
  wandering pacemaker between AV junc-
    tion and, 455
  wandering pacemaker within, 455
Sagittal plane:
  angular measurements of vectors in, 113
  QRS loop in, 116
  vectorcardiogram shown in, 47, 115
Sarcoidosis, 265–266
Scleroderma, 265
Segments, definition of, 58
Semidirect lead hypothesis (local potentials
    hypothesis), vector concept versus, 45–
    46
Sick sinus syndrome, 456–457
Simultaneous tachycardia, 452
Sinoatrial (*see* SA node)
Sinoventricular conduction, 456
  synchronized, 32–33
Sinoventricular rhythm, 456

Sinus arrest or pause, 455–456
Sinus arrhythmias, 454–455
Sinus beats and rhythms, 453
  AV dissociation in, 530–531
  concealment of, 551
  normal, 453
Sinus bradycardia, 453–454
Sinus impulse, 29
Sinus node dysfunction, 456–457
Sinus premature systoles, 425–426
Sinus tachycardia, 453
  paroxysmal reciprocating, 488
Slur, definition of, 64
S₁S₂S₃ syndrome, 369–372
  differential diagnosis of, 165, 369, 625
  RSR' complex in, 165
Spatial vector (see Vectors)
S-T segment, 29, 52, 70–75
  abnormalities, 73–75, 122–127
  area enclosed by T wave and, 90
  in bundle branch block, 125, 127, 182,
    191–194
  in children, 385
  definition of, 6
  differential diagnoses of abnormal, 622–
    623
  with digitalis, 122, 123
  displacement of: in myocardial injury, 14–
    18
    as normal variant, 122, 123
  electrical axis of, determination of, 87
  in hyperpotassemia, 125, 127
  in hypopotassemia, 125, 127
  in ischemia, 307–312
  in myocardial infarction, 244–245
  normal values for, 72
  in pericarditis, 124–127, 320–321
  pseudodepression of, 62, 73
  in subendocardial injury, 123, 124
  in subepicardial injury, 14–18, 123, 124
  in ventricular enlargement: left, 142–146,
    149
    right, 156, 160
  in ventricular strain, 123–124
  (See also specific abnormal conditions)
S-T vector, 112, 116
  abnormalities, 122–127
  in bundle branch block, 127
    left, 193, 197
    right, 186
  with digitalis, 122
  in hyperpotassemia, 127
  in hypopotassemia, 127
  in pericarditis, 124–127

S-T vector (*Cont.*):
  S-T segment displacement and, 122
  in subendocardial injury, 124
  in subepicardial injury, 124
  in ventricular enlargement, left, 143, 147,
    151
  in ventricular strain, 123–124
  (*See also specific abnormal conditions*)
Standard limb leads (see Bipolar limb leads)
Standardization of electrocardiogram, 57
Stenosis:
  aortic, congenital, 391
  idiopathic hypertrophic subaortic, 262, 263,
    373, 391–392
  pulmonic, congenital, 157, 393
S-Tp segment, 52, 62
"Straight back" syndrome:
  electrocardiographic findings, 377
  and pseudoinfarction patterns, 275
  T wave inversion in, 77
ST-T abnormalities, primary: left ventricular
    enlargement and, 149
  right ventricular enlargement and, 168
  (*See also* S-T segment; T wave)
Subarachnoid hemorrhage, spontaneous, 374–
    376
Subendocardial injury, 126
  depolarization and repolarization affected
    by, 18–20
  S-T segment or vector abnormality in, 123–
    124
Subendocardial ischemia, transient, 307–309
Subepicardial injury:
  depolarization and repolarization affected
    by, 14–18
  left bundle branch block with, 291
  pseudo-, in athletes, 272
  QRS, S-T, and T vectors in, relationship
    between, 126
  S-T segment or vector abnormalities in,
    123, 124
  transient, angina pectoris and, 307
Summation beats (see Fusion beats)
Supernormal conduction, 411, 556–562
Supraventricular arrhythmias:
  in exercise testing, 313
  in W-P-W syndrome, 231–233
Supraventricular conduction, 29
Supraventricular paroxysmal tachycardia, dif-
    ferential diagnosis of, 581–597
  capture and reciprocal beats, ventricular,
    593–595
  carotid sinus massage and vagal stimula-
    tion, 591–592

Supraventricular paroxysmal tachycardia, differential diagnosis of (*Cont.*):
  comparison of the QRS complexes during and in the absence of tachycardia, 591
  duration of first ectopic cycle following a capture, 593
  ectopic beats, comparison of, 592–593
  electrophysiological studies, 597
  fusion beats, ventricular, 596–597
  identification of the atrial mechanisms, 589–590
  onset of tachycardia, 585–586
  rate of the tachycardia, 591–592
  termination of the tachycardia, 586
  ventricular QRS complexes, configuration of, 586–589
  ventricular tachycardia, supraventricular tachycardia with abnormal QRS complexes versus, 584–597
Supraventricular tachycardias:
  automatic ectopic, reentrant versus, 486–489
  definition of, 450
  reentrant paroxysmal, 477–480
  (*See also* Supraventricular paroxysmal tachycardia)
Sympathomimetic drugs, electrocardiographic changes produced by, 335
Systole, 80
  premature (*see* Premature systoles)
Systolic overloading of ventricles:
  left, 142, 174
  right, 157, 173

T loop, 111, 112, 116
  (*See also specific abnormal conditions*)
T vector:
  abnormalities of, 119–121
    due to ischemia, 119–120
    metabolic, 119
    primary, 119–120
    secondary, 120
    (*See also specific abnormal conditions*)
  plotting mean spatial, 85
T wave, 29, 75–79
  abnormalities of (changes in), 74, 76–79, 119–121
    functional, 77, 121
    due to ischemia, 119–120
    metabolic, 119
    postextrasystolic, 425, 434
    primary, 13, 119–120
    secondary, 11, 120
    (*See also specific abnormal conditions*)

T wave (*Cont.*):
  area enclosed by S-T segment, and, 90
  in children, 76, 385, 386
  coronary, 244
  cove-plane, 244
  definition of, 6
  differential diagnosis of abnormal, 623–624
  diphasic, 75, 77, 624
  electrical axis of: determination of, 623–624
    mean, 89
  in hyperventilation, 77
  inversion of, 75–79
    in children, 76
    differential diagnosis, 624
    massive, 78–79, 624
  measurement of, 60, 75
  in myocardial infarction, 241, 244–246, 251–254, 257
    with bundle branch block, 290–291, 294
    with fascicular block, 283, 285
  negativity, isolated, 76
  normal values for, 75
  Pardee, 244
  in pericarditis, 320–325
  in precordial leads, 76
  in standard limb leads, 75
  tall, 78
  in unipolar extremity leads, 75–76
  in ventricular enlargement: left, 141–143, 145–146, 149–150
    right, 156, 157, 160, 161, 168
Ta wave (Tp wave), 21, 52, 62
Tachycardias:
  ectopic, 449–453
  idioventricular, 506–508
  nonparoxysmal: AV junctional, 494
    definition of, 450
  parasystolic, ventricular, 514, 518
  paroxysmal (*see* Paroxysmal tachycardia)
  sinus, 453
  supraventricular (*see* Supraventricular tachycardias)
  ventricular (*see* Ventricular tachycardia)
Testing, exercise, 309–314
Tetralogy of Fallot, 155, 393, 394
3:2 SA block, sinus premature systoles versus, 426
Timing of loop, 112
Tocainide hydrochloride, 336
Tosades de pointes, 512–514
Tp wave (Ta wave), 29, 75–79
Transmembrane potential (*see* Potentials, transmembrane)

Transmembrane potential threshold, 406
Transposition of the great vessels:
    complete, 400–401
    congenitally corrected, 389–390
Transsternal leads for monitoring, 101–102
Transverse axis, 94–95
Transverse plane:
    angular measurements of vectors in, 113
    normal vectorcardiogram, 115
    QRS loop in, 113
Tricuspid atresia, 399
Tricuspid valve, 22
Trifascicular blocks, 215–218
    bilateral bundle branch block and, 218–
        219
Trigeminy, 533–535
    concealed, 534, 536
Truncus arteriosus, 401

U wave, 79–80
    abnormality of, 80
        differential diagnosis, 624–625
        (See also specific abnormal conditions)
Unidirectional block:
    macroreentry and, in the AV junction, 412
    without reentry, 412
Unipolar leads, 5–10, 40, 45
    definition of, 5
    precordial (see Precordial leads)
Unipolar limb leads, 36, 38–40, 91
    augmented, 39, 40
    bipolar limb leads and, relationship be-
        tween, 40–41
    derivation of, from FP loop, 116, 117
Uremia, 349

V wave or complex, 106
Vector analysis:
    concept of, 43–46
    electrical axis in frontal plane determined
        by, 83–87
    method of, 47–48
    shortcomings of, 46
Vectorcardiogram:
    abbreviations used in, 112
    angles in, nomenclature of, 113
    derivation of, 50–56
    electrocardiogram and, relation between,
        48
    electrocardiogram derived from, 116–118
    in frontal plane, 47

Vectorcardiogram (Cont.):
    in horizontal plane, 47
    normal, 111–118
        values for, 113
    precordial leads and horizontal plane pro-
        jection, relationship between, 46
    in sagittal plane, 47
    terminology of, 111–112
    (See also specific topics)
Vectorcardiography, cathode-tube, 46–47
Vectorelectrocardiography, 47–48
Vectors:
    addition and subtraction of, 44–45
    angular measurements of planar, 113
    electrical axis and, 82–83
    magnitude of, determining, 111–112
    planar, 113
    plotting of, 85, 86
    (See also specific vectors)
Vena cava, 23
Ventricles:
    depolarization of (see Ventricular depolar-
        ization)
    diastolic overloading of, 142, 158, 173–
        175
    left, 22, 28
        diastolic overloading, 142, 174
        enlargement (see Left ventricular enlarge-
            ment)
        systolic overloading, 142, 173, 174
    repolarization of (see Ventricular repolari-
        zation)
    right, 22, 27, 28
        diastolic overloading, 158, 173–174
        enlargement (see Right ventricular en-
            largement)
        systolic overloading, 157, 173
    single, 399
    systolic overloading of, 142, 157, 173–175
Ventricular aneurysm, 258, 259
Ventricular arrhythmias, 313, 502–514
    in exercise testing, 313
    (See also specific arrhythmias)
Ventricular conduction, aberrant (see Aber-
    rant ventricular conduction)
Ventricular conduction defects, 177–223
    anatomic basis of, 178
    classification of, 177–178
    His bundle electrogram in, 220–221
    recommendations for clinical cardiac pac-
        ing, 222
    (See also Aberrant ventricular conduction;
        Bundle branch block; Fascicular blocks)
Ventricular conduction system, 24

Ventricular depolarization, 26, 28, 29, 33–34, 53–56
  in bundle branch block: left, 191–193
    right, 180, 181
Ventricular dilatation, 166–167
Ventricular ectopy:
  aberrant ventricular conduction and, differential diagnosis between, 448–449
  in atrial fibrillation, 471, 474
  in exercise testing, 313
Ventricular enlargement (ventricular hypertrophy), 140–175
  bundle branch block with: left, 195–196
    right, vectorcardiogram in, 187–189
  combined, 170–173
    diagnosis, 171–172
    vectorcardiogram, 172–173
  differential diagnosis, 236
  left (see Left ventricular enlargement)
  right (see Right ventricular enlargement)
  vectorcardiogram in: combined, 172–173
    with right bundle branch block, 187–189
Ventricular escape beats, 441–442
Ventricular fibrillation, 514, 519
Ventricular flutter, 514
Ventricular fusion beats, 471, 507, 518, 520, 521, 525, 546–548, 603, 606
  diagnosis of, 443–444
Ventricular gradient, 90–91
Ventricular hypertrophy (see Ventricular enlargement)
Ventricular preexcitation (see Wolff-Parkinson-White syndrome)
Ventricular premature beats, concealment of, 554
Ventricular premature systoles (see Premature systoles, ventricular)
Ventricular reciprocal beats, 538–541
Ventricular repolarization, 29, 56, 72
  in bundle branch block: left, 193
    right, 181–182
Ventricular rhythm, 421, 505–506
  accelerated, 506–508
  (See also Fascicular beats and rhythms)
Ventricular septal defect, 397
Ventricular strain:
  left, 142, 146
    QRS, S-T, and T vectors in, relationship between, 126
    S-T segment or vector abnormality in, 123–124
  right, 130, 132, 133
    QRS, S-T, and T vectors in, relationship between, 126

Ventricular strain (Cont.):
  right ventricular enlargement and, 157, 160
  S-T segment or vector abnormality in, 123, 124
Ventricular tachycardia, 504, 506–514
  differential diagnosis between supraventricular paroxysmal tachycardia and, 584–597
  parasystolic, 504, 514, 517, 518
  paroxysmal, 504, 508–513
  polymorphous (torsades de pointes), 512–514
Ventriculophasic sinus arrhythmia, 454
Verapamil hydrochloride, 336
Vulnerable period, 415–417

Wandering pacemaker, 455
Wedensky effect, 556–557
Wedensky facilitation, 556–557
Wedensky inhibition, 412
Wenckebach phenomenon, 580–581
Wilson, central terminal of, 39, 40
Wolff-Parkinson-White (W-P-W) syndrome, 226–239
  classic form of, 226
  classification of, 228–229
    European Study Group new classification of, 228
  clinical significance of, 229–230
  concertina effect in, 231
  diagnosis of, criteria for, 230–231
  differential diagnosis of, 236–237, 267
  electrophysiologic considerations in, 235–236
  His bundle electrogram in, 235
  myocardial infarction and, differential diagnosis between, 267
  theoretical considerations on, 226–228
  Type A, 228–229
    vectorcardiogram, 237–238
  Type B, 228–229, 232
    vectorcardiogram, 238–239
  Type C, 229
  variations of, 231
  vectorcardiogram in, 237–239

X axis, 111
X lead, normal, 44

Y axis, 111
Y lead, normal, 44

Z axis, 111
Z lead, normal, 44